**THIRD EDITION**

# Psychosocial Nursing Care Along the Cancer Continuum

*EDITED BY*

*Nancy Jo Bush, DNP, RN, MN, MA, AOCN®, FAAN*
*Linda M. Gorman, RN, MN, PMHCNS-BC, CHPN, FPCN*

Oncology Nursing Society
Pittsburgh, Pennsylvania

**ONS Publications Department**
Publisher and Director of Publications: William A. Tony, BA, CQIA
Senior Editorial Manager: Lisa M. George, BA
Assistant Editorial Manager: Amy Nicoletti, BA, JD
Acquisitions Editor: John Zaphyr, BA, MEd
Associate Staff Editors: Vanessa Kattouf, BA, Casey S. Kennedy, BA, Andrew Petyak, BA
Design and Production Administrator: Dany Sjoen
Editorial Assistant: Judy Holmes

Copyright © 2018 by the Oncology Nursing Society. All rights reserved. No part of the material protected by this copyright may be reproduced or utilized in any form, electronic or mechanical, including photocopying, recording, or by an information storage and retrieval system, without written permission from the copyright owner. For information, visit www.ons.org/sites/default/files/Publication%20Permissions.pdf, or send an email to pubpermissions@ons.org.

**Library of Congress Cataloging-in-Publication Data**

Names: Bush, Nancy Jo, editor. | Gorman, Linda M., editor. | Oncology Nursing Society, issuing body.
Title: Psychosocial nursing care along the cancer continuum / edited by Nancy Jo Bush, Linda M. Gorman.
Description: Third edition. | Pittsburgh, Pennsylvania : Oncology Nursing Society, [2018] | Preceded by Psychosocial nursing care along the cancer continuum / edited by Rose Mary Carroll-Johnson, Linda M. Gorman, Nancy Jo Bush. 2nd ed. c2006. | Includes bibliographical references and index.
Identifiers: LCCN 2017029342 (print) | LCCN 2017027992 (ebook) | ISBN 9781635930030 | ISBN 9781635930085
Subjects: | MESH: Neoplasms–nursing | Oncology Nursing | Caregivers–psychology | Mental Disorders–nursing | Neoplasms–psychology | Nurse-Patient Relations
Classification: LCC RC266 (ebook) | LCC RC266 (print) | NLM WY 156 | DDC 616.99/40231–dc23
LC record available at https://lccn.loc.gov/2017029342

**Publisher's Note**

This book is published by the Oncology Nursing Society (ONS). ONS neither represents nor guarantees that the practices described herein will, if followed, ensure safe and effective patient care. The recommendations contained in this book reflect ONS's judgment regarding the state of general knowledge and practice in the field as of the date of publication. The recommendations may not be appropriate for use in all circumstances. Those who use this book should make their own determinations regarding specific safe and appropriate patient care practices, taking into account the personnel, equipment, and practices available at the hospital or other facility at which they are located. The editors and publisher cannot be held responsible for any liability incurred as a consequence from the use or application of any of the contents of this book. Figures and tables are used as examples only. They are not meant to be all-inclusive, nor do they represent endorsement of any particular institution by ONS. Mention of specific products and opinions related to those products do not indicate or imply endorsement by ONS. Websites mentioned are provided for information only; the hosts are responsible for their own content and availability. Unless otherwise indicated, dollar amounts reflect U.S. dollars.

ONS publications are originally published in English. Publishers wishing to translate ONS publications must contact ONS about licensing arrangements. ONS publications cannot be translated without obtaining written permission from ONS. (Individual tables and figures that are reprinted or adapted require additional permission from the original source.) Because translations from English may not always be accurate or precise, ONS disclaims any responsibility for inaccuracies in words or meaning that may occur as a result of the translation. Readers relying on precise information should check the original English version.

Printed in the United States of America

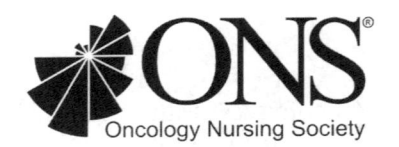

**ONS®**
Oncology Nursing Society

Innovation • Excellence • Advocacy

We dedicate this book to Rose Mary "Rosie" Carroll-Johnson: a mentor, distinguished colleague, and, ultimately, a cherished friend. Rosie was foremost a dedicated mother, loyal wife, daughter, sister, nurse, and friend. She had a tremendous gift of investing herself to help others become the best that they could be. Enrolled in the U.S. Navy, she served our country with great commitment. Rosie began her nursing career at Mount Saint Mary's College in Los Angeles, California. Before it became a specialty, Rosie became an oncology nurse, graduating with a master's degree in nursing from the University of California in 1982. She then began a successful career in publishing, culminating in her position as editor of the *Oncology Nursing Forum* for 20 years. Rosie was coeditor of the first two editions of *Psychosocial Nursing Care Along the Cancer Continuum*. This book was her dream and the essence of what she reflected in her life: comfort of the heart. To those of us who knew her well, Rosie was a warm and gentle soul; each of us are blessed to have been close to her in her life. She was an angel on earth, now a bright star in the heavens. This edition is a reflection of Rosie's spirit living on.

# Contributors

## Editors

**Nancy Jo Bush, DNP, RN, MN, MA, AOCN®, FAAN**
Lecturer/Oncology Nurse Practitioner
UCLA School of Nursing
Los Angeles, California
*Chapter 4. Coping and Adaptation; Chapter 14. Anxiety; Chapter 18. Distress*

**Linda M. Gorman, RN, MN, PMHCNS-BC, CHPN, FPCN**
Clinical Nurse Specialist
Los Angeles, California
*Chapter 1. Psychosocial Impact of Cancer on the Individual, Family, and Society; Chapter 6. Fatigue; Chapter 16. Denial; Chapter 21. Powerlessness; Chapter 25. Therapeutic Modalities in Psychosocial Care; Chapter 26. The Close of Life*

## Authors

**Angela V. Albright, RN, APRN, PhD**
Emeritus Professor
California State University, Dominguez Hills
Carson, California
*Chapter 17. Depression and Suicide*

**Paula J. Anastasia, RN, MN, AOCN®**
Gynecology–Oncology Clinical Nurse Specialist
Cedars-Sinai Medical Center
Los Angeles, California
*Chapter 12. Altered Sexuality*

**Tami Borneman, RN, MSN, CNS, FPCN**
Senior Research Specialist
City of Hope National Medical Center
Duarte, California
*Chapter 7. Hope*

**Deborah A. Boyle, MSN, RN, AOCNS®, FAAN**
Oncology Clinical Nurse Specialist
Advanced Oncology Nursing Resources, Inc.
Huntington Beach, California
*Chapter 2. Survivorship*

**Katherine Brown-Saltzman, RN, MA**
Co-Director
UCLA Health Ethics Center
Assistant Clinical Professor
UCLA School of Nursing
Los Angeles, California
*Chapter 19. Grief*

**Yu-Ping Chang, PhD, RN, FGSA**
Patricia H. and Richard E. Garman Endowed Professor
Associate Professor
Associate Dean for Research and Scholarship
State University of New York at Buffalo School of Nursing
Buffalo, New York
*Chapter 24. Substance Abuse and Addiction*

**Peggy Compton, RN, PhD, FAAN**
Associate Professor
van Ameringen Endowed Chair
Department of Family and Community Health
University of Pennsylvania School of Nursing
Philadelphia, Pennsylvania
*Chapter 24. Substance Abuse and Addiction*

**Liz Cooke, RN, MN, AOCN®, PMHNP-BC, AGPCNP-BC**
City of Hope National Medical Center
Duarte, California
*Chapter 13. Anger and Cancer*

**Rebecca Crane-Okada, PhD, RN, CNS, AOCN®**
Director
Breast Cancer Navigation Program
Willow Sage Wellness Program
Providence Saint John's Health Center
Santa Monica, California
*Chapter 20. Guilt*

**Carol P. Curtiss, MSN, RN-BC**
Clinical Specialist Consultant
Curtiss Consulting
Greenfield, Massachusetts
*Chapter 8. Pain*

**Esther Muscari Desimini, RN, MSN, APRN, BC, MBA**
Vice President/Administrator
Riverside Tappahannock Hospital
Tappahannock, Virginia
*Chapter 3. Cognitive Dysfunction in Cancer; Chapter 11. Altered Mental Status*

**Sheila M. Ferrall, MS, RN, AOCN®**
Senior Director of Nursing
H. Lee Moffitt Cancer Center and Research Institute
Tampa, Florida
*Chapter 28. Caring for the Family*

**Betty R. Ferrell, PhD, FAAN**
Professor, Director
City of Hope National Medical Center
Duarte, California
*Chapter 10. Suffering*

**Margaret I. Fitch, RN, MScN, PhD**
Professor
University of Toronto Faculty of Nursing
Toronto, Ontario, Canada
*Chapter 29. Programmatic Approaches to Psychosocial Support*

**Stacey D. Green, MSN, RN, GNP-BC, AOCNP®**
UCLA Neuro-Oncology Program
UCLA School of Nursing
Los Angeles, California
*Appendix. Psychosocial Support Programs and Resources for People With Cancer and Their Families*

**Rita Hand, RN, MSN, GNP-BC**
Nurse Practitioner
Los Angeles, California
*Chapter 27. Ethical Issues*

**Edith O'Neil-Page, MSN, RN, AOCNS®**
Clinical Nurse Specialist, Palliative Care
Ronald Reagan UCLA Medical Center
Los Angeles, California
*Chapter 6. Fatigue*

**Kathryn E. Pearson, RN, CNS, MN, AOCN®**
Oncology Clinical Nurse Specialist
Fullerton, California
*Chapter 23. Interpersonal and Therapeutic Skills Inherent in Oncology Nursing*

**Marlon Garzo Saria, PhD, RN, AOCNS®, FAAN**
Assistant Professor and Director
Center for Quality and Outcomes Research
Pacific Neuroscience Institute and John Wayne Cancer Institute at Providence Saint John's Health Center
Santa Monica, California
*Chapter 5. Cultural Influences*

**Joan R. Schleper, MS, RN, GNP-BC, CNS**
Clinical Faculty/Guest Lecturer
UCLA School of Nursing
Los Angeles, California
Clinical Educator
Nurses Improving Care for Healthsystem Elders (NICHE)
*Chapter 15. Body Image Disturbance*

**Virginia Sun, PhD, RN**
Assistant Professor
City of Hope National Medical Center
Duarte, California
*Chapter 10. Suffering*

**Elizabeth Johnston Taylor, PhD, RN**
Professor
Loma Linda University School of Nursing
Loma Linda, California
*Chapter 9. Spiritual and Religious Support*

**Sharon M. Valente, RN, APRN, BC, PhD, FAAN**
Assistant Chief
Nursing Research and Evaluation
VA Greater Los Angeles Healthcare System
Los Angeles, California
*Chapter 17. Depression and Suicide*

**Sharon Van Fleet, MS, RN, PMHCNS-BC**
Clinical Nurse Education Specialist
University of North Carolina Hospitals
Chapel Hill, North Carolina
*Chapter 22. Crisis Intervention*

# Disclosure

Editors and authors of books and guidelines provided by the Oncology Nursing Society are expected to disclose to the readers any significant financial interest or other relationships with the manufacturer(s) of any commercial products.

A vested interest may be considered to exist if a contributor is affiliated with or has a financial interest in commercial organizations that may have a direct or indirect interest in the subject matter. A "financial interest" may include, but is not limited to, being a shareholder in the organization; being an employee of the commercial organization; serving on an organization's speakers bureau; or receiving research funding from the organization. An "affiliation" may be holding a position on an advisory board or some other role of benefit to the commercial organization. Vested interest statements appear in the front matter for each publication.

Contributors are expected to disclose any unlabeled or investigational use of products discussed in their content. This information is acknowledged solely for the information of the readers.

The contributors provided the following disclosure and vested interest information:

Paula J. Anastasia, RN, MN, AOCN®: Genentech, Inc., Clovis, Merck & Co., honoraria

Yu-Ping Chang, PhD, RN, FGSA: Fooyin University, Taiwan, consultant or advisory role; State University of New York at Buffalo School of Nursing, Patricia H. Garman Behavioral Health Nursing Endowment Fund, University at Buffalo Institute for Person-Centered Care, National Institutes of Health, research funding

Carol P. Curtiss, MSN, RN-BC: Genentech, Inc., honoraria

Marlon Garzo Saria, PhD, RN, AOCNS®, FAAN: John Wayne Cancer Institute, U.S. Department of the Air Force, Brain Cancer Research Institute, San Diego Brain Tumor Foundation, leadership positions; Cancer Life, consultant; ICU Medical, Inc., honoraria

# Table of Contents

**Preface** ........................................................................................................................................ xv

**Section I. Psychosocial Impact Along the Cancer Continuum** ................................................. 1

**Chapter 1. Psychosocial Impact of Cancer on the Individual, Family, and Society** ................. 3
    Diagnosis .................................................................................................................................. 3
    Cancer Treatment .................................................................................................................... 9
    Recurrence ............................................................................................................................. 13
    Terminal Illness ...................................................................................................................... 16
    Survivorship ........................................................................................................................... 19
    Conclusion ............................................................................................................................. 21
    References ............................................................................................................................. 21

**Chapter 2. Survivorship** ............................................................................................................ 27
    The Paradigm of Extended Survival ..................................................................................... 28
    Fear of Recurrence ................................................................................................................ 29
    Symptom Persistence ........................................................................................................... 31
    Work Reentry ........................................................................................................................ 33
    Caregivers as Secondary Cancer Survivors .......................................................................... 34
    Conclusion ............................................................................................................................. 37
    References ............................................................................................................................. 37

**Section II. Psychosocial Influences** ......................................................................................... 43

**Chapter 3. Cognitive Dysfunction in Cancer** ........................................................................... 45
    Cognitive Impairment in the Oncology Population ............................................................ 45
    Contributing Factors ............................................................................................................. 48
    Indirect Factors ..................................................................................................................... 49
    Assessment ............................................................................................................................ 51
    Implications for Practice ....................................................................................................... 52
    Cognitive Rehabilitation ....................................................................................................... 53
    Conclusion ............................................................................................................................. 54
    References ............................................................................................................................. 54

**Chapter 4. Coping and Adaptation** .......................................................................................... 57
    Definitions of Coping ........................................................................................................... 58
    Coping and Adaptation ........................................................................................................ 60
    Conceptual Framework for Coping Assessment ................................................................. 61
    Coping as a Process .............................................................................................................. 65
    Interventions to Support Coping ......................................................................................... 77
    Conclusion ............................................................................................................................. 82
    References ............................................................................................................................. 83

**Chapter 5. Cultural Influences** ................................................................................................. 91
    Culture in the Nursing Literature ......................................................................................... 92
    Culturally Defined Health Disparities .................................................................................. 94
    Country of Birth and Citizenship ......................................................................................... 94

    Ethnicity and Race .................................................................................................... 95
    Religion ...................................................................................................................... 99
    Gender, Gender Identity, and Sexual Orientation ................................................... 99
    Culturally Competent Care ...................................................................................... 101
    Conclusion ................................................................................................................. 103
    References .................................................................................................................. 103

**Chapter 6. Fatigue** ............................................................................................................. **107**
    Defining Cancer-Related Fatigue .............................................................................. 107
    Epidemiology ............................................................................................................. 108
    Etiology ...................................................................................................................... 110
    Psychosocial Effects of Cancer-Related Fatigue ..................................................... 112
    Management of the Patient With Cancer-Related Fatigue ..................................... 112
    Evidence-Based Practice ........................................................................................... 118
    Conclusion ................................................................................................................. 119
    References .................................................................................................................. 120

**Chapter 7. Hope** ................................................................................................................. **123**
    Hope and Hopelessness ............................................................................................ 124
    Theories and Conceptual Models of Hope .............................................................. 124
    Assessment of Hope in the Clinical Setting ............................................................. 125
    Hope-Fostering Strategies ......................................................................................... 128
    Conclusion ................................................................................................................. 132
    References .................................................................................................................. 132

**Chapter 8. Pain** .................................................................................................................... **137**
    Pain and Quality of Life ............................................................................................ 139
    Developmental Issues Related to Pain Control ...................................................... 142
    The Effects of Culture on Pain and Pain Relief ....................................................... 144
    Promoting Evidence-Based Pain Care ..................................................................... 145
    Conclusion ................................................................................................................. 146
    References .................................................................................................................. 146

**Chapter 9. Spiritual and Religious Support** ...................................................................... **151**
    Concept Descriptions ................................................................................................ 151
    Spiritual Support ....................................................................................................... 152
    Spirituality and Religiosity in Cancer Care: Rationale ........................................... 153
    Spiritual and Religious Responses to Cancer: Evidence ........................................ 154
    Prevalence and Types of Spiritual Needs ................................................................ 154
    Factors Related to Spirituality and Religiosity ....................................................... 155
    Family Caregivers' Spirituality and Religiosity ...................................................... 158
    Spiritual Support: Evidence-Based Approaches ..................................................... 159
    Conclusion ................................................................................................................. 164
    References .................................................................................................................. 164

**Chapter 10. Suffering** ......................................................................................................... **169**
    The Nature of Suffering in Patients With Cancer ................................................... 170
    Sources of Suffering .................................................................................................. 171
    Suffering Across the Cancer Trajectory ................................................................... 172
    Suffering Across the Life Span ................................................................................. 172
    Cultural Considerations ............................................................................................ 174
    Suffering in the Family ............................................................................................. 174
    Nursing Interventions ............................................................................................... 175
    Suffering Among Professionals ................................................................................ 176
    Conclusion ................................................................................................................. 177
    References .................................................................................................................. 178

**Section III. Psychosocial Alterations** ................................................................................. **181**

**Chapter 11. Altered Mental Status** .................................................................................... **183**
    Delirium ..................................................................................................................... 183
    Delirium in Patients With Cancer ............................................................................ 187
    Delirium in Patients With Terminal Cancer ........................................................... 188
    Dementia ................................................................................................................... 188

Nursing Care of Patients With Delirium and Dementia ..................................................................... 189
Psychosocial Response to Delirium and Dementia for the Patient and Family ............................... 196
Healthcare Professionals' Responses to Delirium and Dementia ................................................... 197
Conclusion ........................................................................................................................................ 199
References ........................................................................................................................................ 199

## Chapter 12. Altered Sexuality ............................................................................................................ 203
Important Principles About Sexuality .............................................................................................. 204
Altered Sexuality and Cancer ........................................................................................................... 204
Healthcare Professionals' Responses to Altered Sexuality ............................................................. 212
Nursing Care of Patients Experiencing Altered Sexuality ............................................................... 213
Conclusion ........................................................................................................................................ 223
References ........................................................................................................................................ 223

## Chapter 13. Anger ............................................................................................................................... 229
Theories on Anger ............................................................................................................................ 229
General Expressions of Anger .......................................................................................................... 231
Anger as a Response to Cancer ........................................................................................................ 233
Nurses' Responses to Anger ............................................................................................................. 237
Interventions During an Angry Episode .......................................................................................... 238
Conclusion ........................................................................................................................................ 242
References ........................................................................................................................................ 243

## Chapter 14. Anxiety ............................................................................................................................ 247
Important Principles Related to Anxiety ......................................................................................... 247
Cultural Influences on the Experience and Expression of Anxiety ................................................ 249
Classifications of Anxiety Disorders in Patients With Cancer ........................................................ 250
Anxiety Disorders Caused by Medical Conditions .......................................................................... 252
Post-Traumatic Stress Disorder ....................................................................................................... 253
The Response of Healthcare Professionals to Anxious Patients .................................................... 253
Nursing Care of Patients Experiencing Anxiety .............................................................................. 254
Conclusion ........................................................................................................................................ 261
References ........................................................................................................................................ 262

## Chapter 15. Body Image Disturbance ............................................................................................... 265
Body Image Development ................................................................................................................ 266
Body Image and Illness .................................................................................................................... 269
Body Image and Cancer .................................................................................................................... 271
Specific Cancers and Body Image .................................................................................................... 272
Nursing Care of Patients With Body Image Disturbance ............................................................... 276
Evidence-Based Practice .................................................................................................................. 278
Conclusion ........................................................................................................................................ 282
References ........................................................................................................................................ 282

## Chapter 16. Denial .............................................................................................................................. 289
Denial and Coping ............................................................................................................................ 290
Denial and Illness ............................................................................................................................. 291
Denial and Cancer ............................................................................................................................ 292
Denial and Death .............................................................................................................................. 293
Impact of Denial on the Patient's Family ........................................................................................ 293
Healthcare Professionals' Responses to Denial .............................................................................. 294
Evidence-Based Practice .................................................................................................................. 294
Nursing Care of Patients in Denial .................................................................................................. 295
Conclusion ........................................................................................................................................ 299
References ........................................................................................................................................ 299

## Chapter 17. Depression and Suicide ................................................................................................ 303
Assessment of Depression ............................................................................................................... 303
Depression in Special Populations .................................................................................................. 305
Risk Factors for Depression ............................................................................................................. 305
Differential Diagnosis ...................................................................................................................... 307
Interventions for Depression ........................................................................................................... 308
Assessment and Intervention for Suicide ....................................................................................... 311
Evidence-Based Practice .................................................................................................................. 316

    Conclusion ................................................................................................................................. 319
    References ................................................................................................................................ 319

## Chapter 18. Distress ........................................................................................................................... 323
    Important Principles Related to Distress .................................................................................. 324
    Distress in Patients With Cancer ............................................................................................... 324
    Emergence of Psychosocial Care .............................................................................................. 326
    Distress as the Sixth Vital Sign .................................................................................................. 327
    Screening for Distress ............................................................................................................... 327
    Barriers to Screening ................................................................................................................ 328
    Nursing Care of Patients Experiencing Distress ........................................................................ 329
    Conclusion ................................................................................................................................. 335
    References ................................................................................................................................ 335

## Chapter 19. Grief ................................................................................................................................ 339
    Bereavement and Grief ............................................................................................................. 339
    Theoretical Tasks of Grief ......................................................................................................... 341
    Children and Bereavement ....................................................................................................... 342
    Cultural Issues .......................................................................................................................... 344
    Completion of Case Study ........................................................................................................ 345
    Care of the Grieving Individual ................................................................................................. 346
    Complicated Grief .................................................................................................................... 349
    Anticipatory Grief ..................................................................................................................... 352
    Evidence-Based Practice .......................................................................................................... 353
    When Death Approaches ......................................................................................................... 354
    Unusual Experiences ................................................................................................................ 355
    Professional Grief ..................................................................................................................... 357
    Self-Care ................................................................................................................................... 358
    Conclusion ................................................................................................................................. 359
    References ................................................................................................................................ 360

## Chapter 20. Guilt ................................................................................................................................ 365
    The Nature of Guilt in Cancer ................................................................................................... 366
    Sources of Guilt ........................................................................................................................ 366
    Family Member Guilt ................................................................................................................ 370
    Healthcare Providers and Guilt ................................................................................................ 373
    Conclusion ................................................................................................................................. 375
    References ................................................................................................................................ 375

## Chapter 21. Powerlessness ................................................................................................................ 379
    Powerlessness and Age-Specific Considerations ..................................................................... 381
    Powerlessness and Illness ........................................................................................................ 381
    Powerlessness and Cancer ....................................................................................................... 382
    Evidence-Based Practice .......................................................................................................... 383
    Nursing Care of Patients Experiencing Powerlessness ............................................................ 384
    Clinicians' Experience of Powerlessness .................................................................................. 387
    Conclusion ................................................................................................................................. 388
    References ................................................................................................................................ 388

# Section IV. Psychosocial Interventions ............................................................................................. 391

## Chapter 22. Crisis Intervention ......................................................................................................... 393
    Crisis Assessment ..................................................................................................................... 393
    Interventions ............................................................................................................................ 397
    Cancer as a Crisis ..................................................................................................................... 399
    Evaluation of Interventions Across All Phases of Cancer ......................................................... 401
    Conclusion ................................................................................................................................. 402
    References ................................................................................................................................ 403

## Chapter 23. Interpersonal and Therapeutic Skills Inherent in Oncology Nursing ........................... 407
    Cultural Competence and Communication ............................................................................. 408
    Social Skills ............................................................................................................................... 409
    Communication Skills ............................................................................................................... 410
    Listening Skills .......................................................................................................................... 411

| | |
|---|---|
| Language Skills in Communication | 413 |
| Humor as Communication | 414 |
| Communicating Bad News | 415 |
| Communication to Support Shared Decision Making | 416 |
| Behavioral Therapeutic Techniques | 417 |
| Nurses' Responses to Patient and Family Emotions | 419 |
| Nurses' Roles in Support Groups | 420 |
| The Role of Oncology Nurses in Interprofessional Cancer Care | 422 |
| Conclusion | 422 |
| References | 423 |

### Chapter 24. Substance Abuse and Addiction .................................................. 427
| | |
|---|---|
| Epidemiology | 427 |
| Substance Use Disorders in Oncology Populations | 429 |
| Addictive Disease | 431 |
| Substances of Abuse as Carcinogens | 432 |
| Substance Abuse, Addiction, and Cancer Treatment | 434 |
| Compliance With Cancer Treatment | 435 |
| Assessment for Substance Abuse and Addiction in Patients With Cancer | 436 |
| Approaches to Addiction Treatment in Patients With Cancer | 437 |
| Smoking Cessation | 438 |
| Management of Opioid Abuse and Addiction in Patients With Cancer Pain | 440 |
| Education in Managing Substance Abuse for Oncology Clinicians | 444 |
| Conclusion | 444 |
| References | 445 |

### Chapter 25. Therapeutic Modalities in Psychosocial Care .................................. 451
| | |
|---|---|
| Psychoeducation | 452 |
| Counseling and Psychotherapy | 452 |
| Mind–Body Practices | 456 |
| Behavior Modification Techniques | 458 |
| Other Therapies | 459 |
| The Future of Therapeutic Modalities | 460 |
| Conclusion | 460 |
| References | 460 |

## Section V. Dimensions of Caring .................................................................. 463

### Chapter 26. The Close of Life ............................................................................ 465
| | |
|---|---|
| Initiating Advance Care Planning Conversations | 466 |
| Components of High-Quality End-of-Life Care | 467 |
| End-of-Life Programs | 469 |
| Where People Die | 472 |
| Coping With a Death at Home | 473 |
| Pediatric End-of-Life Care | 474 |
| End-of-Life Nursing | 475 |
| Conclusion | 475 |
| References | 476 |

### Chapter 27. Ethical Issues ................................................................................. 479
| | |
|---|---|
| Defining Ethics | 479 |
| Ethical Nursing Practice | 480 |
| Autonomy, Informed Consent, Truth Telling, and Advance Directives | 481 |
| Medically Inappropriate Treatment: Determining Life and Death | 482 |
| Hastened Death: Assisted Suicide and Euthanasia | 484 |
| The Injustice of Health Disparities | 488 |
| Justice and the Allocation of Health Resources | 490 |
| Conclusion | 491 |
| References | 491 |

### Chapter 28. Caring for the Family ..................................................................... 497
| | |
|---|---|
| Assessment of Caregiver Challenges | 498 |
| Caregiver Quality of Life | 500 |

Strategies to Facilitate Caregiver Coping ........................................................................................ 502
Conclusion .................................................................................................................................... 505
References .................................................................................................................................... 505

**Section VI. Patient Support Systems ..................................................................................... 509**

**Chapter 29. Programmatic Approaches to Psychosocial Support ........................................ 511**
Background Context .................................................................................................................... 512
Helping Patients to Meet Their Psychosocial Needs .................................................................. 515
Programmatic Approaches to Psychosocial Care ....................................................................... 516
Conclusion .................................................................................................................................... 523
References .................................................................................................................................... 524

**Appendix. Psychosocial Support Programs and Resources for People Surviving Cancer
and Their Families** ........................................................................................................................ 531

**Index** ............................................................................................................................................... 559

# Preface

More than 20 years ago, three young oncology nurse colleagues had a dream. This dream became the first edition of this book, published in 1998. In the past 20 years, the world has seen many social, political, and economic changes. In oncology care, so much has changed, yet so much has stayed the same. Technology that influences cancer treatment and research has advanced. Chemotherapy is giving way to targeted treatments, and surgical techniques are using robotics. Rapid changes politically saw the introduction of the Patient Protection and Affordable Care Act increasing access to care, only to see major changes again on the horizon. The Internet has opened the world to endless information, providing patients with educational resources and social support. The world is becoming interconnected and smaller, making it so that we share the pain of others near and far.

Our patients find themselves in a world stage of change and, at the same time, are battling their personal trials with cancer. What has changed in cancer care has been the burgeoning research and clinical attention to psycho-oncology, and what has remained the same is patient and family needs for emotional support. As oncology nurses, we also face challenges of supporting our patients, who are facing adversity in a world of uncertainty.

Within this world stage, cancer plays a major force in the lives of many. The third edition of *Psychosocial Nursing Care Along the Cancer Continuum* reflects the role that nurses play in providing psychosocial care. Content addresses the many emotional challenges that can be experienced with a cancer diagnosis. Along with the physical hardships of the disease, its treatment and aftermath require ongoing psychosocial support. This edition has been expanded with additional topics, updated information, and new case studies. Progress in psycho-oncology and the revised *Diagnostic and Statistical Manual of Mental Disorders* is reflected throughout. The focus is patient-centered care recognizing family caregivers, interpersonal and social relationships, and survivorship issues. Content can assist the nurse at the bedside in providing emotional support or the advanced practice nurse in gaining information on the management of common psychosocial issues.

Psychosocial care is moving to the forefront of care within the realization that mental health is just as essential as physical health. Prior to the first edition, psychosocial oncology texts were not aimed at oncology nursing care. With the success of the first edition, it was another dream to continue to fill that void.

Since publication of the second edition, we have become older and wiser traveling along our own journeys in life. We were profoundly touched by the death of our dear friend and first editor Rose Mary "Rosie" Carroll-Johnson from her own battle with cancer. Nancy Jo's personal battle with cancer and its emotional impact also provided personal and professional lessons. Every oncology nurse is touched by the cancer experience and has given of themselves to share their patients' journeys with hopes of improving the quality of a life by being in a caring presence.

We sincerely hope this new edition provides you with the tools and insight to confidently and compassionately take this journey with your patients. Many thanks to the staff of the Oncology Nursing Society for their dedication to provide a stellar publication. Our thanks to our families and friends, who unselfishly supported our dream, and to our authors, who shared their expertise; we could not have done this without you. No matter the changes across time, we are all working together to bring peace and heart to this battle against cancer.

—Nancy Jo and Linda

# SECTION I

# Psychosocial Impact Along the Cancer Continuum

Chapter 1. Psychosocial Impact of Cancer on the Individual, Family, and Society

Chapter 2. Survivorship

# CHAPTER 1

# Psychosocial Impact of Cancer on the Individual, Family, and Society

*Linda M. Gorman, RN, MN, PMHCNS-BC, CHPN, FPCN*

*We are not ourselves when nature, being oppressed, commands the mind to suffer with the body.*

—William Shakespeare

A cancer diagnosis is a universally stressful experience (Payne, 2014). Psychosocial distress is highly prevalent and diverse at all stages of cancer care and can create as much distress as cancer's physical effects (Holland & Alici, 2010). Psychosocial oncology (also called psycho-oncology) has grown as an interprofessional specialty in recent years to address the emotional effects of cancer and the importance of psychosocial care throughout the disease course. Dr. Jimmie Holland, one of the founders of psycho-oncology, has stressed that the emotional response to cancer can influence both morbidity and mortality (Holland, 2002). A principal goal of psychosocial care in this population is to recognize and address the effects that cancer and its treatment have on the mental status and emotional well-being of patients, families, and professional caregivers (Jacobsen, Holland, & Steensma, 2012). Holland (2003) identified three contributing factors to psychological adaptation: type of cancer, personal coping skills, and society's prevailing attitudes toward the disease.

This chapter will review the psychosocial effects of cancer on the patient and family from initial diagnosis throughout the disease process and will show how the oncology nurse can affect psychosocial patient care throughout the cancer continuum.

## Diagnosis

The word *cancer* evokes fear and shock in most indivivuals. It has been referred to as the "defining plague of our generation" (Mukherjee, 2010). A cancer diagnosis can cause anxiety and uncertainty and disrupt an individual's life by threatening the person's sense of security. In addition, cancer can affect an individual's quality of life by creating negative consequences on physical and psychological well-being (Epplein et al., 2011). Although most cancers are treatable, many maintain profound fears that any cancer diagnosis represents pain, suffering, and death. Holland (2002) noted that no disease has sustained as strong a negative stigma as cancer. Despite advances in earlier detection, treatment, and survivorship, the phrase "you have cancer" is almost always viewed as a death sentence. The prevalence and visibility of cancer are two social factors in the fear of a cancer diagnosis. Most people know someone with cancer and have witnessed the sometimes-devastating effects of the disease and its treatments. Most people also know of someone who has died from cancer (Ferrell & Coyle, 2008).

Whatever the type of cancer, patients are faced with ongoing uncertainty about their future as they deal with the potential for an unpredictable disease trajectory. A cancer diagnosis can lead to a complex set of issues for the patient, including dealing with physical symptoms from the disease and treatment; facing the existential dimension of the illness; and seeking a comforting philosophical, spiritual, or religious belief structure or values that give meaning to life and death (Holland, 2002). It will also affect how the individual views the future (de Vries & Stiefel, 2014).

## Awareness

Prior to a diagnosis, an individual may be aware of body changes that could indicate cancer (e.g., a lump, abnormal bleeding). Nail (2001) called this the Recognition Phase. This awareness creates a state of hyper-alertness in individuals, which eventually leads them to take action and seek medical attention. How quickly this action occurs depends on many variables, including previous experience with cancer in oneself or a family member or friend. An experience with cancer may encourage some to seek quick medical attention. However, this may cause others to avoid medical attention for fear of what the symptoms could mean. Pain or discomfort created by symptoms tends to motivate people to seek medical attention. Other reasons that influence action or inaction include feelings of embarrassment or worry, fatalistic beliefs, financial considerations, inadequate knowledge, and fears regarding dependency or disfigurement (Smith, Pope, & Botha, 2005). In addition, young adults may not have the knowledge or experience to recognize or understand a symptom of cancer (Katz, 2015).

## Receiving the Cancer Diagnosis

In the United States, adherence to the ethical principle of autonomy has resulted in physicians directly telling patients about their cancer diagnosis. The principle of autonomy dictates that individuals have the right to determine their own course of action with a self-determined plan (Beauchamp & Childress, 2012) (see Chapter 27).

In the healthcare field, this means the patient has the right to know and participate in all healthcare decisions. The original *Code of Ethics of the American Medical Association* noted that the physician's duty is to avoid all things that could discourage or depress the spirit (Katz, 1984). This philosophy contributed to physicians receiving limited education about how to deliver bad news (Girgis & Sanson-Fisher, 1995). In 1961, 90% of surveyed physicians preferred not to directly tell patients about their cancer diagnosis (Oken, 1961). In 1977, however, more than 90% of physicians preferred to share this information with their patients (Novack, Plumer, & Smith, 1978). This dramatic change in practice reflected the social changes of the 1960s and 1970s, which encouraged an emphasis on openness. Access to oncology specialists with experience in sharing bad news became widely available during that time. The development of research protocols emphasizing informed consent was another factor (Holland, 2002). Holland and Wiesel (2015) emphasized that the stigma associated with cancer diminished in the late 20th century only when patients began being told their diagnosis.

At times, families still ask that patients not be told about their diagnosis. This creates an ethical dilemma for healthcare providers when obtaining informed consent for treatment. Being pressured by families to use words such as "growth" for the cancer or "special medicine" for chemotherapy makes providing care to these patients more difficult. Dunn, Patterson, and Butow (1993) noted that not being open about the diagnosis will cause patients to become suspicious and believe that their diagnosis must be so horrible that even the healthcare team will not acknowledge it. Avoiding use of the word *cancer* reinforces the fear associated with the word (Holland, 2002, 2003).

If a physician does not tell the patient about the diagnosis, it introduces the risk that a family member or friend will inadvertently disclose the diagnosis to the patient. This can cause the patient to greatly distrust the healthcare team. Dunn et al. (1993) identified the tendency of healthcare professionals and family members to avoid patients who have not been told the truth because of the fear of misspeaking. Openness about the diagnosis and prognosis enables patients to think more realistically about their condition and participate actively in treatment planning. Most individuals are able to adjust to their diagnosis over time (Dunn et al., 1993).

It is important to note that autonomy is not practiced worldwide. Patients and families from other cultures may be unprepared to receive the diagnosis directly. Healthcare professionals need to first address the family's fears about sharing the news and offer suggestions for assisting the patient. Creating a balance between providing some information without alienating the patient or family can be challenging but is important to establish and maintain a trusting relationship.

Delivering bad news is one of the most difficult tasks oncology professionals must undertake (Buckman, 2005). Although nurses may not deliver the initial diagnosis, they often are in a position to reinforce information, provide support, and consult with physicians about sharing the news (Dahlin & Wittenberg, 2015). Figure 1-1 lists some helpful guidelines for sharing the news of a cancer diagnosis. Healthcare professionals, including oncology nurses, need to develop skills in accurately and gently presenting information. In doing so, they can maintain hope regardless of the patient's prognosis. Some studies indicate that the way information is delivered can affect the response and recall of information (Sep, van Osch, van Vliet, Smets, & Bensing, 2014). The timing of delivering bad news to a patient and family can be challenging. If possible, giving information to the patient and family at the same time ensures that everyone involved has been given the same information. Back, Arnold, and Tulsky (2009) have suggested "talking about serious news" rather than the often-used phrase "breaking bad news." The first phrase emphasizes communication rather than just a one-way conversation of giving the information.

The SPIKES model (Setting, Perception, Invitation, Knowledge, Empathy, and Summary and Strategy) is one approach used to present bad news (Buckman, 2005):
- **Setting**—Choose a setting that is private.
- **Perception**—Ask for the patient's perception of the medical situation.
- **Invitation**—Ask what the patient would like to know and his or her wishes in receiving detailed prognostic information.
- **Knowledge**—Give the patient a warning that bad news is coming with a statement such as, "Unfortunately, the news is not what I hoped."
- **Empathy**—Respond to the patient's emotions.
- **Summary and Strategy**—Summarize the discussion and plans for next steps.

Using an effective, organized approach to these conversations can ensure that the professional can effectively communicate with the patient as well as provide support and empathy.

Another communication approach is **Ask, Tell, Ask:** ask permission to present information, tell the patient the information, then check for understanding, and ask for agreement and questions (Back, Arnold, Baile, Tulsky, & Fryer-Edwards, 2005).

As new approaches are being developed, more medical schools and specialty programs are implementing training for physicians in delivering news to their patients in their curriculums and through clinical training (Bousquet et al., 2015; Reed et al., 2015). Advanced practice nurses need to develop skill in this area as well.

## Responding to the Diagnosis

Whether or not a person anticipates the diagnosis, the initial response usually includes disbelief, numbness, and anxiety. Receiving a cancer diagnosis is associated with a peak of negative feelings and distress for many (Nail, 2001). Waves of intense emotions similar to a grief reaction with periods of calmness are common. Following the initial days after receiving the diagnosis, most individuals generally are able to develop a constructive plan of action. Healthcare professionals must remember that no matter how compassionate and skilled they are in delivering bad news, patients may still experience extreme emotional reactions (Shell & Kirsch, 2001). Whether the diagnosis is an early-stage cancer or stage IV disease, the common psychological denominator is the experience of profound life threat and uncertainty (Ganz & Stanton, 2015).

To integrate the idea of having cancer into one's psyche, the patient may feel the need to identify the cause. Asking "Why me?" may be part of this process. Seeking information about the type of cancer and its treatment can give the patient some sense of control. Information seeking is a more common coping mechanism in the early stages of the disease, when

---

- Provide privacy and adequate time to share the information and provide support.
- Ask the patient how much he or she wants to know.
- Encourage the patient to bring a family member to the meeting.
- Consider recording the meeting or providing a written summary of the information.
- Monitor for signs of emotional distress and respond as needed.
- Give the information gradually rather than starting with the diagnosis.
- Listen to the patient's and family's concerns.
- Validate the patient's feelings.
- Assess their understanding of what has been shared throughout the process.
- Develop an alliance with the patient about the treatment plan.
- If needed, ensure that professional interpreters are available.
- If the prognosis is very poor, avoid giving a definite time frame.
- Reinforce information given on subsequent visits and when the patient and family see other healthcare professionals.
- Provide resources for follow-up support.
- Use the key components of the SPIKES model: demonstrate empathy, acknowledge the patient's feelings, explore the patient's understanding and acceptance of the bad news, and provide information about possible interventions. Having a plan of action provides structure for this difficult discussion and helps support all involved.

**Figure 1-1. Guidelines for Giving a Cancer Diagnosis**

*Note.* Based on information from Back et al., 2009; Backman, 2005; Fried et al., 2003; Girgis & Sanson-Fisher, 1995; Kaplan, 2010.

the diagnosis is new and the patient is dealing with a variety of new healthcare professionals (Nail, 2001).

Some individuals initially respond with denial. They cannot allow themselves to think about what will happen if the treatment does not work or how this will affect the family. Denial is a protective mechanism from this tremendous threat. It is a common initial reaction to the overwhelming threat but generally decreases over time. Some individuals forestall any emotional reaction to the news as they research the disease, consider treatment options, and interview physicians. This allows patients to remain more focused on decision making. However, an emotional reaction can surface at any time. See Chapter 16 for more information on denial.

In a landmark study, Weisman and Worden (1976–1977) examined 120 patients in the first 100 days after receiving a cancer diagnosis and described the extreme distress commonly experienced in hearing the news. Intermittent periods of anxiety and depression were common. Some of the factors they found that contributed to poor overall psychosocial adaptation included having more physical symptoms, perceiving the physician as being less helpful, having a psychiatric history, and having a pessimistic view of the world. The most significant variables were a perceived lack of a personal support system, having a more advanced illness, and viewing the physician as being unsupportive. Though prognoses and treatments have improved dramatically, many of the same responses are seen today.

Spittler, Pallikathayil, and Bott (2012) found that after being diagnosed with breast cancer, women commonly are exposed to numerous doctors in a short time span to discuss the disease process, prognosis, and treatment options. For many women, the need to assimilate new information can be overwhelming. The resulting stress adds to a perceived urgency of the circumstances, potentially leading some women to make hasty decisions they later regret, such as their choice of treatment center or drug regimen.

Sherman, Rosedale, and Haber (2012) found that patients with breast cancer exhibited different reactions that were often paradoxical. For example, some patients viewed themselves as victims while viewing others as survivors. After treatment, some patients viewed cancer as an ongoing diagnosis while others viewed it as a past event. Khalili, Farajzadegan, Mokarian, and Bahrami (2013) found that patients with breast cancer often use acceptance, positive thinking, denial, reframing, distraction, and religion as ways to adjust to their diagnosis.

DellaRipa et al. (2015) found that patients with ovarian cancer experienced intensified distress related to witnessing the effect of the diagnosis on those they loved. All were concerned for those around them and found it hard to watch others suffer because of their illness. Baker et al. (2013) studied reactions of patients with a variety of cancers including lung, breast, and prostate. They found that patients early in the cancer trajectory, who had not yet started chemotherapy or radiation therapy, described emotional distress as a temporary and understandable reaction that did not warrant professional intervention.

For many, once a diagnosis is made, the focus shifts quickly to identifying treatment options. This may include going for a second, third, or multiple opinions; joining clinical trials; and researching on the Internet to find the right physician and treatment plan. Patients also need to make decisions about how to communicate the diagnosis to their families and friends. For some, this is a private matter. For others, reaching out for support personally and through social media are viable options. The patient's response to a new diagnosis can also include concealing the diagnosis from others. Gonzalez et al. (2015) found that some patients with lung cancer who concealed the initial diagnosis or recurrence related to more internalized shame regarding the etiology of the cancer.

## Family Reactions

When cancer enters an individual's life, it also enters the lives of family members and close friends. These individuals are sometimes referred to as *informal caregivers*. How these caregivers react will also affect the patient (Rait, 2015). The diagnosis marks a major transition in the family's life (Zaider & Kissane, 2015). A sense of vulnerability and awareness of the inability to protect a loved one can lead to an intense feeling of helplessness. Because family members and patients often share common beliefs, the reactions of family members may parallel those of patients. Denial or blaming others for the diagnosis may occur in close family members. Family members may experience vulnerability with the realization that this could happen to them as well. New demands, role changes, disruption of future plans, and priorities contribute to stress in those close to the patient (Zaider & Kissane, 2015). In addition, family members often oversee the patient's transition into a medical culture, which can be confusing and disarming (Rait, 2015). Role changes can contribute to communication problems if someone is unsure of the usual care routines and schedules. The financial demands of treatment options can create concerns about the need to continue working. The strain of feeling continuously "on duty" to provide physical and emotional support, on top of dealing with their own fears, adds to the pressures already on family members. They also may feel as though they need to conceal their own feelings and fears of what will be expected of them in the future if the disease progresses. Seeing a loved one vulnerable and fearful can create much distress, especially if this is a big change from the patient's personality.

Some family members may assume the role of "cheerleader" to remain upbeat and encourage the patient to remain optimistic. This role can become very draining and lead to resentment if one's own needs are not being recognized or met. Resentment can occur regarding the stress and inconvenience imposed on the family, as well as past behaviors that they attribute to causing the cancer (e.g., smoking, high-stress lifestyle) (Mood, 1996). Some members may take on additional roles, such as assisting with research and treatment decisions, if the patient is paralyzed by anxiety or is too ill to participate.

The family with cancer is a family in transition (Rait, 2015). Multiple challenges can affect all involved in different ways and at different times. Striving to maintain stability of the family system while adapting to the changing needs of the patient are important roles of family members.

Family members play a key role in the support system for most patients. How to provide support to patients and best meet their needs may require a period of trial and error. For example, patients may want to be more independent, whereas family members may feel the need to be protective, leading to resentment and increased stress on both sides. A lack of communication can lead to feeling that one's needs are going unrecognized and feelings of being smothered or isolated from family life. Caregiver stress can lead to changes in caregivers' physical health, immune function, and financial well-being (Northouse, Williams, Given, & McCorkle, 2012).

## Life Span Considerations

A diagnosis of cancer in a child often causes profound shock and disruption among family members. A child's response to a cancer diagnosis of a family member depends on the child's developmental and cognitive levels as well as on how the parents respond (McFresh & Merck, 2011). Parents particularly are overwhelmed with the realization of their child's vulnerability to this disease and may experience high levels of anxiety as they try to protect their child from any distress. In addition to the emotional distress, family members must face the disease-related demands that affect the entire family. During active medical treatment, parents of children and adolescents with cancer face many physical, emotional, and psychosocial challenges. These challenges often generate a need for information regarding medical treatments and a need for psychosocial support (Svavarsdottir & Sigurdardottir, 2013).

During the time of family disruption caused by the diagnosis, the child and siblings may exhibit behavioral and adjustment problems (e.g., problems with school attendance, sleep, aggression) in response to their anxiety. Children with cancer may require complex treatment regimens and multiple hospitalizations, as well as experience late complications, which may require long-term support.

Adolescents and young adults experience a separate set of challenges as a result of the disruptive impact that cancer and its treatment have on normal developmental transitions (Jacobsen et al., 2012). Young adults with cancer often are faced with challenges that put them in more dependent roles at a time when they are striking out on their own. Issues around establishing relationships, fertility, and delays in completing goals (e.g., school, career) are common (Katz, 2015). Individuals diagnosed with cancer during adolescence or young adulthood have the cognitive capacity to understand the severity of their illness and frequently demonstrate persistent distress and anxiety over death, cancer recurrence, or late effects (Zebrack & Isaacson, 2012).

Cancer is increasingly more likely to occur as one ages (Siegel, Miller, & Jemal, 2017). Thus, older adults are more at risk. The majority of cancer survivors are over age 65 (Institute of Medicine [IOM], 2013). In addition, the issues that survivors face can continue into advancing age. One of the major challenges for older adults with cancer is the presence of comorbidities that often complicate treatment and symptom management as well as contribute to more severe side effects (Given & Given, 2015). Other challenges include increasingly complex treatment regimen choices for frail patients. Older patients may have a limited support system, including caregivers that have the same level of limitation as the person with cancer (Meriggi et al., 2014). These concerns need to be incorporated in the decision-making process for cancer treatment. Age alone should not be the deciding factor. Newer treatments with fewer systemic side effects may present more options for the older patient.

## Cancer Treatment

As the diagnostic phase is completed and treatment decisions are made, the patient and family face new experiences that will psychosocially affect them, including hospitalization, surgery, insertion of a central line, starting chemotherapy or other treatments, and frequent doctor visits. An urgency to begin treatment often exists, and no matter how much education the patient receives, he or she still may feel unprepared to enter this unfamiliar world. Each type of treatment creates its own psychosocial impact. Factors that can influence the patient's response to treatment include understanding the necessity of the treatment success rate, potential side effects, and discomforts of the treatment, as well as the relationship with the physician (Puts et al., 2015). Frailty is being recognized as an important factor to be considered in treatment decisions (Ethun et al., 2017).

### Surgery

Surgery is the oldest form of cancer treatment (Mukherjee, 2010). Surgery alone as a cancer treatment may not be associated with the same negative view as other treatments that are more closely aligned to cancer. Patients are more familiar with surgery than other types of cancer treatments because it is routinely performed for noncancerous conditions with positive outcomes. In early stages, surgery may be offered as curative. It is viewed as a way to eliminate the cancer from one's body. However, mastectomies, genital surgeries, head and neck surgeries, and colostomies generally are associated with more distress because of the obvious changes in appearance and body function (Jacobsen, Roth, & Holland, 1998). In women facing primary breast cancer surgery, Miller, Schnur, Weinberger-Litman, and Montgomery (2014) found poor body image was a factor in elevated distress in younger women.

For the individual who receives the news of a cancer diagnosis postoperatively, pain and weakness from the surgery will add to the distress and depression created by the new diagnosis. Psychosocial distress can be related to surgical healing time and the type of procedure (Lester et al., 2015). In the face of advanced cancer, palliative surgery may be chosen as treatment of physical symptoms (Williams, Ferrell, Juarez, & Borneman, 2015).

## Chemotherapy and Targeted Therapies

Most individuals have preconceived ideas about chemotherapy and its side effects. While the patient is still reeling from the diagnosis, starting chemotherapy can intensify the sense of vulnerability to one's already weakened coping reserves. The protective equipment worn by staff members who administer chemotherapy may add to this fear. However, chemotherapy is an active treatment that can give patients a sense of strength as they hope for a cure. Many patients are under the impression that chemotherapy must be given intravenously to be effective. However, many new oral agents, including targeted therapies, with lower side effect profiles are now available. Screening for anxiety during initial chemotherapy is important because it is prevalent (Garcia, 2014). Attention to quality-of-life interventions has been shown to increase completion of chemotherapeutic regimens (Cheville et al., 2015). Because these drugs often have more complex dosing instructions and are managed at home, patients need to understand the importance of self-monitoring (Spoelstra et al., 2013).

Chemotherapy-induced nausea and vomiting is one of the most feared and severe side effects of cancer treatment (Lee et al., 2017). Education about the medications available to control these symptoms can address these concerns. Alopecia has the emotional impact of being a constant reminder of the diagnosis, forcing patients to immediately integrate the diagnosis into their lives. It is a visible reminder to the world that a person has cancer, impeding the opportunity to keep the diagnosis private. Fatigue and risk for infection also contribute to psychosocial distress (see Chapter 6).

Chemotherapy forces the patient and family to adhere to medical appointments and hospitalization schedules and to reallocate family roles because the patient usually cannot meet obligations due to fatigue or other side effects. Seeing the patient in a vulnerable state while coping with the effects of chemotherapy may increase the distress on family members who must watch their loved one suffer. Fatigue and irritability experienced by the patient and family can negatively impact the family system.

## Radiation Therapy

People are taught to fear and avoid radiation. However, the patient is also told that radiation is a treatment for cancer. This dichotomy can create deep-seated anxieties related to the cancer treatment (Greenberg, 1998). Radiation presents many unknowns to the patient. Meeting a new physician and treatment team in the radiation therapy department and lying alone on a table with a large machine overhead can create a sense of isolation and anxiety. Fears about being burned and having visible skin tattoos may contribute to one's distress and create self-consciousness. The patient may have heard myths concerning the side effects of this therapy and needs extensive education about what to expect. Radiation generally involves a longer time commitment of consecutive treatment sessions that can be disruptive in the patient's life, often requiring dependence on others for daily transportation to treatment (Haisfield-Wolfe, McGuire, & Krumm, 2012).

## Palliative Care

Palliative care is a supportive treatment program that is generally for patients with advanced disease but can be appropriate from diagnosis. As defined by the Center to Advance Palliative Care (2015), it is specialized medical care for people with serious illnesses and focuses on providing patients with relief from the symptoms and stress of any serious illness. Palliative care can be provided at any stage of illness along with curative therapy. The goal is to improve quality of life for both the patient and family. The association of palliative care with hospice has led to the misunderstanding that palliative care is an end-of-life program. In 2012, a provisional clinical opinion from the American Society of Clinical Oncology (ASCO) stated that combined standard oncology care and palliative care should be considered early in the course of illness for any patient with metastatic cancer or high symptom burden (Smith et al., 2012). This standard supports bringing palliative care into the forefront of cancer treatment and can be brought in at diagnosis in some patients (IOM, 2015). In 2015, ASCO partnered with the American Academy of Hospice and Palliative Medicine to release a joint statement that established essential palliative care services and set achievable goals for medical oncologists. The established standards identify the basic skills medical oncologists need to provide primary palliative care, including symptom management, advance care planning, and communication and shared decision making.

Palliative care is generally provided by a team either in the hospital, outpatient clinic, or office, as well as in the home for symptom management, emotional support, advance care planning, and resource utilization. The vast majority of programs remain in the hospital, but growth in the other sectors is anticipated. Palliative care can be provided while the patient is still receiving aggressive treatment such as chemotherapy, total parenteral nutrition, and surgery. The presence of palliative care early in the disease trajectory can assist with complex symptom management and advance care planning. Later in the disease process, it can also assist with establishing treatment goals and helping with decision making as the patient is facing treatment choices about level of aggressiveness to pursue. Palliative care also can be a transition to hospice. An interprofessional team approach is generally a key part of palliative care.

The recent growth of the field has been fueled by studies demonstrating the positive impact of palliative care in symptom management, advance care planning, and emotional support (Bakitis, Lyons, Hegel, & Ahles, 2013; Dahlin, Kelley, Jackson, & Temel, 2010; Temel et al., 2010). Bakitis et al. (2013) found that palliative care for patients with cancer generally resulted in positive outcomes except when patients were not ready, lacked preparation for the referral, or equated palliative care with hospice. Temel et al. (2011) studied 151 patients newly diagnosed with non-small cell lung cancer. Those receiving early palliative care significantly improved understanding of their prognosis over time. This, in turn, may affect decision making about care near the end of life.

These patients also experienced improved quality of life and lived longer than the group without palliative care. Rabow et al. (2013) found evidence that palliative care contributed to improved patient satisfaction, symptom control, and quality of life; reduction in healthcare utilization; and longer survival in a population of patients with lung cancer.

Palliative care can provide access to expert symptom management as patients are pursuing curative therapy. If the focus changes to supportive care, then the palliative care team can take a larger role in providing support, managing symptoms, addressing goals, and assisting with plans for the future. Potentially, referral to palliative care will increase access to hospice care earlier in the course of the illness. Outcome measures for palliative care were developed by the National Consensus Project for Quality Palliative Care (2013) to include the following:
- Physical and emotional symptoms
- Support of function and autonomy
- Advance care planning
- Aggressive care near death
- Patient and family satisfaction with care
- Emphasis on quality of life
- Relief of family burden
- Provider continuity and ease of contact
- Bereavement assessment and care planning and support

The Oncology Nursing Society (2014) position statement on palliative care for people with cancer supports that all patients with cancer benefit from palliative care and that oncology nurses are critical participants in the delivery of this care. Pediatric palliative care programs are now available in many settings. The American Academy of Pediatrics (2000) has supported the introduction of palliative care for all children with life-threatening illness at diagnosis and throughout the disease course. Kaye et al. (2015) suggested that possible triggers for pediatric palliative care referrals at diagnosis include stage IV neuroblastoma, metastatic solid tumors, any new diagnosis with complex pain symptoms, and any disease where stem cell transplantation is part of the treatment plan.

With the growth of palliative care, the need for an adequate workforce of professionals to provide all levels of this care is a concern. Educating oncology professionals on the basics of palliative care will help to reach more patients (IOM, 2015). Advanced practice nurses play a key role in providing palliative care and leading many teams. Bedside nurses in many settings who care for patients with cancer will continue to incorporate palliative care principles in patient care (Coyle, 2015; Dahlin, 2015).

## The Patient's and Family's Response to Cancer Treatment

Adjusting to the demands of cancer treatment takes its toll on the patient and family. In addition, many adjustments must continue to be made as treatment continues (Williams & Jeanetta, 2015). For example, treatment side effects may develop, recovery times from procedures may be longer than expected, and outcomes from treatment may be disappointing. Some support needs during treatment include financial resources, information, and spiritual and emotional support (Smith, Hyde, & Stanford, 2014).

The emotional response to treatment has been extensively studied. Baker et al. (2013) found that newly diagnosed patients were less interested in emotional support resources prior to starting cancer treatment but more open to them once treatment had started. They postulated that this was because treatment increased exposure to vulnerability and potential suffering. A study by Sherman et al. (2012) on patients with breast cancer found that treatment challenged women's images of being healthy when looking at their surgical scars or hairless heads. Treatment was associated with a reminder of the potential losses they face, such as loss of roles. During treatment, they were often on high alert to new symptoms that could signify a complication or recurrence of cancer.

The presence of treatment side effects will influence coping. Mortimer and Behrendt (2013) found that symptoms such as hot flashes, sleep disturbance, fatigue, and weight gain related to hormone treatment after breast cancer greatly affected quality of life for some time.

Family and friends are also affected by cancer treatment. With treatment increasingly occurring in the outpatient setting, family members and friends are being asked to take on greater responsibilities for patient care (Jacobsen et al., 2012; Latour, 2014). Cancer treatment leads to changes in responsibilities and roles in loved ones. Family members often assume the caregiving role with little or no preparation and without considering whether they have enough knowledge, resources, or skills (Northouse et al., 2012). These demands can cause changes in their psychological, physical, and financial well-being, especially if the patient or caregiver cannot return to work (Northouse et al., 2012). Duggleby et al. (2015) found that male spouses of patients with breast cancer took on a number of new roles and responsibilities, including as caregivers. They reported better quality of life when they had more hope and less guilt.

Family members need to adjust to the demands of long-term treatment. The patient and family often will transition from the crisis-oriented response of the initial diagnosis to a "new normal" as the treatment schedule and challenges become part of daily life. In long-term treatment, the loved ones need to establish a method of communication to stay informed on the patient's condition without being too intrusive.

## The Oncology Nurse's Role in Cancer Treatment

Patients who are receiving a new diagnosis, starting treatment, and continuing treatment are part of the daily practice of most oncology nurses. These patients and their families are facing one of the biggest crises of their lives. The oncology nurse's role must incorporate an awareness of the tremendous psychosocial implications that exist. Northouse and Northouse (1996) delineated the important interpersonal roles of oncology nurses as imparting information, communicating hope, and dealing with the many emotions that are part of the patient's cancer experience. They viewed the major issues confronting patients as maintaining a sense of control, obtaining information, searching for meaning, and disclosing feelings.

Nurses play an important role in assisting patients in all of these areas. Although nurses are not able to control the disease, they still can provide support in controlling patients' responses to the illness and education about the disease and its treatment. Education will provide patients with the control necessary to deal with side effects and will help them to make the best decisions. Providing education enhances emotional support and fosters hope and the development of a trusting relationship. Nurses should recognize that once hope is taken away, it is very difficult to recapture it. Helping patients to confront intense and confusing emotions is a key role for nurses and an important component of the nurse–patient relationship. Nurses can advise patients about ways to communicate so family and friends can keep abreast of changes without fatiguing the patient.

# Recurrence

With longer survival rates comes the risk of recurrent disease. Because of the unpredictable nature of cancer, many individuals facing a diagnosis and initial treatment eventually must face recurrence or advancing disease in the form of metastasis. Maintaining life balance in the face of new disease and managing pain, fatigue, and other physical and psychological symptoms are major challenges (Ganz & Stanton, 2015). *Recurrence* is the return of the disease after an initial course of treatment with a disease-free period. The disease may recur at the same site, recur near the site, or metastasize to a distant site. The threat of recurrence is one of the reasons why cancer is such a feared disease.

## Psychosocial Response to Recurrence

Individuals move from being short- or long-term survivors of cancer to being patients once more when the cancer returns, and this brings new stresses (Andersen, Shapiro, Farrar, Crespin, & Wells-DiGregorio, 2005; Vivar, Whyte, & McQueen, 2010). Families move from a state of fear of recurrence to one of uncertainty and distress as a result of the new crisis (Vivar, Canga, Canga, & Arantzamendi, 2009). Recurrence brings significant stress, which is not unlike that of the initial diagnosis (Yang, Brothers, & Andersen, 2008).

Research on psychosocial response to recurrence is limited and contradictory. Weisman and Worden (1986) found that the degree of psychological distress at the time of recurrence depended on the degree of symptomatology from the recurrence. Thirty percent of their sample reported less distress with the recurrence. This group was less surprised by the recurrence and had not let themselves believe they were cured. In fact, for some, recurrence was a relief from the distressing uncertainty with which they had been living as they waited for the disease to return. For these patients, the uncertainty can be more distressing than the actual return of disease. With recurrence comes many negative emotions, which are different in that they may be more intense than those after the first diagnosis of cancer. Survivors and their family members have to manage new psychological distress (Vivar et al., 2010). In a study by Schulman-Green et al. (2012), disease progression was as challenging as initial diagnosis of ovarian cancer. Warren (2010) found that diagnosis of metastatic (or secondary) breast cancer was frequently more distressing than the diagnosis of a primary tumor because it indicated the cancer was no longer curable.

Andersen et al. (2005) found that women's previous experiences with a cancer diagnosis may enable them to be emotionally resilient. In this study, patients had less distress with recurrence than with initial diagnosis.

A study by Yang et al. (2008) of women experiencing recurrence of breast cancer found that patients who coped with disengagement strategies such as avoidance, denial, and withdrawal had poorer quality of life. Those who had higher symptom distress experienced more difficulty coping.

Because these patients have already been through some type of cancer treatment, preparing for treatment again may be more difficult because they know what to expect. Patients who experienced severe side effects with the initial treatment may need more encouragement or more aggressive symptom management. These patients also may face decisions regarding more aggressive treatment, such as stem cell transplant, immunotherapy, and/or clinical trials. These treatments may not have been considered the first time around, thus creating more unknowns. In some cases, these therapies may have been offered at the time of initial treatment, and the patient may have decided on a more conservative approach. This can result in feelings of guilt or regret.

The realization that treatment has failed can contribute to depression and a feeling of hopelessness. The patient's sense of hope may have provided the encouragement needed the first time around when a cure was anticipated. The loss of hope may contribute to the realization that the individual must consider the possibility of death. Holland (1998) described the existential crisis of recurrence as the individual having to consider for the first time that death could be the outcome and that one's goals may not be realized. Lamperti et al. (2012) found that depression was higher than anxiety in patients with recurrent brain tumors.

Loss of faith in the medical establishment may be a reaction as the individual realizes the initial treatment did not provide a cure. This can contribute to anger, consideration of alternative therapies, or even refusal of further therapy. Some individuals may experience a sense of personal failure in thinking that they have disappointed their physicians by not being cured. A sense of injustice, noted by a comment such as "It is not fair because I did everything they asked of me," can create more anxiety, anger, and helplessness.

Recurrence may present financial demands if the patient is considering aggressive or experimental treatment. An inability to work, problems with insurance coverage, and a need to relocate may contribute to this challenge and present additional stressors for patients and families. Another fear may be that of facing a more physically disabling illness as the disease progresses and treatment becomes more aggressive.

## The Family's Response to Recurrence

As with the patient, family members must struggle with depression, anger, guilt, and the fear of death. Recurrence creates great suffering in families (Northouse et al., 2002). In a study by Vivar et al. (2010), learning that the cancer had come back was, for most of the families, more devastating than hearing about the initial diagnosis. Signs of shock and suffering were experienced by families as an initial response to recurrence. The new diagnosis often entailed a change in family life. Survivorship period and age also seemed significant in the psychosocial experience of recurrence.

Recurrence may create so much distress that family members and friends will react with detachment because they fear reinvesting in the patient's treatment when the outcome may be less positive. This can be the response when the patient experiences multiple remissions and exacerbations. Maintaining a positive attitude may be more difficult for family members and friends, and providing emotional support to the patient could be more draining. On the other hand, family crises faced at the time of initial diagnosis may have strengthened the family members to better face this new challenge. In the past, spouses or siblings may have thought that they never could have coped with a loved one having cancer, and getting through the initial treatment may have given these individuals confidence in their ability to face whatever happens. At times, the patient may wish to have less contact with family members and friends because of depression or fatigue.

## The Oncology Nurse's Response to Recurrence

Identifying how a patient coped at the time of initial diagnosis is an important early part of the treatment plan that may predict the patient's response to the news of recurrence. Knowing what physicians told the patient also can provide important information to gauge the response. Reinforcement of hope may help to maintain emotional balance. Patients may fear abandonment by the healthcare team after "failing" the first-line treatment. Healthcare professionals often describe it as the patient "failing treatment." In reality, the treatment has failed the patient. By avoiding the association with failure, the nurse can reduce the patient's sense of responsibility for outcomes. Regardless of the treatment goal, physicians and nurses must present a treatment plan that communicates a continued commitment to patients.

Patients experiencing a recurrence will face many choices about treatment and need information to help them make decisions. Making important treatment decisions during a time of emotional upheaval requires patients to have access to a variety of information at different times. Written material may be helpful for patients to review after receiving oral instructions. Access to alternative resources, such as the Internet and cancer information hotlines, may be useful as patients seek more opinions about their options. Awareness of the patient's emotional state, including anxiety and depression, will affect learning; therefore, information needs to be repeated and provided in writing or to a family member or friend to reinforce the content.

Patients and family members need an opportunity to share fears in a safe environment. They may be reluctant to express their deepest fears to one another in order to provide a measure of "protection." The oncology nurse is in a key role to provide this important outlet.

## Terminal Illness

For some, awareness of a terminal illness may come as a gradual realization that the disease is progressing despite aggressive treatment. For others, this realization may be sudden. Some may continue to pursue aggressive treatment until the end, and others may reject treatment at the time of diagnosis. Still others may face life-threatening complications during active treatment. However, when the realization comes, it remains a difficult and emotional journey. At this time, patients and families experience many fears. Death is a threat with many common themes.

### The Patient's Fears

**Fear of the unknown:** Death is one of the strongest fears of all human beings (Rando, 1984), and it presents the greatest "unknown" for many people. Questions concerning what will happen to family, life plans, life's work, and body are difficult to face, and they are also difficult questions for others, such as family members, to hear. Some of these thoughts can be acknowledged by talking about the concerns and preparing to care for loved ones or to achieve a hoped-for goal. Other questions can be acknowledged only in a supportive environment. Spiritual support may provide some comfort.

**Fear of pain and suffering:** Pain is one of the most common and greatest fears for those at the end of life (Breivik et al., 2009; Ng & von Gunten, 1998). Many individuals believe dying must mean terrible pain, loss of dignity, and uncontrollable suffering. Patients may have images of people they have known in the past screaming in torment while dying of cancer. The majority of people with terminal illness can obtain relief (Paice, 2015). Unfortunately, this fear becomes a reality for some when inadequate pain relief is provided. Patients and their caregivers need to be educated about the options for pain control. Pain can produce feelings of guilt for patients who view pain as a cause of suffering for their family. Suffering can be caused by physical symptoms as well as a variety of emotional, social, and spiritual factors. See Chapters 8 and 10 for more information on the psychosocial impact of pain and suffering.

**Fear of abandonment:** As patients weaken and begin to lose some control, the fear that others involved in the care may abandon them can be intense. Patients may particularly fear abandonment by their physicians when the focus of care moves away from aggressive treatment. Physicians may have said, "There is nothing more I can do," which reinforces this fear.

In most cases, physicians' continued involvement during the terminal stage is an important part of supportive care. Even when patients are under hospice care, attending physicians can often remain actively involved. Individuals who feel helpless and anxious around a dying patient may need encouragement to maintain their involvement with the patient to alleviate the patient's fears of being left alone.

**Loss of control:** When advancing cancer causes progressive weakness, fatigue, and confusion, patients have less opportunity to maintain control of their environment and what is happening to them. Because American society places strong value on self-reliance and independence, this loss can be humiliating and provoke anxiety. Loss of control can induce feelings of guilt because patients may feel uncomfortable relying on others and can maintain a belief of needing to be strong. Others can inadvertently add to this fear by taking over decision making and other responsibilities for patients out of a desire to help. Advancing disease that treatment can no longer control represents a loss of patients' power over the cancer. Stopping aggressive treatment may represent a major loss of control as patients feel they are "giving in" to the cancer. This can lead to a fear of becoming a burden to the family (Steele & Davies, 2015). At some point in the dying process, patients may begin detaching from the outside world and becoming withdrawn. At this point, patients give up the struggle to stay invested in controlling aspects of life. This is a self-protective mechanism and is common in the dying process.

Encouraging the completion of advance directives and estate planning to ensure that personal wishes are known by others and will be followed can help patients to maintain a sense of control. Caregivers can be sensitive to the urge to take over for patients when they are still able to complete tasks. Helping patients to conserve energy and establish priorities can enhance a sense of control and allow them to focus on the most important things.

**Loss of identity:** As individuals become weaker, more aspects of self can be lost as they can no longer maintain skills, interests, and relationships. Individuals' abilities often define and affirm who they are, and when this is lost, they can feel more distressed and confused. Loss of dignity as patients become more dependent may increase this fear. Those patients with enough energy can leave a legacy by making video or audio recordings, which helps them to achieve a desired goal and enhances a sense of purpose and identity. For others, maintaining their self-respect and dignity by acknowledging their value as a person can address this fear.

**Loss of body image/self:** Valued physical traits may be lost as weakness and emaciation occur. Patients may be less able to complete normally important personal care routines (e.g., shaving, applying makeup). An individual may no longer be recognized as the same person by others. This can cause patients to feel shame or that they are not lovable. Maintaining patients' dignity, respecting modesty, and assisting with personal care are all important supportive care measures.

**Loss of loved ones:** Perhaps one of the most poignant fears that patients encounter is facing the loss of relationships with loved ones. Just as family members anticipate losing the patient, the patient, too, is anticipating separation and loneliness (Worden, 2000). Because most people cannot truly understand what the patient is facing, terminal illness creates a sense of separation or disconnectedness from others (Borneman & Brown-Saltzman, 2015).

Opportunities to acknowledge the grief, complete unfinished business with important people in their lives, and spend time with loved ones reminiscing about past joys and sorrows can be therapeutic to some patients and family members. Recognizing the limited time one has to right wrongs with a loved one or achieve forgiveness is a struggle for some.

Borneman and Brown-Saltzman (2001) defined forgiveness as letting go of expectations that one will be vindicated for pain and loss. This can provide an opportunity for healing and possible reconciliation. Ferrell (2012) described forgiveness as assisting the person to acknowledge the harm they have done, to feel worthy of being forgiven, and to fully embrace the experience of the other who was involved. Byock (2004) condensed supportive responses to loved ones in four phrases: "Please forgive me," "I forgive you as well," "Thank you," and "I love you."

**Loss of hope:** Hope is a natural part of human existence. Although it is often challenged in the face of terminal illness, hope can also thrive, even with the realization that cure is no longer possible (Cotter & Foxwell, 2015). When hope for a cure is no longer realistic, individuals often are able to alter wishes for the future. The nature of hope can adjust as patients may begin to hope for an easy death, to resolve a conflict with an estranged relative, leave a legacy, or to believe one's spouse will be prepared to face life alone. Reframing hope can be supported by focusing on the present and specifics rather than vague uncertainties in the future. See Chapter 7 for more information about hope and the psychosocial experience.

## The Family's Fears

**Loss of the relationship:** Anticipating the loss of a family member is the beginning of the grieving process, which includes facing sadness, struggling with anger, and anticipating life without this loved one. If the dying person is part of a family member's everyday life, as with a spouse or parent who lives with the family, the loss can be more intense. During the dying process, family members begin to realize what life will be like as the patient weakens, sleeps more, and is less a part of the daily routine. The patient may turn more inward, and there can be less emotional contact for the family. The approach of death may generate an awareness of losing a special relationship (e.g., a daughter losing her father who has always been her protector), loss of a part of oneself (e.g., losing one's wife means giving up a role as husband), or empathy and concern for others (e.g., a man who anticipates losing his lifelong friend and confidant). Corless (2015) described the process of letting go of the relationship as part of the grieving process, but it does not mean cutting off memories of the lost person.

As family members realize that they are losing the relationship, they may fear that if the patient is too sedated to interact, they will be faced with the loss more quickly. Although family members may want the patient to be comfortable, they may try to keep him or her awake out of fear of having to face the painful realization of the loss of the relationship. Helping family members to acknowledge this fear and to reinforce the need to grieve this loss can be helpful along with reassuring them of the patient's need to be comfortable. Chapter 19 discusses the grieving process and ways to manage grief.

**Loss of control:** As with the patient, family members must face a loss of control with the realization that they can do nothing to stop the disease. This can generate many feelings, with anger often being the most pronounced. As a way to maintain some control, this anger may be expressed to physicians for not doing enough for the patient or to nurses whose actions are viewed as unhelpful (e.g., not being able to restart an IV on the first try, not bringing a medication immediately). For individuals who have never faced the death of a loved one, this can be a particularly difficult experience because the sense of loss of control can be overwhelming. Helping family members to face this loss, acknowledging their efforts to advocate for the patient, and helping them to identify ways to maintain some control can be useful interventions. Family members may be facing loss of control in other areas of their lives as schedules are disrupted, sleep is interrupted, and conflicts arise with relatives and friends—all perhaps occurring at the same time. Some family members may need to maintain a job or child care while simultaneously caring for a dying loved one. Giving family members some control in making decisions about care routines or activities can help to reduce the sense of loss of control. See Chapter 21 for more information on loss of control and powerlessness.

**Fear of sorrow:** The growing realization of the impending loss may generate intense emotions that are frightening to some individuals. Family members may have used avoidance as a means of protection from feeling pain. Once it is experienced, depression, anger, preoccupation, irritability, and difficulty making decisions can occur. This is part of the grieving process. As the patient grows more ill and eventually begins to withdraw from day-to-day life, the reality of the impending loss intensifies. This may be felt more strongly if the family member had protected himself or herself by using denial or avoidance. Helping the family member to be open to the grieving process and providing support and acceptance regardless of the reaction are very important.

**Fear of pain and suffering:** Family members may anticipate that the patient will have to endure much suffering during the dying process. This may cause them to seek assistance related to dying, such as physician-assisted suicide or euthanasia. The thought of seeing their loved one suffer can be so overwhelming that some individuals may act rashly to avoid even the remotest possibility of this happening. Education about the dying process must begin early. This should include encouraging family members to express their fears about what they think will happen and then providing information to alleviate those fears. Wright et al. (2008) found that aggressive medical treatment at the end of life was associated with a higher risk of depressive disorder in bereaved caregivers.

### The Oncology Nurse's Role in End-of-Life Care

It is vital for oncology nurses in all settings to be skillful in addressing the fears of patients and families when cancer is progressing. As part of the interprofessional team, the oncology nurse often is a leader in identifying palliative interventions and support needs. Acknowledging emotions, providing a supportive environment, and promoting access to resources of palliative care and hospice are some of the important nursing interventions. Nurses often are the ones who see the patients and family members' raw emotions as they cope with approaching death. Chapter 26 gives more information on end-of-life care.

An additional nursing role is providing information to the patient and family about what to expect in the dying process (Goldsmith, Ferrell, Wittenberg-Lyles, & Ragan, 2013). Information often reduces uncertainty and provides comfort. Family members often model their care of the patient on what they observe from the nurses (Ferrell & Coyle, 2008).

Incorporating discussions about end-of-life wishes is an important role for oncology nurses. Patients who have conversations about their wishes for end-of-life care are more likely to receive care consistent with their preferences (Mack, Weeks, Wright, Block, & Prigerson, 2010).

## Survivorship

Survivorship has become an important area of study for oncology professionals (Hahn & Ganz, 2015). A cancer survivor is any individual who has been diagnosed with cancer, from the time of discovery and for the balance of life, and includes family, friends, and caregivers (National Coalition for Cancer Survivorship, 2013).

Survivors comprise a significant segment of society, especially in light of the advances in early detection and treatment as well as the growth of the aging population (Miller et al., 2016). Survivorship, however, is still a relatively new concept to oncology. Until the 1990s, relatively little research examined this period for patients with cancer, particularly regarding the psychosocial sequelae. This may be because of the assumption that the quality of life of survivors returns to normal after treatment. Leigh (1997) postulated that in the past it was thought that recovery from a once-fatal illness was reward enough, so no need existed to study the quality of survivors' lives. However, growing evidence has suggested that the effects of treatment, both physically and emotionally, remain long after therapy is completed (Dow, 2003). The National Cancer Institute created the Office of Cancer Survivorship in 1996. With advances in treatment, people with a cancer diagnosis are now living longer, and because of the aggressiveness of treatment approaches, physical and psychological aftereffects are common. In 2005, IOM recommended the development of a survivorship care plan and treatment summary to address ongoing needs. Chapter 2 provides more information on survivorship.

Survivorship is a dynamic, lifelong process that is viewed as a continuum or ongoing role rather than an event that occurs at some designated point in time (e.g., five years). The perception of the quality of one's life as a survivor may change over time as new symptoms or treatment effects recede or increase or as one's coping abilities change. This definition not only includes people with no evidence of disease but also those living with cancers not associated with cure or with cancers controlled by treatment but that periodically progress. Along with the long-term effects from the cancer and its treatment, the challenges of survivorship affect many areas of the person's life, including personal relationships, employment, financial security, sexuality, childbearing, and coping style (IOM, 2005).

## Fear of Recurrence

Fear of cancer recurrence remains an ongoing theme for most survivors (Butow, Fardell, & Smith, 2015; Dahl, Wittrup, Væggemose, Petersen, & Blaakaer, 2013; Koch, Jansen, Brenner, & Arndt, 2013). Cancer recurrence is defined as the fear that cancer could return in survivors who have had treatment with a goal of cure (Butow et al., 2015). It has been found that this fear does not necessarily decrease over time for some (Stanton et al., 2002). This chronic uncertainty of health status during and after cancer treatment can be a significant psychological burden (Simard, Savard, & Ivers, 2010; Thewes et al., 2012). Fear of progression (or fear of recurrence) is an appropriate, rational response to the real threat of cancer and cancer treatments. However, elevated levels of fear of progression can become dysfunction, leading to altered well-being, quality of life, and social functioning (Herschbach & Dinkel, 2014). Addressing worry over return of the cancer is the most prevalent unmet supportive care need (Butow et al., 2015; van den Beuken-van Everdingen et al., 2008).

Fear of recurrence often is thought solely as a patient concern, but it concerns caregivers as well and can be contagious in families. Mellon, Northouse, and Weiss (2006) surveyed patients with cancer and their caregivers in a population-based sample. They found that family caregivers reported significantly higher fears of recurrence than patients. A possible explanation for caregivers' higher fear was that they had less contact and communication with health professionals as well as fewer opportunities to get their own questions answered or fears addressed.

### The Oncology Nurse's Role in Survivorship

In whatever nursing setting, cancer survivors will be part of the patient population. In addition to being educators about survivorship issues, oncology nurses need to consider sharing knowledge about the impact of survivorship with non-oncology nurse colleagues—the nurses most likely to see survivors after treatment.

Cancer survivors need information about the psychological changes that will occur, the long-term physical effects of treatment, the challenges of reentering the work world, the financial impact of the disease, and the effect of the disease on the family. Preparing survivors for the anxiety associated with follow-up medical appointments, self-monitoring of symptoms, end of treatment, reactions when returning to work, and anniversary-related emotions can provide important support and reassurance. Providing encouragement to continue medical follow-up and support group involvement is another important nursing role. See Appendix for resource information.

Family members and friends also need preparation and education about the process of survivorship. Members of the patient's support system may assume that life will return to normal after treatment. Nurses need to encourage them to recognize that the individual's ongoing need to share memories or feelings can be important to recovery.

Recognizing the uniqueness of the cancer experience is an important element to remember when assessing survivors. Each individual will respond differently to this process. Some may easily talk about it. Some may avoid bringing up the topic of cancer for fear of "jinxing" themselves, whereas others may become anxious and depressed. Each individual interprets the disease and circumstances around it to fit their perception of the world.

## Conclusion

A cancer diagnosis clearly has significant physical effects on an individual—effects that result from the disease itself and its treatment. Few other diseases, however, wreak the additional psychosocial havoc that cancer does. The psychosocial ramifications are serious, long-lasting, and broad, and they affect not only individuals with cancer but also their extended network of family, friends, and acquaintances. At every stage along the cancer continuum, the care delivered must address physical aspects of the illness in addition to the mental health and coping strengths of the patient and family. The oncology nurse cannot be effective without a respect for and a command of a broad range of psychosocial nursing skills. In no other specialty is nursing quite so instrumental in facilitating psychosocial care. From diagnosis, throughout treatment, and into survivorship, along with the possibility of end-of-life care, the challenges of cancer provide opportunities for oncology nurses to offer support, leadership, and care.

## References

American Academy of Pediatrics. (2000). Palliative care for children. *Pediatrics, 106,* 351–357. Retrieved from http://pediatrics.aappublications.org/content/106/2/351

Andersen, B.L., Shapiro, C.L., Farrar, W.B., Crespin, T., & Wells-DiGregorio, S. (2005). Psychological responses to cancer recurrence: A controlled perspective study. *Cancer, 104,* 1540–1547. doi:10.1002/cncr.21309

Back, A.L., Arnold, R.M., Baile, W.F., Tulsky, J.A., & Fryer-Edwards, K. (2005). Approaching difficult communication tasks in oncology. *CA: A Cancer Journal for Clinicians, 55,* 164–177. doi:10.3322/canjclin.55.3.164

Back, A.L., Arnold, R.M., & Tulsky, J. (2009). *Mastering communication with seriously ill patients: Balancing honesty with empathy and hope.* Cambridge, NY: Cambridge University Press. doi:10.1017/CBO9780511576454

Baker, P., Beesley, H., Dinwoodie, R., Fletcher, I., Ablett, J., Holcombe, C., & Salmon, P. (2013). 'You're putting thoughts into my head': A qualitative study of the readiness of patients with breast, lung or prostate cancer to address emotional needs through the first 18 months after diagnosis. *Psycho-Oncology, 22,* 1402–1410. doi:10.1002/pon.3156

Bakitis, M., Lyons, K.D., Hegel, M.T., & Ahles, T. (2013). Oncologists' perspectives on concurrent palliative care in a National Cancer Institute–designated comprehensive cancer center. *Palliative and Supportive Care, 11,* 415–423. doi:10.1017/S1478951512000673

Beauchamp, T.L., & Childress, J.F. (2012). *Principles of biomedical ethics* (7th ed.). New York, NY: Oxford University Press.

Borneman, T., & Brown-Saltzman, K. (2001). Meaning in illness. In B.R. Ferrell & N. Coyle (Eds.), *Textbook of palliative nursing* (pp. 415–424). New York, NY: Oxford University Press.

Borneman, T., & Brown-Saltzman, K. (2015). Meaning in illness. In B.R. Ferrell, N. Coyle, & J.A. Paice (Eds.), *Oxford textbook of palliative nursing* (4th ed., pp. 554–566). New York, NY: Oxford University Press.

Bousquet, G., Orri, M., Winterman, S., Brugière, C., Verneuil, L., & Revah-Levy, A. (2015). Breaking bad news in oncology: A metasynthesis. *Journal of Clinical Oncology, 33,* 2437–2443. doi:10.1200/JCO.2014.59.6759

Breivik, H., Cherny, N., Collett, B., de Conno, F., Filbet, M., Foubert, A.J., ... Dow, L. (2009). Cancer-related pain: A pan-European survey of prevalence, treatment, and patient attitudes. *Annals of Oncology, 20,* 1420–1433. doi:10.1093/annonc/mdp001

Buckman, R.A. (2005). Breaking bad news: The S-P-I-K-E-S strategy. *Community Oncology, 2,* 138–142. doi:10.1016/S1548-5315(11)70867-1

Butow, P.N., Fardell, J.E., & Smith, A.B. (2015). Fear of cancer recurrence. In J.C. Holland, W.S. Breitbart, P.N. Butow, P.B. Jacobsen, M.J. Loscalzo, & R. McCorkle (Eds.), *Psycho-oncology* (3rd ed., pp. 625–629). New York, NY: Oxford University Press.

Byock, I. (2004). *The four things that matter most: A book about living.* New York, NY: Simon and Schuster.

Center to Advance Palliative Care. (2015). *America's care of serious illness.* Retrieved from https://reportcard.capc.org/

Cheville, A.L., Alberts, S.R., Rummans, T.A., Basford, J.R., Lapid, M.I., Sloan, J.A., ... Clark, M.M. (2015). Improving adherence to cancer treatment by addressing quality of life in patients with advanced gastrointestinal cancers. *Journal of Pain and Symptom Management, 50,* 321–327. doi:10.1016/j.jpainsymman.2015.03.005

Corless, I.B. (2015). Bereavement. In B.R. Ferrell, N. Coyle, & J.A. Paice (Eds.), *Oxford textbook of palliative nursing* (4th ed., pp. 487–499). New York, NY: Oxford University Press.

Cotter, V.T., & Foxwell, A.M. (2015). The meaning of hope in the dying. In B.R. Ferrell, N. Coyle, & J.A. Paice (Eds.), *Oxford textbook of palliative nursing* (4th ed., pp. 475–486). New York, NY: Oxford University Press.

Coyle, N. (2015). Introduction to palliative nursing care. In B.R. Ferrell, N. Coyle, & J.A. Paice (Eds.), *Oxford textbook of palliative nursing* (4th ed., pp. 3–10). New York, NY: Oxford University Press.

Dahl, L., Wittrup, L., Væggemose, U., Petersen, L.K., & Blaakaer, J. (2013). Life after gynecologic cancer—A review of patients quality of life, needs and preferences in regard to follow-up. *International Journal of Gynecological Cancer, 23,* 227–234. doi:10.1097/IGC.0b013e31827f37b0

Dahlin, C.M., (2015). Palliative care: Delivering comprehensive oncology nursing care. *Seminars in Oncology Nursing, 31,* 327–337. doi:10.1016/j.soncn.2015.08.008

Dahlin, C.M., Kelley, J.M., Jackson, V.A., & Temel, J.S. (2010). Early palliative care for lung cancer: Improving quality of life and increasing survival. *International Journal of Palliative Nursing, 16,* 420–423. doi:10.12968/ijpn.2010.16.9.78633

Dahlin, C.M., & Wittenberg, E. (2015). Communication in palliative care: An essential competency for nurses. In B.R. Ferrell, N. Coyle, & J.A. Paice (Eds.), *Oxford textbook of palliative nursing* (4th ed., pp. 81–112). New York, NY: Oxford University Press.

DellaRipa, J., Conlon, J., Lyon, D.E., Ameringer, S.A., Kelly, D.L., & Menzies, V. (2015). Perceptions of distress in women with ovarian cancer. *Oncology Nursing Forum, 42,* 292–300. doi:10.1188/15.ONF.292-300

de Vries, M., & Stiefel, F. (2014). Psycho-oncological interventions and psychotherapy in the oncology setting. In U. Goerling (Ed.), *Psycho-oncology* (pp. 121–135). doi:10.1007/978-3-642-40187-9_9

Dow, K.H. (2003). Challenges and opportunities in cancer survivorship research. *Oncology Nursing Forum, 30,* 455–469. doi:10.1188/03.ONF.455-469

Duggleby, W., Thomas, J., Montford, K.S., Thomas, R., Nekolaichuk, C., Ghosh, S., ... Tonkin, K. (2015). Transitions of male partners of women with breast cancer: Hope, guilt, and quality of life. *Oncology Nursing Forum, 42,* 134–141. doi:10.1188/15.ONF.134-141

Dunn, S.M., Patterson, P.U., & Butow, P.N. (1993). Cancer by any other name: A randomized trial of the effects of euphemism and uncertainty in communicating with cancer patients. *Journal of Clinical Oncology, 11,* 989–996.

Epplein, M., Zheng, Y., Zheng, W., Chen, Z., Gu, K., Penson, D., ... Shu, X. (2011). Quality of life after breast cancer diagnosis and survival. *Journal of Clinical Oncology, 29,* 406–412, doi:10.1200/JCO.2010.30.6951

Ethun, C.G., Bilen, M.A., Jani, A.B., Maithel, S.K., Ogan, K., & Master, V.A. (2017). Frailty and cancer: Implications for oncology surgery, medical oncology, and radiation oncology. *CA: A Cancer Journal for Clinicians, 67,* 362–377. doi:10.3322/caac.21406

Ferrell, B.R. (2012). Forgiveness in palliative nursing. *Journal of Hospice and Palliative Nursing, 14,* 501. doi:10.1097/NJH.0b013e318272e458

Ferrell, B.R., & Coyle, N. (2008). The nature of suffering and the goals of nursing. *Oncology Nursing Forum, 35,* 241–247. doi:10.1188/08.ONF.241-247

Fried, T.R., Bradley, E.H., & O'Leary, J. (2003). Prognosis communication in serious illness: Perceptions of older patients, caregivers, and clinicians. *Journal of the American Geriatrics Society, 51,* 1398–1403. doi:10.1046/j.1532-5415.2003.51457.x

Ganz, P.A., & Stanton, A.L. (2015). Living with metastatic breast cancer. *Advances in Experimental Medicine and Biology, 862,* 243–254. doi:10.1007/978-3-319-16366-6_16

Garcia, S. (2014). The effects education on anxiety levels in patients receiving chemotherapy for the first time: An integrative approach. *Clinical Journal of Oncology Nursing, 18,* 516–521. doi:10.1188/14.CJON.18-05AP

Girgis, A., & Sanson-Fisher, R.W. (1995). Breaking bad news: Consensus guidelines for medical practitioners. *Journal of Clinical Oncology, 13,* 2449–2456.

Given, B., & Given, C.W. (2015). The older patient. In J.C. Holland, W.S. Breitbart, P.N. Butow, P.B. Jacobsen, M.J. Loscalzo, & R. McCorkle (Eds.), *Psycho-oncology* (3rd ed., pp. 541–548). New York, NY: Oxford University Press.

Goldsmith, J., Ferrell, B.R., Wittenberg-Lyles, E., & Ragan, S.L. (2013). Palliative care communication in oncology nursing. *Clinical Journal of Oncology Nursing, 17,* 163–167. doi:10.1188/13.CJON.163-167

Gonzalez, B.D., Jim, H.S., Cessna, J.M., Small, B.J., Sutton, S.K., & Jacobsen, P.D. (2015). Concealment of lung cancer diagnosis: Prevalence and correlates. *Psycho-Oncology, 24,* 1774–1783. doi:10.1002/pon.3793

Greenberg, D.B. (1998). Radiotherapy. In J.C. Holland (Ed.), *Psycho-oncology* (pp. 269–276). New York, NY: Oxford University Press.

Hahn, E.E., & Ganz, P.A. (2015). Implementing the survivorship care plan: A strategy for improving the quality of care for cancer survivors. In J.C. Holland, W.S. Breitbart, P.N. Butow, P.B. Jacobsen, M.J. Loscalzo, & R. McCorkle (Eds.), *Psycho-oncology* (3rd ed., pp. 644–650). New York, NY: Oxford University Press.

Haisfield-Wolfe, M.E., McGuire, D.B., & Krumm, S. (2012). Perspectives on coping among patients with head and neck cancer receiving radiation. *Oncology Nursing Forum, 39,* E249–E257. doi:10.1188/12.ONF.E249-E257

Herschbach, P., & Dinkel, A. (2014). Fear of progression. *Recent Results in Cancer Research, 197,* 11–29. doi:10.1007/978-3-642-40187-9_2

Holland, J.C. (1998). Clinical course of cancer. In J.C. Holland (Ed.), *Psycho-oncology* (pp. 3–15). New York, NY: Oxford University Press.

Holland, J.C. (2002). History of psychosocial oncology: Overcoming attitudinal and conceptual barriers. *Psychosomatic Medicine, 64,* 206–221. doi:10.1097/00006842-200203000-00004

Holland, J.C. (2003). American Cancer Society Award lecture. Psychological care of patients: Psycho-oncology's contribution. *Journal of Clinical Oncology, 21*(Suppl. 23), 253s–5s. doi:10.1200/JCO.2003.09.133

Holland, J.C., & Alici, Y. (2010). Management of distress in cancer patients. *Journal of Supportive Oncology, 8,* 4–12.

Holland, J.C., & Wiesel, T.W. (2015). Introduction: History of psycho-oncology. In J.C. Holland, W.S. Breitbart, P.N. Butow, P.B. Jacobsen, M.J. Loscalzo, & R. McCorkle (Eds.), *Psycho-oncology* (3rd ed., pp. xxv–xxxv). New York, NY: Oxford University Press.

Institute of Medicine. (2005). *From cancer patient to cancer survivor: Lost in transition.* Washington, DC: National Academies Press.

Institute of Medicine. (2013). *Delivering high-quality cancer care: Charting a new course for a system in crisis.* Washington, DC: National Academies Press.

Institute of Medicine. (2015). *Dying in America: Improving quality and honoring individual preferences near the end of life.* Washington, DC: National Academies Press.

Jacobsen, P.B., Holland, J.C., & Steensma, D.P. (2012). Caring for the whole patient: The science of psychosocial care. *Journal of Clinical Oncology, 30,* 1151–1153. doi:10.1200/JCO.2011.41.4078

Jacobsen, P.B., Roth, A.J., & Holland, J.C. (1998). Surgery. In J.C. Holland (Ed.), *Psycho-oncology* (pp. 257–268). New York, NY: Oxford University Press.

Kaplan, M. (2010). SPIKES: A framework for breaking bad news to patients with cancer. *Clinical Journal of Oncology Nursing, 14,* 514–516. doi:10.1188/10.CJON.514-516

Katz, A. (2015). *Meeting the need for psychosocial care in young adults with cancer.* Pittsburgh, PA: Oncology Nursing Society.

Katz, J. (1984). *The silent world of doctor and patient.* New York, NY: The Free Press.

Kaye, E.C., Rubenstein, J., Levine, D., Baker, J.N., Dabbs, D., & Friebert, S.E. (2015). Pediatric palliative care in the community. *CA: A Cancer Journal for Clinicians, 65,* 316–332. doi:10.3322/caac.21280

Khalili, N., Farajzadegan, Z., Mokarian, F., & Bahrami, F. (2013). Coping strategies, quality of life and pain in women with breast cancer. *Iranian Journal of Nursing and Midwifery Research, 18,* 105–111.

Koch, L., Jansen, L., Brenner, H., & Arndt, V. (2013). Fear of recurrence and disease progression in long-term (≥ 5 years) cancer survivors—A systematic review of quantitative studies *Psycho-Oncology, 22,* 1–11. doi:10.1002/pon.3022

Lamperti, E., Pantaleo, G., Finocchiaro, C.Y., Silvani, A., Botturi, A., Gaviani, P., ... Salmaggi, A. (2012). Recurrent brain tumour: The impact of illness on patient's life. *Supportive Care in Cancer, 20,* 1327–1332. doi:10.1007/s00520-011-1220-y

Latour, K. (2014). Surviving caregiving. *Cure, 13,* 44–50.

Lee, J., Cherwin, C., Czaplewski, L.M., Dabbour, R., Doumit, M., Duran, B., ... Whiteside, S. (2017). Putting evidence into practice: Chemotherapy-induced nausea and vomiting. Retrieved from https://www.ons.org/practice-resources/pep/chemotherapy-induced-nausea-and-vomiting

Leigh, S.A. (1997). Quality of life for life: Survivors influencing research. *Quality of Life, 5,* 58–65.

Lester, J., Crosthwaite, K., Stout, R., Jones, R.N., Holloman, C., Shapiro, C., & Andersen, B.L. (2015). Women with breast cancer: Self-reported distress in early survivorship [Online exclusive]. *Oncology Nursing Forum, 42,* E17–E23. doi:10.1188/15.ONF.E17-E23

Mack, J.W., Weeks, J.C., Wright, A.A., Block, S.D., & Prigerson, H.G. (2010). End-of-life discussions, goal attainment, and distress at the end of life: Predictors and outcomes of receipt of care consistent with preferences. *Journal of Clinical Oncology, 28,* 1203–1208. doi:10.1200/JCO.2009.25.4672

McFresh, P.D., & Merck, T.T. (2011). Family-centered care of children with chronic illness or disability. In M.J. Hockenberry, & D. Wilson (Eds.), *Wong's nursing care of infants and children* (9th ed., pp. 844–875). St. Louis, MO: Elsevier Mosby.

Mellon, S., Northouse, L.L., & Weiss, L.K. (2006). A population-based study of the quality of life of cancer survivors and their family caregivers. *Cancer Nursing, 29,* 120–131. doi:10.1097/00002820-200603000-00007

Meriggi, F., Andreis, F., Premi, V., Liborio, N., Codignola, C., Mazzocchi, M., ... Zaniboni, A. (2014). Assessing cancer caregivers' needs for an early targeted psychosocial support project: The experience of the oncology department of the Poliambulanza Foundation. *Palliative and Supportive Care.* Advance online publication. doi:10.1017/S1478951514000753

Miller, K.D., Siegel, R.L., Lin, V.V., Mariotto, A.B., Kramer, J.L., Rowland, J.H., ... Jemal, A. (2016). Cancer treatment and survivorship statistics, 2016. *CA: A Cancer Journal for Clinicians, 66,* 271–289. doi:10.3322/caac.21349

Miller, S.J., Schnur, J.B., Weinberger-Litman, S.L., & Montgomery, G.H. (2014). The relationship between body image, age, and distress in women facing breast cancer surgery. *Palliative and Supportive Care, 12,* 363–367. doi:10.1017/S1478951513000321

Mood, D.W. (1996). The diagnosis of cancer: A life transition. In R. McCorkle, M. Grant, M. Frank-Stromborg, & S.B. Baird (Eds.), *Cancer nursing: A comprehensive textbook* (2nd ed., pp. 298–314). Philadelphia, PA: Saunders.

Mortimer, J., & Behrendt, C.E. (2013). Severe menopausal symptoms are widespread among survivors of breast cancer treatment regardless of time since diagnosis. *Journal of Palliative Medicine, 16,* 1130–1134, doi:10.1089/jpm.2012.0585

Mukherjee, M. (2010). *The emperor of all maladies: A biography of cancer.* New York, NY: Scribner.

Nail, L.M. (2001). I'm coping as fast as I can: Psychosocial adjustment to cancer and cancer treatment. *Oncology Nursing Forum, 28,* 967–970.

National Coalition for Cancer Survivorship. (2013). *History of NCCS.* Retrieved from http://www.canceradvocacy.org/about-us/our-history/

National Consensus Project for Quality Palliative Care. (2013). *Clinical practice guidelines for quality palliative care* (3rd ed.). Pittsburgh, PA: Author.

Ng, K., & von Gunten, C.F. (1998). Symptoms and attitudes of 100 consecutive patients admitted to an acute hospice and palliative care unit. *Journal of Pain and Symptom Management, 16,* 307–316. doi:10.1016/S0885-3924(98)00097-9

Northouse, L.L., Mood, D., Kershaw, T., Schafenacher, A., Mellon, S., Walker, J., ... Decker, V. (2002). Quality of life of women with recurrent breast cancer and their family members. *Journal of Clinical Oncology, 20,* 4450–4464. doi:10.1200/JCO.2002.02.054

Northouse, L.L., & Northouse, P.G. (1996). Interpersonal communication systems. In R. McCorkle, M. Grant, M. Frank-Stromborg, & S.B. Baird (Eds.), *Cancer nursing: A comprehensive textbook* (2nd ed., pp. 1211–1222). Philadelphia, PA: Saunders.

Northouse, L.L., Williams, A., Given, B., & McCorkle, R. (2012). Psychosocial care for family caregivers of patients with cancer. *Journal of Clinical Oncology, 30,* 1227–1234. doi:10.1200/JCO.2011.39.5798

Novack, D.H., Plumer, R., & Smith, R.L. (1978). Changes in physicians' attitudes toward telling the cancer patient. *JAMA, 241,* 897–900. doi:10.1001/jama.1979.03290350017012

Oken, D. (1961). What to tell cancer patients: A study of medical attitudes. *JAMA, 175,* 1120–1128. doi:10.1001/jama.1961.03040130004002

Oncology Nursing Society. (2014). *Palliative care for people with cancer.* Retrieved from https://www.ons.org/advocacy-policy/positions/practice/palliative-care

Paice, J.A. (2015). Pain at the end of life. In B.R. Ferrell, N. Coyle, & J.A. Paice (Eds.), *Oxford textbook of palliative nursing* (4th ed., pp. 135–153). New York, NY: Oxford University Press.

Payne, J.K. (2014). State of the science: Stress, inflammation and cancer. *Oncology Nursing Forum, 41,* 533–540. doi:10.1188/14.ONF.533-540

Puts, M.T., Tapscott, B., Fitch, M., Howell, D., Monette, J., Wan-Chow-Wah, D., ... Alibhai, S.M. (2015). A systematic review of factors influencing older adults' decision to accept or decline cancer treatment. *Cancer Treatment Reviews, 41,* 197–215. doi:10.1016/j.ctrv.2014.12.010

Rabow, M., Kvale, E., Barbour, L., Cassel, J.B., Cohen, S., Jackson, V., ... Weissman, D. (2013). Moving upstream: A review of the evidence of the impact of outpatient palliative care. *Journal of Palliative Medicine, 16,* 1540–1549. doi:10.1089/jpm.2013.0153

Rait, D.S. (2015). A family-centered approach to the patient with cancer. In J.C. Holland, W.S. Breitbart, P.N. Butow, P.B. Jacobsen, M.J. Loscalzo, & R. McCorkle (Eds.), *Psycho-oncology* (3rd ed., pp. 561–566). New York, NY: Oxford University Press.

Rando, T.A. (1984). *Grief, dying, and death.* Champaign, IL: Research Press Company.

Reed, S., Kassis, K., Nagel, R., Verback, N., Mahan, J.D., & Shell, R. (2015). Breaking bad news is a teachable skill in pediatric residents: A feasibility study of an educational intervention. *Patient Education and Counseling, 98,* 748–752. doi:10.1016/j.pec.2015.02.015

Schulman-Green, D., Bradley, E.H., Nicholson, N.R., George, E., Indeck, A., & McCorkle, R. (2012). One step at a time: Self-management and transitions among women with ovarian cancer. *Oncology Nursing Forum, 39,* 354–360. doi:10.1188/12.ONF.354-360

Sep, M.S., van Osch, M., van Vliet, L.M., Smets, E.M., & Bensing, J.M. (2014). The power of clinicians' affective communication: How reassurance about non-abandonment can reduce patients' physiological arousal and increase information recall in bad news consultations. An experimental study using analogue patients. *Patient Education Counseling, 95,* 45–52. doi:10.1016/j.pec.2013.12.022

Shell, J.A., & Kirsch, S. (2001). Psychosocial issues, outcomes, and quality of life. In S.E. Otto (Ed.), *Oncology nursing* (4th ed., pp. 948–972). St. Louis, MO: Mosby.

Sherman, D.W., Rosedale, M., & Haber, J. (2012). Reclaiming life on one's own terms: A grounded theory study of the process of breast cancer survivorship [Online exclusive]. *Oncology Nursing Forum, 39,* E258–E268. doi:10.1188/12.ONF.E258-E268

Siegel, R.L., Miller, K.D., & Jemal, A. (2017). Cancer statistics, 2017. *CA: A Cancer Journal for Clinicians, 67,* 7–30. doi:10.3322/caac.21387

Simard, S., Savard, J., & Ivers, H. (2010). Fear of cancer recurrence: Specific profiles and nature of intrusive thoughts. *Journal of Cancer Survivorship, 4,* 361–371. doi:10.1007/s11764-010-0136-8

Smith, A., Hyde, Y.M., & Stanford, D. (2014). Supportive care needs of cancer patients: A literature review. *Palliative and Supportive Care, 13,* 1013–1017. doi:10.1017/S1478951514000959

Smith, L.K., Pope, C., & Botha, J.L. (2005). Patients' help-seeking experiences and delay in cancer presentation: A qualitative synthesis. *Lancet, 366,* 825–831. doi:10.1016/S0140-6736(05)67030-4

Smith, T.J., Temin, S., Alesi, E.R., Abernathy, A.P., Balboni, T.A., Basch, E.M., ... Von Roenn, J.H. (2012). American Society of Clinical Oncology Provisional Clinical Opinion: The integration of palliative care into standard oncology care. *Journal of Clinical Oncology, 30,* 880–887. doi:10.1200/JCO.2011.38.5161

Spittler, C.A., Pallikathayil, L., & Bott, M. (2012). Exploration of how women make treatment decisions after a breast cancer diagnosis [Online exclusive]. *Oncology Nursing Forum, 39,* E425–E433. doi:10.1188/12.ONF.E425-E433

Spoelstra, S.L., Given, B.A., Given, C.W., Grant, M., Silorskii, A., You, M., & Decker, B. (2013). Issues related to overadherence to oral chemotherapy or targeted agents. *Clinical Journal of Oncology Nursing, 17,* 604–609. doi:10.1188/13.CJON.17-06AP

Stanton, A.L., Danoff-Burg, S., Sworowski, L.A., Collins, C.A., Branstetter, A.D., Rodriguez-Hanley, A., ... Austenfeld, J.L. (2002). Randomized, controlled trial of written emotional expression and benefit finding in breast cancer patients. *Journal of Clinical Oncology, 20,* 4160–4168. doi:10.1200/JCO.2002.08.521

Steele, R., & Davies, B. (2015). Supporting families in palliative care. In B.R. Ferrell, N. Coyle, & J.A. Paice (Eds.), *Oxford textbook of palliative nursing* (4th ed., pp. 500–514). New York, NY: Oxford University Press.

Svavarsdottir, E.K., & Sigurdardottir, A.O. (2013). Benefits of a brief therapeutic conversation intervention for families of children and adolescents in active cancer treatment [Online exclusive]. *Oncology Nursing Forum, 40,* E346–E357. doi:10.1188/13.ONF.E346-E357

Temel, J.S., Greer, J.A., Admane, S., Gallagher, E.R., Jackson, V.A., Lynch, T.J., ... Pirl, W.F. (2010). Longitudinal perceptions of prognosis and goals of therapy in patients with metastatic non-small-cell lung cancer: Results of a randomized study of early palliative care. *Journal of Clinical Oncology, 29,* 2319–2326. doi:10.1200/JCO.2010.32.4459

Temel, J.S., Greer, J.A., Muzikansky, A., Gallagher, E.R., Admane, S., Jackson, V.A., ... Lynch, T.J. (2011). Early palliative care for patients with metastatic non-small cell lung cancer. *New England Journal of Medicine, 363,* 733–742. doi:10.1056/NEJMoa1000678

Thewes, B., Butow, P., Zachariae, R., Christensen, S., Simard, S., & Gotay, C. (2012). Fear of cancer recurrence: A systematic literature review of self-report measures. *Psycho-Oncology, 21,* 571–876. doi:10.1002/pon.2070

van den Beuken-van Everdingen, M.H.J., Peters, M.L., de Rijke, J.M., Schouten, H.C., van Kleef, M., & Patijn, J. (2008). Concerns of former breast cancer patients about disease recurrence: A validation and prevalence study. *Psycho-Oncology, 17,* 1137–1145. doi:10.1002/pon.1340

Vivar, C.G., Canga, N., Canga, A.D., & Arantzamendi, M. (2009). The psychosocial impact of recurrence on cancer survivors and family members: A narrative review. *Journal of Advanced Nursing, 65,* 724–736. doi:10.1111/j.1365-2648.2008.04939.x

Vivar, C.G., Whyte, D.A., & McQueen, A. (2010). Again: The impact of recurrence on survivors of cancer and family members. *Journal of Clinical Nursing, 19,* 2048–2056. doi:10.1111/j.1365-2702.2009.03145.x

Warren, M. (2010). Uncertainty, lack of control and emotional functioning in women with metastatic breast cancer: A review and secondary analysis of the literature using the critical appraisal technique. *European Journal of Cancer Care, 19,* 564–574. doi:10.1111/j.1365-2354.2010.01215.x

Weisman, A.D., & Worden, J.W. (1976–1977). The existential plight in cancer: Significance of the first 100 days. *International Journal of Psychiatry in Medicine, 7,* 1–15. doi:10.2190/UQ2G-UGV1-3PPC-6387

Weisman, A.D., & Worden, J.W. (1986). The emotional impact of recurrent cancer. *Journal of Psychosocial Oncology, 3,* 5–16. doi:10.1300/J077v03n04_03

Williams, A.C., Ferrell, B.R., Juarez, G., & Borneman, T. (2015). The role of nursing in caring for patients undergoing palliative surgery for advanced disease. In B.R. Ferrell, N. Coyle, & J.A. Paice (Eds.), *Oxford textbook of palliative nursing* (4th ed., pp. 793–801). New York, NY: Oxford University Press.

Williams, F., & Jeanetta, S.C. (2015). Lived experiences of breast cancer survivors after diagnosis, treatment and beyond: Qualitative study. *Health Expectations, 19,* 631–642. doi:10.1111/hex.12372

Worden, J.W. (2000). Towards an appropriate death. In T.A. Rando (Ed.), *Clinical dimensions of anticipatory mourning* (pp. 267–277). Champaign, IL: Research Press.

Wright, A.A., Zhang, B., Ray, A., Mack, J.W., Trice, E., Balboni, T., ... Block, S.D. (2008). Associations between end-of-life discussions, patient mental health, medical care near death, and caregiver bereavement adjustment. *JAMA, 300,* 1665–1673. doi:10.1001/jama.300.14.1665

Yang, H.C., Brothers, B.M., & Andersen, B.L. (2008). Stress and quality of life in breast cancer recurrence: Moderation or mediation of coping? *Annals of Behavioral Medicine, 35,* 188–197. doi:10.1007/s12160-008-9016-0

Zaider, T.I., & Kissane, D.W. (2015). Psychosocial interventions for couples and families coping with cancer. In J.C. Holland, W.S. Breitbart, P.N. Butow, P.B. Jacobsen, M.J. Loscalzo, & R. McCorkle (Eds.), *Psycho-oncology* (3rd ed., pp. 526–531). New York, NY: Oxford University Press.

Zebrack, B., & Isaacson, S. (2012). Psychosocial care of adolescents and young adult patients with cancer and survivors. *Journal Clinical Oncology, 30,* 1221–1226. doi:10.1200/JCO.2011.39.5467

# CHAPTER 2

# Survivorship

*Deborah A. Boyle, MSN, RN, AOCNS®, FAAN*

> *Cancer therapists talk in terms of a "five-year survival rate," by which they mean the number of patients with a given tumor who will live five years beyond the time of diagnosis. It is an arbitrary way of measuring human existence but useful for scoring the likelihood of escape from cancer. In mid-March 1980, I tiptoed past the invisible line and into the future.*
>
> —Fitzhugh Mullan, 1983

The American cancer patient mosaic is constantly changing. Central to this change is the current and projected growth in the number of cancer survivors. Although *survivorship* is a term applied to all patients with a diagnosis of cancer, for the purposes of this chapter, it is specifically depicting the psychosocial sequelae of living on after the completion of active cancer therapy.

Earlier diagnosis, improved treatments, and the availability of new technologies and supportive care therapies are major factors in improved cancer survival. When the war on cancer was formally initiated in the early 1970s, five-year survival rates were 49% (American Cancer Society [ACS], 2014). Thirty years later, more than two-thirds of patients (69%) are alive five years following diagnosis (ACS, 2014, 2016). Consider these other defining characteristics of cancer survivors:

- Three malignancies account for 60% of all cancer diagnoses in male survivors: prostate (43%), colorectal (9%), and melanoma (8%).
- Breast (41%), uterine (8%), and colorectal (8%) primaries represent more than half (57%) of all cancer diagnoses in female survivors.
- The majority of cancer survivors (64%) were diagnosed over five years ago; 15% received their cancer diagnoses more than 20 years ago.
- Nearly one-half (46%) of cancer survivors are aged 70 or older, while only 5% are younger than age 40 (ACS, 2014).

Currently, 14.5 million cancer survivors live in the United States (ACS, 2014). By 2026, the number of Americans living with a history of cancer will exceed 20 million (Mayer, Nasso, & Earp, 2017). Hence, not only is the scope of cancer survivorship evolving, but the profile of those living beyond definitive cancer therapy is developing as well.

## The Paradigm of Extended Survival

The concept that a distinct boundary needs to be crossed at a given time frame to differentiate an individual from the role of a "patient" to that of "survivor" was challenged in the 1980s. Mullan (1983), a young physician who was diagnosed with an aggressive cancer, questioned the conventional approach to identifying cancer survivors as those who experienced a "moment of cure" or who "crossed an invisible line" into the new realm of survivorship. He wrote about his emotional angst regarding this quandary:

> During these years, I frequently wondered when I could safely declare victory. When could I say simply that I was cured? Actuarial and population-based figures give us survival estimates for various cancers, but those figures do not speak to the individual patient whose experience is unique and not determined or described by aggregate data. Many patients are "cured" long before they pass the five-year mark, and others go well beyond the five-year point with overt or covert disease that removes them from the ranks of the "cured," no matter how they feel. Survival is a much more useful concept because it is a generic idea that applies to everyone diagnosed as having cancer, regardless of the course of illness. (Mullan, 1983, pp. 270–271)

Refuting the prominent model at that time, Mullan then reconceptualized the cancer trajectory into phases, or what he termed *seasons of survival*. Each phase was distinguished by varied coping requirements aligned with the evolving needs of the individual experiencing cancer at different points in time (Mullan, 1983, 1984, 1985). Table 2-1 delineates these now generally accepted phases of survivorship.

The majority of psychosocial survivor research has targeted patients in the acute survival phase. Existing research addressing the extended and permanent phases of survival are

**Table 2-1. Phases of Cancer Survival and Their Distinguishing Characteristics**

| Survival Phase | Analogous Terms | Timing | Major Coping Issues |
|---|---|---|---|
| Acute | Living with cancer | First year following diagnosis or the period of active treatment | Confronted with own mortality; anticipatory loss; informational confusion; energies focused on coping with the diagnosis and treatment(s); remorse over family disruption caused by illness; concerns about work and finances |
| Extended | Living through cancer | Post-treatment completion up to 3 years | Remission or completion of treatment distances patient from the treatment team, causing separation anxiety; fear of recurrence; uncertainty of how to differentiate new symptoms or changes; ongoing physical limitations; reentry into the workplace and family role |
| Permanent | Living beyond cancer | More than 3 years following treatment completion and beyond | Adaptation to long-term effects; presence of work or insurance discrimination; adaption to permanent relationship changes; death anxiety triggered by the death of others |

*Note.* Based on information from Boyle, 2006; Mullan, 1985.

limited to studies of primarily Caucasian, middle-class, early-stage breast cancer survivors treated at large cancer centers (Boyle, 2015). The absence of heterogeneous study methods and sampling limits the generalizability of findings, especially when considering the importance of ethnicity, age, sociodemographic variables, and setting of cancer care delivery.

Extended survival is best characterized by the survivor's learning to live on after active cancer treatment. Critical to this adaptation is the absence of the close proximity of the cancer treatment team's supportive safety net (Harrison et al., 2012). Infrequent contact with health professionals responsible for the survivor's positive treatment outcomes may prompt feelings of isolation and anxiety as new coping requirements unique to this phase of survival are confronted.

Given the complexity and number of new challenges following active cancer therapy, Stanton, Rowland, and Ganz (2015) recently proposed a further adapted model of post-treatment survivorship divided into three periods: reentry, early survivorship, and long-term survivorship. Irrespective of the nomenclature applied to this trajectory, four themes frequently prompt distress central to the patient and family's adjustment during this time: fear of recurrence, symptom persistence, work reentry, and family caregivers as secondary cancer survivors. These four constructs have been characterized by increased investigation and clinical attention during the past decade.

## Fear of Recurrence

Recurrence is a prohibitive phenomenon in the cancer experience. It challenges patients' hopes that cancer can be cured, provides testimony to the life-threatening nature of the illness, and confirms ambiguity about one's future (Wanat, Boulton, & Watson, 2016). Central to the characterizations of fear of recurrence is the dual phenomenon of managing uncertainty and the reemergence of death anxiety associated with repeated confrontations with potential mortality. Although the personal management of this anxiety is highly varied, worry about the cancer returning is the one unmet need that all cancer survivors expect to experience (Boyle, 2015; Mehnert, Koch, Sundermann, & Dinkel, 2013; Recklitis & Syrjala, 2017).

No consensus exists on a fear of recurrence definition (Simard et al., 2013). Vickberg (2003) described recurrence anxiety as "the fear or worry that the cancer will return or progress in the same organ or in another part of the body" (as cited in Simard, 2010, p. 361). Recurrence anxiety is not simply an emotional reaction but rather a multidimensional construct generated from patient fear of numerous threats. Fear can be generated by internal (i.e., physical) and external (i.e., social, media) cues (Simard, Savard, & Ivers, 2010). It is a complex phenomenon grounded in uncertainty and symptom ambiguity (Miller, 2012).

In an extensive review of quantitative studies on fear of recurrence, Simard et al. (2013) identified the most prominent patient variables associated with the presence of significant fear of recurrence. These variables included younger age and the presence and severity of physical and psychological distress. Lebel, Beattie, Arès, and Bielajew (2013) confirmed younger age as being predictive of heightened recurrence anxiety. Additionally, Crist and Grunfeld (2013) identified factors moderately associated with fear of recurrence as being treatment type, low optimism, presence of family stressors, and few social supports. Relatedly, Savard and Ivers (2013) determined that survivors with poor prognoses (i.e., more advanced cancer or having evidence of recurrent cancer) had increased recurrence anxiety. Also of note was the finding that elevated recurrence anxiety at baseline predicted a continued heightened pattern throughout the remainder of the cancer experience.

Recurrence anxiety is most intense during the first two years following cessation of cancer treatment. Although it often decreases with time, recurrence anxiety may still be experienced up to five years and beyond. This anxiety is characterized by a fluctuating pattern relative to the appearance of triggers (of which there are many) (Koch, Jansen, Brenner, & Arndt, 2013; Mehnert et al., 2013). Triggers include medical follow-up and surveillance, the presence of physical symptoms that mimic symptoms of cancer, media stories related to cancer, deaths of public figures from cancer, a family member's illness, and the occurrence of significant anniversaries (i.e., diagnosis) (Koch et al., 2014; Koch et al., 2013).

The consequences of recurrence anxiety may compromise the survivor's quality of life. Dysfunctional behaviors such as anxious preoccupation, excessive checking for evidence of cancer, and intrusion of negative thoughts may interfere with normal functioning and relationships (Koch et al., 2013; Simard et al., 2010). This is often the case in married or committed relationships where partners possess varying coping styles. For example, a survivor may cope through avoidance or denial, while the partner's coping style may be markedly different, demonstrating hovering behavior, anxiety, and hypervigilance. The differences can be a source of conflict or disruption in the relationship.

Simard et al. (2013) categorized the consequences of recurrence anxiety into two groups. Outcomes on health behaviors included survivors' use of complementary and alternative therapies and positive behavior changes, such as increasing regular checkups, using sunscreen, and adopting a healthy diet. Of note are other findings of complementary and alternative therapy interventions in cancer survivors. Survivors report using these therapies to relieve both stress and the prevalence of cancer-related symptoms (Mao, Palmer, Healy, Desai, & Amsterdam, 2011; Samuel & Faithfull, 2013; Sohl et al., 2014). Another theme addressed reassurance-seeking behaviors, exemplified by making frequent contact with physicians (i.e., scheduling additional office visits and making phone calls to assist with anxiety reduction). Psychological consequences were depicted as experiencing heightened degrees of distress, depression, death anxiety, uncertainty, worry over health problems, and having decisional regret. Of particular note were findings in five studies that family caregivers' recurrence anxiety was higher than the survivor's. In fact, Mellon, Northouse, and Weiss (2006) found that the strongest predictors for family caregivers' quality of life were fear of recurrence and the presence of social support.

A review by Thewes et al. (2012) summarized and evaluated 20 multi-item instruments measuring fear of recurrence. In 2015, Hinz, Mehnert, Ernst, Herschbach, and Schulte published the psychometric properties of their 12-item Fear of Progression Questionnaire (FoP-Q-SF), which documents validity in measuring fear of progression in a sample of adult patients with cancer. Additionally, Costa, Dieng, Cust, Butow, and Kasparian (2016) used an item response theory model to further refine the 42-item Fear of Cancer Recurrence Inventory (Simard & Savard, 2009) in a sample of patients with melanoma. In general, the factor structure of the tool was confirmed. However, problems with discrimination were noted in the domains of reassurance and coping strategies. This evaluation lends credence to the question of generalizability of tools for multiple survivor cohorts. However, results from a total of 2,615 cancer survivors completing the health worries subscale of the Impact of Cancer Scale revealed that generic concerns about one's future health status could be determined (van de Wal, van de Poll-Franse, Prins, & Gielissen, 2016).

The development and utility of short forms for screening will assist oncology nurses involved in survivorship care in identifying those with heightened levels of recurrence anxiety. Custers et al. (2014) investigated the efficacy of the Cancer Worry Scale in screening breast cancer survivors and found it to be an appropriate, nurse-friendly screening instrument in this survivor cohort. Longitudinal studies of recurrence anxiety patterns over time are needed in addition to interventional studies, which currently are few in number. An Australian randomized controlled trial is currently underway to test the efficacy of an intervention that integrates attentional training, detached mindfulness, and metacognitive therapy and values clarification and psychoeducation to augment survivors' responses to recurrence anxiety (Butow et al., 2013).

Evidence-based nursing interventions are needed to plan effective strategies that support survivors and their families across the survivorship trajectory (Boyle, 2013). Of note is that the majority of survivorship care plans do not address psychological health in general nor recurrence anxiety in particular. Few educational materials exist to inform survivors about the prevalence of this phenomenon and how to cope with it (Harrison et al., 2012). As the numbers of adult cancer survivors increase, so will the need and demand for supports and services to ameliorate this common sequela of living beyond cancer.

## Symptom Persistence

Ongoing symptom distress is fast becoming a major factor influencing survivors' quality of life after cancer. Mayer et al. (2017) stated that only a small percentage have no problems with this phenomenon during survivorship. In addition to compromising overall quality of life, the burden of symptom persistence in cancer survivors can deter optimum functioning, impact the resumption of family roles and relationships, delay return to work, lower adherence to medical regimens, and influence suicide risk (Stanton et al., 2015). Although the literature distinguishes between physical and psychosocial distress, they are frequently interrelated. Overwhelming physical symptom distress, for example, can cause deconditioning due to immobility. In turn, this may lead to psychological distress as the survivor may not recover in the time frame as anticipated or be able to engage in activities that previously brought joy and happiness. Zhao, Li, Li, and Balluz (2013) also documented evidence of the interconnectedness between physical and emotional distress. They found that cancer survivors who engaged in physical activity were less likely to report serious psychological distress and receive mental health services. Mellon et al. (2006) determined another link with this construct, noting that quality of life of both the survivors and family caregivers independently contributed to each other.

Numerous aspects of symptom distress have relevance to the cancer survivor. The literature is replete with examples that address symptom prevalence, intensity, tolerability, resolution, and clusters. Some of these may be new symptoms or residual ones (i.e., symptom persistence). Of critical importance is the cumulative effect that considerable symptom distress has on the survivor's ability to live on after the completion of active treatment (i.e., symptom burden).

Wu and Harden (2015) recently noted that an equivalent number of symptoms is often present during both extended survivorship and active treatment. In a longitudinal study of 542 survivors with breast, colorectal, gynecologic, lung, and prostate primaries, Deshields, Potter, Olsen, and Liu (2014) used the Memorial Symptom Assessment Scale to identify that the average number of symptoms survivors experienced at one year was eight. Of the top 10 symptoms experienced overall, three were psychological symptoms (i.e., sadness, worry, irritability). Three others had psychological components (i.e., difficulty concentrating and sleeping, problems with sexual interest or activity). Addressing the early extended survival phase, Shi et al. (2011) focused their research on cancer survivors with high symptom burden to identify risk factors and evaluate this burden on quality of life. They evaluated nearly 5,000 survivors by using ACS's Study of Cancer Survivors–I database. Variables associated with high burden included the presence of metastatic cancer and comorbidity, younger age, inadequate or no insurance, lower income, unemployment, and less education. The symptom cluster of depression, fatigue, and pain had the greatest effect on quality of life. More than one in four cancer survivors had high symptom burden one year following diagnosis. Stanton et al. (2015) and Brant et al. (2011) also identified younger age as a risk factor for debilitating symptom distress into extended survival.

Symptom persistence, as a corollary to symptom burden, can seriously interfere with quality of life. Brant et al. (2011) found that following chemotherapy, symptoms in lymphoma and lung and colorectal primaries persisted for 16 months. Harrington, Hansen, Moskowitz, Todd, and Fuerstein (2010) noted the ongoing presence of anxiety, depression, fatigue, cognitive impairment, insomnia, pain, and sexual difficulties up to 10 years following cancer diagnosis.

The most prominent emotional sequelae during survivorship are depression and anxiety. A meta-analysis by Mitchell, Ferguson, Gill, Paul, and Symonds (2013) reviewed 66 studies with diagnosed major depression in adult cancer survivors in nonpalliative care settings. The studies revealed a 16% prevalence rate, slightly higher than normal controls (10.2%). These findings correlate with psychotropic drug use research in cancer survivors. Punekar, Short, and Moran (2012) reviewed prescription data of cancer survivors from the National Health Interview Survey over a five-year period. Nineteen percent of cancer survivors under age 65 and 16% of survivors age 65 and older used psychotropic medications, namely antidepressants and antianxiety drugs. Pirl, Greer, Temel, Yeap, and Gilman's (2009) evaluation of a large sample of more than 9,000 adults interviewed as part of the National Comorbidity Survey Replication also failed to show a statistically significant increase of depression in cancer survivors. However, these authors explained that, although survivors may not have higher incidences of a major depressive disorder, they may experience greater impairment from the depression than those without a history of cancer.

A diagnosis brings much distress to survivors and their families; therefore, anxiety is a frequent emotional response in cancer survivors (Mitchell et al., 2013). Stafford et al. (2015) conducted a longitudinal study of women with breast and gynecologic malignancies and identified variables most predictive of depression and anxiety as a preexisting condition or history of anxiety or depression and evidence of high neuroticism.

Although psychopathology in cancer survivors is rare, the combined presence of psychological and physical symptoms may cause survivors to episodically experience dimensions of psychological distress well above norms. The period of extended survival is critical to the entire survivorship trajectory, as it sets the stage for long-term recovery. If the patient enters or remains in this phase and is physically and emotionally compromised, overall restoration to health may be difficult and protracted. Because of this, it is imperative that survivors can recognize their individual needs and are able to accept mental health support if necessary.

Normalization of the psychological consequences of cancer should begin with the cancer care team's acknowledgment of these sequelae in discussions with patients. However, a very low proportion of survivors report ever having had a conversation about their psychological needs with a healthcare professional (Forsythe et al., 2013). Whitney, Bell, Bold, and Joseph (2015) found that survivors with cancer and chronic illness had the highest rate of unmet needs specific to mental health services. However, the proportion of survivors who receive counseling or other supportive measures has not increased over time (Buchanan et al., 2013). Emotional support during survivorship prevails as a critical need. Ness et al. (2013) studied the concerns of more than 300 cancer survivors treated at three Mayo Clinic settings. Their study revealed that the fear of recurrence was most common among the cancer survivors (i.e., nearly two-thirds). However, four other emotional concerns experienced by nearly half or greater of the sample were living with uncertainty, managing stress, defining a new sense of normal, and managing difficult emotions, all known corollaries of coping during extended survival.

The prominence of symptom persistence as a potential deterrent to optimal quality of life in cancer survivors creates many options for intervention by oncology nurses. Although definitive research in many areas is lacking, attempts to integrate some preliminary best practices can offer guidance about potential innovation. Figure 2-1 outlines recommendations that address baseline assessment and acknowledgment of emotional distress, screening, recommendations for physical activity, and the integration of complementary and alternative therapies (Shneerson, Taskila, Gale, Greenfield, & Chen, 2013).

## Work Reentry

Patients often regard their return to work as a symbol of recovering and regaining a sense of normality (de Boer et al., 2008). Although 62%–84% of patients diagnosed with cancer return to work, little is known about the support needed to facilitate this transition. What is known is that difficulty returning to work is a major problem for survivors and that healthcare professionals do little to prepare adult patients for work reentry (Recklitis & Syrjala, 2017; Stanton et al., 2015). This represents a pressing need to augment the overall rehabilitation process in adult oncology. A monumental disconnect exists between supports in place in pediatric oncology practice for children returning to school and what is available for adults returning to work (Boyle, 2014). In the childhood realm of cancer care, anticipatory counsel is offered to parents and the school (teachers and other students) about the nature of the child's potential issues and needs upon their return. For adults returning to work, no comparable guidance and assistance exists.

One's ability to work influences self-esteem, income, insurance, and personal indices of productivity. Therefore, it is a critical measure of positive work reentry. Residual cancer bur-

---

- Normalize psychological distress as a prominent issue during survivorship by discussing it and informing the survivor of your interest in knowing about it to the same degree as physical distress.
- Determine a symptom distress monitoring tool to be used at baseline and longitudinally that includes physical and emotional symptom distress.
- Use a brief symptom inventory specific to depression and anxiety to screen for premorbid history (versus a one-item Likert scale).
- Ensure that survivor-specific distress indices are monitored (i.e., fear of recurrence, managing uncertainty, depression, anxiety, elements of work reentry, engagement with social supports).
- Identify resources for referral, especially in community settings (ideally for early intervention).
- Advocate for physical activity and complementary approaches when acceptable (e.g., walking partner, exercise, yoga, meditation, mindfulness, Qigong).
- Participate in mindfulness-based stress reduction.
- Consider use of a survivor coach.

**Figure 2-1. Nursing Interventions That Enhance the Resolution of Symptom Persistence During Ongoing Surveillance/Extended Cancer Survival**

den affects postcancer employment (Tevaarwerk et al., 2013). Cancer-related symptoms such as depression, fatigue, and mobility problems can cause significant interference with work performance. Cognitive limitations such as concentration problems and memory deficits also can affect work capacity (Duijts et al., 2014). Although work expectations considered physically or cognitively demanding are known risk factors for problematic return to work, other aspects of performance have less data to inform anticipatory guidance. Of note is the development of a recent tool to measure the quality of working life of cancer survivors (de Jong, Tamminga, de Boer, & Frings-Dresen, 2016). Use of such an inventory can elucidate the myriad of issues faced by adult cancer survivors returning to the work setting.

A considerable research effort is required to document the landscape of return to work for adult survivors. Needed areas for supplemental evidence include required work adjustments, when and how to exit and return to work, how to manage coworker relationships, and strategies to cope with difficult work scenarios due to physical changes, emotional pressures, and fatigue (Pryce, Munir, & Haslam, 2007). Figure 2-2 proposes potential questions survivors may ask their cancer care team as they embark on the extended survivorship trajectory. Additionally, the potential for rehabilitation, namely, occupational and vocational services, is of particular need of investigation in this cohort (Knott et al., 2014). Identifying vulnerable survivors such as single parents and low-income families also requires special attention.

---

- How will my cancer and its treatment affect my ability to continue working?
- What can I expect when I return to work?
- What limitations could I experience?
- What does my supervisor need to know?
- Should I initially return with reduced hours?
- Are there work accommodations I should ask for or make (i.e., handicapped parking, brief time to rest in the morning and afternoon)?

**Figure 2-2. Suggested Questions for Survivors' Concerns About Work Reentry**

## Caregivers as Secondary Cancer Survivors

Caregiving in the United States is a major public health crisis with emergent implications (Boyle, 2017). Within cancer care, its scope is formidable (Boyle, 2002). Although healthcare providers focus the majority of their efforts and attention on the survivor, a worried, alienated, and "at-risk" family in need of support may be at the bedside. The term *co-survivor*, or secondary cancer survivor, has been applied to the experiences of these caregivers.

Although we can approximate the current number of cancer survivors, it is virtually impossible to quantify the number of caregivers, especially because the broad range of types of caregiving have not yet been clearly distinguished (i.e., varying levels of direct and indirect supportive interventions rendered). Even a modest estimate of every cancer survivor having two caregivers over the course of their illness results in a total of 290 million Americans serving in this role (Boyle, 2002). These caregivers are part of a mostly unrecognized legion who serve as unpaid workers to someone who is ill, disabled, or elderly in the United States. For many, they spend the equivalent of a part-time job (i.e., 20 hours per week or more) providing care to their loved one with cancer (van Ryn et al., 2011). These caregivers may themselves be at increased risk for cancer related to lifestyle, genetics, or toxic exposure (Rowland & Belizzi, 2008). The caregiver role is not usually gender-neutral; the role is usually assumed by a female family member (Kuenzler, Hodgkinson, Zindel, Bargetzi, & Znoj, 2011).

Girgis, Lambert, and Lecathelinais (2011) depicted caregivers' support needs clustering within seven domains: information, emotional/psychological, physical health, healthcare provider and cancer care, relationship with patient, practical support, and legal/financial. Table 2-2 provides examples of these caregiver needs in each cluster. Underscoring this depiction is the reality that lay family caregivers assume the burden of caregiving without structured education and preparation for these new responsibilities—hence adding stress to an already stressful situation.

The distress experienced by family caregivers evolves well into extended survival as needs for monitoring symptoms and managing care during recovery continue. Kim, Spillers, and Hall (2012) acknowledged that one out of seven cancer caregivers is likely to enact the caregiver role many years after the acute phase of survival. Figure 2-3 depicts the multiple social and financial implications of family caregiving that can prevail over time. How family caregivers cope with this protracted strain is important, as family distress during survivorship influences patient coping. Additionally, family member distress may be as high or higher than the survivor's (Turner et al., 2013). Families who are already distressed prior to the cancer experience often remain so for a longer period following treatment (Northouse et al., 2002).

Tools are available to measure family caregiver distress in cancer care. Prue, Santin, and Porter (2015) provided a critical review of seven instruments that assess the needs of informal cancer caregivers. Their review considered psychometric properties, tool length and clinical utility, and tool feasibility across phases of the cancer trajectory. Additionally, two other instruments can be used to evaluate family caregiver experiences: (a) the Family Avoidance of Communication About Cancer (FACC) scale and (b) the Cancer Communication Assessment Tool for Patients and Families (CCAT-PF).

### Table 2-2. Clusters of Family Caregiver Needs

| Cluster | Examples |
| --- | --- |
| Information | Inability to assimilate threatening information; hearing information secondhand (i.e., not always being present during information exchange with cancer care team); not being kept up to date on the most current information; problems interpreting medical information or basing interpretation on others' experiences; fear of asking too many questions or admitting lack of understanding |
| Emotional/psychological | Need to work yet worry about unavailability to help with survivor's needs; assume responsibility for support needs of other family members; ongoing need to minimize stress within family unit |
| Physical health | Placement of own health needs as last priority; need to monitor, assess, and evaluate signs/symptoms in cancer survivor across cancer continuum; potential somatization of distress |
| Healthcare professionals and cancer care | Concern about multiple physicians not communicating with each other; difficulty making sense of conflicting information/advice; potential unavailability to accompany family member to appointments and hear information first-hand |
| Relationship with patient | Reticence to disclose fears and worry about condition; feel responsibility to reduce survivor's stress; worry about impact of information disclosure on patient coping |
| Practical support | Assumption of role of ill family member in addition to usual role; help needed with home maintenance, children, transportation, and meals |

| Financial | Social |
|---|---|
| • Reduced work time<br>• Decreased income<br>• Leave of employment or closure of business<br>• Difficulty with paying bills<br>• Trouble with day-to-day expenses<br>• Additional help needed with childcare or home maintenance<br>• Used up savings<br>• Borrowed money<br>• Loss of sick time and vacation<br>• Additional out-of-pocket expenses associated with parking, travel (i.e., hotel, meals, mileage), medical tests, supplies, therapies, equipment, homecare support, medications not covered by insurance | • Missed events (i.e., children's, social, family, religious)<br>• Lost contact with friends<br>• Potential vacation time influenced by fear of distancing self from cancer treatment team<br>• Isolation from usual support system<br>• "Away time" fraught with worry, guilt<br>• Reduced contact time with other family members<br>• Limited social engagement due to fatigue<br>• Diminished contact with work supports<br>• Conversational isolationism: limited expression of concern and worry through changed communication patterns with support system<br>• Anger toward others deemed insensitive or uncaring |

**Figure 2-3. Potential Indices of the Social and Financial Impact of Cancer Caregiving**

*Note.* Based on information from Carey et al., 2012.

The FACC scale is a five-item measure that addresses the extent to which family members avoid talking about the cancer experience (Mallinger, Griggs, & Shields, 2006; Shin et al., 2015). Originally developed from survey results from a breast cancer cohort, the scale was intended to determine the relationship between open family communication and breast cancer survivors' mental health. CCAT-PF assesses congruence in patient/family communication (Smirnoff, Zyzanski, Rose, & Zhang, 2008). Three themes are targeted in this assessment tool: selective sharing, initiation of communication, and emotional reaction to communication. Lim, Paek, and Shon's (2015) study using this tool revealed the importance of gender in communication sharing, initiation, and reactions. Men were more constrained in their communication styles, limiting disclosure of feelings and needs.

The availability of these instruments has helped determine priority needs of families during survivorship. Using the Supportive Care Needs Survey–Partners and Caregivers, Girgis et al. (2011) identified the top three unmet needs of caregivers with moderate to high intensity (i.e., in responding to, "In the last month, what was your level of need for help with . . . ?") as concern about recurrence, reducing stress for the family member with cancer, and understanding the patient experience. Turner et al. (2013) identified the fear of recurrence as a moderate to high unmet need in one in six study respondents. Mohammed et al. (2015) reported that patient fatigue and spousal depression are associated with caregiver burden. The acuity and morbidity of therapy that the survivor received may also influence caregiver's response. For example, Jin, Li, Chen, and Cao (2015) studied caregiver–survivor dyads within the context of acute leukemia and found that caregivers met more case criteria for post-traumatic stress disorder than survivors (36.8% vs. 18.4%). Hodgkinson et al. (2007) used the Cancer Survivors' Partners Unmet Needs measure to ascertain positive outcomes of caregiving. These included growing as a person, appreciating relationships more, and focusing on important things. These findings could be assistive with resiliency training for family caregivers as an intervention.

Family caregivers are in significant need of education and support as they assume these important roles within cancer care. Making the analogy to the new realm of childbirth for young families, cancer caregivers need preparatory guidance in the form of education and emotional support to help them adjust to unexpected, and at times frightening, responsibilities. Sklenarova et al. (2015) revealed that one in five caregivers had a moderate to high unmet need relating to receiving emotional support for themselves. Psychoeducation, such as what is offered in earlier phases of cancer survivorship, is indicated during extended survival (Leow, Chan, & Chan, 2015). Web-based or virtual support may be particularly amenable to family caregivers who work and are unable to attend onsite programs (Kaltenbaugh et al., 2015). Other technological options offering linkage with the primary cancer team could reduce the angst associated with separation anxiety. The majority of research to date has targeted spousal caregivers. Adult caregivers of older adult parents or siblings require additional study, as the competing demands of caring for one's own family along with an ill parent may be overwhelming. Longitudinal studies can outline the chronology of caregiving and identify triggers of distress over time.

## Conclusion

Although the needs of patients during active cancer therapy have historically received the mainstay of attention in terms of psychosocial support, an increased amount of attention is being paid to the requisite counsel indicated for patients and their loved ones within the extended and permanent phases of cancer survival. A focus on these trajectories is essential, not only because the number of survivors is projected to increase in the coming years, but also because the older adult survivor population will be more prominent in the future, requiring additional care.

An enhanced sensitivity to, and growing knowledge base about, geriatrics will be required to address the majority of the special needs of older adult patients. During extended survival, recurrence anxiety may coexist with worry about the status of other comorbidities. The differentiation of symptoms of cancer and other intercurrent illness may be complicated and complex to discern. Depression, a common corollary of advanced age, could be exaggerated by the imposed burden of ongoing symptom distress following effective cancer treatment. Additionally, older Americans are projected to work longer into their senior years in the coming decades; therefore, employment reentry may continue to be an issue of concern and necessitate intervention. Finally, family issues will prevail as a priority topic. Older survivors who live alone, are caring for an ill spouse, or are in need of help for their ongoing compromise for their comorbid problems or cancer treatment sequelae may be in need of innovative sources of support, as their social situations preclude the availability of adult children to render continued care. These factors position the future cohort of potentially vulnerable cancer survivors to be in need of unique interventions (Stanton et al., 2015).

Cancer survivorship is a nurse-centric phenomenon with a multitude of psychosocial corollaries. Being a critical influence on patients' ability to transition through the cancer trajectory, nurses must increase their sensitivity to the unmet needs of this growing legion of Americans facing a diagnosis of cancer.

## References

American Cancer Society. (2014). *Cancer treatment and survivorship facts and figures, 2014–2015*. Retrieved from https://www.cancer.org/content/dam/cancer-org/research/cancer-facts-and-statistics/cancer-treatment-and-survivorship-facts-and-figures/cancer-treatment-and-survivorship-facts-and-figures-2014-2015.pdf

American Cancer Society. (2016). *Cancer facts and figures 2016.* Retrieved from https://www.cancer.org/content/dam/cancer-org/research/cancer-facts-and-statistics/annual-cancer-facts-and-figures/2016/cancer-facts-and-figures-2016.pdf

Boyle, D.A. (2002). Families facing cancer: The forgotten majority. *Clinical Journal of Oncology Nursing, 6,* 69–70. doi:10.1188/02.CJON.69-70

Boyle, D.A. (2006). Survivorship. In R.M. Carroll-Johnson, L.M. Gorman, & N.J. Bush (Eds.), *Psychosocial nursing care along the cancer continuum* (2nd ed., pp. 25–51). Pittsburgh, PA: Oncology Nursing Society.

Boyle, D.A. (2013). Those dreaded words: "It's back" [Web blog post]. Retrieved from http://www.theonc.org/author.asp?section_id=1845&doc_id=267009

Boyle, D.A. (2014). Beyond the initial return to work: Enduring problems for cancer survivors. Retrieved from http://www.theonc.org/author.asp?section_id=1845&doc_id=272646

Boyle, D.A. (2015). Emotional struggles while surviving cancer: The script unfolds. Retrieved from http://www.theonc.org/messages.asp?piddl_msgthreadid=282135

Boyle, D.A. (2017). The caregiving quandary. *Clinical Journal of Oncology Nursing, 21,* 139. doi:10.1188/17.CJON.139

Brant, J.M., Beck, S., Dudley, W.N., Cobb, P., Pepper, G., & Miaskowski, C. (2011). Symptom trajectories in post-treatment cancer survivors. *Cancer Nursing, 34,* 67–77. doi:10.1097/NCC.0b013e3181f04ae9

Buchanan, N.D., King, J.B., Rodriguez, J.L., White, A., Trivers, K.F., Forsythe, L.P., ... Sabatino, S.A. (2013). Changes among U.S. cancer survivors: Comparing demographic, diagnostic, and health care findings from the 1992 and 2010 National Health Interview Surveys. *International Scholarly Research Notices, 2013,* 1–9. doi:10.1155/2013/238017

Butow, P.N., Bell, M.L., Smith, A.B., Fardell, J.E., Thewes, B., Turner, J., ... Mihalopoulos, C. (2013). Conquer fear: Protocol of a randomized controlled trial of a psychological intervention to reduce fear of recurrence. *BMC Cancer, 13,* 201. doi:10.1186/1471-2407-13-201

Carey, M., Paul, C., Cameron, E., Lynagh, M., Hall, A., & Tzelepis, F. (2012). Financial and social impact of supporting a hematological cancer survivor. *European Journal of Cancer Care, 21,* 169–176. doi:10.1111/j.1365-2354.2011.01302.x

Costa, D.J., Dieng, M., Cust, A.E., Butow, P.N., & Kasparian, N.A. (2016). Psychometric properties of the Fear of Recurrence Inventory: An item response theory approach. *Psycho-Oncology, 25,* 832–838. doi:10.1002/pon.4018

Crist, J.V., & Grunfeld, E.A. (2013). Factors reported to influence fear of recurrence in cancer patients: A systematic review. *Psycho-Oncology, 22,* 978–986. doi:10.1002/pon.3114

Custers, J.A., van den Berg, S.W., van Laarhoven, H.W., Bleiker, E.M., Gielissen, M.F., & Prins, J.B. (2014). The cancer worry scale. *Cancer Nursing, 37,* E44–E50. doi:10.1097/NCC.0b013e3182813a17

de Boer, A., Verbeek, J.H., Spelten, E.R., Uitterhoeve, A.L., Ansink, A.C., de Reijke, T.M., ... van Dijk, F.J. (2008). Work ability and return to work in cancer patients. *British Journal of Cancer, 98,* 1342–1347. doi:10.1038/sj.bjc.6604302

de Jong, M., Tamminga, S.J., de Boer, A.G., & Frings-Dresen, M.H. (2016). Quality of working life of cancer survivors: Development of a cancer-specific questionnaire. *Journal of Cancer Survivorship, 10,* 394–405. doi:10.1007/s11764-015-0485-4

Deshields, T.L., Potter, P., Olsen, S., & Liu, J. (2014). The persistence of symptom burden: Symptom experience and quality of life of cancer patients across one year. *Supportive Care in Cancer, 22,* 1089–1096. doi:10.1007/s00520-013-2049-3

Duijts, S.F., van Egmond, M.P., Spelten, E., van Muijen, P., Anema, J.R., & van der Beek, A.J. (2014). Physical and psychosocial problems in cancer survivors beyond return to work: A systematic review. *Psycho-Oncology, 23,* 481–492. doi:10.1002/pon.3467

Forsythe, L., Kent, E., Weaver, K., Buchanan, N., Hawkins, N.A., Rodriguez, J.L., ... Rowland, J.R. (2013). Receipt of psychosocial care among cancer survivors in the United States. *Journal of Clinical Oncology, 31,* 1961–1969. doi:10.1200/JCO.2012.46.2101

Girgis, A., Lambert, S., & Lecathelinais, C. (2011). The supportive care needs survey for partners and caregivers of cancer survivors: Development and psychometric evaluation. *Psycho-Oncology, 20,* 387–393. doi:10.1002/pon.1740

Harrington, C.B., Hansen, J.A., Moskowitz, M., Todd, B.L., & Fuerstein, M. (2010). It's not over when it's over: Long-term symptoms in cancer survivors—A systematic review. *International Journal of Psychiatry in Medicine, 40,* 163–181. doi:10.2190/PM.40.2.c

Harrison, S.E., Watson, E.K., Ward, A.M., Khan, N.F., Turner, D., Adams, E., ... Rose, P.W. (2012). Cancer survivors' experiences of discharge from hospital follow-up. *European Journal of Cancer Care, 21,* 390–397. doi:10.1111/j.1365-2354.2011.01312.x

Hinz, A., Mehnert, A., Ernst, J., Herschbach, P., & Schulte, T. (2015). Fear of progression in patients six months after cancer rehabilitation—A validation study of the fear of progression questionnaire FoP-Q-12. *Supportive Care in Cancer, 23,* 1579–1587. doi:10.1007/s00520-014-2516-5

Hodgkinson, K., Butow, P., Hobbs, K.M., Hunt, G.E., Lo, S.K., & Wain, G. (2007). Assessing unmet supportive care needs in partners of cancer survivors: The development and evaluation of the Cancer Survivors' Partners Unmet Needs measure (CaSPUN). *Psycho-Oncology, 16,* 805–813. doi.10.1002/pon.1138

Jin, M., Li., J., Chen, C., & Cao, F. (2015). Post-traumatic stress disorder symptoms in family caregivers of adult patients with acute leukemia from a dyadic perspective. *Psycho-Oncology, 24,* 1754–1760. doi.10.1002/pon.3851

Kaltenbaugh, D.J., Klem, M.L., Hu, L., Turi, E., Haines, A.J., & Lingler, J.H. (2015). Using web-based interventions to support caregivers of patients with cancer: A systematic review. *Oncology Nursing Forum, 42,* 156–164. doi.10.1188/15.ONF.156-164

Kim, Y., Spillers, R.L., & Hall, D.L. (2012). Quality of life of family caregivers five years after a relative's cancer diagnosis: Follow-up of the national quality of life survey for caregivers. *Psycho-Oncology, 21,* 273–281. doi.10.1002/pon.1888

Knott, V., Zrim, S., Shanahan, M., Anastassiadis, P., Lawn, S., Kichenadasse, G., ... Koczwara, B. (2014). Returning to work following curative chemotherapy: A qualitative study of return to work barriers and preferences for intervention. *Supportive Care in Cancer, 22,* 3263–3273. doi.10.1007/s00520-014-2324-y

Koch, L., Bertram, H., Eberle, A., Holleczek, B., Schmid-Höpfner, S., Waldman, A., ... Arndt, V. (2014). Fear of recurrence in long-term breast cancer survivors—Still an issue. Results on prevalence, determinants, and the association with quality of life and depression from the cancer survivorship—A multi-regional population-based study. *Psycho-Oncology, 23,* 547–554. doi.10.1002/pon.3452

Koch, L., Jansen, L., Brenner, H., & Arndt, V. (2013). Fear of recurrence and disease progression in long-term (≥ 5 years) cancer survivors—A systematic review of quantitative studies. *Psycho-Oncology, 22,* 1–11. doi.10.1002/pon.3022

Kuenzler, A., Hodgkinson, K., Zindel, A., Bargetzi, M., & Znoj, H.J. (2011). Who cares, who bears, who benefits? Female spouses vicariously carry the burden after cancer diagnosis. *Psychological Health, 26,* 337–352. doi.10.1080/08870440903418877

Lebel, S., Beattie, S., Arès, I., & Bielajew, C. (2013). Young and worried: Age and fear of recurrence in breast cancer survivors. *Health Psychology, 32,* 695–705. doi.10.1037/a0030186

Leow, M., Chan, S., & Chan, M.F. (2015). A pilot randomized, controlled trial of the effectiveness of a psychoeducational intervention on family caregivers of patients with advanced cancer [Online exclusive]. *Oncology Nursing Forum, 42,* E63–E72. doi.10.1188/15.ONF.E63-E72

Lim, J., Paek, M., & Shon, E. (2015). Gender and role differences in couples' communication during survivorship. *Cancer Nursing, 38,* E51–E60. doi.10.1097/NCC.0000000000000191

Mallinger, J.B., Griggs, J.J., & Shields, C.G. (2006). Family communication and mental health after breast cancer. *European Journal of Cancer Care, 15,* 355–361. doi.10.1111/j.1365-2354.2006.00666.x

Mao, J.J., Palmer, C., Healy, K.E., Desai, K., & Amsterdam, J. (2011). Complementary and alternative medicine use among cancer survivors: A population-based study. *Journal of Cancer Survivorship, 5,* 8–17. doi.10.1007/s11764-010-0153-7

Mayer, D.K., Nasso, S.F., & Earp, J.A. (2017). Defining cancer survivors, their needs, and perspectives on survivorship health care in the USA. *Lancet Oncology, 18,* E11–E18. doi:10.1016/S1470-2045(16)30573-3

Mehnert, A., Koch, U., Sundermann, C., & Dinkel, A. (2013). Predictors of fear of recurrence in patients one year after cancer rehabilitation: A prospective study. *Acta Oncologica, 52,* 1102–1109. doi.10.3109/0284186X.2013.765063

Mellon, S., Northouse, L.L., & Weiss, L.K. (2006). A population-based study of the quality of life of cancer survivors and their family caregivers. *Cancer Nursing, 29,* 120–131. doi.10.1097/00002820-200603000-00007

Miller, L.E. (2012). Sources of uncertainty in cancer survivorship. *Journal of Cancer Survivorship, 6,* 431–440. doi.10.1007/s11764-012-0229-7

Mitchell, A.J., Ferguson, D.W., Gill, J., Paul, J., & Symonds, P. (2013). Depression and anxiety in long-term cancer survivors compared with spouses and healthy controls: A systematic review and meta-analysis. *Lancet Oncology, 14,* 721–732. doi.10.1016/S1470-2045(13)70244-4

Mohammad, N.H., Walter, A.W., van Oijen, M.G., Hulshof, M.C., Bergman, J.J., Anderegg, M.C., ... van Laarhoven, H.W. (2015). Burden of spousal caregivers of stage II and III esophageal cancer survivors 3 years after treatment with curative intent. *Supportive Care in Cancer, 23,* 3589–3598. doi.10.1007/s00520-015-2727-4

Mullan, F. (1983). *Vital signs: A young doctor's struggle with cancer.* New York, NY: Laurel Books.

Mullan, F. (1984). Re-entry: The educational needs of the cancer survivor. *Health Education Quarterly, 10*(Suppl. 10), 88–94.

Mullan, F. (1985). Seasons of survival: Reflections of a physician with cancer. *New England Journal of Medicine, 313,* 270–273. doi.10.1056/NEJM198507253130421

Ness, S., Kokal, J., Fee-Schroeder, K., Novotny, P., Satele, D., & Barton, D. (2013). Concerns across the cancer trajectory: Results from a survey of cancer survivors. *Oncology Nursing Forum, 40,* 35–42. doi.10.1188/13.ONF.35-42

Northouse, L.L., Mood, D., Kershaw, T., Schafenacker, A., Mellon, S., Walker, J., ... Decker, V. (2002). Quality of life of women with recurrent breast cancer and their family members. *Journal of Clinical Oncology, 20,* 4050–4064. doi.10.1200/JCO.2002.02.054

Pirl, W.F., Greer, J., Temel, J.S., Yeap, B.Y., & Gilman, S.E. (2009). Major depressive disorder in long-term cancer survivors: Analysis of the National Comorbidity Survey Replication. *Journal of Clinical Oncology, 27,* 4130–4134. doi.10.1200/JCO.2008.16.2784

Prue, G., Santin, O., & Porter, S. (2015). Assessing the needs of informal caregivers to cancer survivors: A review of instruments. *Psycho-Oncology, 24,* 121–129. doi.10.1002/pon.3609

Pryce, J., Munir, F., & Haslam, C. (2007). Cancer survivorship and work: Symptoms, supervisor response, coworker disclosure and work adjustment. *Journal of Occupational Rehabilitation, 17,* 83–92. doi.10.1007/s10926-006-9040-5

Punekar, R.S., Short, P.F., & Moran, J.R. (2012). Use of psychotropic medications by U.S. cancer survivors. *Psycho-Oncology, 21,* 1237–1243. doi.10.1002/pon.2039

Recklitis, C.J., & Syrjala, K.L. (2017). Provision of integrated psychosocial services for cancer survivors post-treatment. *Lancet Oncology, 18,* E39–E50. doi:10.1016/S1470-2045(16)30659-3

Rowland, J.H., & Belizzi, K.M. (2008). Cancer survivors and survivorship research: A reflection on today's successes and tomorrow's challenges. *Hematology/Oncology Clinics of North America, 22,* 181–200. doi:10.1016/j.hoc.2008.01.008

Samuel, C.A., & Faithfull, S. (2013). Complementary therapy support in cancer survivorship: A survey of complementary and alternative medicine practitioners' provision and perception of skills. *European Journal of Cancer Care, 23,* 180–188. doi.10.1111/ecc.12099

Savard, J., & Ivers, H. (2013). The evolution of fear of recurrence during the cancer care trajectory and its relationship with cancer characteristics. *Journal of Psychosomatic Research, 74,* 354–360. doi.10.1016/j.jpsychores.2012.12.013

Shi, Q., Smith, T.G., Michonski, J.D., Stein, K.D., Kaw, C.K., & Cleeland, C.S. (2011). Symptom burden in cancer survivors one year after diagnosis: A report from the American Cancer Society's studies of cancer survivors. *Cancer, 117,* 2779–2790. doi.10.1002/cncr.26146

Shin, D.W., Shin, J., Kim, S.Y., Yang, H.K., Cho, J., Youm, J.H., ... Park, J.H. (2015). Family avoidance of communication about cancer: A dyadic examination. *Cancer Research Treatment, 48,* 384–392. doi:10.4143/crt.2014.280

Shneerson, C., Taskila, T., Gale, N., Greenfield, S., & Chen, Y.F. (2013). The effect of complementary and alternative medicine on the quality of life of cancer survivors: A systematic review and meta-analyses. *Complementary Therapies in Medicine, 4,* 417–429. doi.10.1016/j.ctim.2013.05.003

Simard, S., & Savard, J. (2009). Fear of Cancer Recurrence Inventory: Development and initial validation of a multidimensional measure of fear of recurrence. *Supportive Care in Cancer, 17,* 241–251. doi:10.1007/s00520-008-0444-y

Simard, S., Savard, J., & Ivers, H. (2010). Fear of cancer recurrence: Specific profiles and the nature of intrusive thoughts. *Journal of Cancer Survivorship, 4,* 361–371. doi.10.1007/s11764-010-0136-8

Simard, S., Thewes, B., Humphris, G., Dixon, M., Hayden, C., Mireskandari, S., & Ozakinci, G. (2013). Fear of cancer recurrence in adult cancer survivors: A systematic review of quantitative studies. *Journal of Cancer Survivorship, 7,* 300–322. doi.10.1007/s11764-013-0272-z

Sklenarova, H., Krümpelmann, A., Haun, M.W., Friederich, H.C., Huber, J., Thomas, M., ... Hartmann, M. (2015). When do we need to care about the caregiver? Supportive care needs, anxiety, and depression among informal caregivers of patients with cancer and cancer survivors. *Cancer, 121,* 1513–1519. doi.10.1002/cncr.29223

Smirnoff, L.A., Zyzanski, S.J., Rose, J.H., & Zhang, A.Y. (2008). The cancer communication assessment tool for patients and families (CCAT-PF): A new measure. *Psycho-Oncology, 17,* 1216–1224. doi.10.1002/pon.1350

Sohl, S.J., Weaver, K.E., Birdee, G., Kent, E.E., Danhauer, S.C., & Hamilton, A.S. (2014). Characteristics associated with the use of complementary health approaches among long-term cancer survivors. *Supportive Care in Cancer, 22,* 927–936. doi.10.1007/s00520-013-2040-z

Stafford, L., Judd, F., Gibson, P., Komiti, A., Mann, G.B., & Quinn, M. (2015). Anxiety and depression symptoms in the 2 years following diagnosis of breast or gynaecologic cancer: Prevalence, course and determinants of outcome. *Supportive Care in Cancer, 23,* 2215–2224. doi.10.1007/s00520-014-2571-y

Stanton, A.L., Rowland, J.H., & Ganz, P.A. (2015). Life after diagnosis and treatment of cancer in adulthood: Contributions of psychosocial oncology research. *American Psychologist, 70,* 159–174. doi.10.1037/a0037875

Tevaarwerk, A.J., Lee, J.W., Sesto, M.E., Buhr, K.A., Cleeland, C.S., Manola, J., ... Fisch, M.J. (2013). Employment outcomes among survivors of common cancers: The Symptom Outcomes and Practice Patterns (SOAPP) study. *Journal of Cancer Survivorship, 7,* 191–202. doi.10.1007/s11764-012-0258-2

Thewes, B., Butow, P., Zachariae, R., Christensen, S., Simard, S., & Gotay, C. (2012). Fear of cancer recurrence: A systematic literature review of self-report measures. *Psycho-Oncology, 21,* 571–587. doi.10.1002/pon.2070

Turner, D., Adams, E., Boulton, M., Harrison, S., Khan, N., Rose, P., ... Watson, E.K. (2013). Partners and close family members of long-term cancer survivors: Health status, psychosocial well-being, and unmet supportive care needs. *Psycho-Oncology, 22,* 12–19. doi.10.1002/pon.2050

van de Wal, M., van de Poll-Franse, L., Prins, J., & Gielissen, M. (2016). Does fear of recurrence differ between cancer types? A study from the population-based PROFILES registry. *Psycho-Oncology, 25,* 772–778. doi.10.1002/pon.4002

van Ryn, M., Sanders, S., Kahn, K., van Houtven, C., Griffin, J.M., Martin, M., ... Rowland, J. (2011). Objective burden, resources, and other stressors among informal cancer caregivers: A hidden quality issue? *Psycho-Oncology, 20,* 44–52. doi.10.1002/pon.1703

Vickberg, S.M. (2003). The concerns about recurrence scale (CARS): A systematic measure of women's fears about the possibility of breast cancer recurrence. *Annals of Behavioral Medicine, 25,* 16–24. doi.10.1207/S15324796ABM2501_03

Wanat, M., Boulton, M., & Watson, E. (2016). Patients' experience with cancer recurrence: A meta-ethnography. *Psycho-Oncology, 25,* 242–252. doi.10.1002/pon.3908

Whitney, R., Bell, J., Bold, R., & Joseph, J.G. (2015). Mental health needs and service use in a national sample of adult cancer survivors in the U.S.: Has psychosocial care improved? *Psycho-Oncology, 24,* 80–88. doi.10.1002/pon.3569

Wu, H.S., & Harden, J.K. (2015). Symptom burden and quality of life in survivorship. *Cancer Nursing, 38,* E29–E54. doi.10.1097/NCC.0000000000000135

Zhao, G., Li., C., Li, J., & Balluz, L.S. (2013). Physical activity, psychological distress, and receipt of mental healthcare services among cancer survivors. *Journal of Cancer Survivorship, 7,* 131–139. doi.10.1007/s11764-012-0254-6

# SECTION II

# Psychosocial Influences

Chapter 3. Cognitive Dysfunction in Cancer
Chapter 4. Coping and Adaptation
Chapter 5. Cultural Influences
Chapter 6. Fatigue
Chapter 7. Hope
Chapter 8. Pain
Chapter 9. Spiritual and Religious Support
Chapter 10. Suffering

CHAPTER 3

# Cognitive Dysfunction in Cancer

*Esther Muscari Desimini, RN, MSN, APRN, BC, MBA*

> *If one loves me for my judgment, memory, he does not love me, for I can lose these qualities without losing myself.*
>
> —Blaise Pascal

Cognitive functioning is the aspect of behavior that involves the processes or domains of attention, concentration, learning and memory; sensory perceptual function; executive function abilities; psychomotor efficiency and manual dexterity; visuospatial ability; and general intelligence. Many of these processes or domains are highly interrelated and multidimensional. Language can be affected either in comprehension or expression. *Visuospatial ability* is the comprehension and effective manipulation of nonverbal, graphic, or geographic information, and executive function refers to the ability to plan, perform abstract reasoning, solve problems, focus despite distractions, and shift focus when appropriate.

Kolb and Wishaw (2009) described *cognitive functioning* as higher-order information processing that begins with the foundation of attention, concentration, and memory. When these are intact, the executive cognitive functions of psychomotor skills, processing speed, planning, decision making, and judgment are supported (Baxter, Dulworth, & Smith, 2011). Impairment can be evident in a number of behaviors. For example, attention allows people to select information from the environment, concentrate on that information, exclude irrelevant information or simultaneous stimuli, and sustain their attention on that selected information. Learning and memory are multidimensional and include short- and long-term memory. Memory is either contextual (i.e., information stored within the context of other information, such as being part of a greater story or memory) or noncontextual (i.e., information committed to memory without other information). Short-term memory involves everything associated with the present or recent hours or days. Long-term memory involves information storage that extends back years.

## Cognitive Impairment in the Oncology Population

Cognitive impairment was first reported in the 1980s in women with breast cancer (Dow, 2003). In the 1990s, it received a surge of attention when the National Coalition for Cancer

Survivorship recognized cognitive impairment as a challenge for patients who had undergone chemotherapy. Early studies of cognitive impairment were cross-sectional and showed a wide range of incidence (16%–75%), with some effects persisting up to 10 years after therapy (Hedayati, Schedin, Nyman, Alinaghizadeh, & Albertsson, 2011). Research primarily focused on cognitive performance of people younger than age 65, without association to specific tumor types or cancer diagnoses. Although research has since expanded to other solid tumors, breast cancer studies are more prevalent in understanding the experience of cognitive impairment.

Cancer-associated cognitive dysfunction (CACD) is characterized as deficits in areas of cognition, including memory, attention, concentration, and executive function. Highly prevalent, CACD can be detected in up to 20%–30% of patients prior to chemotherapy, up to 75% of patients during treatment, and may still be present in up to 35% of patients several years following treatment (Janelsins et al., 2012; Root, Ryan, & Ahles, 2015). Reports of impairment, with higher complaints of memory impairment, have been associated with the combination of chemotherapy and radiation treatments (Ganz et al., 2013). Quality of life and decision making can be affected by cognitive impairment. Causes associated with impaired cognitive functioning include the individual's characteristics, immune function, neural toxicity from treatment, and baseline genetics. Prevention research is limited, with more of an emphasis on interventional research to assist patients to respond and manage their care in order to maintain and maximize function (Janelsins, Kesler, Ahles, & Morrow, 2014). In addition, subtle cognitive changes may be intensified by fatigue, anxiety, or depression, often symptoms associated with cancer and its treatment (Janelsins et al., 2014).

The most frequently documented impairments to cognition in the oncology population are altered attention span, decreased concentration, inability to stay focused, mental fogginess, and short-term memory loss. Other impairments that have been reported from alterations in cognitive domains include disorganization, difficulty with arithmetic skills, and altered language skills (Andreano, Waisman, Donely, & Cahill, 2012; Baxter et al., 2011; Galica, Rajacich, Kane, & Pond, 2012; Hedayati et al., 2011; Joly, Rigal, Noal, & Giffard, 2011). Problems may fluctuate, with patients reporting good and bad days. On assessment, individuals may note that cognition is worse when they are multitasking, fatigued, or stressed.

## Controversial Research

The major limitations of early research studies were the use of cross-sectional, post-treatment–only designs and the inability to extrapolate to non–breast cancer populations (Kurita, Meyerowitz, Hall, & Gatz, 2011; Vardy & Tannock, 2007). Pretreatment assessment was not included in many of the early studies, which is needed to accurately assess changes over time. When considering pretreatment assessment, a potential confounding factor to acknowledge is that the anxiety and stress associated with a new diagnosis and the impending onset of treatment can influence the assessment (Joly et al., 2011). Within early study designs, the specifics of individual antineoplastic agents and disease sites also need to be considered to identify which are more toxic to cognitive function and to what degree.

Inconsistency in choice of neuropsychological tests, time periods in the disease continuum identified for testing, lack of baseline data prior to diagnosis, lack of standardized guidelines for assessment and management, and absence of longitudinal studies may all complicate the ability to fully and accurately comprehend the incidence, extent, and causes associated with cognitive impairment (Joly et al., 2011; Kurita et al., 2011). Because CACD has been reported years beyond treatment completion, and cancer survivorship has been consistently improving, mastering an understanding of cognitive impairment for cancer survivors is a significant concern (Kvale, 2009; Raffa, 2013; Schuurs & Green, 2013).

IQ and education level have not been controlled for in past studies. Both contribute to the challenge of extrapolating past results because of their influence on neuropsychological test scores. Additionally, having a higher IQ may reduce the negative impact of trauma to the brain, a concept known as *cognitive reserve*. Cognitive reserve refers to greater synaptic density associated with enriched cognitive stimulation that has developed over many years and has been examined in patients with Alzheimer disease (Stern, 2012). It has not been examined in the oncology population but most likely will be considered as the mechanisms of impairment are studied and researchers begin to consider why some patients develop cognitive impairment when others do not.

## Subjective Versus Objective Reports

CACD is perceived and described by patients as having difficulties with their ability to remember, think, find the right words, concentrate, and/or learn new material and comprehend what they are reading.

Patients may describe their difficulties as "chemobrain," "chemo fog," or "chemo clutter" (Brem & Kumar, 2011; Galica et al., 2011; Raffa, 2013). Self-report rates have been noted to be as high as 70% following cancer treatment, contributing to the challenge of distinguishing subjective changes from objective findings (Schuurs & Green, 2013; Shilling & Jenkins, 2007). Subjective patient experiences are important because they influence quality of life; however, studies support discrepancies between patients' perceptions and objective testing (Potrata, Cavet, Blair, & Molassiotis, 2010). Subjective perception of cognitive impairment after chemotherapy varies. Personality traits, along with sociodemographic and psychological characteristics, influence subjective perception. Additionally, the individual's characteristics can influence the perception of the degree of disruption caused by CACD.

In a qualitative study of multiple myeloma patients, people subjectively described their problems with recall of experiences or information, inability to focus attention without becoming distracted, and short-term recent memory loss (Potrata et al., 2010). Objective testing can be done via neuropsychological tests and magnetic resonance imaging (MRI) and positron-emission tomography (PET) scans. Neuropsychological testing measures psychological function linked to a particular part of the brain. Examples of neuropsychological testing include the Mini-Mental State Examination, the Mini-Cog™, the Montreal Cognitive Assessment, and the High Sensitivity Cognitive Screen (Root et al., 2015). These tests aim to compare the individual's score to that of a population with similar characteristics in order to provide an assessment of the individual's current cognitive function. Different tests can assess the different domains of cognition: intelligence, memory, language, executive function, and visuospatial.

Brain imaging via MRI or PET scans can assess changes in brain function or structure, thus contributing to understanding the biology of cognitive function and the effect of cancer treatment. Recently, gray and white matter changes in patients with breast cancer who were exposed to chemotherapy aligned with neuropsychological test results, supporting patients' experiences that underlying cerebral changes could be affecting functioning (Deprez et al., 2012; McDonald, Conroy, Ahles, West, & Saykin, 2010).

Older studies may not have supported a correlation with cerebral changes and neuropsychological testing, possibly because of a lack of specificity of assessment tools (Ganz et al., 2013). Also, neuropsychological tests were initially developed for patients suffering from brain injuries, such as stroke, head injury, or brain disease. Despite high self-report incidence rates of cognitive impairment six months after treatment completion, no correlation with objective testing was found.

## Contributing Factors

Factors contributing to CACD can be separated into direct (disease-related) factors and indirect (treatment-related) factors. Direct causes include primary or metastatic cancer and personal characteristics, such as age and intelligence. The list of indirect causes is extensive (see Figure 3-1).

- Depression
- Anxiety
- Fatigue
- Cytokines
- Inflammatory markers
- Treatment-induced menopause
- Hormonal manipulation
- Chemotherapeutic agents
- Side effects from other medications
- Sleep disturbance

**Figure 3-1. Indirect Causes of Cancer-Associated Cognitive Dysfunction**

### Age

Cognitive function is influenced by age. As adults age, they can experience a progressive decline in cognitive function. Declines do not develop uniformly but rather depend on the cognitive function affected, the rate of change, and when changes become apparent within or across cognitive domains. Because aging is highly individualized, no assumptions should be made about cognitive functioning based on chronologic age.

Some predictable changes occur with age in performance on neuropsychological tests, with differences noted in short-term memory and the inability to learn new information. This minimal cognitive impairment is normal age-associated mental impairment, as opposed to a disease process such as dementia. Memory loss associated with the natural aging process and other coexisting health conditions is difficult to isolate or separate from cancer-related causes.

As the population ages, the incidence of dementia increases. With increasing life expectancies and a growing aging population, the prevalence and risk for dementia increases as well. *Dementia* is a general term for a group of cognitive disorders, with Alzheimer disease being the most common (Centers for Disease Control and Prevention [CDC], 2015). The risk for Alzheimer disease doubles every five years, starting at the age of 65, coinciding with the increased incidence of cancer diagnoses. By age 85, 25%–50% of people will have Alzheimer disease (CDC, 2015) (see Chapter 11 for additional information on dementia).

In addition to dementia, cognitive loss can be caused by delirium and depression as well as CACD. Cognitive impairment in older adults because of disease or treatment can be subdivided into acute reversible and chronic irreversible forms. Because older adults are more likely to suffer from comorbidities that impair cognition (e.g., vascular disease) and are more affected by cancer treatment toxicities, age is a contributing factor in the assessment of cognitive impairment in the older adult survivor of cancer.

# Indirect Factors

## Chemotherapy

The majority of cognitive impairment research with cancer has involved patients with breast cancer. Only recently have other cancer diagnoses and their association with cognitive impairment from chemotherapy been investigated (Ek, Almkvist, Wiberg, Stragliotto, & Smits, 2010; Galica et al., 2012; Joly et al., 2011; Kurita et al., 2011; Whiting et al., 2012). In an early review of the evidence, Ahles and Saykin (2002) evaluated the prevalence of cognitive deficits in women receiving chemotherapy for breast cancer compared to healthy individuals. The need for long-term, longitudinal studies along with pretreatment neuropsychological assessments was noted. Ahles et al. (2002) compared patients with lymphoma or breast cancer treated with systemic therapy to matching populations receiving local therapy only. Global cognitive deficits that affect a wide range of higher-order cognitive performance domains were associated with systemic chemotherapy, with significant differences in the specific domains of verbal memory and psychomotor functioning. Patients were, on average, 10 years out from chemotherapy, supporting the belief that deficits seen up to two years after treatment can continue for the long term. These early findings set the stage for further study to define the extent of cognitive deficits, the percentage of patients actually affected, and the factors that contribute to the risk of long-term cognitive deterioration.

After conducting a review of original studies between 2000 and 2010, Joly et al. (2011) noted early associations between cognitive impairment and chemotherapy in the breast cancer population. The authors substantiated that the association with chemotherapy and subtle, transient cognitive dysfunctions were detectable only with neuropsychological testing. The domains most commonly affected were memory, concentration, and speed of information processing. In addition, the broad range of chemotherapy doses used in the different studies could explain the variation in the responses of cognitive impairment (Joly et al., 2011). The researchers summarized that, because of limited data, the prevention, evaluation, and management of chemotherapy-induced cognitive impairment necessitated longitudinal studies to evaluate influence on quality of life.

## Radiation Therapy

Cognitive impairment is a late adverse effect of cranial radiation for primary and metastatic tumors, affecting 40%–50% of patients who live longer than six months after treatment (Whiting et al., 2012; Zhang, Yang, & Tian, 2015). However, Ek et al. (2010) found that adults treated with radiation therapy for brain tumors had cognitive deficits that were evident at baseline and not the result of radiation effects. Cognitive impairment was noted to be associated with large tumors in the left frontal lobe, affecting predominantly young males. Cognitive impairments after primary brain tumor diagnosis are prevalent in almost 90% of patients and have been noted in the domains of attention, memory, executive function, and language (Gehring, Aaronson, Taphoorn, & Sitskoorn,

2010). Because the effects of disease progression are difficult to differentiate from the effects of radiation therapy, this raises the question of how to follow patients for the long term. These findings also raise the issue of what role patients' overall condition plays in cognitive performance.

## Hormonal Influences

Artificially induced hormonal changes have been linked to cognitive impairments (Janelsins et al., 2011). Estrogen deficits and alterations in cytokines related to postmenopausal status have been implicated as potential contributing factors in cognitive deficits (Janelsins et al., 2011). Therefore, greater cognitive impairment has been noted in women treated with both chemotherapy and specific estrogen receptor modulators than those receiving chemotherapy alone. Greater cognitive impairment has also been observed in women who experience a treatment-induced menopause (Bender et al., 2006; Jenkins et al., 2006). Larger studies are needed to confirm these results and to investigate the combined effects of chemotherapy and endocrine therapy on cognitive function (Janelsins et al., 2011).

Within the male population, Heather et al. (2010) noted greater overall cognitive impairment among men who had received luteinizing hormone–releasing hormone agonists and surgery for prostate cancer than healthy matched counterparts. Recommendations from this work consisted of longitudinal studies that included measurements before and after surgical and hormonal treatment for prostate cancer.

## Cytokines

Abnormal concentrations of cytokines and chemokines can lead to cognitive impairment by affecting the integrity of neurons. This is observed in some neurodegenerative diseases such as Alzheimer. The degree to which this occurs in the patient receiving chemotherapy is not well understood. Chemotherapy has been associated with increased levels of proinflammatory cytokines in the breast cancer population, which has also been studied for the incidence of cognitive impairment. When studying the relationship between cytokine levels and different chemotherapy agents in early-stage breast cancer regimens, Janelsins et al. (2012) noted different responses in cytokines/chemokines along with self-reported cognitive changes. The findings pointed to the need for further study to conduct neuropsychological testing at baseline prior to chemotherapy administration and longitudinally as cytokine levels are monitored.

## Psychological Factors

A patient's response to a cancer diagnosis may explain cognitive dysfunction prior to therapy. Stress, anxiety, and depression can interfere with cognition (Klein, Reijneveld, & Heimans, 2008). Andreano et al. (2012) assessed the influence of glucocorticoid and ovarian disruption on cognitive dysfunction. Their results supported the idea that a disruption of the enhancement of memory by stress may contribute to cognitive difficulties following breast cancer treatment.

The traumatic nature of the diagnosis can cause alterations in memory, attention, and emotional relationships, leading to anxiety and depression. It can also cause a major disruption in overall functioning, as well as impede goals, as it generates a discontinuity from past, present, and future events. It is unknown to what degree a person's psychological adjustment to the cancer and treatment has on cognitive impairment (Galica et al., 2012).

## Multifactorial Etiology

Assessment and interpretation of CACD in patients with cancer is difficult, and at times, it is self-limiting to the population at hand because of the multifactorial nature of the impairments. The interrelationship between the contributing factors compounds the challenge of identifying one specific etiology (Brem & Kumar, 2011; Ek et al., 2010).

## Assessment

When meeting with patients, first indications of cognitive impairment, if not volunteered by the patient, are sometimes apparent in conversation. Repeated questions, difficulty following directions, searching for a word, or inability to remember the sequence of past events since the last appointment may raise suspicions in the healthcare provider. Inquiring how patients arrived at the clinic, how they adapt when outside their home in an unfamiliar setting, or what recent decisions they have made can indicate a need for more in-depth evaluation.

During the health history, pertinent questions, such as whether the onset was sudden or acute, can help in identifying an underlying acute medical condition (e.g., infection, trauma, small stroke). Delirium or confusion might be present in older adults who recently have been discharged from the hospital or are recovering from an acute infection or surgery. To support assessment, age adjustment and age-adjusted norms need to be incorporated into standardized neuropsychological testing.

Patients might volunteer unsolicited examples of changes in cognitive function. They may describe short-term memory difficulty or trouble with word recall, which can lead to further evaluation and possibly formal neuropsychological testing. Patients or family members may disclose that their participation in social activities has decreased and that they have been giving up hobbies or avoiding situations, people, or events that they previously enjoyed (Ek et al., 2010). Finances, housework, or meals may go unattended as patients become unable to carry out normal daily activities.

Agitation, paranoia, and irritability are indicators of possible cognitive impairment. Patients can become suspicious during the early stages of impairment because they have a subtle awareness of deficits or "changes" occurring within themselves. Healthcare providers should note patients' decreased ability to concentrate on the questioning, their emotional responses, and any unkempt outward appearance because these could be indicative of problems.

The Mini-Mental State Examination (MMSE), developed from the more extensive cognitive mental status examination, suggests a first-line assessment tool that can be used in any clinical setting (Folstein, Folstein, & McHugh, 1975). The MMSE separates patients with cognitive disturbances from those without such disturbances. It includes 11 questions and requires 10 minutes to administer. The MMSE does not require the administrator to have special training and is therefore very practical to use routinely and serially. It concentrates on the cognitive aspects of mental functions and excludes questions pertaining to mood, abnormal mental experiences, and process of thinking. It tests patients' short-term memory, ability to spell forward and backward, ability to perform simple math equations, and the capacity to recall three unrelated words. The MMSE is not intended to diagnose but rather raise awareness that further testing is needed. MMSE failures on orientation, memory, reading, and writing have clear implications for patients with cancer who are trying to care for themselves, make decisions in their care, and move forward in their lives. A challenge of the MMSE may be its lack of sensitivity for mild cognitive impairment, which may not be detected with this traditional screening tool.

Neuropsychological testing examines the brain-behavior relationship. Assessment is standardized and crosses multiple domains. Assessment areas commonly tested include attention, verbal and visual learning and memory; critical reasoning; complex problem solving; processing speed and mental efficiency; language comprehension and fluency; reaction time; motor dexterity; and sensory functioning. The testing aspect of assessment includes an array of tests that often are lengthy in nature (four to seven hours) and require a trained administrator. The assessment usually requires more than one test to capture all potentially affected domains; therefore, these tests are not conducive to administration in the clinical oncology setting.

Neurocognitive testing addresses various thinking abilities, encompassing domains of attention and concentration, abstract reasoning, cognitive processing speed, language, visuospatial and visuoconstruction, executive functions, learning and memory, and sensorimotor functions. The necessary tests are different than those used for neuropsychological testing.

Baxter et al. (2011) suggested routine screening as part of occupational therapy evaluations using the Montreal Cognitive Assessment (MoCA) tool after noting a 36% prevalence rate in their study group. MoCA requires approximately 10 minutes to administer and has high sensitivity, test–retest reliability, and consistency for determining mild cognitive impairment in the oncology survivorship population. The tool assists in determining the areas of cognitive functioning causing difficulty. Because of the lack of concise, practical, standardized neuropsychological tests in clinical oncology, the MoCA may fill the gap. Root et al. (2015) provided a list of commonly used neurocognitive and neuropsychological function assessment tools, most of which require a considerable amount of testing time and administration by an expert professional.

## Implications for Practice

Patients' abilities to care for themselves, recall daily responsibilities and events, and maintain their roles within their family and professional lives are dependent on cognitive abilities. An alteration in any of these abilities potentially affects satisfaction with life and, ultimately, quality of life (Summers, 2012). As the research literature increases, a better understanding of the cognitive domains most often affected and by which treatment modalities will be a great asset to clinicians and can contribute to a more tailored neurocognitive assessment. As healthcare providers learn more about cognitive impairment, patients' risks for impairment and which potential domain will be affected can be determined before patients experience deficits. Patient and family education can then be tailored to specific risks (as determined by the cancer site, treatment modality, age, hormonal status, and education level). Although cognitive training, which involves performing tasks that improve attention and short-term memory, can help patients and families, research is insufficient to support approaches that prevent or treat thinking and memory problems (Von Ah, Jansen, & Allen, 2014).

Clinician awareness of the commonly affected domains can lead to appropriate tools to empower patients. Visual materials for home use can help patients to respond to short-term memory losses so that the deficits are not as debilitating. Maximizing patients' potential for optimal functioning can be achieved through frequently reviewing medication profiles, managing possible comorbid conditions, treating emotional/mood disorders, and maintaining normal laboratory profiles. Optimal symptom management contributes to minimizing any distraction to maximal attention and concentration, efficiency of thinking, and multitasking.

Because it is common for patients to fear that their brain is not working well or that they are "losing their mind," it is important that their experiences are consistently and frequently validated (Breitbart, Gibson, & Tremblay, 2002). Knowing that cognitive deficits exist within specific domains and do not necessarily impair all mental functions can help patients to feel less vulnerable to changes and that they have some control over other aspects of their life.

Clinicians will need to be confident that patients experiencing cognitive impairment have provided true informed consent. This particularly is important in patients' decision-making capacity to provide consent for research (Casarett, Karlawish, & Hirschman, 2003). Patients might need more than one informative session, written materials, and assistance from a family member to learn about the clinical plan and to help them to adhere to the appointments.

# Cognitive Rehabilitation

The Society for Cognitive Rehabilitation (2013) defines *cognitive rehabilitation therapy* as a process of relearning cognitive skills that have been lost or altered as a result of damage to brain cells or brain chemistry. If skills cannot be relearned, then new ones can be learned to help the person compensate for lost cognitive functions.

Because the cognitive impairments experienced by most patients with cancer do not stop them from engaging in activities of daily living (ADLs) and the pharmacologic approach remains limited, cognitive rehabilitation is gaining increased attention, use, and investigation (Brem & Kumar, 2011; Gehring et al., 2010; Joly et al., 2011). Improved objective and subjective cognition with formalized cognitive rehabilitation programs have been reported, with noted improvements in overall cognition, immediate memory, delayed memory, and visuospatial/visuoconstructional performance (Ferguson et al., 2007; Schuurs & Green, 2013; Smith et al., 2009). Cognitive rehabilitation is intended to improve the independence level of patients, with vocational rehabilitation focused on improving productivity in their volunteer or professional efforts and ADLs. Cognitive rehabilitation begins with identifying and validating the patient's deficits.

Tailored programs for cognitive rehabilitation can include education about the different types and causes of memory changes. It is a relief for some to understand that what they are experiencing is a focused, specific aspect from treatment and not an indication of a more global condition such as Alzheimer disease. Describing to patients how the cancer therapy causes cognitive impairment and affects their thinking is the first step. Explaining how individuals will experience the impairment in daily life can be integral to rehabilitation:

- **A short attention span** will increase the amount of time needed to learn a new task or, for example, the time it takes to assist with a child's homework.
- **Spatial performance deficits** will cause difficulty envisioning or describing the route between their home and work.

- **Short-term memory deficits** will affect appointments and responsibilities; word-recall problems will cause people to find themselves in the middle of a sentence struggling to say a word they have used many times.
- **Number sequencing** and math skills difficulties may decrease their ability to balance a checkbook.

In an extensive research review, Von Ah et al. (2014) reported that cognitive training, either individually or within a group, has the greatest impact in providing patients with the most improvement after experiencing cognitive impairment caused by cancer. The Oncology Nursing Society defines *cognitive training* as "any intervention aimed at improving, maintaining, or restoring mental function through the repeated and structured practice of tasks which pose an inherent problem or mental challenge. Group cognitive training is provided to individuals in a group setting" (Von Ah et al., 2016). Research surrounding other practices is insufficient or unsupportive. These practices range from exercise to ginkgo biloba and erythropoiesis.

Once patients can see the specifics of how their cognition is impaired, they feel reassured that they are not "losing their mind" and can focus their attention on the identified areas to bolster and support themselves. Working with an individual to develop a structured, methodic approach to daily routines, situations, and problem solving is part of cognitive rehabilitation. For example, regular use of a daily electronic or paper calendar that has built-in alerts or reminders can assist with memory. Smartphone applications can also help with memory and organization. Placing a small calculator in a checkbook can assist with arithmetic skills. Limiting activities to short, frequent periods, if energy levels allow, can lessen difficulty with attention. Focusing on improving independence level, performing ADLs, and engaging in vocational rehabilitation can empower cognitively impaired patients to function at their potential. A focus should be placed on time management and energy conservation in order to minimize contributing factors and maximize sleep habits.

# Conclusion

Cognitive impairment can be frightening to patients, families, and even caregivers because it is the ability to think, problem solve, follow directions, and make decisions that helps to define who we are as individuals. When cognition is altered, it places a person in a position of vulnerability. Nurses are in an optimal position, by virtue of the many roles within oncology, to have an impact on patients and their family members who are at risk for or are actively experiencing cognitive impairment. Therefore, identifying risk factors and understanding and differentiating the domains that process information allows for an assessment that produces interventions and assistance specific to the area of thinking affected. Rather than feeling vulnerable or overwhelmed with fear, patients and families can be encouraged and function at levels satisfying to their quality of life.

# References

Ahles, T., & Saykin, A. (2002). Breast cancer chemotherapy-related cognitive dysfunction. *Clinical Breast Cancer, 3*(Suppl. 3), S84–S89. doi:10.3816/CBC.2002.s.018

Ahles, T., Saykin, A., Furstenberg, C., Cole, B., Mott, L., Skalla, K., ... Silberfarb, P.M. (2002). Neuropsychologic impact of standard-dose systemic chemotherapy in long-term survivors of breast cancer and lymphoma. *Journal of Clinical Oncology, 20,* 485–493. doi:10.1200/JCO.20.2.485

Andreano, J.M., Waisman, J., Donley, L., & Cahill, L. (2012). Effects of breast cancer treatment on the hormonal and cognitive consequences of acute stress. *Psycho-Oncology, 21,* 1091–1098. doi:10.1002/pon.2006

Baxter, M.F., Dulworth, A.N., & Smith, T.M. (2011). Identification of mild cognitive impairments in cancer survivors. *Occupational Therapy in Health Care, 25,* 26–37. doi:10.3109/07380577.2010.533251

Bender, C., Sereika, S.M., Berga, S.L., Vogel, V.G., Brufsky, A.M., Paraska, K.K., & Ryan, C.M. (2006). Cognitive impairment associated with adjuvant therapy in breast cancer. *Psycho-Oncology, 15,* 422–430. doi:10.1002/pon.964

Breitbart, W., Gibson, C., & Tremblay, A. (2002). The delirium experience: Delirium recall and delirium-related distress in hospitalized patients with cancer, their spouses/caregivers, and their nurses. *Psychosomatics, 43,* 183–194. doi:10.1002/pon.964

Brem, S., & Kumar, N. (2011). Management of treatment-related symptoms in patients with breast cancer: Current strategies and future directions. *Clinical Journal of Oncology Nursing, 15,* 63–71. doi:10.1188/11.CJON.63-71

Casarett, D., Karlawish, J., & Hirschman, K. (2003). Identifying ambulatory cancer patients at risk of impaired capacity to consent to research. *Journal of Pain and Symptom Management, 26,* 615–622. doi:10.1016/S0885-3924(03)00221-5

Centers for Disease Control and Prevention. (2015). Dementia/Alzheimer's disease. Retrieved from https://www.cdc.gov/aging/aginginfo/alzheimers.htm

Deprez, S., Amant, F., Smeets, A., Peeters, R., Leemans, A., Van Hecke, W., … Sunaert, S. (2012). Longitudinal assessment of chemotherapy-induced structural changes in cerebral white matter and its correlation with impaired cognitive functioning. *Journal of Clinical Oncology, 30,* 274–281. doi:10.1200/JCO/2011.36.8571

Dow, K.H. (2003). Challenges and opportunities in cancer survivorship research. *Oncology Nursing Forum, 30,* 455–469. doi:10.1188/03.ONF.455-469

Ek, L., Almkvist, O., Wiberg, M.K., Stragliotto, G., & Smits, A. (2010). Early cognitive impairment in a subset of patients with presumed low-grade glioma. *Psychology Press, 16,* 503–511. doi:10.1080/13554791003730634

Ferguson, R.J., Ahles, T.A., Saykin, A.J., McDonald, B.C., Furstenberg, C.T., Cole, B.F., & Mott, L.A. (2007). Cognitive-behavioral management of chemotherapy-related cognitive change. *Psycho-Oncology, 16,* 772–777. doi:10.1002/pon.1133

Folstein, M., Folstein, S., & McHugh, P. (1975). "Mini-mental state": A practical method for grading the cognitive state of patients for the clinician. *Journal of Psychiatric Research, 12,* 189–198. doi:10.1016/0022-3956(75)90026-6

Galica, J., Rajacich, D., Kane, D., & Pond, G. (2012). The impact of chemotherapy-induced cognitive impairment on the psychosocial adjustment of patients with non-metastatic colorectal cancer. *Clinical Journal of Oncology Nursing, 16,* 163–169. doi:10.1188/12.CJON.163-169

Ganz, P.A., Kwan, L., Castellon, S.A., Oppenheim, A., Bower, J.E., Silverman, D.H.S., … Belin, T.R. (2013). Cognitive complaints after breast cancer treatments: Examining the relationship with neuropsychological test performance. *Journal of the National Cancer Institute, 10,* 1–11. doi:10.1093/jnci/djt073

Gehring, K., Aaronson, N.K., Taphoorn, M.J., & Sitskoorn, M.M. (2010). Interventions for cognitive deficits in patients with a brain tumor: An update. *Expert Review of Anticancer Therapy, 10,* 1779–1795. doi:10.1586/era.10.163

Heather, S., Jim, L., Small, B.J., Patterson, S., Salup, R., & Jacobsen, P. (2010). Cognitive impairment in men treated with luteinizing hormone-releasing hormone agonists for prostate cancer: A controlled comparison. *Supportive Care in Cancer, 18,* 21–27. doi:10.1007/s00520-009-0625-3

Hedayati, E., Schedin, A., Nyman, H., Alinaghizadeh, H., & Albertsson, M. (2011). The effects of breast cancer diagnosis and surgery on cognitive functions. *Acta Oncologica, 50,* 1027–1036. doi:10.3109/0284186X.2011.572911

Janelsins, M.C., Kesler, S.R., Ahles, T.A., & Morrow, G.R. (2014). Prevalence, mechanisms, and management of cancer-related cognitive impairment. *International Review of Psychiatry, 26,* 102–113. doi:10.3109/09540261.2013.864260

Janelsins, M.C., Kohli, S., Mohile, S.G., Usuki, K., Ahles, T.A., & Morow, G.R. (2011). An update on cancer- and chemotherapy-related cognitive dysfunction: Current status. *Seminars in Oncology, 38,* 431–438. doi:10.1053/j.seminoncol.2011.03.014

Janelsins, M.C., Mustian, K.M., Palesh, O.G., Mohile, S.G., Peppone, L.J., Sprod, L.K., … Morrow, G.R. (2012). Differential expression of cytokines in breast cancer patients receiving different chemotherapies: Implications for cognitive impairment research. *Supportive Care in Cancer, 20,* 831–839. doi:10.1007/s00520-011-1158-0

Jenkins, V., Shilling, V., Deutsch, G., Bloomfield, D., Morris, R., Allan, S., … Winstanley, J. (2006). A 3-year prospective study of the effects of adjuvant treatments on cognition in women with early stage breast cancer. *British Journal of Cancer, 94,* 828–834. doi:10.1038/sj.bjc.6603029

Joly, F., Rigal, O., Noal, S., & Giffard, B. (2011). Cognitive dysfunction and cancer: Which consequences in terms of disease management? *Psycho-Oncology, 20,* 1251–1258. doi:10.1002/pon.1903

Klein, M., Reijneveld, J., & Heimans, J. (2008). Subjective ratings vs. objective measurement of cognitive function. *International Journal of Radiation Oncology, Biology, Physics, 70,* 961–962. doi:10.1016/j.ijrobp.2007.09.031

Kolb, B., & Whishaw, I.Q. (2009). *The development of neuropsychology. Fundamentals of human neuropsychology* (6th ed.). New York, NY: Worth Publishers.

Kurita, K., Meyerowitz, B., Hall, P., & Gatz, M. (2011). Long-term cognitive impairment in older adult twins discordant for gynecologic cancer treatment. *Journals of Gerontology, 66A,* 1343–1349. doi:10.1093/gerona/glr140

Kvale, E.A. (2009). Cognitive speed of processing and functional declines in older cancer survivors: An analysis of data from the ACTIVE trial. *European Journal of Cancer Care, 19,* 110–117. doi:10.1111/j.1365-2354.2008.01018.x

McDonald, B.C., Conroy, S.K., Ahles, T.A., West, J.D., & Saykin, A.J. (2010). Gray matter reduction associated with systemic chemotherapy for breast cancer: A prospective MRI study. *Breast Cancer Research and Treatment, 123,* 819–828. doi:10.1007/s10549-010-1088-4

Potrata, B., Cavet, J., Blair, S., & Molassiotis, A. (2010). Like a sieve: An exploratory study on cognitive impairments in patients with multiple myeloma. *European Journal of Cancer Care, 19,* 721–728. doi:10.1111/j.1365-2354.2009.01145.x

Raffa, R.B. (2013). Cancer "survivor-care": II. Disruption of prefrontal brain activation top down control of working memory capacity as possible mechanism for chemo-fog/brain (chemotherapy associated cognitive impairment). *Journal of Clinical Pharmacy and Therapeutics, 38,* 265–268. doi:10.1111/jcpt.12071

Root, J.C., Ryan, E., & Ahles, T.A. (2015). Screening and assessment for cognitive problems. In J.C. Holland, W.S. Breitbart, P.N. Butow, P.B. Jacobsen, M.J. Loscalzo, & R. McCorkle (Eds.), *Psycho-oncology* (3rd ed., pp. 405–410). New York, NY: Oxford University Press.

Schuurs, A., & Green, H.J. (2013). A feasibility study of group cognitive rehabilitation for cancer survivors: Enchancing cognitive function and quality of life. *Psycho-Oncology, 22,* 1043–1049. doi:10.1002/pon.3102

Shilling, V., & Jenkins, V. (2007). Self-reported cognitive problems in women receiving adjuvant therapy for breast cancer. *European Journal of Oncology Nursing, 11,* 6–15. doi:10.1016/j.ejon.2006.02.005

Smith, G.E., Housen, P., Yaffe, K., Ruff, R., Kennison, R.F., Mahncke, H.W., & Zelinski, E.M. (2009). A cognitive training program based on principles of brain plasticity: Results from the improvement in memory with plasticity-based adaptive cognitive training (IMPACT) study. *Journal of the American Geriatrics Society, 57,* 594–603. doi:10.1111/j.1532-5415.2008.02167.x

Society for Cognitive Rehabilitation. (2013). What is cognitive rehabilitation therapy? Retrieved from http://www.societyforcognitiverehab.org/about-scr-and-cognitive-rehab/about.php

Stern, Y. (2012). Cognitive reserve in ageing and Alzheimer's disease. *Lancet Neurology, 11,* 1006–1012. doi:10.1016/S1474-4422(12)70191-6

Summers, L.E. (2012). Effects of chemotherapy on patients' cognitive function. *Cancer Nursing Practice, 11,* 27–31. doi:10.7748/cnp2012.10.11.8.27.c9356

Vardy, J., & Tannock, I. (2007). Cognitive function after chemotherapy in adults with solid tumors. *Critical Reviews in Oncology/Hematology, 63,* 183–202. doi:10.1016/j.critrevonc.2007.06.001

Von Ah, D., Allen, D.H., Jansen, C.E., Merriman, J.D., Myers, J.S., & Wulff, J. (2016). Putting Evidence into Practice: Cognitive impairment. Retrieved from https://www.ons.org/practice-resources/pep/cognitive-impairment

Von Ah, D., Jansen, C.E., & Allen, D.A. (2014). Evidence-based interventions for cancer- and treatment-related cognitive impairment. *Clinical Journal of Oncology Nursing, 18*(Suppl. 6), 17–24 doi:10.1188/14.CJON.S3.17-25

Whiting, D.L., Simpson, G.K., Kosh, E., Wright, K.M., Simpson, T., & Firth, R. (2012). A multi-tiered intervention to address behavioural and cognitive changes after diagnosis of primary brain tumour: A feasibility study. *Brain Injury, 26,* 950–961. doi:10.3109/02699052.2012.661912

Zhang, L., Yang, H., & Tian, Y. (2015). Radiation-induced cognitive impairment. *Therapeutic Targets for Neurologic Diseases, 2,* E837. doi:10.14800/ttnd.837

# CHAPTER 4

# Coping and Adaptation

*Nancy Jo Bush, DNP, RN, MN, MA, AOCN®, FAAN*

> *Every tear I ever cried,*
> *turned to pearl before it died.*
> *Every pain that in me burned,*
> *turned to wisdom I had earned.*
>
> —Joan Walsh Anglund

Coping is an integral part of everyday life. As people deal with daily hassles in their environment, they cope on many different levels. Hassles are those mundane, everyday challenges that can be considered minor annoyances or serious pressures. Coping is the response that people employ in an attempt to adapt to the internal and external demands of stressful events (Arnold, 2016; Folkman, 2013; Kohn, 1996). Daily stressors may comprise work dissatisfaction, family dysfunction, time pressures, and various other demands. These mundane stressors can adversely affect health, and, if cumulative, they may have a negative impact on physical and psychological well-being exceeding that of major life-changing stressors. Therefore, the continuum of coping can range from confronting the stresses of everyday life to facing a chronic, life-threatening illness such as cancer (Maybery, Neale, Arentz, & Jones-Ellis, 2007). The patient experiencing cancer is attempting to cope not only with the daily stressors of living but, at the same time, is trying to integrate and adapt to a life-threatening illness (Nail, 2001; Tallman, 2013). Normal demands of everyday life, such as child care, family and job responsibilities, and financial pressures, will be exaggerated in a time of crisis. For example, if marital discontent already exists, a cancer diagnosis may put additional pressure on the relationship, exceeding the personal coping resources the couple has available (Lewis, 2004, 2010; Traa, DeVries, Bodenmann, & Den Oudsten, 2015). Individuals and families confronting cancer experience many changes in their day-to-day lives, incorporating illness and treatment-related demands into daily routines that may already be overwhelmed with hassles and everyday stressors (Nail, 2001). Coping in the context of cancer is the ability of the patient and family to adapt functionally to the stress of diagnosis and treatment as well as to the long-term adjustments that cancer brings (Sivesind & Paire, 2009).

Coping responses are complex phenomena. Many variables affect the way in which people respond to stress. The situation or context of the stressor is one important variable, in addition to personality traits. When conceptualizing coping, contextual approaches look at coping as a dynamic process that changes over time as the individual confronts different stressful demands (Arnold, 2016; Holahan, Moos, & Schaefer, 1996; Nail, 2001). The intensity of stress incurred when juggling career and home is different than when these daily demands are combined with chemotherapy treatments for cancer. The challenges a person faces at the diagnostic stage of cancer will be different from those faced during treatment or at end of life. Therefore, the context of the stress will influence the individual's and family's coping responses. In addition, the coping responses that people habitually apply are influenced by their personality characteristics and past experiences. Coping also has been conceptualized from a dispositional approach, taking into account the consistent manner by which individuals adapt when confronted with stress (Holahan et al., 1996; Kohn, 1996; Nail, 2001). For example, if one is prone to anxiety, confronting a stressful situation will heighten this emotional response (Levin & Alici, 2010).

Characteristics of personality and coping develop over a lifetime as a person moves toward emotional maturity. Cancer can strike, often without warning, anywhere along the continuum of psychosocial development. Although the individual confronts cancer with a preset repertoire of coping skills, these skills may not be adequate for the specific situation, or the cancer experience may tax the individual's emotional resources. In addition, the cancer diagnosis may be the first life-threatening stressor that the individual and family have had to face, calling upon the need for reinforcement of past coping styles and the need to form new coping strategies that fit the demands of the situation. Therefore, coping is a complex, changing process influenced by the situation (context), individual differences (personality traits), and previous experiences. There is no "right" or "wrong" way to cope (Nail, 2001).

> Every person brings unique characteristics to dealing with illness; a particular personality, a way of coping, a set of beliefs and values, and a way of looking at the world. The goal is to take these qualities into consideration and make sure that they work in favor of the person at each point along the cancer journey. (Holland & Lewis, 2000, p. 3)

## Definitions of Coping

Historically, coping had been viewed as an unconscious defense in response to intrapsychic conflict. Coping has been conceptualized as an active, conscious response to stress (Lazarus, 2000). Several specific definitions exist to describe the function of coping mechanisms. Historically, *coping* has been defined as a stabilizing factor that promotes adaptive functioning during stressful periods (Holahan et al., 1996) and as "any effort to manage external or internal demands that are appraised as negative or challenging" (Maes, Leventhal, & de Ridder, 1996, p. 226). Additional concepts have been added to reflect the complexity of coping. The construct of coping has been interchanged with concepts such as adaptation, mastery, resiliency, and adjustment (Arnold, 2016; Henderson, Gore, Davis, & Condon, 2003). Coping is an adaptive response to stress; a person attempts to restore equilibrium in response to stressful life events such as cancer (Henderson et al., 2003). Within the framework of a self-regulation model of coping, Spencer, Carver, and Price (1998) defined *coping* as those behaviors and cognitive activities aimed at responding to and overcoming adversity. *Engagement coping strategies* have been defined as active, goal-directed behaviors aimed to either reduce the impact of the stressor itself or influence the emotional responses or efforts needed to adapt to the stressor and include problem solving, seeking support, acceptance, and positive reframing (Yu & Sherman, 2015). Adaptation is the result of effective coping and is a state of equilibrium, reflecting the individual's return to life activities, goals, and social functioning. Ineffective coping is disengagement from, or the inability to return to, the normal activities of life (Spencer et al., 1998). Disengagement coping strategies are coping efforts that take attention away from the stressor and include emotional, cognitive, and behavioral avoidance, such as denial, substance abuse, and self-blame (Yu & Sherman, 2015).

## Situational Coping

Coping efforts aim to reduce or eliminate the stressful conditions one is facing in an attempt to minimize the inherent emotional distress that one is experiencing. Thus, coping strategies are behavioral and cognitive efforts that are shaped by context (Folkman, 2013; Lazarus, 1993). Therefore, coping effectiveness is best evaluated within the context of the challenges faced by the individual and family (Rait, 2015). These context-driven or contextual definitions of coping are based on the stressors (e.g., cancer) and the situational factors (e.g., chemotherapy, radiation) that shape an individual's coping mechanisms. When coping is assessed in relation to a specific context, the assessments become problem specific, and outcomes are measured in regard to specific stressors (e.g., confronting the cancer, dealing with treatment) (Arnold, 2016; Somerfield & Curbow, 1992). Within this framework, evaluation of coping effectiveness can be based on outcomes rather than coping strategies per se, and interventions to enhance coping can focus on a modifiable stressor (Nail, 2001).

## Dispositional Coping

Coping also has been defined within the framework of an individual's personality or habitual way of responding to stress, in other words, their coping style. Dispositional approaches to defining coping behaviors are based on evaluating the individual's inherently stable person-based traits or resources that influence the coping mechanisms chosen when facing stress (Holahan et al., 1996; Wynn, 2015). Personality variables, such as optimism and pessimism, attitude or "fighting spirit," and locus of control, influence the coping strategies one chooses when confronting stress (Hoffman, Lent, & Raque-Bogdan, 2013; Somerfield & Curbow, 1992; Spencer et al., 1998; Wilkes, O'Baugh, Luke, & George, 2003). Families also have personalities or traits that influence coping. The family stress theory contends that the family is a social system; stress in one family member has a reverberating effect on each family member in the system (Friedman, Bowden, & Jones, 2003; Lewis, 2010). Families develop basic and unique strengths to protect their members from adverse events. Family communication, problem solving, and interpersonal relationships influence how families cope and adapt to stressful life experiences (Friedman et al., 2003; McCubbin & McCubbin, 1996; Rait, 2015).

## Summary

Two distinct ways of conceptualizing coping emerge: (a) a disposition or trait that becomes a mode or pattern of coping for the person and family or (b) a process that the person and family carry out in response to a specific stressful experience (Cohen & Lazarus, 1979; Holahan et al., 1996). Inherently, one influences the other. Coping outcomes are based on individual experiences and coping traits, and coping is a process that changes over time (Nail, 2001), dependent on the challenges faced. Coping can be conceptualized within a framework of adaptation—a positive, adaptive resource of all human beings (Rowland, 1989a). When faced with stressful experiences, an individual and family evaluate the stressors as challenges to be mastered to bring about adaptation and equilibrium.

## Coping and Adaptation

Defining coping within an adaptational framework challenges healthcare professionals to identify and promote effective coping strategies that strengthen physical and psychosocial adaptation (Rowland, 1989a). In the 1970s, White (1974) described mastery as the successful conclusion of adaptive efforts. Mastery becomes a major goal when coping is conceptualized as a positive, conscious attempt toward resolution and adaptation (Pearlin & Schooler, 1978). Adapting to a cancer diagnosis has been known to present greater challenges than other life-threatening and debilitating diseases because of the negative connotations that society has placed on the illness. Cancer is thought of as a synonym for death—the catastrophic "big C" (Nail, 2001; Neilson-Clayton & Brownlee, 2002). Therefore, applying stress and coping theories to the experience of cancer often is limited and daunting. Nail (2001) warned that clinical application based on coping research is challenging because of the diversity and complexity of conceptual coping models, assumptions underlying coping research, and a lack of clear implications for evidence-based interventions. Lewis (2004) concurred in a review of family-focused oncology nursing research. As an example, coping behaviors that underlie stress and adaptation theory have not always proved to be predictive of how the family actually responds and adjusts to the experience of breast cancer (Lewis, 2004). Conceptual theories provide a framework for the assessment of coping with cancer, yet one must proceed with caution.

For oncology nurses, it is imperative to understand how coping has been defined within the broader realm of human experience, to recognize the limitations of research and application, and then to evaluate the patient's and family's coping efficacy based on outcomes rather than adherence to a specific set of coping theories or strategies (Nail, 2001). For many patients, the experience of cancer is a crisis with such demands that their past coping repertoire is not sufficient to support them. It is no longer sufficient to assess patients' past coping mechanisms or coping habits and expect this pattern to fit the new and often threatening challenges they face. Patients facing cancer often have to problem solve in an entirely new context (Jacobsen et al., 2014). Personality-based traits must be evaluated yet reinforced with social and psychological resources that fit the situation or crisis. This demands not only an assessment of the contextual component of coping but also application of a developmental approach to evaluate effective responses.

In the past, many authors (Holland, 1989; Mages & Mendelsohn, 1979; Rait, 2015; Sales, 1991; Sales, Schulz, & Biegel, 1992) have conceptualized coping as a developmental process in which individuals and families respond to the different demands and tasks inherent in the various stages of cancer. Yet, the experience of living with and surviving cancer may not fit into clearly defined transition points, such as diagnosis, treatment, recurrence, and palliation (Lethborg, Kissane, Burns, & Snyder, 2000). Cessation of active cancer treatment brings forth its own set of stressors, such as the fear of recurrence (Butow, Fardell, & Smith, 2015; Lethborg et al., 2000), and coping responses in the prediagnosis phase is an area that has not been investigated (Nail, 2001). The important issue concerns the "pattern of distress" over the course of the cancer trajectory (Spencer et al., 1998). Disease-related variables, such as the type of cancer, treatment requirements, and prognosis, also are important determinants to how individuals and families cope. If coping is a process that changes over time, then coping effectiveness will vary depending on the different clinical stages of cancer and the different illness-related demands. For example, denial and avoidant coping may be effective during the early stages of cancer to temper the threat and prevent the individual from becoming overwhelmed with anxiety. Avoidant coping may represent unconscious patterns that the patient uses to protect the self from full awareness of a challenging or conflicted situation (Arnold, 2016). This coping strategy is less effective or maladaptive if prolonged into later stages of the disease continuum because the avoidant behavior delays action and compromises trust (Arnold, 2016; Somerfield & Curbow, 1992; Spencer et al., 1998).

For many, the experience of cancer may be a crisis added to another life-changing event (e.g., a comorbid illness, the recent death of a family member). Because of an accumulation of stressors combined with a depleted level of psychosocial coping resources, these additional circumstances may overwhelm the patient and family. In contrast, success in coping effectively with previous life stressors likely may influence adaptation and subsequent coping with the next stressful life event (Spencer et al., 1998; Wynn, 2015). The chronicity of cancer leaves patients and families at risk for long-term depletion of emotional, social, and financial resources. Family-focused research has indicated that family relationships may worsen with long-term survival. Without appropriate interventions, family members may wear out over time or become "stuck" (Kornblith, 1998; Lewis, 2004, 2010). Some individuals have described the cancer experience as one that has added meaning and perspective to their lives (Stanton, 2015; Tallman, 2013; Taylor, 1995). Others may view the journey as a challenging but positive life-changing event (Schnoll, Knowles, & Harlow, 2002; Stanton, 2015; Tallman, 2013).

Being aware of the dispositional, contextual, and developmental mechanisms underlying coping strategies prevents professionals from defining effective or adaptive coping for patients. Instead, a knowledge base about coping variables assists professionals in helping patients to identify their own coping strengths and weaknesses and to identify and provide appropriate resources (Nail, 2001). Oncology nurses are in a pivotal position to assess, intervene, and help strengthen coping mechanisms and, if necessary, refer patients for psychological counseling. A major goal when intervening is to promote adaptation by ensuring that patients and families move along the cancer continuum with the education, compassion, and support needed to secure or reinforce their own coping abilities. Thus, by helping patients to gain mastery over the challenges of the cancer experience, nurses can be instrumental in guiding patients to create strategies that can promote effective coping and bring adaptation to chronic illness.

# Conceptual Framework for Coping Assessment

## Coping Strategies

A classic and commonly cited model for coping is the stress-coping framework (Lazarus, 2000; Lazarus & Folkman, 1984). This model presents coping as a dynamic process of appraisal and response that changes over time as individuals interact and confront stressors in their environment (Arnold, 2016; Somerfield & Curbow, 1992). The underlying principle of the Lazarus-Folkman model is that an individual's emotional or behavioral responses to stress are determined by how the person evaluates or appraises the stressor (Arnold, 2016; Hoffman et al., 2013; Maes et al., 1996). Lazarus (1982) asserted that people apply cognitive activities (e.g., evaluative perceptions, inferences) to interpret stressful experiences and that these evaluations guide their adaptational interchange with the environment. Within this framework, three major functions of coping have been identified: appraisal-focused coping, problem-focused or instrumental coping, and emotion-focused or palliative coping (Arnold, 2016; Hoffman et al., 2013; Maes et al., 1996; Rowland, 1989a). After appraisal of the stressor, coping is categorized as either problem focused or emotion focused. Problem-focused coping targets modifying and solving the problem at hand (e.g., seeking advice), whereas emotion-focused coping deals with managing the emotional distress associated with the problem (e.g., seeking emotional support) (Cho, Park, & Blank, 2013). Additionally, researchers have recognized avoidance-focused coping as a function of withdrawing from a threat (Arnold, 2016; Spencer et al., 1998). Positive emotions result if the person appraises the stressor as a challenge; negative emotions occur if the stressor is appraised as threatening (Maes et al., 1996). Most often, the person confronting cancer experiences a roller coaster of positive and negative emotions depending on the circumstances (Wilkes et al., 2003). People with cancer often appraise situations as both threatening (potential for harm) and challenging (potential for mastery) at the same time (Nail, 2001). Therefore, a combination of coping strategies that are individualized and driven by the patient's appraisal of the stressors often is the most effective method. Appraisal of the stressors from cancer may also contribute to what has been termed *anticipated post-traumatic growth*, possibly another coping process when confronting life-threatening illness (Tallman, 2013).

**Appraisal-focused coping:** The appraisal or evaluation of a stressful event is a major determinant of coping responses. Lazarus and Folkman (1984) identified two types of appraisal processes: primary appraisal and secondary appraisal. Primary appraisal addresses the personal meaning of the stressful event and whether the threat is interpreted as negative or challenging. Primary appraisal is shaped by the person's belief system, values, and life goals (Folkman, 2013). Most often, illnesses such as cancer are appraised as stressful and threatening; the threats of harm and loss, such as loss in self-esteem, role function, and independence, are anticipatory fears of most patients confronting cancer (Barry, 2002a). Cancer affects every aspect of the individual's life: physical, psychological, interpersonal, vocational, and spiritual (Aziz, 2007; Hoffman et al., 2013). The ultimate threat is the fear of dying, especially in pain (Nail, 2001). "Cognitive appraisal of one's cancer has been related to anxiety and adjustment in that the higher the perceived threat, the lower level of well-being and the greater level of distress" (Hoffman et al., 2013, p. 247). Secondary appraisal incorporates the person's evaluation of their capability to reduce the threat or damage caused by the stressor. Secondary appraisal is the person's evaluation of their options for coping (Folkman, 2013). These options are determined by the situation and other factors, including the person's physical, psychological, material, and spiritual resources for coping (Folkman, 2013). A common question is, "What can I do about it?" (Barry, 2002a). For the patient with cancer, the question is often, "How can I take control of the situation?" (Wilkes et al., 2003). The individual's past experiences (e.g., with cancer) and personality (e.g., coping style) will influence how he or she will appraise the stressor. The appraisal of stress, and the subsequent need for coping strategies, may also be influenced by age, with older patients potentially appraising the stressor of cancer differently than younger patients (Hoffman et al., 2013; Lifford et al., 2015). The diagnosis of cancer at a younger age has been attributed to negative psychosocial adjustment and ongoing distress (Hoffman et al., 2013). Other personality variables, such as self-efficacy, influence the appraisal process. The role of self-efficacy, individuals' confidence in their ability to carry out appropriate behaviors and skills, has been shown not only to influence the appraisal of a stressor but also to improve coping skills (Baider & Balducci, 2011; Devins & Binik, 1996).

**Problem-focused coping:** Once the stressful situation is appraised, the patient directs problem-focused coping at the external event (e.g., cancer, chemotherapy). To problem solve, the person attempts to change the stressful situation by changing either their actions or the environment (Arnold, 2016; Maes et al., 1996). Problem-focused coping is action oriented, and the goal is to solve the problem or resolve the stressor at hand (Hoffman et al., 2013). Problem-focused coping is viewed as the most effective coping mechanism (Nezu, Nezu, & Salber, 2015). Two methods of problem-focused coping are information seeking and direct action. Information seeking serves as a basis for action (e.g., problem solving) by providing the knowledge necessary for a coping decision or for reappraisal of the threat. A cancer diagnosis is extremely threatening, but if the individual gains knowledge regarding the actual stage, treatment, and prognosis of the cancer, this information can be applied to the person's emotional reactions (e.g., dispelling the myths and fears with concrete information). Patients and families differ in the timing, type, and amount of information needed to support their coping efforts. Problem-focused coping often begins with seeking an accurate diagnosis, gathering information, seeking second opinions, and making treatment decisions. All of these behaviors correlate with emotional well-being in the early stages of cancer (Hoffman et al., 2013). Research has found that different informational coping styles exist (Nikoletti, Kristjanson, Tataryn, McPhee, & Burt, 2003). For example, much of the information imparted to patients at diagnosis is standard, disease-related content, is impersonal, and is given at a time when patients and families feel overwhelmed with anxiety and fear (Delbar & Benor, 2001). Information supports effective problem solving when it is tailored to the individual patient and family based upon their history, life experiences, emotional needs, education, and culture (Delbar & Benor, 2001; Grassi, Nanni, Donovan, & Jacobsen, 2015; Nail, 2001; Nikoletti et al., 2003). Disparity between the amount of information given and the individual's coping style can lead to increased distress (Nikoletti et al., 2003).

*Direct action* includes any actions the person carries out, excluding cognitive means, to minimize the threat or danger of the stressor. The patient experiencing a breast lump may take direct action by obtaining a mammogram and following through with a breast biopsy. Taking direct action to confront the stressor gives patients confidence in their ability to control the situation, based on knowing "what to expect" and "what to do if" (Delbar & Benor, 2001). Inherent in problem-solving coping is patients' and families' need to feel empowered and in control of the challenge at hand. Patients' taking control has been linked to having a positive attitude when fighting cancer (Wilkes et al., 2003). Understanding the concept of control is essential to support coping, but the individual's feeling of control will be personal and situational (Nail, 2001). For example, a patient who has a trusting relationship with their physician may seek the physician's advice and allow the physician to make the treatment decision while the patient still maintains a sense of control (Nail, 2001). Overall, patients and families have reported that learning to control symptoms, reduce pain and discomfort, and improve quality of life creates a sense of control that enables them to believe in their ability to cope (Delbar & Benor, 2001; Redinbaugh, Baum, Tarbell, & Arnold, 2003). Supporting problem-focused strategies can help patients and families to feel in control and prevent them from feeling helpless or powerless, but resources must be made available to supplement their coping abilities. Perceived control may become challenged by the ongoing side effects from treatment, setbacks, and recurrences that can occur along the cancer continuum (Hoffman et al., 2013) (see Chapter 21 for information on powerlessness).

**Emotion-focused coping:** Maintaining emotional equilibrium is another function of coping. Emotion-focused coping relies on *intrapsychic processes*, the varied cognitive processes that influence emotional responses (e.g., feelings, concerns, worries regarding the cancer) (Maes et al., 1996). To regulate emotional distress, the person attempts to manage the subjective and somatic components of stress-related emotions. In contrast to problem-focused and active coping, emotion-focused coping is viewed as passive or palliative coping. This does not imply that emotion-focused coping is negative or maladaptive. Emotional expression, such as crying, is a palliative coping measure that appropriately can serve the goal of regaining emotional balance. Expressing feelings, such as anger and fear, is important for healing, and studies have found diversions such as humor to be positive coping tactics (Jacobsen et al., 2014; Johnson, 2002; Lethborg et al., 2000; Spencer et al., 1998). Recent research has delineated two types of emotion-focused coping under the umbrella of emotional approach coping: emotional processing and emotional expression. Emotional processing is helpful in promoting positive adjustments in women with cancer, and emotional expression is helpful in reducing negative adjustments in men (Cho et al., 2013). Emotion-focused coping also encompasses defense mechanisms, such as denial, that a person may apply to seek emotional insulation from a threat. Nurses may mistakenly diagnose denial as unhealthy coping (Jacobsen et al., 2014). A newly diagnosed patient with cancer can become overwhelmed with fear and anxiety. Denial early in the cancer experience is a common protective mechanism that allows the patient time to integrate emotionally to what is happening. This defense can be adaptive in the short run, but avoidance coping must be evaluated based on the situation. For example, if a patient with cancer states that he or she is avoiding thinking about the disease in order to move forward, the nurse must determine whether this is denial or avoidant coping (Spencer et al., 1998). In palliative care, the patient may state, "I believe in miracles." By understanding that these types of statements often do not reflect a dense denial but rather serve as an effective coping strategy that defends against a painful reality, the nurse can better support the patient (Jacobsen et al., 2014) (see Chapter 16 for information on denial and coping).

**Avoidance-focused coping:** Researchers have identified this method of coping as the person's attempt to disengage mentally or even physically from a threatening situation (Kohn, 1996; Spencer et al., 1998). Avoidance coping is the inhibition of action that may hamper coping effectiveness. Cognitive and behavioral escape–avoidance has been associated with more emotional distress (Cho et al., 2013). The fear of cancer or fearing "the worst" may cause an individual to delay seeking medical advice. For patients with cancer, prolonging a diagnosis or refusing necessary treatment out of fear are inherently risky behaviors. Lack of communication about sensitive topics (e.g., feelings related to having cancer, sexuality concerns, fears about disease progression and death) has been found to be a type of disengagement avoidance among couples that contributes to anxiety, depression, and stress in the partner with cancer (Yu & Sherman, 2015). Hopman and Rijken (2015) found when investigating the effect of illness characteristics and coping, more passive coping was applied by patients with cancer who perceived their illness as long-lasting, more emotionally burdensome, and having more negative consequences on their life. Conceptually, avoidance-focused coping and denial are difficult to apply across gender, age, and cultural populations; the function these behaviors serve must be evaluated on an individual basis and within the context of each individual situation.

**Post-traumatic growth:** Researchers have recently begun to investigate positive growth or benefits that result from the cancer experience (Tallman, 2013). Post-traumatic growth has been defined as "a positive psychological change resulting from a traumatic life event" (Tallman, 2013, p. 72). Cordova (2008) outlined characteristics that affected the individual's positive growth after the cancer experience.

First, because of the fear of recurrent disease, patients with cancer may begin to evaluate their lives differently, questioning and changing their priorities. Second, because of the need to adapt to the physical and psychological ramifications that a diagnosis of cancer brings, patients find themselves developing a "new normal" regarding everyday life. Third, patients with cancer often are required to become more dependent on others for both tangible and emotional support, causing them to reevaluate their relationships. Lastly, cancer brings forth an existential crisis, demanding that individuals confront their mortality. This crisis often brings about introspection regarding one's religious and spiritual beliefs and how one views the world (Cordova, 2008; Stanton, 2015; Tallman, 2013). The theory of stress and coping (Lazarus & Folkman, 1984) plays a role in the conceptualization of post-traumatic growth, as theories of growth after cancer incorporate coping or coping style (Tallman, 2013).

## Summary

Research has shown that problem-focused coping strategies, such as changing one's lifestyle (e.g., smoking cessation) in response to the diagnosis, facilitate adaptation among patients with cancer and survivors alike (Nezu et al., 2015; Schnoll et al., 2002). Patients most often employ problem-focused coping in response to stressful experiences that are perceived as changeable (Kohn, 1996; Rowland, 1989a). The other two methods of coping, appraisal and emotion focused, commonly are implemented in situations appraised as uncontrollable, as often is the case when confronted with cancer (Rowland, 1989a). Although the diagnosis of cancer is not changeable, the inherent challenges can be modified, controlled, and met with courage and perseverance (Nezu et al., 2015). Cancer demands the reordering of one's priorities and the revision of one's goals, often contributing to reappraisal of the event as an opportunity for growth rather than only as a loss (Nolen-Hoeksema, 2000; Stanton, 2015; Tallman, 2013).

## Coping as a Process

Coping is not a static event; it is an ever-changing and expanding process that develops and changes over time (Folkman, 2013). When dealing with a stressful, life-threatening illness such as cancer, flexibility in coping will promote adaptation at different transition points during the illness (Cohen & Lazarus, 1979; Nail, 2001). Coping may be best conceptualized as a process of "two steps forward, one step back" (Murphy, 1974), or one that is influenced by constantly changing variables. "Coping is not a single act but rather a constellation of many acts and thoughts, triggered by a complex set of demands that change with time" (Cohen & Lazarus, 1979, p. 225). Coping must be assessed within the reality of the illness and, most importantly, by accepting the reality of the person undergoing the experience (Mages & Mendelsohn, 1979; Nail, 2001). Furthermore, assessment must recognize the interpersonal relationships supporting the patient (e.g., family, social support). Understanding the many variables that follow and how they influence coping responses is vital for accurate assessment and to plan interventions based on the individual coping needs of the patient and family.

### Nature of the Illness

Included in the contextual and personality-based dimensions that influence coping, researchers have identified specific variables that are important determinants of how one may cope with a stressful situation (see Figure 4-1). When discussing coping with cancer,

- Nature of the illness
- Phases of illness
- Personality dimensions
- Coping styles
- Cultural, socioeconomic, and gender dimensions
- Developmental life stage
- Social networks and support
- Family coping
- Personal meaning, spirituality, and hope
- Specific coping challenges

**Figure 4-1. Variables That Influence Coping**

Rowland (1989a) stated that the primary influence on coping is the nature of the stress. When evaluating how the individual is coping with a cancer diagnosis, determining the site, stage, and type of cancer; the course of treatment; and the prognosis is of the utmost importance. Research highlights the fact that the optimal nature of coping efficacy and its associated skills may depend on the type of cancer and its treatment (Hoffman et al., 2013). A woman diagnosed with stage I breast cancer will have a different coping response than a woman diagnosed with stage III disease that requires chemotherapy and radiation. The general stressor—confronting cancer—is the same, but the realities and the threat of each specific case will be entirely different. Disease and treatment variables, such as chemotherapy side effects, have been shown to change an individual's perception and experience of the illness (Lethborg et al., 2000; Maes et al., 1996). The stressful array of physical symptoms (e.g., alopecia, total body hair loss) have been reported to cause psychological trauma (Lethborg et al., 2000). Table 4-1 outlines the side effects of cancer and treatment that influence coping.

Studies have reported numerous objective stressors that affect patients and families when attempting to cope with cancer. These include disease prognosis (Howell, Fitch, & Deane, 2003), caregiving demands, the duration of the illness, and the patient's distress (Borneman

**Table 4-1. Treatment-Related Variables Influencing Coping**

| Treatment | Stressor | Coping Challenge |
|---|---|---|
| Surgery | Preoperative anxiety and fear<br>Loss of body part<br>Loss of body function | Integrate the functional and cosmetic deficits of surgery into body image, self-esteem, and sexuality. |
| Chemotherapy | Systemic side effects: nausea and vomiting, diarrhea, stomatitis, alopecia, and fatigue<br>Length of treatment | Continue with role function and family/job responsibilities while undergoing treatment.<br>Integrate changes in body image. |
| Radiation | Skin markings (tattooing)<br>Site-specific side effects: nausea and vomiting, diarrhea, stomatitis, alopecia, and fatigue<br>Length of treatment | Cope with visual signs of cancer.<br>Continue with role function and family/job responsibilities while undergoing treatment. |
| Biotherapy/hormone therapy | Side effects: fever, fatigue, malaise, and muscle/joint tenderness<br>Neurologic effects: mood disturbances and changes in cognition | Incorporate rest periods into daily routine.<br>Continue with role function and family/job responsibilities while undergoing treatment.<br>Cope with mood changes, fatigue, and cognitive effects. |

et al., 2003; Given, Given, & Kozachik, 2001; Haley, 2003; Redinbaugh et al., 2003; Sales et al., 1992). Research indicates that caregiver strain correlates with helping patients with self-care and physical needs and with managing their treatments and symptoms. Also, the longer the duration of the illness, the more evidence of distress. When the continuum of cancer extends over long periods of time, personal and social resources needed to cope effectively may be depleted (Lewis, 2004; Rowland, 1989a).

## Phases of Illness

Different stages or phases of the cancer continuum will present specific coping challenges (Hoffman et al., 2013). These phases most often are categorized as diagnostic, treatment, remission, recurrence, and terminal. Anxiety and worry are common emotional responses during the diagnostic phase of cancer. Weisman and Worden (1976–1977) noted the first 100 days after diagnosis as the "existential plight in cancer." Fear may give way to shock, numbness, and denial when a cancer is confirmed (Cloutier & Ferrall, 1996). A multitude of emotions may follow—sadness, anger, depression, and personal grief—but gradually, reality must be incorporated into the person's psyche (Fawzy, Fawzy, Hyun, & Wheeler, 1997). The treatment phase will bring a variety of emotional reactions, and the management of treatment side effects becomes a major coping challenge. Surgery can generate fear related to changes in body image or loss of bodily functions. Chemotherapy and radiation may cause anticipatory fear resulting from a lack of knowledge about the treatment (e.g., it is common for patients to fear that external radiation may cause them to be radioactive). Common side effects of treatment (e.g., relentless fatigue, nausea and vomiting, alopecia, the disruption of normal lifestyle) leave the patient vulnerable to feelings of anxiety and depression.

When treatment ends, patients may enter the remission phase with uncertainty. Feelings of fear and ambivalence regarding the future may surface at this time. The patient may feel a loss of control over the cancer when active treatment has ended and may feel that nothing is being done to keep the cancer at bay. The literature has described this transition point as being "cast adrift" (Lethborg et al., 2000). Fears of recurrence threaten cancer survivors, especially patients who have been treated for more advanced disease (Butow et al., 2015; Kornblith, 1998). If the fear becomes reality, the recurrence phase of cancer is especially difficult for patients and families. At this stage, the initial hope for cure is gone. Many of the feelings—shock, disbelief, anxiety, anger, and depression—are similar to those experienced in the diagnostic phase but usually are more intense (Borneman et al., 2003; Fawzy et al., 1997). Women experiencing recurrent ovarian cancer have reported a sense of desperation and difficulties coping with the side effects of progressive disease (Howell et al., 2003).

Even if the recurrence is limited and asymptomatic, the patient's hope, confidence, and future plans are shaken (Weisman & Worden, 1986). The coping challenge in the advanced or terminal phase is the evident progression of disease and the inevitable awareness of mortality (Borneman et al., 2003). "Helping patients calibrate their hopes and develop an accurate awareness of prognosis should be, when the disease allows, a gentle process" (Jacobsen et al., 2014, p. 464). As the cancer progresses, issues surrounding intimacy and dependency may cause patients to feel helpless (Cloutier & Ferrall, 1996). Hope shifts from cure to a hope for relief from suffering (Borneman et al., 2003). Fears of abandonment, pain, and loss of dignity are common in the terminal phase of cancer (Fawzy et al., 1997).

Hoffman et al. (2013) noted that some of the variation in psychological symptoms over time may be due, in part, to premorbid vulnerabilities, such as mood disorders, or other factors, such as age, level of personal resources (e.g., optimism, perceived control), and social support. In regard to the effect of cancer on the patient's family, Rait (2015) condensed the course of cancer into three broad stages: acute, chronic, and resolution. Many of the same emotional responses experienced by the patient will be shared by the family. These stages of illness define the issues that the patient and the family will face; therefore, it helps to anticipate points of psychological distress (Rait, 2015). These transition points include treatment, end of treatment, remission, and recurrent disease.

## Personality Dimensions

The personal meanings of illness and cancer will be incorporated into the person's appraisal of the diagnosis. Past experiences with cancer, a prior psychiatric history, and other individual variables, such as values, beliefs, and religious preferences, will affect coping responses (Rowland, 1989a; Spencer et al., 1998). The individual may perceive the cancer diagnosis as punishment for wrongdoing or as a sign of weakness and failure. Some people confront cancer with a fighting spirit, interpreting the disease as the "enemy" and the treatment as the "battlefield" (Rowland, 1989a). Fighting spirit has been reported to positively influence adaptation in patients with cancer (Spencer et al., 1998). Intrinsic to these perceptual differences are the person's basic personality structure and life experiences (Wynn, 2015).

One's personality includes the emotional or internal resources and cognitive characteristics that influence the appraisal and coping processes. Certain personality traits will affect how people appraise life events, how they perceive their coping efficacy, and how they manage coping strategies (Hoffman et al., 2013). Examples of such traits that may influence psychological adjustment to cancer include the individual's proneness to anxiety and depression, locus of control, optimism, hardiness, and ego strength. It has been reported that individuals who have a prior history of significant anxiety or depression are at the highest risk for emotional instability when confronting cancer (Pasacreta, Minarik, & Nield-Anderson, 2001; Pasacreta, Minarik, Nield-Anderson, & Paice, 2015). If a person has trait anxiety, he or she is predisposed to more frequent and intense reactions to stressful events (Levin & Alici, 2010), and the normal anxieties experienced with cancer (e.g., apprehension, tension, nervousness, worry) may become exacerbated.

Along with anxiety, depression has been described as one of the most common psychosocial responses to the cancer experience. Depression is a normal response to perceived loss. When assessing the losses incurred by cancer, an adjustment disorder with depressed mood is not an uncommon finding. This diagnosis must be differentiated from a predisposition to depression or a past history of depressive episodes that may be intensified by the illness. Depressed individuals are more likely to use emotional and avoidance-style coping strategies (Zeidner & Saklofske, 1996). Therefore, individuals with a history of anxiety and depression may be at a greater risk for appraising the stressor of cancer as more threatening and overwhelming than individuals without such a history (see Chapters 14 and 17 for more information on anxiety and depression).

Locus of control is a personality construct that has been applied to evaluating health outcomes. Internal locus of control has been defined as the belief that people have internal control or responsibility for their perception of life events and their reactions to them (Fernsler & Miller, 2000). When confronted with ambiguous or overwhelming situations, the individual with an internal locus of control is more likely to appraise the situation as challenging and controllable (Barsevick, Much, & Sweeney, 2000). Patients experiencing cancer who have an internal locus of control may be more likely to be active participants in their care plan and use problem-focused coping. External locus of control is the individual's belief that life events and consequences are beyond personal control or are external to the individual (Fernsler & Miller, 2000). This trait in patients with cancer may cause them to displace blame for the onset of illness and displace responsibility for the success of treatment. The characteristic of internal–external locus of control can be compared to the construct of control versus helplessness/hopelessness, and hopelessness is a major determinant for ineffective coping (Barry, 2002b).

Another innate trait reported to influence coping is optimism (Aspinwall & Brunhart, 2000; Hoffman et al., 2013; Nail, 2001; Schnoll et al., 2002). *Optimism* refers to a person's generalized confidence and positive expectations of the future. Optimistic patients are more likely to cope in active, problem-focused ways, whereas pessimistic patients are more likely to apply passive or avoidant forms of coping (Aspinwall & Brunhart, 2000; Maes et al., 1996). Past research has pointed to a relationship between optimism and a fighting spirit and positive outcomes of coping (Parle & Maguire, 1995; Spencer et al., 1998). Most recent research has found higher levels of optimism to be associated not only with lower levels of avoidant coping but also with overall improvement in mental and physical health, higher levels of social support, and emotional well-being (Hoffman et al., 2013; Schnoll et al., 2002). Another personality characteristic, described as good ego strength (Rowland, 1989a), may buffer the effects of stressful life events and contribute positively to an individual's psychological hardiness or resilience to stress. Resiliency is a relatively new concept that addresses the ability to withstand and rebound from crises and adversity (Arnold & Boggs, 2016; Nolen-Hoeksema, 2000). Resilience encompasses the use of effective coping styles (e.g., problem focused, emotion focused) and how one remains relatively stable and functional despite enduring stress (Arnold & Boggs, 2016). In the area of developmental psychology, resilient children have been observed to be flexible in adapting their coping styles to specific situations and evaluating the effectiveness of their coping efforts (Hawley & DeHaan, 1996). These same characteristics of resiliency can apply to adults. Ego strength is a resiliency trait that has been defined as an intrapsychic and unconscious response. It involves the use of defense mechanisms that the ego engages to master the stress being confronted (Barry, 2002b). If coping fails, self-control and ego strength give way to defenses such as displacement, heightened alertness, anxiety, panic attacks, and loss of control (Barry, 2002b). Rowland (1989a) pointed out that characteristics used to describe emotionally healthy individuals, or people with strong egos, are most likely the same personality traits that accompany the use of effective coping strategies and a more positive adaptation to illness. Researchers have described resiliency in families as consisting of action-oriented behaviors aimed to reduce stress, obtain resources, and manage tension within the family system when confronting stress and crises (Friedman et al., 2003; McCubbin & McCubbin, 1996). Current thinking in the field of family therapy is to focus on the resilience of family in the face of cancer, not on deficit and pathology (Zaider & Kissane, 2010). Resilient families accept whatever the level of threat, thus developing confidence in their ability to respond (Zaider & Kissane, 2010).

## Coping Styles

Certain personality characteristics, such as optimism and anxiety, have been found to contribute to habitual ways or styles of coping (see Figure 4-2). Research supports that avoidant and passive styles of coping, such as helplessness/hopelessness, correlate with poor disease outcomes (Aspinwall & Brunhart, 2000; Watson & Greer, 1998). Problem-solving coping, which includes characteristics such as having a fighting spirit, has been correlated with positive disease outcomes (Cho et al., 2013; Watson & Greer, 1998). Studies have demonstrated that an optimistic personality is associated with good health related to the optimists' more active coping efforts and lower levels of avoidant coping (Aspinwall & Brunhart, 2000).

**Fighting spirit**—An active problem-solving coping style. Patient accepts the disease, is determined to fight, and actively takes part in treatment decisions. This style is associated with optimism.

**Approach coping**—Problem-focused and emotion-focused coping strategies (e.g., seeking social support) that focus on reducing the stressor at hand. Related to better self-esteem and positive effect.

**Avoidance (denial)**—An avoidance-style of coping in which the patient refuses to accept the diagnosis, denies the seriousness of the illness, or avoids thinking about it. This style involves disengagement and cognitive avoidance and is related to worse psychological and physical functioning.

**Fatalism (stoic acceptance)**—A passive style of coping in which the patient accepts the diagnosis and becomes resigned and fatalistic in attitude.

**Anxious preoccupation**—An emotion-focused style of coping in which the patient anxiously worries about the cancer and is preoccupied with fears that any physical ailment is the return of the disease. The patient requires constant reassurance. This style may be associated with preexisting anxiety.

**Hopelessness/helplessness**—An emotion-focused coping style in which the patient feels overwhelmed and is engulfed by the illness and feels like giving up. This style is associated with pessimism.

**Figure 4-2. Coping Styles**

*Note.* Based on information from Benedict & Penedo, 2013; Watson & Greer, 1998.

## Cultural, Socioeconomic, and Gender Dimensions

A person's culture has been described as the lens through which he or she perceives the world (Barsevick et al., 2000). Cultural beliefs play a complex role in the stress-coping response (Helman, 2001). Different cultural groups exposed to similar stressors will appraise the situation through their worldview (Helman, 2001), although cancer is one of the most feared diseases in every culture (Die-Trill, 1998). Culturally ascribed norms will influence the behaviors associated with coping (e.g., health-seeking behaviors) and the resources used for social support (e.g., family, community) (Barsevick et al., 2000). Culture also may influence the psychological response to a cancer diagnosis, presence or absence of psychopathology (e.g., anxiety or depression), awareness and knowledge of treatment options, and acceptance of psychological interventions (Grassi et al., 2015). Current research has demonstrated differences in cancer-related concerns across different cultural groups (Grassi et al., 2015). Past research supports that both African American and Caucasian women seek social support as a coping strategy, yet the sources of support differ between the two groups (Bourjolly & Hirschman, 2001; Henderson et al., 2003). African American women reported that God, prayer, and spirituality are their main sources of emotional support, while Caucasian women reported relying more on their spouses, children, and friends (Bourjolly & Hirschman, 2001; Henderson et al., 2003). In a qualitative study of breast cancer across different ethnic groups (African Americans, Asians, Latinos, and Caucasians), differences related to psychosocial issues were found and included choices of treatment, language barriers, worries about children and family burden, spiritual beliefs, and coping (Ashing-Giwa et al., 2004).

To provide culturally competent care, nurses must recognize the differences that exist when the experience of coping with cancer is framed within the cultural belief system of the individual. As with patients, family attitudes also are shaped by the cultural beliefs about the specific illness. Beliefs about cancer causation, communication and language barriers, truth-telling practices, and family roles in cancer care will differ across culturally diverse populations (Die-Trill, 1998; Grassi et al., 2015). To provide culturally sensitive patient care, continued oncology nursing research is needed to address healthcare behaviors and disparities in cultural groups (Cope, 2015).

Socioeconomic status is linked closely to the cultural dimensions of coping. Minority populations have fewer financial and educational resources, and these factors will influence the appraisal and coping strategies employed by patients with fewer socioeconomic means (Barsevick et al., 2000; Fernandes-Taylor & Bloom, 2015). Factors that negatively influence coping responses include limited access to care, lack of education, unemployment, and limited insurance. Socioeconomic status and level of education may be predictors of the type of support available to minority populations (Bourjolly & Hirschman, 2001). Despite overall cancer outcomes improving in the past two decades, patients with lower socioeconomic status have not improved as quickly as those with higher socioeconomic status (Fernandes-Taylor & Bloom, 2015). As for the influence of education on coping, individuals with more education are better equipped to navigate the bureaucracies of health care and are more likely to have better information processing and literacy skills, greater health-related knowledge, and better relationships with healthcare providers (Fernandes-Taylor & Bloom, 2015). Economic resources (e.g., wealth) lead to better health via access to health-promoting venues: nutrition, housing, and healthcare materials (Fernandes-Taylor & Bloom, 2015). Low-income carries the risk of chronic stressors (e.g., unemployment, finances), exposure to carcinogens in the home and workplace, and fewer social supports, adversely affecting health (Fernandes-Taylor & Bloom, 2015). Therefore, demographic and clinical variables shown to support coping have included higher income and level of education and a positive perception of one's health (Schnoll et al., 2002). Low socioeconomic status is predictive of avoidance-style coping, which may result in higher levels of emotional distress (Spencer et al., 1998). Therefore, healthcare providers must aim interventions to support coping at the socioeconomic limitations faced by many minority groups, such as providing bus tokens or cab vouchers for transportation to treatment and free, culturally sensitive educational programs and support groups (Bourjolly & Hirschman, 2001).

Limitations in research and practice present additional barriers to appreciating the coping process across different disease sites and different genders. The majority of research has focused on women's adaptation to breast cancer, leaving a dearth of information necessary to understand coping strategies for other malignancies, and even less is known about adaptation for male patients (Cho et al., 2013; McGovern, Heyman, & Resnick, 2002; Spencer et al., 1998). Men may be at higher risk for poor adjustment to cancer. For example, research on coping has revealed that men tend to use more withdrawal behaviors, such as avoiding feelings, not reaching out for social support, and attempting to hide the level of stress they are facing from others (Friedman et al., 2003). Men may be more unwilling to attend support groups (McGovern et al., 2002). In a study regarding coping with incontinence after prostate surgery, only a minority of the men studied were able to explicitly describe the emotional effects of incontinence (e.g., depression) in comparison to the participants' ability to address the physical and practical problems they encountered (Palmer, Fogarty, Somerfield, & Powel, 2003). Further research is needed to elucidate not only gender differences in adjustment and coping but also gender differences related to specific malignancies and treatments (Cho et al., 2013; Kornblith, 1998).

It should be noted that little research has been conducted to address sexual and gender minorities, such as the lesbian, gay, bisexual, and transgender population (Kim, Loscalzo, & Clark, 2015).

## Developmental Life Stage

Cancer can strike at any point in an individual's life cycle. Erikson (1963) described psychosocial development and the inherent tasks or challenges that the person must resolve at each stage of emotional growth. Disruption of these tasks will affect the ability to cope (Rowland, 1989a). Although the prescribed ages within Erikson's theoretical framework must be adapted to current societal norms, the identified stages and tasks are still pertinent (Barry, 2002b). For example, the task for puberty and adolescence is defined as "ego identity versus role confusion." Ego identity answers the question "Who am I?" A basic conflict of this psychosocial stage is the adolescent's identity formation contrasted with identity confusion. The late adolescent is asserting independence and confronting social demands, and these tasks will be challenged with a cancer diagnosis. Dependency on parents, interruptions of social and role functions because of treatment, and the effects of body-image changes on sexuality are just a few examples of the identity confusion that can result when the adolescent faces cancer. For each psychosocial stage of development, from infancy to late adulthood, cancer can disrupt emotional development and the resolution of life goals. If cancer strikes in child-bearing years, the potential of treatment-induced infertility can create emotional distress and marital problems (Kornblith, 1998). Research has identified that in this aspect and in others (e.g., physical health, finances, employment), young people experiencing cancer reported greater adjustment problems and poorer quality of life than older people with cancer. This age demographic is often described as medically and psychologically vulnerable (Barsevick et al., 2000; Munoz et al., 2016). Cancer is a disease of the aging population, and older adults have special needs that must be met to ensure quality of care (Given & Given, 2015; Wiesel & Alici, 2015). Psychosocial care of older adults must address comorbid illnesses, social and financial resources, family caregiving, and special considerations, such as dementia, delirium, depression, and existential concerns (Wiesel & Alici, 2015).

## Social Networks and Support

Social support is another significant variable believed to be positively associated with coping and adapting to the stress of cancer (Benedict & Penedo, 2013; Blanchard, Albrecht, Ruckdeschel, Grant, & Hemmick, 1995; Hoffman et al., 2013; Schnoll et al., 2002). Social support encompasses family, personal relationships, community, church, and larger social systems (e.g., culture) (Guidry, Aday, Zhang, & Winn, 1997). Social support can buffer the negative impact of cancer and influence the manner in which individuals cope (Benedict & Penedo, 2013; Pierce, Sarason, & Sarason, 1996; Thoits, 1986). It also can assist with coping by helping patients to reappraise the situation as less threatening, by assisting patients in problem solving and making decisions, and by providing direct intervention through physical and emotional support (Rowland, 1989b; Schnoll et al., 2002). Table 4-2 outlines the principal domains of social support. When evaluating social support for patients, it is important to remember that what and how strongly patients perceive their social support are critical factors (Hudek-Knezevic, Kardum, & Pahljina, 2002). For example, a patient may attend a cancer support group but feel it does not meet their personal needs, which is not an uncommon finding for minority populations (Henderson et al., 2003).

Social support has been classified in terms of *structural* and *functional* (Hoffman et al., 2013). Structural support comprises one's social network, social integration, and marital status (Helgeson & McUmber, 2010). Functional support has been defined as the quality of supportive resources, including emotional, instrumental, and informational support (Helgeson & McUmber, 2010; Hoffman et al., 2013). Overall, seeking out social support as a coping strategy is vital to coping with cancer. Schnoll et al. (2002) found that in the four domains of social support (informational, companionship, instrumental, and esteem) assessed by the Interpersonal Support Evaluation List tool, all four correlated strongly with positive adaptation to cancer survivorship—sexual, extended family, social, and psychological adjustment. Therapeutic support in the form of psychoeducational support has

### Table 4-2. Functions and Components of Social Support

| Functions of Support | Components of Support |
| --- | --- |
| Informational/ educational | Provides necessary information, knowledge, and skills for decision making and coping |
| Emotional/ affectional | Interpersonal relationships that provide love, nurturance, acceptance, intimacy, and caring support |
| Tangible/ instrumental | Provides financial assistance, physical goods, or services |
| Affirmational | Provides the sense that one's feelings are accepted and understood |
| Affiliational | Provides a sense of belonging or social identity |
| Appraisal | Provides supportive feedback and validation to the patient |

*Note.* Based on information from Hudek-Knezevic et al., 2002; Rowland, 1989b.

been shown to positively enhance psychological and physical well-being (Edelman, Craig, & Kidman, 2000; Neilson-Clayton & Brownlee, 2002), as well as strenghten the immune system (Fagundes, Lindgren, & Kielcolt-Glaser, 2013; Fawzy & Fawzy, 2011; Fawzy, Fawzy, Arndt, & Pasnau, 1995).

When evaluating the effectiveness of social support, consider intervening variables. First, the dynamics of family functioning and social support will vary across cultural groups. Oncology nurses need to understand and respect the diversity among ethnic populations and be aware that social support will be defined within their cultural perspective (Grassi et al., 2015). For example, in Native American culture, the entire "family" is actively involved with the patient's treatment and recovery. In the Native American community, family is not restricted to blood relatives; therefore, from the Native Americans' perspective, family support comes from interpersonal ties and the "adoption" of extended fathers, mothers, sisters, and cousins (Burhansstipanov & Hollow, 2001). Minority populations may be unaware of support resources available to them. When investigating preferences for psychosocial interventions in a multiethnic population, Gotay and Lau (2003) found that only 10% of patients studied had received information about psychosocial counseling; mental health professionals were not routinely incorporated in the cancer care system for these patients. Notable gaps exist in the literature regarding the benefits of psychosocial interventions for ethnic and racial minorities and how these interventions should be tailored (Benedict & Penedo, 2013) (see Chapter 5 for information on culture).

Lastly, oncology nurses must recognize that different forms of social support are helpful for some patients and not for others, especially when taking into account different family functioning and gender differences in coping. Lewis (2004) pointed out that spouses coping with breast cancer have differing views of what constitutes supportive behavior (e.g., the husband may feel that trying to reassure his wife or cheer her up is the most helpful, whereas the wife may find that these behaviors avoid dealing with her emotions). Diminished social support from family and friends over time has been found to be a distressing hardship of long-term survivors (Kornblith, 1998). After the crises of diagnosis and treatment, many family and friends do not understand the residual physical and psychological effects of cancer and may unknowingly desire for the patient to "return to normal." But as one patient with cancer poignantly expressed, returning to normalcy does not mean returning to the same place or identity (Lethborg et al., 2000). The family's adjustment can positively or negatively support the patient's coping, depending on the level of family functioning.

## Dyadic and Family Coping

Adapting to the strain and ever-changing demands of cancer is as much a task for families as for patients. Although stress and coping have traditionally been examined at the individual level, growing attention is being given to the relational context of coping with cancer, often referred to as *dyadic coping* (Regan et al., 2014, Traa et al., 2015; Zaider & Kissane, 2010). Having a supportive spouse can buffer the stressful impact of cancer, yet the partner's stress often parallels that of the patient and at times has been found to be more intense (Regan et al., 2015). The Systemic–Transactional Model has been used to conceptualize dyadic coping as a reciprocal system based on the couples' shared appraisals of stress and coping (Regan et al., 2014). As stress is communicated from one partner to the other, either a positive or negative dyadic coping response is initiated. Positive responses occur when partners engage in joint emotion or problem-focused coping, whereas negative dyadic coping occurs if a response is ambivalent, hostile, superficial, or lacks emotional warmth or empathy (Regan et al., 2014). Essentially, coping among patient and partner is interdependent and mutually influences their adjustment process (Rottman et al., 2015). The same can be said for other members of the family.

The emotional distress experienced by family members is not just caused by the patient's illness-related stressors but also results from redefined relationships and roles and the increased stress placed on the family system (Given et al., 2001; Lewis, 2004; Neilson-Clayton & Brownlee, 2002; Rait, 2015). In a review of family-focused oncology nursing research, Lewis (2004) outlined pertinent findings that may be contrary to what professionals would expect regarding family adaptation to breast cancer. A major finding was that long-term adjustment to breast cancer negatively affected marital quality, family members' ability to cope, the child's self-esteem, and the quality of the child–parent relationship. Lewis found that the coping behaviors of the family remained stable over time regardless of illness demands. Evidence of family burnout existed when confronted with long-term stressors. Past research of other cancer sites (e.g., head and neck) supports this worsening of family relationships caused by the chronic nature of illness demands (Kornblith, 1998). However, "the individual's and family's responses to cancer can be viewed as efforts to master a crisis, or a series of crises, and to restore order in the face of continual life threat, rather than signs of incipient psychopathology" (Rait, 2015, p. 563).

Using a family systems approach to cancer care will enhance both patient and family coping (Rait, 2015). Similar to the patient's experience, the family's emotions range from shock to despair, anxiety to anguish. Research shows that cancer affects couple functioning and parent–child relationships (Duhamel & Dupuis, 2004; Rait, 2015). "The family with cancer is a family in transition, as the illness presents the patient and family with challenges at every level of functioning, from practical to existential" (Rait, 2015, p. 562). When applying a family systems' perspective, healthy functioning occurs only when family needs are met. In family assessment, the family should be approached as a unique cultural system including ethnicity, race, religion, and social class (Rait, 2015). Assessment of family functioning also should include the family's developmental level, history, and relationships (Rait, 2015).

Family members most often feel isolated and alone in their feelings and tend to rank their own emotional needs and physical health as a low priority (Nikoletti et al., 2003). Studies have found that perceived health is lower and depression is greater in family caregivers than in the general population. The social impact of cancer on the family includes interpersonal losses of outside relationships, activities, and paid employment (Haley, 2003).

Family dynamics have been found to influence problem solving and treatment decision making (Lewis, 2010; Zhang & Siminoff, 2003). Family caregivers who are emotionally involved with patients have been found to show empathy and support for patient decisions, whereas noncohesive or "disengaged" families display more discordance about treatment decisions (Rait, 2015; Zhang & Siminoff, 2003). To support family coping, nurses must be aware of disparity between the patient's and family's emotions and needs and validate each person's feelings. Duhamel and Dupuis (2004) have identified four elements as essential for effective family coping: acknowledging the family's existence, experience, expertise, and their need to maintain hope amid the losses they are experiencing. The patient's coping responses are interdependent with the family's coping responses—one cannot be separated from the other.

## Personal Meaning, Spirituality, and Hope

An important variable influencing coping and adaptation to cancer is that patients can find some positive meaning for their cancer when answering the question, "Why me?" (Hoffman et al., 2013; Taylor, 1995). The search for meaning is a significant part of the cancer experience, and most often, the majority of patients with cancer ascribe positive meanings to their experience (Stanton, 2015; Tallman, 2013). These include reprioritization of life goals, changed lifestyles and personal values, increased appreciation for life, and spiritual development (Tallman, 2013; Taylor, 1995). Gaining insight into the meaning of life and having resilience and strength in the face of adversity can support coping in family members (Nolen-Hoeksema, 2000).

Appraisal of what cancer may mean and its impact on valued goals—life roles, changed self-image, and fundamental beliefs of one's life purpose—may occur (Hoffman et al., 2013). Park and Folkman (1977) referred to this type of appraisal-focused coping as "meaning making." Hoffman et al. (2013) discussed that meaning making is inherent in the appraisal process as patients experiencing cancer aim to interpret the meaning of the experience in their lives. This process has been linked to emotional and social well-being. Meaning-centered psychotherapy, based on the work of Viktor Frankl, has been developed to address this patient need (Lichtenthal, Applebaum, & Breitbart, 2015).

Confronting the existential issues brought about by cancer can be a profound emotional experience that contributes to these changed perspectives. Research has indicated that spirituality (defined as the metaphysical or transcendent aspects of life related to supernatural forces) may have a positive impact on the emotional adjustment of patients with cancer (Canada & Fitchett, 2015; Jenkins & Pargament, 1995). Spirituality encompasses organized religion in addition to the belief in a "higher power" or other philosophies. The role of religion and spirituality in the appraisal process of coping may lead to both cognitive (e.g., appraising an illness as part of God's plan) and behavioral (e.g., praying or attending religious services) aspects of coping (Thune-Boyle, 2013). Religious practice and strong spirituality may promote effective coping by decreasing the intensity of symptoms (e.g., pain, anxiety), social isolation (Jenkins & Pargament, 1995), and psychological distress (Schreiber, 2011). However, research has also documented that feeling punished or abandoned by God was associated with higher levels of anxiety and depression (Canada & Fitchett, 2015). Hope or hopefulness is another variable thought to positively influence the cancer experience. Studies have associated a sense of hope with spiritual healing, improved quality of life, and more effective coping (Felder, 2004; Jacobsen et al., 2014; Post-White et al., 1996). Folkman (2013) illustrated the dynamic, interdependent relationship between hope and coping and stated that at times it is difficult, if not impossible, to have one without the other. Although defining the dimensions of personal meaning, spirituality, and hope is difficult, healthcare professionals should evaluate the influence of these variables on emotional responses for each patient and family experiencing cancer (see Chapters 7 and 9 for more information on hope and spirituality).

## Specific Coping Challenges With Cancer

Different physiologic and psychological demands along the cancer continuum will present specific coping challenges. These demands may be illness- or treatment-related: fatigue, pain, cognitive changes, medication side effects, and grief and loss.

Unrelenting fatigue has been the most frequently reported symptom of cancer and treatment, and patients have identified fatigue as having a negative effect on quality of life (Mock, 2001; National Comprehensive Cancer Network®, 2017). Fatigue can increase patients' feelings of distress while undergoing cancer treatment, can have a negative effect on cognitive function, and can contribute to anxiety and depression, hopelessness, and overall psychological distress (Alici, Bower, & Breitbart, 2015) (see Chapter 6 for more information on fatigue).

Unmanaged pain is another subjective phenomenon that influences coping. Cancer-related pain has major effects on psychological distress, and psychiatric diagnoses (e.g., adjustment disorder with depressed or anxious mood, major depression) increase in patients with cancer and uncontrolled pain (Breitbart & Payne, 1998; Tickoo, Key, & Breitbart, 2015). Severe pain increases anxiety, which increases the perception of pain (Pasacreta et al., 2001; Tickoo et al., 2015). "Pain can overwhelm a person's ability to adaptively cope, resulting in behavior suggestive of psychiatric disorders, which disappears once the pain is relieved" (Tickoo et al., 2015, p. 180). Uncontrolled pain is also a major risk factor for cancer-related suicide (Breitbart & Payne, 1998; Dees, Vernooij-Dassen, Dekkers, Vissers, & van Weel, 2011) (see Chapters 8 and 17 for information on pain, depression, and suicide).

Cognitive changes in patients with cancer are a distressing challenge and may be the direct (e.g., primary brain tumors or metastatic disease) or indirect (e.g., metabolic or electrolyte imbalances, drug or radiation side effects, infection) effects of disease or treatment on the central nervous system. Research has supported declines in cognitive abilities in individuals diagnosed and treated for non–central nervous system cancer, including breast and prostate cancer (Ahles, Andreotti, & Correa, 2015). Certain chemotherapeutic agents (e.g., vinca alkaloids) may contribute to depression and mood changes in addition to affecting cognition. Alcohol and drug abuse also may compromise the patient's cognitive abilities. Cognitive changes can impair general appearance and behavior, mood, affect, and thought content and can lead to more serious psychiatric diagnoses, such as dementia or delirium. Cognitive disabilities that range from the inability to concentrate to loss of memory and symptoms of dementia can contribute to feelings of powerlessness and loss of control and dignity (see Chapter 3 for more information on cognitive dysfunction).

Finally, grief and loss throughout the cancer continuum are major coping challenges. Beginning with diagnosis, patients constantly confront physical and psychological losses that must be successfully grieved to enable individuals to cope effectively. Physical changes, such as loss of a body part or function, will affect body image and self-esteem. Successful mourning must take place to enable the individual to incorporate a new sense of self. Psychological losses involve changes in role function, job security, financial security, and, if cancer recurs, constant readjustment of lifestyle and future goals. A necessary challenge for patients and families is to reorganize and readjust as they face the continued demands of chronic illness (Lewis, 2004). If resolution of loss does not happen, patients are vulnerable to psychiatric complications, such as major depression. The ultimate challenge is the anticipatory grieving experienced by patients and families when death is imminent. Healthcare professionals are in a unique position to help patients and families through anticipatory grieving, resolution of conflicts, and preparation for bereavement (Chockinov & Holland, 1989; Johansson & Grimby, 2012; Neimeyer, 2011; Nolen-Hoeksema, 2000; Redinbaugh et al., 2003) (see Chapter 26 on the close of life).

## Interventions to Support Coping

Psychosocial support should be an inseparable entity of the cancer treatment plan (Adler & Page, 2008; Guidry et al., 1997). If not addressed, the acute and chronic stress associated with cancer can cause emotional distress for patients, interfere with life goals, and contribute to a lower quality of life (Anderson, 2003). When planning interventions, nurses must recognize that (a) no single coping response is more effective than another, (b) interventions must be individualized for the specific needs of the patient and family, and (c) it may be necessary to provide a variety of resources to meet different challenges as they emerge (Nail, 2001; Pearlin & Schooler, 1978; Rait, 2015; Walsh, 1996). Nurses should base interventions on a thorough psychosocial assessment of the many variables that influence coping behaviors (see Figure 4-1). Interventions should target patients at high risk for coping difficulties (e.g., trait anxiety) and at points of time when they are most needed (e.g., recurrence) (Nail, 2001). Healthcare professionals must assess patients' emotional reactions to cancer at the outset of the cancer experience. Research has shown that early reactions often are predictive of individuals at risk for later adaptation and psychiatric problems (e.g., anxiety, depression) (Pasacreta et al., 2001; Pasacreta et al., 2015).

Benedict and Penedo (2013) recommended a "stepped care approach" to psychosocial interventions. This is a collaborative approach in which the cancer survivor is involved in the treatment planning, and therapeutic resources are used based on the systematic assessment and monitoring of the individual's psychosocial well-being.

A major goal of supporting patient and family coping is to promote adaptation. The adaptive tasks of chronic illness include reducing environmental threats, tolerating negative events, maintaining a positive self-image, maintaining emotional equilibrium, and positively staying involved in interpersonal relationships (Cohen & Lazarus, 1979). Figure 4-3 outlines assessment criteria and interventions that support effective coping and adaptation for patients and families. The hallmark of successful adaptation has been described as "engagement": a full and enthusiastic return to the normal activities of life (Spencer et al., 1998). The "engaged" patient underlies a more patient-centered system of care (Golant, Buzaglo, & Thiboldeaux, 2015). Interventions directed toward adaptation focus on assisting patients and families with choosing effective coping strategies, helping them to regain preillness equilibrium, and, if possible, aiding them to integrate and find meaning in the experience. Overcoming the challenges of cancer can lead to emotional growth and can contribute to a positive change in self-perception and one's life (Nolen-Hoeksema, 2000; Stanton, 2015; Tallman, 2013). Nurses can support this healing process by identifying how each patient and family define what coping means to them, moving toward what Lewis (2004) poignantly called "relational-focused care."

To meet and adjust to the physical and emotional demands of cancer, patients and families must constantly reappraise the meaning of the experience in relation to their beliefs, values, and life goals. Nurses can support this appraisal-focused coping by encouraging patients

**Assessment Criteria for Patient and Family Coping**
- Understand the patient's and family's appraisal of the situation; identify what is appraised as threatening and what is appraised as challenging.
- Identify the stressors confronting the individual and family as perceived by them, within their reality, and within the context of their situations/lives.
- Assess coping efficacy based on their individual and family experiences, strengths, and coping traits.
- Acknowledge the patient's and family's experience of the illness. Allow them to tell their story and discover their feelings and the meaning that each person ascribes to the experience.
- Assessment should take into account the patterns and representations related to the patient's and family's culture, including language, thoughts, beliefs, traditions, and values.

**Interventions to Promote Effective Coping and Adaptation**
- Incorporate a family systems approach. Acknowledge the family's existence, experience, and expertise, as well as their need to maintain hope.
- Communicate basic but necessary information to support coping: your name, your credentials, your role in their care, and how and when they can contact you.
- Use simple gestures that acknowledge their presence. Address the patient and family by name, shake their hands, and include them in conversations.
- Recognize and respect cultural and religious belief systems in the delivery of care.
- Provide clear, concise information regarding the care plan, what patient-active approach is expected of the individual, and what the patient can expect of you.
- Enhance confidence and hope. Note the patient's and family's strengths and abilities, and support and reinforce their unique coping styles.
- Use evidence-based interventions appropriate to the goal of care and the individual situation.
- Do not overload the patient and family with information. Assess readiness to learn, and recognize that information seeking is different for each patient and family.
- Be aware of your professional presence and role and its effect on the patient.
- Communicate positivism. Encourage the patient and family to be positive; do not tell them. Respect the patient's and family's attitudes and perceptions.
- Validate your assessment of the situation with the patient and family. Do not assume that your evaluation is correct and in line with the patient's and family's perspectives.
- Evaluate outcomes based on the individual's and family's coping efficacy and values, and not on preconceived notions of what constitutes effective coping.

**Figure 4-3. Assessment Criteria and Interventions to Support Effective Coping and Adaptation for the Patient and Family**

*Note.* Based on information from Arnold & Boggs, 2016; Duhamel & Dupuis, 2004; Grassi et al., 2015; Nail, 2001; Wilkes et al., 2003.

and families to examine their internal feelings—thoughts and impulses that are influencing their emotional responses. A wide variety of interventions can help reduce the anxiety and fears that patients with cancer most often experience, thus allowing more emotional energy to be directed toward cognitive restructuring and problem solving. Interventions used to manage emotional stress include relaxation training, guided imagery, hypnosis, exercise, and music and art therapy (see Chapter 25). Encouraging a positive and optimistic attitude also will promote adaptive coping. Exploring positive emotions has been shown to elicit positive affect and promote resilience (Jacobsen et al., 2014). Encouraging patients and family members to focus on short-term, attainable goals will help them to positively reframe what they find threatening and uncontrollable. Role modeling a positive and optimistic attitude will not only promote more effective coping (Wilkes et al., 2003) but also will allow patients and families to define what these concepts mean to them. For example, is optimism seen as hope for cure, pain relief, or quality time with those they love? The meaning of a hopeful, fighting spirit—like coping—will be dynamic and change over the continuum of the disease (Folkman, 2013). Hopefulness can be present no matter what the stage of disease or the goals for cure (Nail, 2001). Inherent risks are involved if supportive resources are not provided for emotion-focused coping. Coping behaviors can remain unchanged over time, not meeting the emotional needs of those involved (Lewis, 2004).

In addition, coping interventions should be evidence based. Research has demonstrated that strategies promoting active problem-solving behaviors, in contrast to passive or avoidant styles, have consistently proved to be more effective (Nezu et al., 2015; Schnoll et al., 2002). For example, encouraging the patient to become an active and informed part of the treatment plan will promote effective coping behaviors and increase the patient's sense of control. Information seeking is an identified coping strategy that provides patients and families with the knowledge needed for decision making. Independent of where patients are on the cancer continuum, health education regarding the disease and treatment is vital. Coping failure most often begins with a lack of the knowledge, skills, or experience needed to make competent decisions (Lazarus & Folkman, 1984). If the educational component of cancer care is missing, patients will feel overwhelmed and confused, leading to feelings of powerlessness (see Chapter 21). In a review of stress research and quality-of-life interventions, Anderson (2003) found that education stood out as a significant intervention for improvement in both physical and mental health for patients. Another coping strategy, direct action (e.g., deciding to enter a clinical trial), cannot take place without adequate knowledge and an understanding of personal risks and benefits involved. When providing information to patients and families, nurses must take into account information-coping styles and readiness to learn. Education also must be balanced with emotional support to help patients and families deal effectively with the information and its implications (Nikoletti et al., 2003).

Helping patients develop new strategies as they move along the cancer continuum is another necessity. Research has shown that individuals who have exhibited more flexibility in their coping efforts have been more resilient and better able to cope (Aspinwall & Brunhart, 2000). The same is true for families—optimal functioning is characterized by flexibility (Rait, 2015). It is important to provide patients and families with choices and alternatives, recognizing that just because one intervention is frequently used does not mean it is effective across the board (Nail, 2001). An understanding of what feeling in control means for patients and families is critical to support their coping (Nail, 2001). For example, employing simple but challenging interventions in a busy healthcare setting (e.g., allowing the patient to choose appointment times, structuring chemotherapy sessions for family members to be present) can be the difference between patients and family members feeling in control and supported or frustrated and unheard. Interventions should target the most pressing stressor, focusing on what can and cannot be changed. If the stressor cannot be changed or identified, then interventions should be directed toward modifying the response to the stressor (Nail, 2001). A cancer diagnosis cannot be changed, but symptom management during treatment can modify the impact on patients' quality of life. During crisis-free periods, the nurse can encourage patients to recognize and celebrate times of stability. "Eliciting joy and happiness is an important part of coping support" (Jacobsen et al., 2014, p. 465). Nursing interventions using a self-care approach have been found to improve patients' coping abilities (Delbar & Benor, 2001). Teaching patients how to predict and manage their own symptoms promotes independence and an internal locus of control.

To be successful, coping interventions should be constructed within a systems framework—incorporating family, community, and social support—while maintaining sensitivity to cultural and spiritual beliefs. Caring for the family supports the greatest resource the patient has in striving to cope with and adapt to cancer (Rait, 2015). In the construct of appraisal-focused coping, it has been found that family caregivers who are hopeful are better equipped to find meaning in their lives amid the challenges of cancer (Borneman et al., 2003). To support problem solving in families, nurses can facilitate communication between the patient and family members. Long-standing family roles and communication patterns influence the different perceptions of care needs and the different emotional responses of the patient and family during the cancer trajectory (Given et al., 2001; Rait, 2015). If these family roles and communication patterns go unrecognized, research has found that they can contribute to the caregiver's sense of burden, adding to family conflict and caregiver distress (Given et al., 2001). Lewis (2004) has proposed a "healing paradigm" for evidence-based understanding and intervention to promote family coping (see Figure 4-4). Caregivers who are able to "reframe" coping by accepting their loved one's illness and who can redefine the illness demands in a more manageable way feel more capable to meet these challenges and thus experience less caregiver stress (Redinbaugh et al., 2003) (see Chapter 28 for information on caring for the family).

---

- Help the family to stabilize and maintain its core functions during stressful times.
- Sustain or enhance relationships among family members—as a family "unit," not as a family with cancer.
- Nurture the needs of individual members within the family, despite the cancer.
- Add to the family members' competencies; promote confidence to manage illness-related challenges based on the family's definition of the stressor and their perception of the situation, not on the professional's assumptions.
- Help the family to reorganize routines around treatment, symptom management, long-term care, and survivorship while protecting "quality" family time apart from the cancer experience.
- Support family relationships by reconfiguring, stabilizing, protecting, and enhancing communication, especially for children and in the parent-child relationship.
- Provide safety for family members to express their feelings and thoughts about the cancer experience over time, and validate and normalize their feelings.

**Figure 4-4. Healing Paradigm for Family Coping**

*Note.* Based on information from Lewis, 2004.

---

Finally, reinforcing social support strongly influences patients' and families' capacity to cope. Fawzy and Fawzy (2011) recommended implementation of structured psychosocial interventions for patients early in the course of cancer diagnosis and treatment. Figure 4-5 outlines components of a structured psychiatric intervention program for newly diagnosed patients and those in late stages of treatment. Enhancing problem-solving capabilities should include training in (a) how to identify the most pressing stressor/problem, (b) how to brainstorm possible solutions, (c) how to select and implement appropriate strategies, and (d) how to evaluate outcomes and reappraise the situation (Fawzy et al., 1997; Fawzy & Fawzy, 2011). Skills training should include characteristics of effective coping styles (e.g., optimism, practicality, flexibility, resourcefulness). Support groups and psychoeducational support programs are examples of structured interventions that can provide patients with tools to enhance problem-focused coping. Resources such as the Cancer Support Community provide support for both patients and families. The philosophy of this community is patient empowerment by knowledge, strength by action, and sustainment by community. With appropriate education and support, patients are less apt to use avoidance-focused styles of coping.

Psychological support for patients can be provided in the form of crisis intervention, counseling, and psychotherapy. Crisis intervention models frequently are applied in the area

**Newly Diagnosed or Early Treatment Stage**
- Health education
- Stress management and behavioral training
- Coping strategies, including problem solving
- Psychosocial group support

**Advanced Metastatic Disease or Late Treatment Stage**
- Weekly group support programs
- Focus on daily coping
- Pain management, symptom management
- Existential issues related to death and dying

**Figure 4-5. Components of Structured Psychiatric Interventions**

*Note.* Based on information from Fawzy & Fawzy, 2011; Fawzy et al., 1995.

of oncology (Chase, 2013) (see Chapter 22 for information on crisis intervention). This type of practice model is short term and involves (a) defining the threatening events, (b) assessing the patient's interpretation of the stressors, (c) assessing the patient's coping efforts and the resources available, and (d) assessing the patient's level of functioning. Family crisis interventions follow the same principles to mobilize family coping capabilities as a whole (Friedman et al., 2003). Most often, patients experiencing cancer must deal with specific crisis events (e.g., diagnosis, recurrence), and the most beneficial interventions aim to help patients and families deal effectively with the most pressing challenges.

More in-depth interpersonal interventions, such as counseling and psychotherapy, may be warranted if particular dynamics of the individual are not solved by crisis intervention or structured psychoeducational support. If an individual has difficulty coping because of underlying conflicts or personal agenda, interventions aimed at general populations may be inadequate (Lazarus & Folkman, 1984; Pasacreta et al., 2001; Pasacreta et al., 2015). Individual therapy provides a safe forum for patients to work out intrapsychic conflicts that may be interfering with effective coping behaviors. If the patient has overwhelming anxiety or depression or a past history of psychiatric disorders, referral for psychotherapy is necessary. Massie, Holland, and Straker (1989) first described the goals of psychotherapy with a patient who had cancer to focus on the illness and its consequences, exploring only the past and present issues that affect coping and adaptation to cancer. Today, psychotherapeutic goals range from teaching problem-solving skills (Nezu et al., 2015) to helping the patient find meaning in the experience of cancer (Lichtenhal et al., 2015; Stanton, 2015). Cognitive behavioral therapy is a form of psychotherapy that places cognition (thoughts, beliefs, emotions, and behaviors) at the forefront, helping patients to reframe negative thoughts, problem solve, and choose more effective coping (Moorey & Watson, 2015). Psychopharmacologic management of emotional distress, psychiatric symptoms (e.g., anxiety, depression), and disease-related symptoms (e.g., insomnia, pain) also play an important role in the treatment plan (Massie & Lesko, 1989; Pasacreta et al., 2001; Pasacreta et al., 2015) (see Chapter 25).

Social support and psychological resources must be a consistent and ongoing component of cancer care (see Appendix). Patients continue to process cancer as a major life experience, even after completion of treatment and recovery. Some have expressed a perceived reduction in supportive networks as they ask themselves "What shall I do with my life now?" (Bush, 2009, 2010; Lethborg et al., 2000; Stanton, 2012). At end of treatment, feelings of apprehension, vulnerability, and abandonment can ensue (Harrison et al., 2012). Other patients have expressed that at stressful transition points, such as recurrence, communication and support between themselves and healthcare providers became strained, causing them to feel helpless and abandoned (Howell et al., 2003). Stanton, Rowland, and Ganz (2015) noted that the fear of recurrence is challenging for healthcare professionals to manage. The need for social support for men also must be recognized. Gender differences exist, and men have different yet equally pressing needs for social support networks (Poole et al., 2001). Men in support groups have been found to use coping styles with less hopelessness and helplessness and with more fighting spirit (McGovern et al., 2002). Cultural differences exist as well, and social support networks should be made available to meet the needs of racially and ethnically diverse populations (Bourjolly & Hirschman, 2001; Gotay & Lau, 2003; Munoz et al., 2016).

Social support should use a family systems approach. Each family is a unique cultural system influenced by ethnicity, race, religion, and social class (Rait, 2015). Solution-focused brief therapy was suggested as a viable approach with families (Neilson-Clayton & Brownlee, 2002). This approach helps families recognize their strengths, coping abilities, and hopefulness toward solving problems and moving into the future (Neilson-Clayton & Brownlee, 2002). Northouse et al. (2002) studied the effectiveness of a family-based intervention program that incorporated both the Lazarus and Folkman (1984) stress-coping model and the McCubbin and McCubbin (1996) family stress and resiliency model. This family-based program outlines nursing interventions tailored to address each component of the FOCUS program—family involvement, optimistic attitude, coping effectiveness, uncertainty reduction, and symptom management. The core content of the program was tailored to meet the particular needs and strengths of each family. The program incorporated an essential principle that should underlie all interventions to enhance coping, which is to identify and base interventions on how patients and families function and cope within their "reality," not on how theories predict they should (Lewis, 2004; Nail, 2001). The FOCUS program is a relationship enhancement and prevention program that applies a supportive and educative approach to enhance communication, coping, and self-care, as well as manage the uncertainty that cancer brings (Zaider & Kissane, 2015). Nail (2001) stressed the importance of evaluating outcomes based on the coping efficacy of patients and family members, not on the specific coping strategies they employ. A family-centered approach recognizes the family as a system in transition across the disease continuum and considers the developmental stage of the family members in assessment (Rait, 2015). This approach to care is vital because the family is the major social support network for the patient, and the family and patient are interdependent in functioning (see Chapter 28 for information on caring for the family).

# Conclusion

Nursing plays an integral role in helping patients and families to cope and adapt to cancer. The crux of nursing is a humanistic approach and nurturance of the human potential (Friedman et al., 2003). Supporting patient coping is congruent with the goals of oncology nursing care. From nurses at the bedside to those in advanced practice, nursing interventions to enhance coping occur across the cancer continuum. Interventions include patient and family education, symptom management, supporting and reinforcing effective coping strategies, and referring patients and families to appropriate resources if ineffective coping is identified. Intrinsic to all coping interventions are the goals of empowering patients and families and providing hope. Empowerment occurs when the necessary information, skills, and problem-solving methods are provided to build the self-esteem and self-confidence of patients and family members to successfully meet the challenges they face (Friedman et al., 2003; Golant et al., 2015). Hope is a far less tangible goal, but one that may be an essential ingredient for coping effectively with cancer (Folkman, 2013; Reading, 2004). Even during the terminal stage of illness, patients can hope for life goals, such as having the resources to finish their life business, being free of pain, and dying with dignity. Martocchio (1985) succinctly summed up the relationship between hope and coping: "Hoping is coping" (p. 297).

# References

Adler, N.E., & Page, A.E.K. (Eds.). (2008). *Cancer care for the whole patient: Meeting psychosocial health needs*. Washington, DC: National Academies Press.

Ahles, T.A., Andreotti, C., & Correa, D.D. (2015). Neuropsychological impact of cancer and cancer treatments. In J.C. Holland, W.S. Breitbart, P.N. Butow, P.B. Jacobsen, M.J. Loscalzo, & R. McCorkle (Eds.), *Psycho-oncology* (3rd ed., pp. 225–238). New York, NY: Oxford University Press.

Alici, Y., Bower, J.E., & Breitbart, W.S. (2015). Fatigue. In J.C. Holland, W.S. Breitbart, P.N. Butow, P.B. Jacobsen, M.J. Loscalzo, & R. McCorkle (Eds.), *Psycho-oncology* (3rd ed., pp. 209–219). New York, NY: Oxford University Press.

Anderson, B.L. (2003). Psychological interventions for cancer patients. In C.W. Given, B. Given, V.L. Champion, S. Kozachik, & D.N. DeVoss (Eds.), *Evidence-based cancer care and prevention: Behavioral interventions* (pp. 179–217). New York, NY: Springer.

Arnold, E.C. (2016). Empowerment oriented communication strategies to reduce stress. In E.C. Arnold & K.U. Boggs (Eds.), *Interpersonal relationships: Professional communication skills for nurses* (pp. 309–332). St. Louis, MO: Elsevier.

Arnold, E.C., & Boggs, K.U. (2016). *Interpersonal relationships: Professional communication skills for nurses* (7th ed.). St. Louis, MO: Elsevier.

Ashing-Giwa, K.T., Padilla, G., Tejero, J., Kraemer, J., Wright, K., Coscarelli, A., ... Hills, D. (2004). Understanding the breast cancer experience of women: A qualitative study of African American, Asian American, Latina and Caucasian cancer survivors. *Psycho-Oncology, 13,* 408–428. doi:10.1002/pon.750

Aspinwall, L.G., & Brunhart, S.M. (2000). What I do know won't hurt me: Optimism, attention to negative information, coping, and health. In J.E. Gillham (Ed.), *The science of optimism and hope: Research essays in honor of Martin E.P. Seligman* (pp. 163–200). Philadelphia, PA: Templeton Foundation Press.

Aziz, N.M. (2007). Late effects of treatment. In P.A. Ganz (Ed.), *Cancer survivorship: Today and tomorrow* (pp. 54–76). New York, NY: Springer.

Baider, L., & Balducci, L. (2011). Psychosocial interventions for elderly cancer patients: How old would you be if you did not know how old you are? In M. Watson & D. Kissane (Eds.), *Handbook of psychotherapy in cancer care* (pp. 233–246). Hoboken, NJ: Wiley-Blackwell.

Barry, P.D. (2002a). Stress: Effective coping and adaptation. In P.D. Barry (Ed.), *Mental health and mental illness* (7th ed., pp. 157–170). Philadelphia, PA: Lippincott Williams & Wilkins.

Barry, P.D. (2002b). Theories and stages of personality development. In P.D. Barry (Ed.), *Mental health and mental illness* (7th ed., pp. 85–105). Philadelphia, PA: Lippincott Williams & Wilkins.

Barsevick, A.M., Much, J., & Sweeney, C. (2000). Psychosocial responses to cancer. In C.H. Yarbro, M.H. Frogge, M. Goodman, & S.L. Groenwald (Eds.), *Cancer nursing: Principles and practice* (5th ed., pp. 1529–1549). Burlington, MA: Jones & Bartlett Learning.

Benedict, C., & Penedo, F.J. (2013). Psychosocial interventions in cancer. In B.I. Carr & J. Steel (Eds.), *Psychological aspects of cancer: A guide to emotional and psychological consequences of cancer, their causes and management* (pp. 221–253). New York, NY: Springer.

Blanchard, C.G., Albrecht, T.L., Ruckdeschel, J.C., Grant, C.H., & Hemmick, R.M. (1995). The role of social support in adaptation to cancer and to survival. *Journal of Psychosocial Oncology, 13,* 75–95. doi:10.1300/J077V13N01_05

Borneman, T., Chu, D.Z.J., Wagman, L., Ferrell, B., Juarez, G., McCahill, L.E., & Uman, G. (2003). Concerns of family caregivers of patients with cancer facing palliative surgery for advanced malignancies. *Oncology Nursing Forum, 30,* 997–1005. doi:10.1188/03.ONF.997-1005

Bourjolly, J.N., & Hirschman, K.B. (2001). Similarities in coping strategies but differences in sources of support among African American women coping with breast cancer. *Journal of Psychosocial Oncology, 19*(2), 17–38. doi:10.1300/J077v19n02_02

Breitbart, W., & Payne, D.K. (1998). Pain. In J.C. Holland (Ed.), *Psycho-oncology* (pp. 451–467). New York, NY: Oxford University Press.

Burhansstipanov, L., & Hollow, W. (2001). Native American cultural aspects of oncology nursing care. *Seminars in Oncology Nursing, 17,* 206–219. doi:10.1053/sonu.2001.25950

Bush, N.J. (2009). Post-traumatic stress disorder related to the cancer experience. *Oncology Nursing Forum, 36,* 395–400. doi:10.1188/09.ONF.395-400

Bush, N.J. (2010). Post-traumatic stress disorder related to cancer: Hope, healing, and recovery [Online exclusive]. *Oncology Nursing Forum, 37,* E331–343. doi:10.1188/10.ONF.E331-E343

Butow, P.N., Fardell, J.E., & Smith, A.B. (2015). Fear of cancer recurrence. In J.C. Holland, W.S. Breitbart, P.N. Butow, P.B. Jacobsen, M.J. Loscalzo, & R. McCorkle (Eds.), *Psycho-oncology* (3rd ed., pp. 625–629). New York, NY: Oxford University Press.

Canada, A.L., & Fitchett, G. (2015). Religion/spirituality and cancer: A brief update of selected research. In J.C. Holland, W.S. Breitbart, P.N. Butow, P.B. Jacobsen, M.J. Loscalzo, & R. McCorkle (Eds.), *Psycho-oncology* (3rd ed., pp. 503–508). New York, NY: Oxford University Press.

Chase, E. (2013). Crisis intervention for nurses. *Clinical Journal of Oncology Nursing, 17,* 337–339. doi:10.1188/13.CJON.337-339

Cho, D., Park, C.L., & Blank, T.O. (2013). Emotional approach coping: Gender differences on psychological adjustment in young to middle-aged cancer survivors. *Psychology and Health, 28,* 874–894. doi:10.1080/08870446.2012.762979

Chockinov, H., & Holland, J.C. (1989). Bereavement: A special issue in oncology. In J.C. Holland & J.H. Rowland (Eds.), *Handbook of psychooncology: Psychological care of the patient with cancer* (pp. 612–627). New York, NY: Oxford University Press.

Cloutier, A., & Ferrall, S. (1996). Psychosocial aspects of complex responses to cancer. In P.D. Barry (Ed.), *Psychosocial nursing care of physically ill patients and their families* (pp. 412–433). Philadelphia, PA: Lippincott Williams & Wilkins.

Cohen, F., & Lazarus, R.S. (1979). Coping with the stresses of illness. In G.C. Stone, F. Cohen, & N.E. Adler (Eds.), *Health psychology: A handbook. Theories, applications, and challenges of a psychological approach to the health care system* (pp. 217–254). San Francisco, CA: Jossey-Bass.

Cope, D.G. (2015). Cultural competency in nursing research. *Oncology Nursing Forum, 42,* 305–307. doi:10.1188/15.ONF.305-307

Cordova, M.J. (2008). Facilitating posttraumatic growth following cancer. In S. Joseph & P.A. Linley (Eds.), *Trauma, recovery, and growth: Positive psychological perspectives on posttraumatic stress* (pp. 185–206). Hoboken, NJ: John Wiley & Sons.

Dees, M.V.D., Vernooij-Dassen, M.J., Dekkers, W.J., Vissers, K.C., & van Weel, C. (2011). 'Unbearable suffering': A qualitative study on the perspectives of patients who request assistance in dying. *Journal of Medical Ethics, 37,* 727–734. doi:10.1136/jme.2011.045492

Delbar, V., & Benor, D.E. (2001). Impact of a nursing intervention on cancer patients' ability to cope. *Journal of Psychosocial Oncology, 19,* 57–74. doi:10.1300/J077v19n02_04

Devins, G.M., & Binik, Y.M. (1996). Facilitating coping with chronic physical illness. In M. Zeidner & N.S. Endler (Eds.), *Handbook of coping: Theory, research, applications* (pp. 640–696). New York, NY: John Wiley.

Die-Trill, M. (1998). The patient from a different culture. In J.C. Holland (Ed.), *Psycho-oncology* (pp. 857–866). New York, NY: Oxford University Press.

Duhamel, F., & Dupuis, F. (2004). Guaranteed returns: Investing in conversations with families of patients with cancer. *Clinical Journal of Oncology Nursing, 8,* 68–71. doi:10.1188/04.CJON.68-71

Edelman, S., Craig, A., & Kidman, A.D. (2000). Group interventions with cancer patients: Efficacy of psychoeducational versus supportive groups. *Journal of Psychosocial Oncology, 18,* 67–85. doi:10.1300/J077v18n03_05

Erikson, E. (1963). *Childhood and society* (2nd ed.). New York, NY: Norton.

Fagundes, C.P., Lindgren, M.E., & Kiecolt-Glaser, J.K. (2013). Psychoneuroimmunology and cancer: Incidence, progression, and quality of life. In B.I. Carr & J. Steel (Eds.), *Psychological aspects of cancer: A guide to emotional and psychological consequences of cancer, their causes and management* (pp. 1–11). New York, NY: Springer.

Fawzy, F.I., & Fawzy, N.W. (2011). A short term, structured, psychoeducational intervention for newly diagnosed cancer patients. In M. Watson & D. Kissane (Eds.), *Handbook of psychotherapy in cancer care* (pp. 119–135). Hoboken, NJ: Wiley-Blackwell.

Fawzy, F.I., Fawzy, N.W., Arndt, L.A., & Pasnau, R.O. (1995). Critical review of psychosocial interventions in cancer care. *Archives of General Psychiatry, 52,* 100–113. doi:10.1001/archpsyc.1995.03950140018003

Fawzy, F.I., Fawzy, N.W., Hyun, C.S., & Wheeler, J.G. (1997). Brief, coping-oriented therapy for patients with malignant melanoma. In J.L. Spira (Ed.), *Group therapy for medically ill patients* (pp. 133–163). New York, NY: Guilford Press.

Felder, B.E. (2004). Hope and coping in patients with cancer diagnoses. *Cancer Nursing, 27,* 320–324. doi:10.1097/00002820-200407000-00009

Fernandes-Taylor, S., & Bloom, J.R. (2015). A psychosocial perspective on socioeconomic disparities in cancer. In J.C. Holland, W.S. Breitbart, P.N. Butow, P.B. Jacobsen, M.J. Loscalzo, & R. McCorkle (Eds.), *Psycho-oncology* (3rd ed., pp. 28–34). New York, NY: Oxford University Press.

Fernsler, J.I., & Miller, M.A. (2000). Factors affecting health behavior. In C.H. Yarbro, M.H. Frogge, M. Goodman, & S.L. Groenwald (Eds.), *Cancer nursing: Principles and practice* (5th ed., pp. 85–99). Burlington, MA: Jones & Bartlett Learning.

Folkman, S. (2013). Stress, coping, and hope. In B.I. Carr & J. Steel (Eds.), *Psychological aspects of cancer: A guide to emotional and psychological consequences of cancer, their causes and management* (pp. 119–127). New York, NY: Springer.

Friedman, M.M., Bowden, V.R., & Jones, E.G. (2003). *Family nursing: Research, theory, and practice* (5th ed.). Upper Saddle River, NJ: Prentice Hall.

Given, B.A., & Given, C.W. (2015). The older patient. In J.C. Holland, W.S. Breitbart, P.N. Butow, P.B. Jacobsen, M.J. Loscalzo, & R. McCorkle (Eds.), *Psycho-oncology* (3rd ed., pp. 541–548). New York, NY: Oxford University Press.

Given, B.A., Given, C.W., & Kozachik, S. (2001). Family support in advanced cancer. *CA: A Cancer Journal for Clinicians, 51,* 213–231. doi:10.3322/canjclin.51.4.213

Golant, M., Buzaglo, J., & Thiboldeaux, K. (2015). The engaged patient: The cancer support community's integrative model of evidence-based psychosocial programs, services, and research. In J.C. Holland, W.S. Breitbart, P.N. Butow, P.B. Jacobsen, M.J. Loscalzo, & R. McCorkle (Eds.), *Psycho-oncology* (3rd ed., pp. 710–716). New York, NY: Oxford University Press.

Gorman, L.M., Raines, M.L., & Sultan, D.F. (2002). *Psychosocial nursing for general patient care* (2nd ed.). Philadelphia, PA: F.A. Davis.

Gotay, C.C., & Lau, A.K. (2003). Preferences for psychosocial interventions among newly diagnosed cancer patients from a multiethnic population. *Journal of Psychosocial Oncology, 20*(4), 23–37. doi:10.1300/J077v20n04_02

Grassi, L., Nanni, M.G., Donovan, K.A., & Jacobsen, P.B. (2015). Cross-cultural considerations in screening and assessment. In J.C. Holland, W.S. Breitbart, P.N. Butow, P.B. Jacobsen, M.J. Loscalzo, & R. McCorkle (Eds.), *Psycho-oncology* (3rd ed., pp. 411–416). New York, NY: Oxford University Press.

Guidry, J.J., Aday, L.A., Zhang, D., & Winn, R.J. (1997). The role of informal and formal social support networks for patients with cancer. *Cancer Practice, 5,* 241–246.

Haley, W.E. (2003). Family caregivers of elderly patients with cancer: Understanding and minimizing the burden of care. *Journal of Supportive Oncology, 1*(4 Suppl. 2), 25–29.

Harrison, S.E., Watson, E.K., Ward, A.M., Khan, N.F., Turner, D., Adams, E., ... Rose, P.W. (2012). Cancer survivors' experiences of discharge from hospital follow-up. *European Journal of Cancer Care, 21,* 390–397. doi:10.1111/j.1365-2354.2011.01312.x

Hawley, D.R., & DeHaan, L. (1996). Toward a definition of family resilience: Integrating life-span and family perspectives. *Family Process, 35,* 283–298. doi:10.1111/j.1545-5300.1996.00283.x

Helgeson, V.S., & McUmber, A.L. (2010). Social environment and cancer. In J.C. Holland, W.S. Breitbart, P.B. Jacobsen, M.S. Lederberg, M.J. Loscalzo, & R. McCorkle (Eds.), *Psycho-oncology* (2nd ed., pp. 62–68). New York, NY: Oxford University Press.

Helman, C.G. (2001). *Culture, health, and illness* (4th ed.). London, England: Hodder Arnold Publications.

Henderson, P.D., Gore, S.V., Davis, B.L., & Condon, E.H. (2003). African American women coping with breast cancer: A qualitative analysis. *Oncology Nursing Forum, 30,* 641–647. doi:10.1188/03.ONF.641-647

Hoffman, M.A., Lent, R.W., & Raque-Bogdan, T.L. (2013). A social cognitive perspective on coping with cancer: Theory, research and intervention. *Counseling Psychologist, 41,* 240–267. doi:10.1177/0011000012461378

Holahan, C.J., Moos, R.H., & Schaefer, J.A. (1996). Coping, stress resistance, and growth: Conceptualizing adaptive functioning. In M. Zeidner & N.S. Endler (Eds.), *Handbook of coping: Theory, research, applications* (pp. 24–43). New York, NY: John Wiley.

Holland, J.C. (1989). Clinical course of cancer. In J.C. Holland & J.H. Rowland (Eds.), *Handbook of psychooncology: Psychological care of the patient with cancer* (pp. 75–100). New York, NY: Oxford University Press.

Holland, J.C., & Lewis, S. (2000). *The human side of cancer: Living with hope, coping with uncertainty.* New York, NY: HarperCollins.

Hopman, P., & Rijken, M. (2015). Illness perceptions of cancer patients: Relationships with illness characteristics and coping. *Psycho-Oncology, 24,* 11–18. doi:10.1002/pon.3591

Howell, D., Fitch, M.I., & Deane, K.A. (2003). Women's experiences with recurrent ovarian cancer. *Cancer Nursing, 26,* 10–17. doi:10.1097/00002820-200302000-00002

Hudek-Knezevic, J., Kardum, I., & Pahljina, R. (2002). Relations among social support, coping, and negative affect in hospitalized and nonhospitalized cancer patients. *Journal of Psychosocial Oncology, 20,* 45–63. doi:10.1300/J077v20n02_03

Jacobsen, J., Kvale, E., Rabow, M., Rinaldi, S., Cohen, S., Weissman, D., & Jackson, V. (2014). Helping patients with serious illness live well through the promotion of adaptive coping: A report from the Improving Outpatient Palliative Care (IPAL-OP) Initiative. *Journal of Palliative Medicine, 17,* 463–468. doi:10.1089/jpm.2013.0254

Jenkins, R.A., & Pargament, K.I. (1995). Religion and spirituality as resources for coping with cancer. *Journal of Psychosocial Oncology, 13,* 51–74. doi:10.1300/J077V13N01_04

Johansson, A.K., & Grimby, A. (2012). Anticipatory grief among close relatives of patients in hospice and palliative wards. *American Journal of Hospice and Palliative Medicine, 29,* 134–138. doi:10.1177/1049909111409021

Johnson, P. (2002). The use of humor and its influence on spirituality and coping in breast cancer survivors. *Oncology Nursing Forum, 29,* 691–695. doi:10.1188/02.ONF.691-695

Kim, Y., Loscalzo, M.J., & Clark, K. (2015). Sexual minority health in psycho-oncology. In J.C. Holland, W.S. Breitbart, P.N. Butow, P.B. Jacobsen, M.J. Loscalzo, & R. McCorkle (Eds.), *Psycho-oncology* (3rd ed., pp. 574–578). New York, NY: Oxford University Press.

Kohn, P.M. (1996). On coping adaptively with daily hassles. In M. Zeidner & N.S. Endler (Eds.), *Handbook of coping: Theory, research, applications* (pp. 181–201). New York, NY: John Wiley.

Kornblith, A.B. (1998). Psychosocial adaptation of cancer survivors. In J.C. Holland (Ed.), *Psycho-oncology* (pp. 223–254). New York, NY: Oxford University Press.

Lazarus, R.S. (1982). Stress and coping as factors in health and illness. In J. Cohen, J. Cullen, & T.R. Martin (Eds.), *Psychosocial aspects of coping* (pp. 163–190). New York, NY: Raven Press.

Lazarus, R.S. (1993). Coping theory and research: Past, present, and future. *Psychosomatic Medicine, 55,* 234–247. doi:10.1097/00006842-199305000-00002

Lazarus, R.S. (2000). Evolution of a model of stress, coping, and discrete emotions. In V.H. Rice (Ed.), *Handbook of stress, coping, and health: Implications for nursing research, theory, and practice* (pp. 195–222). Thousand Oaks, CA: Sage Publications.

Lazarus, R.S., & Folkman, S. (1984). *Stress, appraisal, and coping.* New York, NY: Springer.

Lethborg, C.E., Kissane, D., Burns, W.I., & Snyder, R. (2000). "Cast adrift": The experience of completing treatment among women with early stage breast cancer. *Journal of Psychosocial Oncology, 18,* 73–90. doi:10.1300/J077v18n04_05

Levin, T.T., & Alici, Y. (2010). Anxiety disorders. In J.C. Holland, W.S. Breitbart, P.B. Jacobsen, M.S. Lederberg, M.J. Loscalzo, & R. McCorkle (Eds.), *Psycho-oncology* (2nd ed., pp. 324–339). New York, NY: Oxford University Press.

Lewis, F.M. (2004). Family-focused oncology nursing research. *Oncology Nursing Forum, 31,* 288–292. doi:10.1188/04.ONF.288-292

Lewis, F.M. (2010). The family's "stuck points" in adjusting to cancer. In J.C. Holland, W.S. Breitbart, P.B. Jacobsen, M.S. Lederberg, M.J. Loscalzo, & R. McCorkle (Eds.), *Psycho-oncology* (2nd ed., pp. 11–515). New York, NY: Oxford University Press.

Lichtenthal, W.G., Applebaum, A.J., & Breitbart, W.S. (2015). Meaning-centered psychotherapy. In J.C. Holland, W.S. Breitbart, P.N. Butow, P.B. Jacobsen, M.J. Loscalzo, & R. McCorkle (Eds.), *Psycho-oncology* (3rd ed., pp. 475–479). New York, NY: Oxford University Press.

Lifford, K.J., Witt, J., Burton, M., Collins, K., Caldon, L., Edwards, A., ... Brain, K. (2015). Understanding older women's decision making and coping in the context of breast cancer treatment. *BMC Medical Informatics and Decision Making, 15,* 45–56. doi:10.1186/s12911-015-0167-1

Maes, S., Leventhal, H., & de Ridder, D. (1996). Coping with chronic diseases. In M. Zeidner & N.S. Endler (Eds.), *Handbook of coping: Theory, research, applications* (pp. 221–251). New York, NY: John Wiley.

Mages, N.L., & Mendelsohn, G.A. (1979). Effects of cancer on patients' lives: A personological approach. In G.C. Stone, F. Cohen, & N.E. Adler (Eds.), *Health psychology: A handbook. Theories, applications, and challenges of a psychological approach to the health care system* (pp. 255–284). San Francisco, CA: Jossey-Bass.

Martocchio, B.C. (1985). Family coping: Helping families help themselves. *Seminars in Oncology Nursing, 1,* 292–297. doi:10.1016/0749-2081(85)90010-5

Massie, M.J., Holland, J.C., & Straker, N. (1989). Psychotherapeutic interventions. In J.C. Holland & J.H. Rowland (Eds.), *Handbook of psychooncology: Psychological care of the patient with cancer* (pp. 455–469). New York, NY: Oxford University Press.

Massie, M.J., & Lesko, L.M. (1989). Psychopharmacological management. In J.C. Holland & J.H. Rowland (Eds.), *Handbook of psychooncology: Psychological care of the patient with cancer* (pp. 470–491). New York, NY: Oxford University Press.

Maybery, D.J., Neale, J., Arentz, A., & Jones-Ellis, J. (2007). The negative event scale: Measuring frequency and intensity of adult hassles. *Anxiety Stress Coping, 20,* 163–176. doi:10.1080/10615800701217654

McCubbin, M.A., & McCubbin, H.I. (1996). Resiliency in families: A conceptual model of family adjustment and adaptation in response to stress and crises. In H.I. McCubbin, A.I. Thompson, & M.A. McCubbin (Eds.), *Family assessment: Resiliency, coping, and adaptation: Inventories for research and practice* (pp. 1–64). Madison, WI: University of Wisconsin.

McGovern, R.J., Heyman, E.N., & Resnick, M.I. (2002). An examination of coping style and quality of life of cancer patients who attend a prostate cancer support group. *Journal of Psychosocial Oncology, 20,* 57–68. doi:10.1300/J077v20n03_04

Mock, V. (2001). Fatigue management. *Cancer, 92*(Suppl. 6), 1699–1707. doi:10.1002/1097-0142(20010915)92:6+<1699::AID-CNCR1500>3.0.CO;2-9

Moorey, S., & Watson, M. (2015). Cognitive therapy. In J.C. Holland, W.S. Breitbart, P.N. Butow, P.B. Jacobsen, M.J. Loscalzo, & R. McCorkle (Eds.), *Psycho-oncology* (3rd ed., pp. 458–463). New York, NY: Oxford University Press.

Munoz, A.R., Kaiser, K., Yanez, B., Victorson, D., Garcia, S.F., Snyder, M.A., & Salsman, J.M. (2016). Cancer experiences and health-related quality of life among racial and ethnic survivors of young adult cancer: A mixed methods study. *Supportive Care in Cancer, 24,* 4861–4870. doi:10.1007/s00520-016-3340-x

Murphy, L.B. (1974). Coping, vulnerability, and resilience in childhood. In G.V. Coelho, D.A. Hamburg, & J.E. Adams (Eds.), *Coping and adaptation* (pp. 69–100). New York, NY: Basic Books.

Nail, L.M. (2001). I'm coping as fast as I can: Psychosocial adjustment to cancer and cancer treatment. *Oncology Nursing Forum, 6,* 967–970.

National Comprehensive Cancer Network. (2017). *NCCN Clinical Practice Guidelines in Oncology (NCCN Guidelines®): Cancer-related fatigue* [v.1.2017]. Retrieved from http://www.nccn.org/professionals/physician_gls/pdf/fatigue.pdf

Neilson-Clayton, H., & Brownlee, K. (2002). Solution-focused brief therapy with cancer patients and their families. *Journal of Psychosocial Oncology, 20,* 1–13. doi:10.1300/J077v20n01_01

Neimeyer, R.A. (2011). Reconstructing meaning in bereavement. In M. Watson & D. Kissane (Eds.), *Handbook of psychotherapy in cancer care* (pp. 247–257). Hoboken, NJ: Wiley-Blackwell.

Nezu, A.M., Nezu, C.M., & Salber, K.E. (2015). Building problem-solving skills. In J.C. Holland, W.S. Breitbart, P.N. Butow, P.B. Jacobsen, M.J. Loscalzo, & R. McCorkle (Eds.), *Psycho-oncology* (3rd ed., pp. 470–474). New York, NY: Oxford University Press.

Nikoletti, S., Kristjanson, L.J., Tataryn, D., McPhee, R., & Burt, L. (2003). Information needs and coping styles of primary family caregivers of women following breast cancer surgery. *Oncology Nursing Forum, 30,* 987–996. doi:10.1188/03.ONF.987-996

Nolen-Hoeksema, S. (2000). Growth and resilience among bereaved people. In J.E. Gillham (Ed.), *The science of optimism and hope: Research essays in honor of Martin E.P. Seligman* (pp. 107–127). Philadelphia, PA: Templeton Foundation Press.

Northouse, L.L., Walker, J., Schafenacker, A., Mood, D., Mellon, S., Galvin, E., … Freeman-Gibb, L. (2002). A family-based program of care for women with recurrent breast cancer and their family members. *Oncology Nursing Forum, 29,* 1411–1419. doi:10.1188/02.ONF.1411-1419

Palmer, M.H., Fogarty, L.A., Somerfield, M.R., & Powel, L.L. (2003). Incontinence after prostatectomy: Coping with incontinence after prostate cancer surgery. *Oncology Nursing Forum, 30,* 229–238. doi:10.1188/03.ONF.229-238

Park, C.L., & Folkman, S. (1977). Meaning in the context of stress and coping. *Review of General Psychology, 76,* 863–875.

Parle, M., & Maguire, P. (1995). Exploring relationships between cancer, coping, and mental health. *Journal of Psychosocial Oncology, 13*(1/2), 27–50. doi:10.1300/J077V13N01_03

Pasacreta, J.V., Minarik, P.A., & Nield-Anderson, L. (2001). Anxiety and depression. In B.R. Ferrell & N. Coyle (Eds.), *Textbook of palliative nursing* (pp. 269–289). New York, NY: Oxford University Press.

Pasacreta, J.V., Minarik, P.A., Nield-Anderson, L., & Paice, J.A. (2015). Anxiety and depression. In B.R. Ferrell, N. Coyle, & J.A. Paice (Eds.), *Oxford textbook of palliative nursing* (4th ed., pp. 366–384). New York, NY: Oxford University Press.

Pearlin, L.I., & Schooler, C. (1978). The structure of coping. *Journal of Health and Social Behavior, 19,* 2–21. doi:10.2307/2136319

Pierce, G.R., Sarason, I.G., & Sarason, B.R. (1996). Coping and social support. In M. Zeidner & N.S. Endler (Eds.), *Handbook of coping: Theory, research, applications* (pp. 434–451). New York, NY: John Wiley.

Poole, G., Poon, C., Achille, M., White, K., Franz, N., Jittler, S., … Doll, R. (2001). Social support for patients with prostate cancer: The effect of support groups. *Journal of Psychosocial Oncology, 19*(2), 1–16. doi:10.1300/J077v19n02_01

Post-White, J., Ceronsky, C., Kreitzer, M.J., Drew, D., Mackey, K.W., Koopmeiners, L., & Gutknecht, S. (1996). Hope, spirituality, sense of coherence, and quality of life in patients with cancer. *Oncology Nursing Forum, 23,* 1571–1579.

Rait, D.S. (2015). A family-centered approach to the patient with cancer. In J.C. Holland, W.S. Breitbart, P.N. Butow, P.B. Jacobsen, M.J. Loscalzo, & R. McCorkle (Eds.), *Psycho-oncology* (3rd ed., pp. 561–566). New York, NY: Oxford University Press.

Reading, A. (2004). *Hope and despair: How perceptions of the future shape human behavior.* Baltimore, MD: Johns Hopkins University Press.

Redinbaugh, E.M., Baum, A., Tarbell, S., & Arnold, R. (2003). End-of-life caregiving: What helps family caregivers cope? *Journal of Palliative Medicine, 6,* 901–909. doi:10.1089/109662103322654785

Regan, T.W., Lambert, S.D., Kelly, B., Falconier, M., Kissane, D., & Levesque, J.V. (2015). Couples coping with cancer: Exploration of theoretical frameworks from dyadic studies. *Psycho-Oncology, 24,* 1605–1617. doi:10.1002/pon.3854

Regan, T.W., Lambert, S.D., Kelly, B., McElduff, P., Girgis, A., Kayser, K., & Turner, J. (2014). Cross-sectional relationships between dyadic coping and anxiety, depression and relationship satisfaction for patients with prostate cancer and their spouses. *Patient Education and Counseling, 96,* 120–127. doi:10.1016/j.pec.2014.04.010

Rottman, N., Hansen, D.G., Nicolaisen, A., Johansen, C., Larsen, P.V., Flyger, H., & Hagedoorn, M. (2015). Dyadic coping within couples dealing with breast cancer: A longitudinal, population-based study. *Health Psychology, 34,* 486–495. doi:10.1037/hea0000218

Rowland, J.H. (1989a). Intrapersonal resources: Coping. In J.C. Holland & J.H. Rowland (Eds.), *Handbook of psychooncology: Psychological care of the patient with cancer* (pp. 44–57). New York, NY: Oxford University Press.

Rowland, J.H. (1989b). Intrapersonal resources: Social support. In J.C. Holland & J.H. Rowland (Eds.), *Handbook of psychooncology: Psychological care of the patient with cancer* (pp. 58–71). New York, NY: Oxford University Press.

Sales, E. (1991). Psychosocial impact of the phase of cancer on the family: An updated review. *Journal of Psychosocial Oncology, 9*(4), 1–17. doi:10.1300/J077v09n04_01

Sales, E., Schulz, R., & Biegel, D. (1992). Predictors of strain in families of cancer patients: A review of the literature. *Journal of Psychosocial Oncology, 10*(2), 1–26. doi:10.1300/J077v10n02_01

Schnoll, R.A., Knowles, J.C., & Harlow, L. (2002). Correlates of adjustment among cancer survivors. *Journal of Psychosocial Oncology, 20*(1), 37–59. doi:10.1300/J077v20n01_03

Schreiber, J.A. (2011). Image of God: Effect on coping and psychospiritual outcomes in early breast cancer survivors. *Oncology Nursing Forum, 38,* 293–301. doi:10.1188/11.ONF.293-301

Sivesind, D.M., & Paire, S. (2009). Coping with cancer: Patient and family issues. In C.C. Burke (Ed.), *Psychosocial dimensions of oncology nursing care* (2nd ed., pp. 1–28). Pittsburgh, PA: Oncology Nursing Society.

Somerfield, M., & Curbow, B. (1992). Methodological issues and research strategies in the study of coping with cancer. *Social Science and Medicine, 34,* 1203–1216. doi:10.1016/0277-9536(92)90313-F

Spencer, S.M., Carver, C.S., & Price, A.A. (1998). Psychological and social factors in adaptation. In J.C. Holland (Ed.), *Psycho-oncology* (pp. 211–219). New York, NY: Oxford University Press.

Stanton, A.L. (2012). What happens now? Psychosocial care for cancer survivors after medical treatment completion. *Journal of Clinical Oncology, 30,* 1215–1220. doi:10.1200/JCO.2011.39.7406

Stanton, A.L. (2015). Positive consequences of the experience of cancer: Perceptions of growth and meaning. In J.C. Holland, W.S. Breitbart, P.N. Butow, P.B. Jacobsen, M.J. Loscalzo, & R. McCorkle (Eds.), *Psycho-oncology* (3rd ed., pp. 630–634). New York, NY: Oxford University Press.

Stanton, A.L., Rowland, J.H., & Ganz, P.A. (2015). Life after diagnosis and treatment of cancer in adulthood: Contributions from psychosocial oncology research. *American Psychologist, 70,* 159–174. doi:10.1037/a0037875

Tallman, B.A. (2013). Anticipated posttraumatic growth from cancer: The role of adaptive and maladaptive coping strategies. *Counseling Psychology Quarterly, 26,* 72–88. doi:10.1080/09515070.2012.728762

Taylor, E.J. (1995). Whys and wherefores: Adult patient perspectives of the meaning of cancer. *Seminars in Oncology Nursing, 11,* 32–40. doi:10.1016/S0749-2081(95)80040-9

Thoits, P.A. (1986). Social support as coping assistance. *Journal of Consulting and Clinical Psychology, 54,* 416–423. doi:10.1037/0022-006X.54.4.416

Thune-Boyle, I.C.V. (2013). Religiousness and spirituality in coping with cancer. In B.I. Carr & J. Steel (Eds.), *Psychological aspects of cancer: A guide to emotional and psychological consequences of cancer, their causes and management* (pp. 129–155). New York, NY: Springer.

Tickoo, R.S., Key, R.K., & Breitbart, W.S. (2015). Cancer-related pain. In J.C. Holland, W.S. Breitbart, P.N. Butow, P.B. Jacobsen, M.J. Loscalzo, & R. McCorkle (Eds.), *Psycho-oncology* (3rd ed., pp. 171–198). New York, NY: Oxford University Press.

Traa, M.J., De Vries, J., Bodenmann, G., & Den Oudsten, B.L. (2015). Dyadic coping and relationship functioning in couples coping with cancer: A systematic review. *British Journal of Health Psychology, 20,* 85–114. doi:10.1111/bjhp.12094

Walch, S.E., Ahles, T.A., & Saykin, A.J. (1998). Neuropsychological impact of cancer and cancer treatments. In J.C. Holland (Ed.), *Psycho-oncology* (pp. 500–505). New York, NY: Oxford University Press.

Walsh, F. (1996). The concept of family resilience: Crisis and challenge. *Family Process, 35,* 261–281. doi:10.1111/j.1545-5300.1996.00261.x

Watson, M., & Greer, S. (1998). Personality and coping. In J.C. Holland (Ed.), *Psycho-oncology* (pp. 91–98). New York, NY: Oxford University Press.

Weisman, A.D., & Worden, J.W. (1976–1977). The existential plight in cancer: Significance of the first 100 days. *International Journal of Psychiatry in Medicine, 7,* 1–15. doi:10.2190/UQ2G-UGV1-3PPC-6387

Weisman, A.D., & Worden, J.W. (1986). The emotional impact of recurrent cancer. *Journal of Psychosocial Oncology, 3*(4), 5–16. doi:10.1300/J077v03n04_03

White, R.W. (1974). Strategies of adaptation: An attempt at systematic description. In G.V. Coelho, D.A. Hamburg, & J.E. Adams (Eds.), *Coping and adaptation* (pp. 47–68). New York, NY: Basic Books.

Wiesel, T.W., & Alici, Y. (2015). Special considerations in older adults with cancer. What psycho-oncologists should know. In J.C. Holland, W.S. Breitbart, P.N. Butow, P.B. Jacobsen, M.J. Loscalzo, & R. McCorkle (Eds.), *Psycho-oncology* (3rd ed., pp. 549–553). New York, NY: Oxford University Press.

Wilkes, L.M., O'Baugh, J., Luke, S., & George, A. (2003). Positive attitude in cancer: Patients' perspectives. *Oncology Nursing Forum, 30,* 412–416. doi:10.1188/03.ONF.412-416

Wynn, J.D. (2015). Difficult personality traits and disorders in oncology. In J.C. Holland, W.S. Breitbart, P.N. Butow, P.B. Jacobsen, M.J. Loscalzo, & R. McCorkle (Eds.), *Psycho-oncology* (3rd ed., pp. 356–366). New York, NY: Oxford University Press.

Yu, Y., & Sherman, K.A. (2015). Communication avoidance, coping, and psychological distress of women with breast cancer. *Journal of Behavioral Medicine, 38,* 565–577. doi:10.1007/s10865-015-9636-3

Zaider, T.I., & Kissane, D.W. (2010). Psychosocial interventions for couples and families coping with cancer. In J.C. Holland, W.S. Breitbart, P.B. Jacobsen, M.S. Lederberg, M.J. Loscalzo, & R. McCorkle (Eds.), *Psycho-oncology* (2nd ed., pp. 483–487). New York, NY: Oxford University Press.

Zaider, T.I., & Kissane, D.W. (2015). Psychosocial interventions for couples and families coping with cancer. In J.C. Holland, W.S. Breitbart, P.N. Butow, P.B. Jacobsen, M.J. Loscalzo, & R. McCorkle (Eds.), *Psycho-oncology* (3rd ed., pp. 526–531). New York, NY: Oxford University Press.

Zeidner, M., & Saklofske, D. (1996). Adaptive and maladaptive coping. In M. Zeidner & N.S. Endler (Eds.), *Handbook of coping: Theory, research, applications* (pp. 505–531). New York, NY: John Wiley.

Zhang, A.Y., & Siminoff, L.A. (2003). The role of the family in treatment decision making by patients with cancer. *Oncology Nursing Forum, 30,* 1022–1028. doi:10.1188/03.ONF.1022-1028

# CHAPTER 5

# Cultural Influences

*Marlon Garzo Saria, PhD, RN, AOCNS®, FAAN*

> *If we are to achieve a richer culture, rich in contrasting values, we must recognize the whole gamut of human potentialities, and so weave a less arbitrary social fabric, one in which each diverse gift will find a fitting place.*
>
> —Margaret Meade

Culture is more than demographics. Edward Burnett Tylor, an English anthropologist, first used the term *culture* in the context of learned human behavior patterns in his book, *Primitive Culture*, published in 1871. He defined culture as "that complex whole which includes knowledge, belief, art, law, morals, custom, and any other capabilities and habits acquired by man as a member of society" (p. 1). In his attempt to describe the nature of culture, Herskovits (1955) stated that culture is the "man-made part of the environment" (p. 17). He supports this by making the following paradoxical statements: (1) Culture is universal in man's experience, yet each local or regional manifestation of it is unique; (2) culture is stable, yet is also dynamic, and manifests constant change; and (3) culture fills and largely determines the course of our lives, yet rarely intrudes into conscious thought (Herskovits, 1955).

Of all those invisible threads and sympathetic fibers that connect one life to another, culture is, perhaps, the most ubiquitous. Culture affects every action and response to the exigencies of life. Cultural fibers are the invisible threads that influence how individuals respond to a cancer diagnosis, treatment, side effects of treatment, living with the disease, and facing death.

Nishimoto and Foley (2001) noted that it is the empathetic appreciation of the patient's background and way of life that supports and enables the provision of culturally competent care. What the cancer experience means to patients and their families cannot be interpreted or understood in isolation; rather, it must be viewed from the cultural context that frames responses to the cancer experience. In many ways, culture functions as a tool for the creation of one's reality and the definition of one's purpose in life within that reality. Culture plays a pivotal role in defining the proper way to behave in a particular situation to maintain integrity and self-respect (Kagawa-Singer, 1998).

The cultural background of an ethnic or racial group influences the knowledge, attitudes, and practices of the group members that, in large part, determine the way members respond to disease prevention, treatment, and health care. When oncology nursing fails to attend to patients' culture and ethnicity, patients can interpret the care as insensitive and inappropriate (Guidry & Walker, 1999).

People form beliefs about health and illness from their unique cultural/racial background and experience. Therefore, knowledge of the cultural identity of patients with cancer and concomitant skill in providing culturally competent care are key. Without understanding how culture and race affect patients' behavioral responses, oncology nurses cannot provide appropriate, competent care.

## Culture in the Nursing Literature

Nursing has distinguished itself as a profession through a legacy of upholding and defending the dignity of every individual. In *Textbook of the Principles and Practice of Nursing*, which is regarded as the first scholarly textbook for nursing, Harmer (1922) described an essential quality of a nurse as "a democratic spirit which leaves class and race prejudice behind. In a hospital it is the aim to give the same kind of care to men, women, and children, to all colors and creeds, rich and poor, enemies and friends" (p. 7). Madeleine Leininger, nursing's foremost authority in cultural care and founder of the worldwide transcultural nursing movement, succinctly stated that "culture refers to a way of life belonging to a designated group of people" (Leininger, 1990, p. 54). *Code of Ethics for Nurses With Interpretive Statements* (American Nurses Association, 2015) leaves no room for doubt about the fundamental principle woven through nursing practice: "respect for the inherent dignity, worth, unique attributes, and human rights of all individuals. The need for and right to health care is universal, transcending all individual differences" (p. 1).

In the time between the publication of Tylor's book in 1871 and the revised *Code of Ethics for Nurses*, a large body of evidence on the profound influence of culture on healthcare experience has been published. In addition, professional organizations have strategically examined issues related to culture. The American Academy of Nursing commissioned an expert panel on culturally competent care from which three monographs, published between 1995 and 1997, expanded the view of culture beyond race and ethnicity and included an emphasis on a spectrum of marginalized and disenfranchised groups that include women, older adults, and sexual minorities (Gray & Thomas, 2005). In their critical analysis of culture, Gray and Thomas (2005) identified a number of common assumptions predominant in the nursing literature (see Figure 5-1).

Historically, provision of care occurred in communities where healthcare professionals and patients belonged to similar racial and ethnic backgrounds. However, the U.S. Census Bureau (2012) projected that the population will be considerably older and more racially and ethnically diverse by 2060:
- The population of adults aged 65 and older is expected to more than double between 2012 and 2060 (43.1 million to 92 million).
- Those aged 85 and older are projected to more than triple (5.9 million to 18.2 million).
- Although the non-Hispanic White population will remain the single largest group, no group will be considered the majority.
- The non-Hispanic White population is projected to peak in 2024 at 199.6 million and slowly decrease, falling by nearly 20.6 million until 2060.
- The Hispanic population would more than double between 2012 and 2016 (53.3 million to 128.8 million).

- All people belong to and are influenced by various features of culture; thus, culture is assumed to be a universal phenomenon.
- Culture exists independently of our perceptions of it; it is an essential feature of human beings and human association.
- Culture is a dynamic and ever-changing process.
- Cultural practices are neutral and inclusive.
- An individual can identify with multiple cultural groups.
- Culture is learned rather than considered an innate or genetic feature of human life; ways of learning about culture are extensive and both overt and covert.
- Cultural groups can be identified and constituted based on distinct characteristics that differentiate one group from another.
- Although there may be some variation within a culture, significant common patterns of cultural expression exist within a given culture.
- Culture can only be understood through knowing similarities and differences between groups.
- Culture can be represented in cultural guidebooks outlining information about a given geographic region or geopolitical entity (e.g., locations, religions, languages, ethnic compositions, ethnic or race-specific diseases, infant feeding practices, child rearing practices).
- Culture has a major effect on health and illness.

**Figure 5-1. Common Cultural Assumptions Predominant in Nursing Literature**

*Note.* Based on information from Gray & Thomas, 2005.

- The African American population is expected to increase from 41.2 million to 61.8 million.
- The Asian population is projected to more than double, from 15.9 million in 2012 to 34.4 million over the same period.
- Minorities, now 37% of the U.S. population, are projected to comprise 57% of the population by 2060.

In order to effectively address the needs of patients, healthcare providers must appreciate the influence of culture on health care. It is indispensable to approach every healthcare encounter with a conscious effort to recognize cultural variations in the individual response to health and illness. Every encounter between providers and recipients of care presents the opportunity for the interface of different cultures. Weaving together multiple cultures influences healthcare behavior that ultimately affects adherence to the plan of care, satisfaction, healthcare use, and outcomes (Bussey-Jones & Genao, 2003).

The U.S. population is a fluid and dynamic mix of cultural and ethnic groups. Diversity within groups, variance in levels of acculturation and adaptation, socioeconomic status, and religious backgrounds also contribute to this rich mosaic. As a result, oncology nurses will inevitably work with patients and clients from diverse cultural and ethnic backgrounds. Although this is exciting, it also is challenging because the population is ever growing, both in number and diversity.

Globalization has fostered diversity around the world, particularly in the United States, the world's leading destination country for immigrants since the 19th century. This unique characteristic of a country being constantly built and rebuilt by immigrants has earned it the description of a "permanently unfinished country." The United States often has been referred to as "the great melting pot," a metaphor that describes the integration of many cultures, languages, and demographics into a single American identity. This metaphor, however, fails to capture the slow, arduous, and often contentious process by which individuals of diverse backgrounds blend in with the U.S. society (U.S. Department of State, 2010). The processes by which individuals become part of a society are outlined in Figure 5-2.

- **Socialization** is the process by which members become part of a society by learning what is important and acceptable within a society, such as how to live, work, and become an accepted member. Socialization to the norms of the middle and upper class has significant impact on health status and access to health in many countries.
- **Enculturation** is a natural process of learning accepted cultural norms, values, and roles in society, and achieving competence in one's culture. Enculturation can be through formal educational apprenticeship, mentorship, role modeling, and so forth.
- **Acculturation** involves changes when people from different cultures interact with each other over time. Changes occur in both directions, although the newcomer will usually change more than the people in the established culture. Successful adaptation to the new culture by learning the appropriate behavior of the host culture can take time.
- **Assimilation** is a blending of cultural heritage and the new host culture. It involves developing a new cultural identity, and one takes on the worldview of the new culture over time.

**Figure 5-2. Processes by Which Individuals Become Part of Society**

*Note.* Based on information from Andrews et al., 2010.

## Culturally Defined Health Disparities

It generally is believed that identity development with respect to social categories (e.g., ethnicity and race, gender, religion) is socially constructed and not transcendent or innately acquired. Cultures have an arbitrary and unique way of classifying members into different social categories, usually involving customs and traditions that dictate how to move individuals between categories (i.e., rites of passage) (Andrews et al., 2010). Governments and states construct social categories that can be contested and remain variable over time, as in the case of the use of national census that prescribes social categories, some of which may not be congruent with an individual's self-identification (Andrews et al., 2010). These social categories are often included as variables in health services research to identify not only social inequities in health but also the differences in human responses to health. They have been explored to identify inequalities in the full health–illness continuum across the lifespan. Specific to cancer, an abundance of reports establish inequalities in the primary prevention, early detection and secondary prevention, diagnosis and treatment, and palliative care for cancer and other cancer-related health conditions and behaviors that affect health services outcomes and effectiveness (e.g., economics and cost-effectiveness, epidemiology, survival, burden of cancer).

## Country of Birth and Citizenship

In 2013, foreign-born residents and citizens of the United States made up 12.9% of the population (U.S. Census Bureau, 2013). Although disparities in health outcomes between foreign-born and U.S.-born residents (also categorized as immigrants and non-immigrants) have been documented in the literature, the extent to which foreign-born or immigrant status contribute to these disparities is not clearly understood. Siddiqi, Zuberi, and Nguyen (2009) examined the relationship between known disparities in healthcare access and insurance between immigrants and non-immigrants in the United States and concluded that health insurance is a critical factor for explaining disparities in access to health care between immigrants and non-immigrants. Within the immigrant population, disparities related to citizenship status have also been documented. "Immigrants who are not U.S. citizens are less likely to receive employer-sponsored health insurance or government coverage." (Carrasquillo, Carrasquillo, & Shea, 2000; Singh, Rodriguez-Lainz, & Kogan, 2013). With respect to average annual medical expenditures, Ku (2009) reported that, although immigrants were less likely than non-immigrants to be publicly insured, they had lower public and private medical expenditures. In addition, immigrants had lower medical utilization (i.e., they had fewer medical visits, inpatient admissions, outpatient hospital visits, and emergency medical visits) (Ku, 2009).

Foreign birth has been explored as one of the variables that contribute to disparities in U.S. cancer screening. Considering this, screening rates of foreign-born residents will become increasingly important as the proportion of foreign-born residents who belong to the age group recommended to be screened for breast and colorectal cancers (Reyes & Miranda, 2015). A study by Goel et al. (2003) suggested that foreign birth might explain the disparities in cancer screening previously attributed to race and ethnicity. Another study reported that one of the consistent findings among different ethnic groups in California was the association of longer time in the United States with increased use of breast and cervical cancer screening (Chawla, Breen, Liu, Lee, & Kagawa-Singer, 2015). A recent study exploring the role of tumor biology did not detect any difference in survival with foreign-born and U.S.-born women with estrogen receptor/progesterone receptor–positive (ER/PR-positive) breast cancer; however, survival was significantly worse for foreign-born women with ER/PR-negative breast cancer compared to those born in the United States. Although no significant differences were found in treatment options and tumor size that may account for decreased survival among ER/PR-negative foreign-born women, stage at diagnosis was significantly more advanced, reflecting issues related to access to care, screening, or appropriate insurance coverage (Camacho-Rivera, Kalwar, Sanmugarajah, Shapira, & Taioli, 2014).

In 2010, the Patient Protection and Affordable Care Act (ACA), which was designed to improve healthcare access for all legal U.S. residents, was signed into law. Implementation of the ACA resulted in a decrease of 16 million nonelderly uninsured legal U.S. residents by 2016 and provided expanded healthcare access for millions more. By eliminating access barriers, the ACA is presumed to increase the availability and use of preventive and treatment services, contributing to achieving the goal of better health outcomes and reduced health disparities that disproportionately affect minorities (O'Keefe, Meltzer, & Bethea, 2015). As of the time of this publication, the future of the ACA remains to be determined.

# Ethnicity and Race

Andrews et al. (2010) distinguished ethnicity from race by describing it as more than biologic identification that involves commitment and participation in cultural customs and rituals. *Ethnicity* is defined as the perception of belonging to a single or multiple ethnic groups. *Race* is the category used to classify people in groups based on skin color. Data on ethnicity and race are still collected by federal agencies (census) and in clinical trials, despite being recognized as nonanthropologic or non-scientifically-based designations (see Figure 5-3). Additionally, the Human Genome Project, an international scientific research project, publicized as early as 2000 that no genetic basis existed for race and that only 0.01% of genetic variations accounted for differences between humans (Andrews et al., 2010).

Ethnic and racial differences in health care have been well established, prompting U.S. Congress in 1999 to commission the Health and Medicine Division of the National Acade-

**Categories for Race**
- **American Indian or Alaska Native**—A person having origins in any of the original peoples of North and South America (including Central America), and who maintains tribal affiliation or community attachment.
- **Asian**—A person having origins in any of the original peoples of the Far East, Southeast Asia, or the Indian subcontinent including, for example, Cambodia, China, India, Japan, Korea, Malaysia, Pakistan, the Philippine Islands, Thailand, and Vietnam.
- **African American**—A person having origins in any of the black racial groups or Africa. Terms such as *Haitian* or *Negro* can be used in addition to *Black* or *African American*.
- **Caucasian**—A person having origins in any of the original peoples of Europe, the Middle East, or North Africa.
- **Native Hawaiian and Other Pacific Islander**—A person having origins in any of the original peoples of Hawaii, Guam, Samoa, or other Pacific Islands.

**Categories for Ethnicity**
- **Hispanic or Latino**—A person of Cuban, Mexican, Puerto Rican, South or Central American, of other Spanish culture or origin, regardless of race. The term *Spanish origin* can be used in addition to *Hispanic* or *Latino*.
- **Not Hispanic or Latino**—A person who is not of Hispanic, Latino, or Spanish origin.

**Figure 5-3. Revised Standards for the Classification of Federal Data on Race and Ethnicity**

*Note.* Based on information from Smedley et al., 2003.

mies of Sciences, Engineering, and Medicine (formerly the Institute of Medicine [IOM]) to explore the extent of disparities that cannot be attributed to other factors. These additional factors included access-related issues or clinical needs, preferences, and appropriateness of intervention (Smedley, Stith, & Nelson, 2003). Unfortunately, health disparities have persisted, and in some cases, have increased in recent years. In a study exploring the reasons for disparities in breast cancer mortality in Chicago, Smedley et al. (2003) reported that breast cancer mortality among African American women in Chicago has not decreased since 1980. As a matter of fact, it has increased compared to the large decrease in mortality seen in New York City and the United States in general. Furthermore, Ansell et al. (2009) stated that "the growing Black/White breast cancer mortality disparity in Chicago cannot be easily attributed to biologic or comorbid differences between Blacks and Whites but suggests that differential screening and treatment are contributors" (p. 1686). A study in Florida found strong evidence of racial disparities in non-small cell lung cancer survival; however, results were atypical in that Asians had better survival when compared to Caucasians (Tannenbaum, Koru-Sengul, Zhao, Miao, & Byrne, 2014).

The National Institutes of Health has stepped up its efforts to eliminate health disparities and uphold equality among all people by promoting the inclusion of minorities and underserved groups in clinical trials. It is important to include people from all racial and ethnic groups in cancer studies, as this will provide more data on culturally appropriate interventions that could reduce racial and ethnic disparities in healthcare (Salman, Nguyen, Lee, & Cooksey-James, 2015).

## American Indian or Alaska Native

Compared with the general population, disparities in health status and mortality have persisted among the American Indian/Alaska Native (AIAN) populations. Overall cancer mortality was higher, mostly influenced by lung cancer death rates, which have shown minimal improvement among AIANs compared to Caucasians (White et al., 2014). Data on mortality from colorectal cancer also revealed regional disparities, with Alaska Natives experiencing a threefold greater mortality rate than AIANs in the southwest. When examined as a whole, no measurable progress was found in colorectal cancer death rates among AIANs compared to the improvement in colorectal cancer death rates among Caucasians (White et al., 2014). It also has been noted that colorectal cancer screening disparities have persisted among AIANs compared to Caucasians and African Americans even after accounting for factors related to access to care (Johnson-Jennings, Tarraf, Hill, & González, 2014). Breast cancer outcomes have been reported to be worse among AIANs, as evidenced by higher death rates in Alaska and the Southern Plains, lack of improvement in breast cancer death rate trends, and poorer survival indicators. All of these factors may be associated with the lower prevalence of mammography use among AIAN women compared to Caucasian women (White et al., 2014).

Although AIAN men were less likely to develop prostate cancer, their mortality rate was higher compared to Caucasian men. Increased screening services for cervical cancer has greatly reduced mortality among AIANs, and efforts to further improve screening practices and expand the use of human papillomavirus vaccines are expected to contribute to this success (White et al., 2014).

## Asians

Asians are one of the fastest growing ethnic minority groups in the United States. Healthcare disparities observed among this group have been attributed to multiple factors, including sociocultural orientation, poorer continuity of care, previous experiences across the healthcare system, expectations, and culturally mediated response behavior (Palmer et al., 2014). Asians are also one of the most ethnically diverse groups (Chang, Chan, & Han, 2014). Asians have been reported to have comparable education, socioeconomic status, and income to non-Hispanic Whites. Statistically significant differences in cancer health disparities between the groups were found to be of little clinical significance. One study found evidence of statistically significant better cancer-specific survival in Asians even after adjusting for factors known to affect survival outcomes (Trinh et al., 2015). Asian Americans have also been reported to have the lowest mortality rate from breast, colorectal, lung, and prostate cancer (Aizer et al., 2014).

Among the different subgroups, certain healthcare behaviors may influence the perceived or actual disparities. One example is how Chinese patients view their physicians, as authority makes these patients less inclined to ask a question or to question their recommendations. This can lead to potentially unmet needs that affect their perception of the quality of care they receive (Palmer et al., 2014). A qualitative study documented the fatalism in some Asian subcultures; quietly accepting a breast cancer diagnosis reflected as a seemingly passive involvement in their own care. In the same study, the investigators explored the role of patient–provider communication in perceived quality of care and found that, although improving communication between physicians and patients can help improve perceived quality of care, addressing communication alone would not be enough to close the disparities gap (Palmer et al., 2014).

Asians, along with Blacks/African Americans, have been reported to be disproportionately underscreened for colorectal cancer despite recommendations for screening in all Americans over 50 years of age. Although data showed that Asian Americans were more likely to forego screening, further analysis revealed that nonadherence was mainly attributed to the lack of screening recommendation from the providers (May, Almario, Ponce, & Spiegel, 2015).

## African Americans

Factors such as a decrease in smoking prevalence rates, increased cancer screening, and more effective cancer treatments contributed to a decline in cancer mortality by gender and race in the United States between 2000 and 2010; however, African American men and women were reported to have higher age-adjusted mortality rates for breast, colorectal, lung, and prostate cancers, with the exception of lower lung cancer mortality in women, when compared with Caucasians (O'Keefe et al., 2015). Similar to the data presented for other ethnic groups, healthcare disparities have been reported in African Americans, even after adjusting for other demographic and treatment variables. Among all major ethnic groups, these disparities do not appear to be diminishing when examined over time (1988–2007) (Aizer et al., 2014).

One study examining the disparities in stage at diagnosis, delivery of definitive therapy, and cancer-specific mortality in head and neck cancers found that African Americans were significantly more likely to present with metastatic cancer, less likely to receive definitive treatment, and have a higher risk of head and neck cancer–specific mortality compared to the rest of the study participants (Mahal, Inverso, Aizer, Bruce Donoff, & Chuang, 2014). Another study examining the disparity in prostate cancer–specific mortality among African Americans found a 12% increased relative risk for prostate cancer–specific mortality compared with Caucasian men even after adjusting for sociodemographic factors and known prostate cancer prognostic factors. Despite the higher risk, African Americans received treatment with the intent to cure less often (18%) than compared to Caucasian men. This magnitude of disparity did not change over time in the study (Aizer et al., 2014; Mahal, Aizer, et al., 2014).

A review of multiple studies exploring symptom severity in relation to ethnicity revealed inconclusive evidence. Some studies showed that African American cancer survivors tended to report less symptom distress. Other studies reported that African American men were more likely to report more severe symptoms when compared to Caucasians. Still, other studies reported no ethnic differences in symptom scores among the major ethnic groups (Finney et al., 2015).

It has been suggested that later stage at diagnosis and less adherence or acceptance of proposed treatment options have contributed to the observed disparities. These factors (i.e., delayed presentation and variability in treatment decision making among African Americans) need to be explicated in future studies (O'Keefe et al., 2015).

## Native Hawaiians and Other Pacific Islanders

Cancer disparities among Native Hawaiians and Other Pacific Islanders (NHOPI) have been explored, but the lack of annual population estimates for specific subgroups within the NHOPI population serves as a barrier in understanding the burden of cancer for this ethnic group. Liu et al. (2013) reviewed the data for nearly 20,000 Native Hawaiian, Samoan, and Guamanian/Chamorro cancer cases from 13 Surveillance, Epidemiology, and End Results program registries from 1990–2008 and reported the following key findings: (a) notable differences were found in cancer incidence rates between NHOPI subgroups and Caucasians, (b) cancer-specific incidence trends vary by degree and direction within NHOPI subgroups, (c) cancer trends continue to rise among Samoans and Guamanians/Chamorros, and (d) observed differences were found in cancer incidence rates between Native Hawaiians in Hawaii and those on the mainland.

When compared to Caucasians, NHOPIs were reported to share the same burden of common cancers (i.e., breast, colorectal, lung, and prostate). However, data have consistently shown higher risks for stomach, liver, and uterus cancers in the NHOPI population (Liu et al., 2013). Additionally, cancer survival rates were worse among Pacific Islanders, an observation that has been associated with the lower socioeconomic status of Pacific Islanders. Similarly, Samoans were found to have poorer cancer survival and higher stage at diagnosis, even after adjusting for disease severity, a finding that may indicate delayed diagnosis and suboptimal treatment after diagnosis (Goggins & Wong, 2007). For primary cancer prevention, a study describing the attitudes of Samoan women toward mammography and breast cancer found that Samoans view cancer as a death sentence and sickness as unpreventable and noted their use of traditional healers. These factors may contribute to less adherence to screening recommendations and less attention to early warning signs of cancer (Goggins & Wong, 2007).

Disparities among NHOPIs are consistent with known data on their socioeconomic status; that is, NHOPIs are economically and educationally disadvantaged compared to Caucasians; however, the relationship of their socioeconomic status compared to African Americans and Native Americans is less clear (Goggins & Wong, 2007).

## Religion

Although the population of U.S. adults grew from 227 million in 2007 to 245 million in 2014, the percentage of adults identifying as Christians declined from 178 million (78% of the population in 2007) to 173 million. Meanwhile, 56 million adults now identify as religiously unaffiliated, an increase of about 19 million since 2007, making them second only to Evangelical Protestants in size and more numerous than Catholics or mainline Protestants (Pew Research Center, 2017). It has been reported that one of the factors for the growth of the religiously unaffiliated group is generational replacement. As more millennials enter adulthood, they display a significantly lower level of religious affiliation, with 36% of young millennials (ages 18–24) and 34% of older millennials (ages 25–33) identifying as religiously unaffiliated. In addition, approximately 25% of Gen Xers do not identify with any particular religion or describe themselves as atheists or agnostics, representing an increase of 4% in seven years. Likewise, some baby boomers have been identified as religiously unaffiliated in recent years (Pew Research Center, 2017).

Patients with cancer use their religious beliefs to cope with the cancer diagnosis and the reality of living with cancer. Some may view religion as a mediator to diminish disease burden and facilitate healthy coping. In addition, the more tangible benefit from religion is the social support obtained from fellow believers. It has been documented that cancer patients find meaning in their suffering and believe that prayers are helpful, despite having doubts when prayers are considered unanswered (Caplan, Sawyer, Holt, & Brown, 2014). In a study that explored the potential influence of fatalistic beliefs and religion on cancer screening among Hispanic Catholics of Puerto Rican and Dominican origin, the investigators reported that fatalistic attitudes were infrequently expressed and that Catholic doctrine encouraged health behaviors and supported the use of health care (Leyva et al., 2014). Another study looking at the association between the rates of Pap testing and religion-related factors in American Muslim women reported that negative religious coping (view of illness as punishment from God) is associated with lower rates of Pap testing (Caplan et al., 2014).

## Gender, Gender Identity, and Sexual Orientation

One of the significant public health omissions linked to culture is the enduring lack of national surveillance data on cancer among sexual minorities. In 2011, IOM called attention to the inadequacy of national data, estimating cancer incidence and prevalence among lesbian, gay, bisexual, transgender, and queer/questioning (LGBTQ) individuals. IOM published a report that highlighted the absence of cancer data in the lesbian population (Rosario et al., 2014). For the purpose of this chapter, definitions for terms such as *sex, gender, gender identity, gender expression*, and *sexual orientation* can be found in Figure 5-4.

Gender differences in health behavior have long been established. Studies have shown that healthcare utilization of women, including both well and sick visits, is higher compared to men. These differences have been attributed to many factors, including distinct services (e.g., reproductive health needs), higher levels of morbidity, illness perception, and health-seeking behaviors (Everett & Mollborn, 2014). However, even when sex differences in healthcare needs have been accounted for, gender disparities still persist. Disparities cannot directly be attributed to biologic factors but are in part the product of social factors associated with gender identity and performance (Everett & Mollborn, 2014).

The estimated 5%–10% of the U.S. population that identifies as LGBTQ faces disparities in health care associated with denial of their civil and human rights, discrimination, increased incidence of violence and victimization, and societal stigma (Brown & Mayer, 2015; Grant, 2010; U.S. Department of Health and Human Services, 2017). Access to health care; increased incidence of anxiety, depression, and suicide; higher rates of sexually transmitted diseases; predisposition to cigarette smoking, alcohol abuse, and recreational drug use; and lower rates of cancer screening are some of the measurable outcomes of healthcare disparities faced by the LGBTQ community (Brown & Mayer, 2015; Joint Commission, 2014; Quinn, Schabath, Sanchez, Sutton, & Green, 2015).

Gender disparities have been recorded among those in the LGBTQ community as well. Women in the LGBTQ community are more likely to report unmet medical needs com-

---

- **Sex** refers to a person's biological status and is typically categorized as male, female, or intersex (i.e., atypical combinations of features that usually distinguish male from female). There are a number of indicators for biological sex, including sex chromosomes, gonads, internal reproductive organs, and external genitalia.
- **Gender** refers to the attitudes, feelings, and behaviors that a given culture associates with a person's biological sex. Behavior that is compatible with cultural expectations is referred to as gender normative; behaviors that are viewed as incompatible with these expectations constitute gender nonconformity.
- **Gender identity** refers to "one's sense of oneself as male, female, or transgender" (APA, 2006). When one's gender identity and biological sex are not congruent, the individual may identify as transsexual or as another transgender category.
- **Gender expression** refers to the "way in which a person acts to communicate gender within a given culture; for example, in terms of clothing, communication patterns, and interests. A person's gender expression may or may not be consistent with socially prescribed gender roles, and may or may not reflect his or her gender identity" (APA, 2008, p. 28).
- **Sexual orientation** refers to the sex of those to whom one is sexually and romantically attracted. Categories of sexual orientation typically have included attraction to members of one's own sex (gay men or lesbians), attraction to members of the other sex (heterosexuals), and attraction to members of both sexes (bisexuals). Although these categories continue to be widely used, research has suggested that sexual orientation does not always appear in such definable categories and instead occurs on a continuum. In addition, some research indicates that sexual orientation is fluid for some people; this may be especially true for women.

**Figure 5-4. Definitions of Terms**

APA—American Psychological Association

*Note.* From "Guidelines for Psychological Practice With Lesbian, Gay, and Bisexual Clients," by American Psychological Association, 2012, *American Psychologist, 67,* p. 11. Copyright 2011 by American Psychological Association. Reprinted with permission.

pared to heterosexual women. There have been no differences reported between sexual minority and heterosexual men (Everett & Mollborn, 2014). It also has been reported in the literature that healthcare use by gender can vary across sexual orientation identities. A study on healthcare use revealed that women who identify with a feminine gender identity are more likely to make regular gynecologic visits than lesbians who identify with a more masculine gender identity (Everett & Mollborn, 2014).

Certain cancer risk behaviors are reported to be higher among sexual minorities. These behaviors likely may have developed during adolescence and persisted through behavioral reinforcement and neurobiologic reward circuits over the years. Risk categories found to be higher among sexual minority youths include substance abuse, sexual behaviors, diet, and physical activity (Rosario et al., 2014).

Among transgender individuals, cancer incidence rates are largely unknown. Cancer screening requires a modified approach, as most recommendations lack information specific or relevant to transgender individuals (Levitt, 2015). In addition, transgender patients may find healthcare navigation more complex as a result of healthcare providers' consistent use of gendered language and documentation, lack of specialized knowledge about surgery and hormones, and gender-segregated systems, which can be exacerbated by issues with insurance coverage for gender-specific care (Levitt, 2015).

The healthcare industry is recognizing the unique needs of sexual minorities, and progress is being made, albeit slowly. In 2014, the Joint Commission released a field guide to help facilitate patient and family engagement and foster effective communication between healthcare providers and sexual minorities (available at www.jointcommission.org/lgbt). In February 2015, the American Academy of Nursing expert panel on LGBTQ—whose members (known as "fellows") are nursing's most accomplished leaders in education, management, practice, and research—published a policy brief titled "Same-Sex Partnership Rights: Health Care Decision Making and Hospital Visitation" in which the organization declared its strong support for the rights of LGBTQ people in hospital visitation for their partners and children. In April 2015, the Oncology Nursing Society, a professional organization of more than 39,000 members committed to promoting excellence in oncology nursing and the transformation of cancer care, endorsed this policy brief.

## Culturally Competent Care

In the current landscape, cultural competence is viewed as an indispensable tool in providing patient-centered care; however, this has not always been the case. In the 1970s, cultural competence was missing from virtually all government policies, regulatory standards, academic curricula, or professional practice (Palos, 2015).

The role of culture in the lives of individuals is undisputedly significant. Many trivial day-to-day and transformative life-changing decisions are affected by culture and the perspective that it has imprinted on the individual (Delgado et al., 2013). Culturally competent care, comprising awareness, communication, and respect, should be inherent to all providers of care (Muñoz-Antonia, 2014). Cultural competence expands to providers having an "attitude of empathy for others, an attitude of curiosity, an attitude of basic respect for self and others, and an acknowledgment of the intrinsic value of all humans" (Delgado et al., 2013, p. 204).

Within the landscape of changing demographics and cancer healthcare disparities, oncology nurses need to maintain competence in providing culturally appropriate care. Culture is important in determining patients' responses to the cancer experience. It must be included as part of valid assessment. No care provider is exempt from responsibility and accountability to give culturally competent care. Cultural assessment is not merely an assessment of patients but an assessment of self, family, and support for people who may be involved in the care. Nurses need to explore their own worldviews and examine their personal cultural beliefs, values, biases, and prejudices before attempting to understand their patients (Ali, 1996). The need to increase diversity within the oncology nursing workforce has never been greater. That fact notwithstanding, oncology nurses from all cultural backgrounds must develop cultural assessment skills to communicate in culturally appropriate ways. Table 5-1 presents guidelines for practicing culturally competent nursing care (Douglas et al., 2014).

### Table 5-1. Guidelines for the Practice of Culturally Competent Nursing Care

| Guideline | Description |
| --- | --- |
| 1. Knowledge of Cultures | Nurses shall gain an understanding of the perspectives, traditions, values, practices, and family systems of culturally diverse individuals, families, communities, and populations they care for, as well as knowledge of the complex variables that affect the achievement of health and well being. |
| 2. Education and Training in Culturally Competent Care | Nurses shall be educationally prepared to provide culturally congruent health care. Knowledge and skills necessary for assuring that nursing care is culturally congruent shall be included in global health care agendas that mandate formal education and clinical training, as well as required ongoing, continuing education for all practicing nurses. |
| 3. Critical Reflection | Nurses shall engage in critical reflection of their own values, beliefs, and cultural heritage in order to have an awareness of how these qualities and issues can impact culturally congruent nursing care. |
| 4. Cross-Cultural Communication | Nurses shall use culturally competent verbal and nonverbal communication skills to identify client's values, beliefs, practices, perceptions, and unique health care needs. |
| 5. Culturally Competent Practice | Nurses shall utilize cross-cultural knowledge and culturally sensitive skills in implementing culturally congruent nursing care. |
| 6. Cultural Competence in Health Care Systems and Organizations | Health care organizations should provide the structure and resources necessary to evaluate and meet the cultural and language needs of their diverse clients. |
| 7. Patient Advocacy and Empowerment | Nurses shall recognize the effect of health care policies, delivery systems, and resources on their patient populations, and shall empower and advocate for their patients as indicated. Nurses shall advocate for the inclusion of their patient's cultural beliefs and practices in all dimensions of their health care. |
| 8. Multicultural Workforce | Nurses shall actively engage in the effort to ensure a multicultural workforce in health care settings. One measure to achieve a multicultural workforce is through strengthening of recruitment and retention efforts in the hospitals, clinics, and academic settings. |

*(Continued on next page)*

| Guideline | Description |
|---|---|
| 9. Cross-Cultural Leadership | Nurses shall have the ability to influence individuals, groups, and systems to achieve outcomes of culturally competent care for diverse populations. Nurses shall have the knowledge and skills to work with public and private organizations, professional associations, and communities to establish policies and guidelines for comprehensive implementation and evaluation of culturally competent care. |
| 10. Evidence-Based Practice and Research | Nurses shall base their practice on interventions that have been systematically tested and shown to be the most effective for the culturally diverse populations that they serve. In areas where there is a lack of evidence of efficacy, nurse researchers shall investigate and test interventions that may be the most effective in reducing the disparities in health outcomes. |

Table 5-1. Guidelines for the Practice of Culturally Competent Nursing Care *(Continued)*

*Note.* From "Guidelines for Implementing Culturally Competent Nursing Care," by M.K. Douglas, M. Rosenkoetter, D.F. Pacquiao, L.C. Callister, M. Hattar-Pollara, J. Lauderdale, ... L. Purnell, 2014, *Journal of Transcultural Nursing, 25,* p. 110. Copyright 2014 by The Authors. Reprinted with permission from SAGE Publications.

## Conclusion

It is impossible to overemphasize the importance of culture in determining patients' responses to the cancer experience; culture cannot be even minimally understood without careful, valid assessment. No care provider is exempt from responsibility and accountability to give culturally competent care. The need to increase diversity in the oncology nursing workforce is ever before us. Oncology nurses from all cultural backgrounds must hone and develop cultural assessment skills to communicate in culturally appropriate ways.

Oncology nurses who adopt the principles of culturally competent care will be less vulnerable to the natural tendencies of ethnocentrism and stereotyping. They will be more likely to engage in ongoing, open communication that fosters valid assessment of culture and its relative influence on patients' responses to the cancer experience. As the diversity of the United States increases, the need for culturally competent care is even more critical. Oncology nurses must resolve to do things differently to make culturally competent care in oncology nursing practice a priority and a reality for all people with cancer.

*The author would like to acknowledge DeLois P. Weekes, RN, BS, MS, DNSc, for her contribution to this chapter from the previous edition of this book.*

## References

Aizer, A.A., Wilhite, T.J., Chen, M.H., Graham, P.L., Choueiri, T.K., Hoffman, K.E., ... Nguyen, P.L. (2014). Lack of reduction in racial disparities in cancer-specific mortality over a 20-year period. *Cancer, 120,* 1532–1539. doi:10.1002/cncr.28617

Ali, N.S. (1996). Providing culturally sensitive care to Egyptians with cancer. *Cancer Practice, 4,* 212–215.

American Nurses Association. (2015). *Code of ethics for nurses with interpretive statements*. Silver Spring, MD: Author.
American Psychological Association. (2006). Answers to your questions about transgender individuals and gender identity. Retrieved from http://www.apa.org/topics/transgender.html
American Psychological Association. (2008). *Report of the APA Task Force on Gender Identity and Gender Variance*. Retrieved from http://www.apa.org/pi/lgbt/resources/policy/gender-identity-report.pdf
Andrews, M., Backstrand, J.R., Boyle, J.S., Campinha-Bacote, J., Davidhizar, R.E., Doutrich, D., ... Zoucha, R. (2010). Chapter 3. Theoretical basis for transcultural care. *Journal of Transcultural Nursing, 21*(Suppl. 4), 53S–136S. doi:10.1177/1043659610374321
Ansell, D., Grabler, P., Whitman, S., Ferrans, C., Burgess-Bishop, J., Murray, L.R., ... Marcus, E. (2009). A community effort to reduce the black/white breast cancer mortality disparity in Chicago. *Cancer Causes and Control, 20*, 1681–1688. doi:10.1007/s10552-009-9419-7
Brown, C., & Mayer, D.K. (2015). Are we doing enough to address the cancer care needs of the LGBT community? *Clinical Journal of Oncology Nursing, 19*, 242–243. doi:10.1188/15.CJON.242-243
Bussey-Jones, J., & Genao, I. (2003). Impact of culture on health care. *JAMA, 95*, 732–735.
Camacho-Rivera, M., Kalwar, T., Sanmugarajah, J., Shapira, I., & Taioli, E. (2014). Heterogeneity of breast cancer clinical characteristics and outcome in US black women—effect of place of birth. *Breast Journal, 20*, 489–495. doi:10.1111/tbj.12302
Caplan, L., Sawyer, P., Holt, C., & Brown, C.J. (2014). Religiosity after a diagnosis of cancer among older adults. *Journal of Religion, Spirituality, and Aging, 26*, 357–369. doi:10.1080/15528030.2014.928922
Carrasquillo, O., Carrasquillo, A.I., & Shea, S. (2000). Health insurance coverage of immigrants living in the United States: Differences by citizenship status and country of origin. *American Journal of Public Health, 90*, 917–923. doi:10.2105/AJPH.90.6.917
Chang, E., Chan, K.S., & Han, H.-R. (2014). Factors associated with having a usual source of care in an ethnically diverse sample of Asian American adults. *Medical Care, 52*, 833–841. doi:10.1097/MLR.0000000000000187
Chawla, N., Breen, N., Liu, B., Lee, R., & Kagawa-Singer, M. (2015). Asian American women in California: A pooled analysis of predictors for breast and cervical cancer screening. *American Journal of Public Health, 105*, e98–e109. doi:10.2105/AJPH.2014.302250
Delgado, D.A., Ness, S., Ferguson, K., Engstrom, P.L., Gannon, T.M., & Gillett, C. (2013). Cultural competence training for clinical staff: Measuring the effect of a one-hour class on cultural competence. *Journal of Transcultural Nursing, 24*, 204–213. doi:10.1177/1043659612472059
Douglas, M.K., Rosenkoetter, M., Pacquiao, D.F., Callister, L.C., Hattar-Pollara, M., Lauderdale, J., ... Purnell, L. (2014). Guidelines for implementing culturally competent nursing care. *Journal of Transcultural Nursing, 25*, 109–121. doi:10.1177/1043659614520998
Everett, B.G., & Mollborn, S. (2014). Examining sexual orientation disparities in unmet medical needs among men and women. *Population Research and Policy Review, 33*, 553–577. doi:10.1007/s11113-013-9282-9
Finney, J.M., Hamilton, J.B., Hodges, E.A., Pierre-Louis, B.J., Crandell, J.L., & Muss, H.B. (2015). African American cancer survivors: Do cultural factors influence symptom distress? *Journal of Transcultural Nursing, 26*, 294–300. doi:10.1177/1043659614524251
Goel, M.S., Wee, C.C., McCarthy, E.P., Davis, R.B., Ngo-Metzger, Q., & Phillips, R.S. (2003). Racial and ethnic disparities in cancer screening: The importance of foreign birth as a barrier to care. *Journal of General Internal Medicine, 18*, 1028–1035. doi:10.1111/j.1525-1497.2003.20807.x
Goggins, W.B., & Wong, G.K. (2007). Poor survival for US Pacific Islander cancer patients: Evidence from the Surveillance, Epidemiology, and End Results database: 1991 to 2004. *Journal of Clinical Oncology, 25*, 5738–5741. doi:10.1200/JCO.2007.13.8271
Grant, J. (2010). *Outing age 2010: Public policy issues affecting lesbian, gay, bisexual and transgender elders*. New York, NY: National Gay and Lesbian Task Force Policy Institute.
Gray, D.P., & Thomas, D. (2005). Critical analysis of "culture" in nursing literature: Implications for nursing education in the United States. *Annual Review of Nursing Education, 3*, 249–270.
Guidry, J.J., & Walker, V.D. (1999). Assessing cultural sensitivity in printed cancer materials. *Cancer Practice, 7*, 291–296. doi:10.1046/j.1523-5394.1999.76005.x
Harmer, B. (1922). *Textbook of the principles and practice of nursing*. New York, NY: MacMillan.
Herskovits, M.J. (1955). *Cultural anthropology*. New York, NY: Random House.
Johnson-Jennings, M.D., Tarraf, W., Hill, K.X., & González, H.M. (2014). United States colorectal cancer screening practices among American Indians/Alaska Natives, blacks, and non-Hispanic whites in the new millennium (2001 to 2010). *Cancer, 120*, 3192–3299. doi:10.1002/cncr.28855
Joint Commission. (2014). *Advancing effective communication, cultural competence, and patient- and family-centered care for the lesbian, gay, bisexual, and transgender (LGBT) community*. Retrieved from http://www.jointcommission.org/assets/1/18/LGBTFieldGuide.pdf

Kagawa-Singer, M. (1998). The cultural context of death rituals and mourning practices. *Oncology Nursing Forum, 25,* 1752–1756.

Ku, L. (2009). Health insurance coverage and medical expenditures of immigrants and native-born citizens in the United States. *American Journal of Public Health, 99,* 1322–1328. doi:10.2105/AJPH.2008.144733

Leininger, M.M. (1990). The significance of cultural concepts in nursing. *Journal of Transcultural Nursing, 2,* 52–59. doi:10.1177/104365969000200108

Levitt, N. (2015). Clinical nursing care for transgender patients with cancer. *Clinical Journal of Oncology Nursing, 19,* 362–366. doi:10.1188/15.CJON.362-366

Leyva, B., Allen, J.D., Tom, L.S., Ospino, H., Torres, M.I., & Abraido-Lanza, A.F. (2014). Religion, fatalism, and cancer control: A qualitative study among Hispanic Catholics. *American Journal of Health Behavior, 38,* 839–849. doi:10.5993/AJHB.38.6.6

Liu, L., Noone, A.M., Gomez, S.L., Scoppa, S., Gibson, J.T., Lichtensztajn, D., … Miller, B.A. (2013). Cancer incidence trends among native Hawaiians and other Pacific Islanders in the United States, 1990–2008. *Journal of the National Cancer Institute, 105,* 1086–1095. doi:10.1093/jnci/djt156

Mahal, B.A., Aizer, A.A., Ziehr, D.R., Hyatt, A.S., Sammon, J.D., Schmid, M., … Nguyen, P.L. (2014). Trends in disparate treatment of African American men with localized prostate cancer across National Comprehensive Cancer Network risk groups. *Urology, 84,* 386–392. doi:10.1016/j.urology.2014.05.009

Mahal, B.A., Inverso, G., Aizer, A.A., Bruce Donoff, R., & Chuang, S.K. (2014). Impact of African-American race on presentation, treatment, and survival of head and neck cancer. *Oral Oncology, 50,* 1177–1181. doi:10.1016/j.oraloncology.2014.09.004

May, F.P., Almario, C.V., Ponce, N., & Spiegel, B.M. (2015). Racial minorities are more likely than Whites to report lack of provider recommendation for colon cancer screening. *American Journal of Gastroenterology, 110,* 1388–1394. doi:10.1038/ajg.2015.138

Muñoz-Antonia, T. (2014). Don't neglect cultural diversity in oncology care. *Journal of the National Comprehensive Cancer Network, 12*(Suppl. 5), 836–837.

Nishimoto, P.W., & Foley, J. (2001). Cultural beliefs of Asian Americans associated with terminal illness and death. *Seminars in Oncology Nursing, 17,* 179–189. doi:10.1053/sonu.2001.25947

O'Keefe, E.B., Meltzer, J.P., & Bethea, T.N. (2015). Health disparities and cancer: Racial disparities in cancer mortality in the United States, 2000–2010. *Frontiers in Public Health, 3,* 51. doi:10.3389/fpubh.2015.00051

Palmer, N.R., Kent, E.E., Forsythe, L.P., Arora, N.K., Rowland, J.H., Aziz, N.M., … Weaver, K.E. (2014). Racial and ethnic disparities in patient-provider communication, quality-of-care ratings, and patient activation among long-term cancer survivors. *Journal of Clinical Oncology, 32,* 4087–4094. doi:10.1200/JCO.2014.55.5060

Palos, G.R. (2015). Celebrating ONS's 40th anniversary and its commitment to cultural competency, diversity, and inclusiveness. *Clinical Journal of Oncology Nursing, 19,* 228–229. doi:10.1188/15.CJON.228-229

Pew Research Center. (2017). America's changing religious landscape. Retrieved from http://www.pewforum.org/2015/05/12/americas-changing-religious-landscape

Quinn, G.P., Schabath, M.B., Sanchez, J.A., Sutton, S.K., & Green, B.L. (2015). The importance of disclosure: Lesbian, gay, bisexual, transgender/transsexual, queer/questioning, and intersex individuals and the cancer continuum. *Cancer, 121,* 1160–1163. doi:10.1002/cncr.29203

Reyes, A.M., & Miranda, P.Y. (2015). Trends in cancer screening by citizenship and health insurance, 2000–2010. *Journal of Immigrant and Minority Health, 17,* 644–651. doi:10.1007/s10903-014-0091-y

Rosario, M., Corliss, H.L., Everett, B.G., Reisner, S.L., Austin, S.B., Buchting, F.O., & Birkett, M. (2014). Sexual orientation disparities in cancer-related risk behaviors of tobacco, alcohol, sexual behaviors, and diet and physical activity: Pooled youth risk behavior surveys. *American Journal of Public Health, 104,* 245–254. doi:10.2105/AJPH.2013.301506

Salman, A., Nguyen, C., Lee, Y.H., & Cooksey-James, T. (2015). A review of barriers to minorities' participation in cancer clinical trials: Implications for future cancer research. *Journal of Immigrant and Minority Health, 18,* 447–453. doi:10.1007/s10903-015-0198-9

Siddiqi, A., Zuberi, D., & Nguyen, Q.C. (2009). The role of health insurance in explaining immigrant versus nonimmigrant disparities in access to health care: Comparing the United States to Canada. *Social Science and Medicine, 69,* 1452–1459. doi:10.1016/j.socscimed.2009.08.030

Singh, G.K., Rodriguez-Lainz, A., & Kogan, M.D. (2013). Immigrant health inequalities in the United States: Use of eight major national data systems. *Scientific World Journal, 2013,* 1–21. doi:10.1155/2013/512313

Smedley, B.D., Stith, A.Y., & Nelson, A.R. (Eds.). (2003). *Unequal treatment: Confronting racial and ethnic disparities in health care.* Washington, DC: National Academies Press.

Tannenbaum, S.L., Koru-Sengul, T., Zhao, W., Miao, F., & Byrne, M.M. (2014). Survival disparities in non-small cell lung cancer by race, ethnicity, and socioeconomic status. *Cancer Journal, 20,* 237–245. doi:10.1097/PPO.0000000000000058

Trinh, Q.D., Nguyen, P.L., Leow, J.J., Dalela, D., Chao, G.F., Mahal, B.A., ... Aizer, A.A. (2015). Cancer-specific mortality of Asian Americans diagnosed with cancer: A nationwide population-based assessment. *Journal of the National Cancer Institute, 107*(6), djv054. doi:10.1093/jnci/djv054

Tylor, E.B. (1871). *Primitive culture: Researches into the development of mythology, philosophy, religion, art, and custom.* London, England: Bradbury and Evans.

U.S. Census Bureau. (2012). U.S. Census Bureau projections show a slower growing, older, more diverse nation a half century from now. Retrieved from http://www.census.gov/newsroom/releases/archives/population/cb12-243.html

U.S. Census Bureau. (2013). Selected social characteristics in the United States: 2009–2013: American community survey 5-year estimates. Retrieved from http://factfinder.census.gov/faces/tableservices/jsf/pages/productview.xhtml?pid=ACS_13_5YR_DP02&src=pt

U.S. Department of Health and Human Services. (2017). Healthy People 2020: Lesbian, gay, bisexual, and transgender health. Retrieved from https://www.healthypeople.gov/2020/topics-objectives/topic/lesbian-gay-bisexual-and-transgender-health

U.S. Department of State. (2010). Becoming American: Beyond the melting pot. *eJournalUSA, 15*(9). Retrieved from http://photos.state.gov/libraries/amgov/30145/publications-english/EJ-immigration0110.pdf

White, M.C., Espey, D.K., Swan, J., Wiggins, C.L., Eheman, C., & Kaur, J.S. (2014). Disparities in cancer mortality and incidence among American Indians and Alaska Natives in the United States. *American Journal of Public Health, 104*(Suppl. 3), S377–S387. doi:10.2105/AJPH.2013.301673

**CHAPTER 6**

# Fatigue

*Edith O'Neil-Page, MSN, RN, AOCNS®, and
Linda M. Gorman, RN, MN, PMHCNS-BC, CHPN, FPCN*

> *Sometimes I wonder who I am anymore. I am so tired. I don't have the energy to get up or get dressed, let alone go to work or care for my family. Cancer changes everything!*
>
> —Patient with cancer during treatment

Cancer-related fatigue (CRF) is a universal experience of people with cancer that has been clinically researched and explored. Forty percent of patients report CRF at diagnosis. It frequently is the first symptom identified and often motivates patients to seek medical consultation (Hofman, Ryan, Figueroa-Moseley, Jean-Pierre, & Morrow, 2007). Throughout the diagnosis and treatment process, fatigue often continues and may intensify. The degree of fatigue experienced by the person with cancer varies. For some, fatigue may simply be a bothersome symptom; for others, it may be completely debilitating. It negatively affects well-being and quality of life and requires recognition as part of psychosocial and physical care. Because of the devastating impact of CRF, oncology practitioners need to incorporate assessments and interventions for fatigue (just as is expected for pain or anemia).

## Defining Cancer-Related Fatigue

Before defining CRF, it is important to differentiate it from fatigue unrelated to cancer. In a healthy population, general fatigue is a protective response to physical or psychological stress in that it promotes and stimulates restorative rest (Neefjes, van der Vorst, Blauwhoff-Buskermolen, & Verheul, 2013). General fatigue may be chronic or acute. Although significant, it generally does not affect quality of life to the same extent as CRF (Tralongo, Respini, & Ferraù, 2003). Fatigue as an acute symptom generally includes having a rapid onset associated with physical stressors. This is accompanied by symptoms of short duration and often relieved by rest and/or medication. Chronic fatigue may exhibit physical or mental symptoms and may be difficult to relieve (Tralongo et al., 2003).

The National Comprehensive Cancer Network® (NCCN®, 2017b) defines *CRF* as "a distressing, persistent, subjective sense of physical, emotional, and/or cognitive tiredness or exhaustion related to cancer or cancer treatment that is not proportional to recent activity and interferes with usual functioning" (p. 1).

CRF is of greater magnitude than what one would expect and is generally not relieved by rest—leaving the patient with an overwhelming and sustained sense of exhaustion. CRF may persist longer than the diagnosis and treatment of cancer itself (Neefjes et al., 2013). It continues for months and even years following completion of treatment in approximately one-third of patients with cancer (Hofman et al., 2007; Jones et al., 2016). In addition to rest or sleep not relieving fatigue, some patients report an inability to sleep thus experiencing shortened, interrupted sleep (Horneber, Fischer, Dimeo, Rüffer, & Weis, 2012).

CRF is qualitatively different from the fatigue experienced by the general population. Unlike fatigue, CRF occurs in the absence of physical exertion (Morrow, Andrews, Hickok, Roscoe, & Matteson, 2002). Symptoms of CRF develop over time and may result from the cumulative effects of treatment (e.g., chemotherapy, radiation, surgery), which can continue for years following active treatment (Mitchell, 2010). CRF is also associated with emotional distress, depression, anxiety, insomnia, and diminished physical capabilities. Loss or diminished cognitive function may result in functional disabilities and lead to a reduction or loss of employment, which could significantly affect economic and family relationships (Keeney & Head, 2011).

CRF significantly affects quality of life (Alici, Bower, & Breitbart, 2015; Barsevick, Frost, Zwinderman, Hall, & Halyard, 2010; Weis, 2011). CRF contributes to physical and mental fatigue, reduced activity and motivation, and decreased social function. All of these fall within the domain of quality of life. Patients often report fatigue as the most distressing experience, outweighing even pain (Barsevick et al., 2010; Berger et al., 2015). With cancer survivors living longer, the effect of ongoing fatigue is a major concern.

Statements used to describe CRF often convey feelings (e.g., "I do not care what happens."), cognitive impact (e.g., "I am so tired I cannot think."), or perceived condition (e.g., "I do not have enough energy to eat."). Because some descriptors of fatigue can be vague or very subjective, CRF can remain an elusive symptom. Because of its prolonged nature, it can be ubiquitous, leading to clinicians not always addressing it as they would acute symptoms such as pain (Stasi, Abriani, Beccaglia, Terzoli, & Amadori, 2003). Research related to CRF can be very challenging because of its elusive nature, poor recognition by providers, and a lack of consensus in definition and treatment (Aaronson et al., 2014). Alici et al. (2015) suggested that CRF is a multidimensional symptom involving the entire person and affecting every facet of daily life. It can progressively interfere with a patient's physical and social activities, resulting in withdrawal from normal activities. The experience of CRF may be as part of a symptom cluster, which may include a variety of other distressing symptoms, such as nausea and depression. CRF has a motivational component in addition to the physical and psychological factors, which adds to the challenge of defining it (Alici et al., 2015).

# Epidemiology

CRF is the most common reported symptom among patients with cancer. It is highly prevalent in all cancer populations and nearly universal in patients receiving cancer treatment (Hofman et al., 2007; NCCN, 2017b). CRF is a distressing cancer-related symptom with a greater negative effect on daily activities and quality of life than other cancer-related symptoms, including pain and depression (Jones et al., 2016). A majority of patients diagnosed and treated for cancer report fatigue symptoms at some point along the continuum. Many patients experience the psychosocial effects of fatigue as an extremely frustrating loss of identity. CRF knows no boundaries, affecting all ages and populations. A majority of patients with cancer experience fatigue as a response to disease or treatment in all cancer diagnoses. This fatigue has a profound effect on both physical and psychosocial function (Aaronson et al., 2014). Jones et al. (2016) studied breast, colorectal, and prostate populations and found that patients with breast and colorectal cancer had significantly higher levels of fatigue. Bower (2014) reported the strongest and most consistent predictor of post-treatment fatigue to be pretreatment fatigue. In 2006, Bower et al. found approximately 34% of study participants reported significant fatigue at 5–10 years after diagnosis. Fatigue also is a major contributor to increased dependence in older adults (Luciani et al., 2008).

Despite oncology professionals being aware of the wide-ranging effects of fatigue on patients and their families, it continues to be often unrecognized and undertreated (Mitchell et al., 2014; NCCN, 2017b). The absence of a clear, consistent definition of CRF and its prolonged nature can delay initiation of appropriate treatment modalities.

## Older Adults

In comparing CRF to fatigue in the general population, Butt et al. (2010) investigated the effect of age and cancer diagnosis on ratings of fatigue. They used the Functional Assessment of Chronic Illness Therapy–Fatigue (FACIT-F) to measure the fatigue experience and its effect on daily life using a scale of 0 (severe fatigue) to 52 (no fatigue) on a sample size of 1,075 participants. Results indicated that the patient with cancer experienced more severe fatigue than the general population. Across the overall sample of patients with cancer and the general population, age showed a statistically significant but somewhat modest increase in fatigue. This study also demonstrated that patients with advanced cancer ranked fatigue as the most important symptom they experienced. One commonality of fatigue is anemia. The older adult patient with cancer is particularly vulnerable to fatigue, with a greater likelihood of comorbidities and frailty. Giacalone et al. (2013) found that only a few studies have specifically examined the effect of fatigue on this population.

## Pediatric Issues

The treatment of cancer in children has expanded rapidly; progress and technological advances have extended life expectancy through an increasing number of treatments. Fatigue is a major issue for both children and adolescents with cancer (Erickson et al., 2010; Nunes, Jacob, Adlard, Secola, & Nascimento, 2015). Treatments may lead to numerous side effects, of which fatigue is most common. CRF may cause physical and/or psychosocial problems in children due to their limited energy and resultant inability to play games and engage with others. This negatively affects growth and development. CRF also can cause irritability and depression, as well as problems with concentration. Additional effects of fatigue include altered muscle metabolism, endocrine dysfunction, circadian disruption, and anemia (Miller, Jacob, & Hockenberry, 2011). Although fatigue is most common, more attention is often paid to more obvious, uncomfortable symptoms, such as nausea, vomiting, pain, hair loss, and decreased appetite. Healthcare professionals identify signs of fatigue as symptom clusters in children; mood changes, lethargy, decreased appetite, exhaustion, and disinterest may be indicators of fatigue (Yilmaz, Taş, Muslu, Başbakkal, & Kantar, 2010). Research identifies cancer treatment (chemotherapy, radiation, and bone marrow transplantation) as critical factors in inducing fatigue in children. Assessment of CRF in children and adolescents remains challenging and significant because of its effect on quality of life.

# Etiology

The etiology of CRF can be linked to cancer biology as well as the result of treatment—both negatively influencing quality of life (Barsevick et al., 2010). CRF in patients with cancer is multifactorial and may be influenced by a variety of demographic, medical, psychosocial, behavioral, and biologic factors (Bower, 2014).

# Pathophysiology

### Biology

The exact mechanism that causes CRF is unknown (Alici et al., 2015; Hofman et al., 2007). Through the examination of anemia research, a number of biologic and genetic pathways have been identified to clarify and further differentiate biologic markers from behavioral ones (Barsevick et al., 2010). Some potential mechanisms of CRF include inflammatory processes, disruption of the hypothalamic-pituitary-adrenal axis (HPA), metabolic disturbances, and physical deconditioning. Barsevick et al. (2013) noted that the inflammatory process contributing to CRF is by far the most studied mechanism. Tariman and Dhorajiwala (2016) found in their review that inflammatory and immune response pathways, including the neurologic proinflammatory cytokine pathway, have statistically significant association with CRF. Additional biologic mechanisms that may be involved include cytokine and serotonin dysregulation, alterations of adenosine triphosphate (ATP), circadian rhythm disruption, and vagal nerve activation. Cytokine dysregulation can contribute to anemia, cachexia, anorexia, fever, infection, and depression—all of which are associated with fatigue. HPA controls the secretion of cortisol in response to stress and influences the development of immune cells, cytokine production, and the diurnal cycle. Because of inhibition by exposure to cytokines from cancer and cancer therapies, fatigue is associated with low levels of cortisol production.

Another hypothesis on the biologic nature of fatigue addresses the increase of serotonin, or 5-hydroxytryptamine (5-HT), by using a mechanism of proinflammatory cytokines. This complex interaction produces a sensation of decreased activity. ATP is an energy source of muscle mass and dysregulation that can result in peripheral or muscular fatigue. Circadian rhythms play an important role in sleep–wake cycles. Disruption of these cycles can play a significant role in the etiology of fatigue.

### Impaired Muscle Function

This impairment occurs from changes in metabolism, prolonged disuse, muscle wasting, or treatment-related changes (e.g., radiation can alter cell membranes affecting ion transportation). The relationship between neuromuscular function and fatigue in patients with prostate cancer undergoing radiation therapy is supported by Barsevick et al. (2013). The reduced oxygen delivery to muscle cells and the subsequent limitation in the availability of ATP to the mitochondria induced anaerobic metabolism, thus increasing energy expenditure. Subsequently, neuromuscular output decreased with an ensuing accumulation of toxins. Therefore, because the supply of oxygen to mitochondrial muscle fibers is a critical factor in the regulation of energy production, a decreased supply may contribute to the pathogenesis of fatigue (Tralongo et al., 2003).

### *Anemia*

Anemia is highly prevalent in patients with cancer, with more than 40% affected (Knight, Wade, & Balducci, 2004). Anemia may be the direct result of malignancy through suppression of hematopoiesis or because of bleeding, hemolysis, hereditary disease, or any such combination (Knight et al., 2004; NCCN, 2017a). Anemia also is associated with myelosuppressive chemotherapy or radiation therapy by directly impairing hematopoiesis in the bone marrow. NCCN guidelines (2017a) recommend assessment for anemia for patients with a hemoglobin level of 11 g/dl or less.

Anemia related to disease and treatment is a well-researched cause of fatigue (NCCN, 2017a, 2017b). Data in multiple studies have consistently demonstrated a significant and positive relationship between hemoglobin rise and reduction in fatigue. In one study where randomized patients received darbepoetin alfa, erythropoietin, or a placebo, results indicated significant hemoglobin improvement of at least 2 g/dl over a 12-week span was associated with meaningful improvement in fatigue (Cella, Kallich, McDermott, & Xu, 2004).

## Other Causes of Fatigue

### *Cancer Treatment Effects*

Cancer treatment may contribute to CRF. Some examples include opioids for pain, radiation therapy to bone marrow–producing sites, chemotherapy, and side effects of many other medications. The presence of pain also is associated with the increased incidence of fatigue. As pain and fatigue are subjective, complex symptoms, they also have much in common (Alici et al., 2015).

### *Sleep Patterns*

Fatigue may be associated with or caused by altered sleep patterns for patients with cancer (Bower, 2014; NCCN, 2017b). Factors contributing to sleep disturbances include alterations in circadian rhythms, stress and anxiety, and side effects of treatment. Ancoli-Israel, Moore, and Jones (2001) performed a review of the state of the literature examining the relationship between CRF and sleep. Their appraisal attested inadequate or unrefreshing sleep and its possible importance to expression of fatigue to the patients' quality of life and tolerance to treatment. In addition, fatigue resulting from sleep disruption may influence the development of mood disorders and clinical depression (Bower, 2014).

### *Psychosocial Factors*

The symptoms of depression and anxiety may contribute to fatigue. The emotional consequences of a cancer diagnosis and its ensuing treatments can influence and deplete many of the patient's coping resources, leading to poor sleep, poor diet, emotional withdrawal, draining of emotional reserves. Emotional distress (e.g., anxiety, fear, anger, sadness, depression) contributes to patients feeling fatigued (Gélinas & Fillion, 2004). Bower (2014) reported that the tendency to "catastrophize" around the cancer diagnosis may also contribute to CRF. Physical symptoms of CRF can directly and indirectly influence the psychological symptoms associated with quality of life (Duijts et al., 2014; So et al., 2009). Family stress may also influence fatigue. Emotional consequences and psychological burden of fatigue can influence many aspects of the patient's life—from family and social life to work and recreation. For example, patients may experience conflict from the desire or necessity to return to work at the same or previous level of function as soon as possible, weighing desire and necessity with ability prior to diagnosis and treatment. The inability to assume a previous work or role capacity may result in significant loss of self-esteem (Duijts et al., 2014).

## Psychosocial Effects of Cancer-Related Fatigue

Fatigue can affect anything—from financial worries, to a loss of emotional energy and sexual functioning, to sleep. It is a multidimensional symptom affecting all aspects of the patient's life along the cancer trajectory. The magnitude of CRF includes the timing of the experience (temporal dimension), the emotional meaning of fatigue (affective dimension), the physical and psychological symptoms of fatigue (sensory dimension), and the psychosocial effect of the experience (severity dimension) (Ream & Richardson, 1999). One seminal theoretical framework for CRF was proposed by Piper (1997), which led to the development of the Piper Fatigue Scale (PFS). PFS measures fatigue in a variety of subscales. Over the years, its revision as a shorter version is supported in multiple studies across a variety of cancer diagnoses, patient ages, and cultural backgrounds (Piper et al., 1998; Reeve et al., 2012). In addition, Ream and Richardson (1999) provided insight into the multidimensional facets of the fatigue experience for patients. These resources can assist oncology nurses in understanding the psychosocial effect of this symptom. Nursing-oriented models of fatigue in the literature also can be helpful for the oncology nurse to identify the patient's perception of CRF and guide interventions to screen, manage, and reduce this life-altering symptom.

Greenberg (1998) eloquently expressed the emotional effect of the fatigue experience along the cancer continuum. The anxiety and fear common at diagnosis can drain the patient's energy, contributing to fatigue. During treatment, the patient hopes that the loss of energy and endurance are a time-limited price for cure. At other times, fatigue may raise fears that the cancer has recurred or progressed. Most distressing, fatigue may symbolize "progressive debility and waning of life" (Greenberg, 1998, p. 485).

Depression is a common comorbidity with a cancer diagnosis, and fatigue can be a symptom of depression or an outcome of it. Symptom overlap between the two can include sleep disturbance, change in eating patterns, poor concentration, and memory loss. It is important to remember that CRF and depression can occur at the same time (Alici et al., 2015). Depression is usually more associated with hopelessness and feelings of worthlessness, which may not be part of the fatigue picture.

Sexual activity may decrease in patients with cancer for a variety of reasons, including fatigue. Fatigue is a major factor contributing to a general lack of interest or the fear of becoming more fatigued. One survey of patients with ovarian cancer cited lack of interest, physical limitation, and fatigue as reasons why they were sexually inactive (Carmack Taylor, Basen-Engquist, Shinn, & Bodurka, 2004; NCCN, 2017b) (see Chapter 12 for more information on altered sexuality).

## Management of the Patient With Cancer-Related Fatigue

### Assessment

Assessment and screening of fatigue begins at initial diagnosis and continues throughout the cancer continuum, from active treatment through survivorship. The initial assessment includes the whole person: mind, body, and spirit. The interpretation of fatigue is not unlike pain and expressed as a subjective interpretation of stimuli (Alici et al., 2015; Hauser, Rybicki, & Walsh, 2010). In clinical practice, fatigue may be neglected or underdetected because it is a subjective experience assessed by patient self-report (Butt et al., 2013).

NCCN guidelines (2017b) delineate a process for evaluation and treatment. The guidelines recognize that fatigue is a subjective experience that requires assessment using a self-report along with other sources of data. Guidelines for assessment include fatigue screening using a numerical score of 0–10 (much like the numerical pain scale) followed by a focused history and physical examination; assessment of concurrent symptoms and treatable contributing factors; and the presence or absence of comorbidities, including depression, sleep disturbances, poor sleep hygiene, and a poor or inadequate diet.

NCCN identified the following barriers to effective treatment: (a) patient not reporting the symptom due to a belief that it is expected, (b) fear that reporting it will affect cancer treatment, and (c) healthcare professionals not including CRF in the assessment because of a lack of knowledge about treatment. Additional barriers include an overall lack of standardization for the assessment and treatment of this multidimensional symptom (NCCN, 2017b).

A thorough history as part of the assessment uses open-ended questions to identify the patient's perception of the disease, treatment(s), concurrent symptoms, and underlying etiologies. This is followed by a thorough physical examination to identify specific physical causes of fatigue (Borneman, 2013). Because the fatigue experience is subjective, it is important to hear the patient's description of the fatigue and its effect on their life rather than relying on checklists. Symptoms should not be viewed individually but as a part of a cluster of interrelated symptoms (Aaronson et al., 2014). An extensive history allows exploration of all facets of contributing factors of fatigue. Additionally, discussion and assessment of the patient's knowledge of symptoms and openness to ideas of self-management interventions (e.g., adoption of healthier lifestyles such as exercise) are important (Aaronson et al., 2014). Reflection and clarification of self-report during the interview helps to illuminate the patient's fatigue experience and provides an opportunity to identify any associated symptoms (e.g., dyspnea, weakness, somnolence). CRF may be exacerbated by or contribute to other known prevalent symptoms related to cancer, such as pain and psychological distress (NCCN, 2017b).

A pertinent fatigue history should include evaluation of the onset (timing), duration (days versus weeks or months), characteristics (physical, mental, emotional, and spiritual), aggravating and alleviating factors (anxiety, rest), and treatments for fatigue (exercise, medications) that the patient has experienced. The onset and duration of fatigue are especially important to determine the effect on quality of life. The patient should be asked if the fatigue experience is interfering with work, family, or activities of daily living.

The history should assess quality and quantity of rest and sleep patterns to determine if rest and sleep are restorative. Inquiring about sleep aids and other medications (e.g., narcotics, anxiolytics, antiemetics) is important because medications within the treatment profile may contribute to or exacerbate CRF. The nurse needs to inquire about other pharmacologic agents as well, including alcohol, herbal remedies, and recreational drugs. The history must reflect daily activities at home, at work, and socially. It is important to address exercise patterns. Nursing awareness and inquiry of performance status and the use of self-reporting tools measuring mobility and exercise are imperative.

A comprehensive fatigue assessment also includes a thorough review of systems based on current literature, with an evaluation of undiagnosed or unmanaged comorbidities (e.g., cardiac, pulmonary, renal, neurologic, endocrine diseases). Other possible contributing factors (e.g., medications; nutritional status; fluid, electrolyte, and metabolic balance) must be evaluated using a standardized self-reporting tool.

Many screening tools are available to identify fatigue (see Table 6-1). The 0–10 fatigue scale can be readily incorporated in an assessment (NCCN, 2017b). More in-depth tools that address various dimensions of fatigue beyond its severity may also be used (e.g., PFS) (Piper et al., 2008). The patient should be placed at the forefront of the assessment process, as they require continuous evaluation to ensure accurate measurement.

Whitehead (2009) reviewed fatigue measures, the populations using the scales, and the evaluation criteria to assist in clinical decision-making. It is important that nursing professionals become familiar with tools for the evaluation of fatigue and understand the critical value of what and how measurement affects treatment.

Chan, Yates, and McCarthy (2016) found that patients with advanced cancers want to use a number for behaviors to control their fatigue. This study emphasized that self-management strategies be focused on advanced as well as early-stage cancers.

Finally, it is important to include evaluation of symptoms of nausea, vomiting, anorexia, diarrhea, bleeding, pain, menopausal symptoms, anxiety, and depression in the history—all symptoms that may compound the fatigue experience. Other complaints, such as poor concentration or alteration in work or social function, require documentation as well as evaluation of any associated cognitive changes.

**Table 6-1. Fatigue Scales**

| Screening Tool | Dimensions | General Information |
| --- | --- | --- |
| Brief Fatigue Inventory | Severity | Easy to use |
| Visual Analogue Fatigue Scale | Severity | Easy to use |
| Functional Assessment of Chronic Illness Therapy–Fatigue (FACIT-F) | Physical, social, emotional, functional | Longer tool but relatively simple to use. Measures change over time. |
| Piper Fatigue Score-12 | Sensory, behavioral/severity, affective meaning, cognitive/mood | First validated multidimensional scale. Shortened version of original currently in clinical use |
| Schwartz Cancer Fatigue Scale (revised) | Physical/perceptual | This revised tool is shorter than original. |
| Multidimensional Fatigue Symptom Inventory | Physical/perceptual | Long and short versions are available. |

*Note.* Based on information from National Comprehensive Cancer Network, 2017b.

## Treatment

No gold standard currently exists for CRF treatment because of a poor understanding of its etiology. Multifactorial clinical manifestations of CRF involve both psychological and physical components (Butt et al., 2013). Clinical management should aim to correct anemia and other physiologic causes, improve nutrition, manage pain and depression, provide psychosocial support, and introduce an appropriate exercise or activity program. See Figure 6-1 for a list of interventions that the Oncology Nursing Society has found likely to be effective.

- Cognitive behavioral interventions/approach for sleep
- Energy conservation and activity management
- Ginseng
- Management of concurrent symptoms
- Massage/aromatherapy massage
- Mindfulness-based stress reduction
- Multicomponent rehabilitative intervention
- Psychoeducation/psychoeducational interventions
- Yoga

**Figure 6-1. Oncology Nursing Society Putting Evidence Into Practice Interventions: Likely to Be Effective for Fatigue Management**

*Note.* From "Putting Evidence Into Practice: Fatigue," by S.A. Mitchell, T.A. Albrecht, M.O. Alkaiyat, K. Browne, J.C. Clark, R.M. DeGennaro, ... B.M. Weisbrod, 2016. Retrieved from https://www.ons.org/practice-resources/pep/fatigue. Copyright 2016 by Oncology Nursing Society. Reprinted with permission.

## *Pharmacologic Interventions*

Pharmacologic interventions include psychostimulants (e.g., methylphenidate), antidepressants (e.g., paroxetine), wakefulness-promoting agents (e.g., modafinil), and corticosteroids. Methylphenidate has shown mixed results. Bruera et al. (2013) found no difference from placebo; however, NCCN (2017b) recommended its inclusion if other causes of fatigue are ruled out.

According to some studies, the treatment of anemia using erythropoietin appears to have an effect on reducing fatigue through the increase of hemoglobin-stimulating factors. Use of hemoglobin-stimulating factors continues to remain controversial, as it is related to possible adverse events (e.g., promotion of tumor growth and/or emboli). As a result, guidelines include recommendations to defer administration until hemoglobin is less than 10 g/dl.

Use of complementary, alternative medicines, including supplements and herbs, is currently undergoing study. Ginseng is shown to produce some benefit (Fouladbakhsh, Balneaves, & Jenuwine, 2013; Mitchell et al., 2016; NCCN, 2017b). CRF is also emerging as a dose-limiting toxicity associated with established and newer therapies, including targeted agents such as tyrosine kinase inhibitors, that can ultimately limit the effectiveness of treatment (Cornelison, Jabbour, & Welch, 2012).

## *Nonpharmacologic Interventions*

Nonpharmacologic interventions include physical activity and psychosocial therapies. Mitchell et al. (2016) noted that exercise is the only intervention with solid evidence of benefits. Physical activity enhancement involves some form of exercise, either walking or movement. Effectiveness increases with intensity and timing. Programs include both supervised and home-based programs; some reports indicate that supervised programs have improved results (Berger et al., 2015). Findings demonstrate positive results with inclusion of psychosocial interventions of stress management, psychoeducation, cognitive behavioral therapy, and supportive therapies used for patients with CRF (Alici et al., 2015).

In addition, mind–body interventions have also been found useful (Appling, Scarvalone, MacDonald, McBeth, & Helzlsouer, 2012; NCCN, 2017b). These interventions can include relaxation, mindfulness, yoga, and therapeutic touch (Aghabati, Mohammadi, & Esmaiel, 2010). Chan et al. (2016) found that their study group used self-management approaches of distraction, relaxation, and resting during the day without falling asleep.

## Nursing Management of Cancer-Related Fatigue

Nursing interventions need to include a comprehensive assessment that comprises screening for risk factors. Nursing management incorporates a variety of educational and supportive approaches to address fatigue.

### *Education*

The primary intervention for fatigue should always be education. Prior to beginning fatigue-inducing treatments, NCCN guidelines (2017b) recommend educating all patients about the expected pattern and duration of fatigue associated with their specific illness state and treatment(s). Every patient receiving treatment requires education and information that some degree of fatigue may occur during therapy. Symptom interpretation is not to be associated with disease progression or treatment inadequacy or failure. In addition, fatigue is a real and multidimensional experience requiring identification and treatment.

By incorporating education and counseling regarding the patterns of fatigue that typically occur during specific treatment protocols, patients are likely to be less stressed by the fatigue and better equipped to cope with it (Mock, 2001). Education also needs to include information regarding treatments.

### *Evaluation and Treatment of Anemia*

Oncology practitioners treating anemia must investigate different causes such as bleeding, hematologic toxicity from cancer treatment, vitamin or mineral deficiencies, or anemia of chronic disease. A more accurate investigation requires a complete blood count; peripheral blood cytology; vitamin $B_{12}$ assay; folate, iron, transferrin, ferritin, and erythropoietin levels; and a Coombs direct and indirect test. If inconclusive, a bone marrow biopsy may be required. Therapeutic interventions may include blood transfusions, administration of recombinant human erythropoietin, and interventions to support patient symptoms (Hurter & Bush, 2007). If treatment of anemia does not resolve the patient's experience of fatigue and no other physiologic cause can be identified (e.g., sleep deprivation), then nonpharmacologic behavioral interventions should be initiated (Mock, 2001).

### *Nutritional Evaluation*

A full nutrition consultation and evaluation by a registered dietitian can provide management strategies to improve overall nutritional status. Strategies can manage deficiency states resulting from symptoms of anorexia, nausea, vomiting, diarrhea, or constipation. Approaches that may prove helpful include suggestions of frequent small meals or drinks, proposing alternative eating times or places, encouraging healthy shopping and cooking habits, and providing education on high-protein supplements.

### *Restorative Therapy*

Restorative therapy activity focuses on the sensory dimension of the fatigue experience (Mock, 2001). These interventions prevent "attentional fatigue" (e.g., inability to concentrate, focus attention, or problem solve). Relaxation activities such as walking or sitting in a natural environment, tending plants and gardening, bird-watching, or viewing nature can improve recovery and promote healing through tension and fatigue reduction (Valdres, Escalante, & Manzullo, 2001). Similar activities such as listening to music, watching television, or reading may be helpful in combating fatigue through relaxation and distraction (Mock, 2001). Meditation may reduce stress that contributes to CRF. Bower et al. (2015) found mindful meditation to be helpful in the relief of fatigue in breast cancer survivors.

Restorative yoga is also receiving recognition by enhancing concentration as well as providing stress relief. The nurse can promote these restorative activities on a regular basis through primary and group experience programs.

### *Energy Conservation*

Oncology nurses can educate and counsel patients on how to conserve energy, especially during peak treatment times, such as the first few days after chemotherapy or several weeks into radiation treatment. Energy conservation is the deliberate and planned management of one's personal energy resources to prevent depletion (NCCN, 2017b). Energy conservation strategies include planning, delegating, setting priorities, pacing, resting, and scheduling activities that require high energy use at times of peak energy. Balancing rest and activity during times of high fatigue allows for maintenance of adequate energy to perform valued activities and reach important goals (Mitchell et al., 2016). Nurses can help patients to prioritize their activities by scheduling high-priority activities at times when energy levels are at their highest (e.g., early morning) and scheduling rest and nap periods during the day when appropriate. Delegating high-energy responsibilities to others includes giving the patient permission to ask for needed help and support from family members and friends.

### *Sleep Hygiene*

Sleep patterns should be included in the assessment, and sleep hygiene should be part of standardized teaching when patients report fatigue or sleep difficulties. Daytime napping may be a strategy but should be limited to less than one hour a day so as not to interfere with nighttime sleep (NCCN, 2017b). Nonpharmacologic interventions for insomnia include avoidance of caffeine and other stimulants, relaxation measures, cognitive behavioral approaches (e.g., challenging negative thoughts), and analysis of the sleep environment. These can be incorporated into the patient's routine.

### *Exercise*

Exercise can reduce CRF among patients during and following cancer treatment (Mitchell et al., 2016; NCCN, 2017b; Puetz & Herring, 2012). Extensive studies indicate the benefit of exercise in randomized controlled trials and indicate effective treatment of fatigue.

Recommendations by NCCN (2017b) include individualized exercise programs that take into account the patient's age, type of cancer, and fitness level. Nurses are instrumental to patient education and exercise and are responsible for assisting patients to problem solve and establish a workable exercise routine. All exercise programs need to take into consideration the patient's condition, comorbidities, and any treatment-related complications, such as bone metastasis or thrombocytopenia, that may require alterations in the recommendations. Most beneficial to the patient may be the recommendation to remain active by carrying out usual activities such as household chores and walking, and then tailoring an increase in exercise based on pretreatment levels, age, and interest (Ream & Richardson, 1999). Although patients may intuitively want to rest to relieve fatigue, the opposite appears to be true (Keeney & Head, 2011). Nurses may assist in personal activity plans to promote gradual increase in activity.

### *Recognition of Depression*

Clinically, depression contributes to both physical and emotional fatigue. It is vital for the oncology nurse to assess separately, then together, the common signs and symptoms of both depression and CRF and the possible interface for each patient who presents with overlapping complaints (e.g., insomnia, anorexia, stress, anxiety). When clinical depression is suspected, the underlying problem should be treated with continued evaluation of fatigue as the patient's mood lifts with supportive therapy. Greenberg (1998) provided a simple example to help differentiate depression from CRF. If the patient states, "I'm too tired," then this implies that the patient has the desire but does not feel that they have the stamina required to carry out an activity. This is most likely related to fatigue versus a depressive state, where the patient lacks the desire because of anhedonia, loss of interest, and resultant fatigue. Antidepressants may be effective in increasing depressed mood, which may increase energy. See Chapter 17 for more interventions on depression. Use of cognitive behavioral approaches can provide structure to challenge negative thoughts and support positive behaviors.

### *Emotional Support*

NCCN (2017b) guidelines recommend counseling patients with cancer and referring them to available resources for the management of stress, depression, anxiety, and other emotions that can aggravate fatigue. Recommended resources include support groups, individual counseling, psychoeducational programs that teach coping strategies, stress management training, and tailored behavioral interventions (e.g., I Can Cope®). The cause-and-effect interrelationships between fatigue, emotional distress, insomnia, and depression and anxiety are not clearly defined, yet the correlation between fatigue and emotional distress in patients with cancer is positive (Mock, 2001). Participating in supportive group therapy or learning new coping strategies should be encouraged as fatigue may decrease perception and experience. Along with coping skills training and imagery/hypnosis, cognitive behavioral therapy has improved the cancer-related symptoms of pain, fatigue, and sleep disturbance by challenging negative thoughts (Borneman, 2013).

## Evidence-Based Practice

Balneaves et al. (2014) studied nine women, all breast cancer survivors, who undertook a 24-week exercise program (focus group) for weight reduction. The study interventions included a lifestyle intervention focused on reframing dietary habits and exercise. Participants received a reduced-calorie diet and an exercise program of 150 minutes per week of moderate to vigorous aerobics. Although the purpose of the study was to promote weight loss, the results indicated increased aerobic fitness, strength, stamina, and energy levels. Whether or not they met the weight loss goal, all women reported improved physical benefits. Although this study did not specifically set out to measure fatigue, the results may indicate an improvement toward that end. Griffie and Godfroy (2014) implemented a walking track in their outpatient cancer center to offer easy access to exercise in a supervised environment. Their project led to improved assessment and documentation of disease states.

Fatigue may also improve with psychological support. A small study by Ream, Gargaro, Barsevick, and Richardson (2015) found that providing motivational interviewing by telephone to patients with cancer reduced fatigue severity and distress. A pilot study by Nooner, Dwyer, DeShea, and Yeo (2016) also demonstrated that the use of relaxation and guided imagery can lead to improvement in fatigue and sleep disturbances in patients with cancer.

## Case Study

Ruth is a single 40-year-old woman who works as a schoolteacher with a challenging group of fifth graders. After beginning cancer treatment for her stage II breast cancer, Ruth struggles to keep up her usual lifestyle and responsibilities. She leaves school each day to drive through traffic to get to her radiation therapy appointment on time. When she returns home to plan the next day's lesson, she frequently falls asleep at her desk at 3 am. Because of her fatigue, she begins to decline all social events and stops exercising. She finds that she sleeps more but does not awake refreshed. The radiation therapy advanced practice nurse (APN) notices that Ruth appears tense and harried on each visit. The APN makes an appointment with Ruth after one of her treatments to better identify coping skills and to determine the effect the radiation has had on Ruth's lifestyle. Ruth reports her level of fatigue as 9 out of 10. When the APN expresses concern about this, Ruth believes she just has to push through and everything will improve when radiation is completed. An additional four weeks of radiation therapy is scheduled.

### Discussion

Ruth was struggling with fatigue related to her cancer treatment. She did not incorporate any lifestyle changes to help her better cope with it. The APN provided education on the cause of the fatigue and discussed the need to incorporate fatigue management into her lifestyle rather than avoiding it. Primarily, Ruth was encouraged to seek out some assistance at her school to ease her workload. By not sharing her situation and needs, colleagues did not offer any assistance.

After Ruth informed a few of her colleagues of her situation and they began offering to drive her to her radiation therapy appointments, she found she could conserve her energy and have more free time at home. Her colleagues were more than eager to help once they knew what she was going through. By involving others, Ruth could incorporate regular short walks on the weekend and sometimes during her lunch hour. Some strategies to improve her sleep included decompressing an hour prior to bedtime rather than working on schoolwork. By addressing her fatigue, Ruth was also able to verbalize her need for social support to face the cancer and its treatment, which is important in coping with the cancer.

## Conclusion

CRF is the most common symptom associated with the diagnosis of cancer. Research shows significant improvements in the recognition, treatment, and management of CRF; however, further studies are necessary to identify the unique complex mechanisms and pathways to identify treatment targets.

Patients continue to experience the physical effects of CRF from diagnosis through treatment and often long after treatment ends. CRF is a consequential problem interfering with physical, psychological, emotional, social, and economic function. It requires early recognition and identification of symptoms combined with education and support that effects necessary lifestyle changes. Exercise is a major component in successful relief of fatigue. Oncology nurses play important roles in the assessment, treatment, intervention, education, and support for successful management of CRF. In addition, continued clinical research is necessary to identify both physiologic and behavioral components of CRF and its effect on the quality of life of patients.

*The authors would like to acknowledge Mady C. Stovall, RN, MSN, ONP, OCN®, and Mercedes K. Young, RN, MSN, ONP, for their contributions to this chapter from the previous edition of this book.*

# References

Aaronson, N.K., Mattioli, V., Minton, O., Weis, J., Johansen, C., Dalton, S.O., ... van de Poll-Franse, L.V. (2014). Beyond treatment—Psychosocial and behavioural issues in cancer survivorship research and practice. *European Journal of Cancer Supplements, 12,* 54–64. doi:10.1016/j.ejcsup.2014.03.005

Aghabati, N., Mohammadi, E., & Esmaiel, Z.P. (2010). The effect of therapeutic touch on pain and fatigue of cancer patients undergoing chemotherapy. *Evidence-Based Complementary and Alternative Medicine, 7,* 375–381. doi:10.1093/ecam/nen006

Alici, Y., Bower, J.E., & Breitbart, W.S. (2015). Fatigue. In J.C. Holland, W.S. Breitbart, P.N. Butow, P.B. Jacobsen, M.J. Loscalzo, & R. McCorkle (Eds.), *Psycho-oncology* (3rd ed., pp. 209–219). New York, NY: Oxford University Press.

Ancoli-Israel, S., Moore, P., & Jones, V. (2001). The relationship between fatigue and sleep in cancer patients: A review. *European Journal of Cancer Care, 10,* 245–255. doi:10.1007/s00520-005-0861-0

Appling, S.E., Scarvalone, S., MacDonald, R., McBeth, M., & Helzlsouer, K.J. (2012). Fatigue in breast cancer survivors: The impact of a mind-body medicine intervention. *Oncology Nursing Forum, 39,* 278–286. doi:10.1188/12.ONF.278-286

Balneaves, L.G., Van Patten, C., Truant, T.L.O., Kelly, M.T., Neil, S.E., & Campbell, K.L. (2014). Breast cancer survivors' perspectives on a weight loss and physical activity lifestyle intervention. *Supportive Care in Cancer, 22,* 2057–2065. doi:10.1007/s00520-014-2185-4

Barsevick, A.M., Frost, M., Zwinderman, A., Hall, P., & Halyard, M. (2010). I'm so tired: Biological and genetic mechanisms of cancer-related fatigue. *Quality of Life Research, 19,* 1419–1427. doi:10.1007/s11136-010-9757-7

Barsevick, A.M., Irwin, M.R., Hinds, P., Miller, A., Berger, A., Jacobsen, P., ... Cella, D. (2013). Recommendations for high-priority research on cancer-related fatigue in children and adults. *Journal of the National Cancer Institute, 105,* 1432–1440. doi:10.1093/jnci/djt242

Berger, A.M., Mooney, K., Alvarez-Perez, A., Breitbart, W.S., Carpenter, K.M., Cella, D., ... Smith, C. (2015). Cancer-related fatigue, version 2.2015. *Journal of the National Comprehensive Cancer Network, 13,* 1012–1039.

Borneman, T. (2013). Assessment and management of cancer-related fatigue. *Journal of Hospice and Palliative Nursing, 15,* 77–86. doi:10.1097/NJH.0b013e318286dc19

Bower, J.E. (2007). Cancer-related fatigue: Links with inflammation in cancer patients and survivors. *Brain Behavior Immunology, 21,* 863–871. doi:10.1016/j.bbi.2007.03.013

Bower, J.E. (2014). Cancer-related fatigue: Mechanisms, risk factors, and treatments. *Nature Reviews Clinical Oncology, 11,* 597–609. doi:10.1038/nrclinonc.2014.127

Bower, J.E., Crosswell, A.D., Stanton, A.L., Crespi, C.M., Winston, D., Arevalo, J., ... Ganz, P.A. (2015). Mindfulness meditation for younger breast cancer survivors: A randomized controlled trial. *Cancer, 121,* 1231–1240. doi:10.1002/cncr.29194

Bower, J.E., Ganz, P.A., Desmond, K.A., Bernards, C., Rowland, J.H., Meyerowitz, B.E., & Belin, T.R. (2006). Fatigue in long-term breast carcinoma survivors: A longitudinal investigation. *Cancer, 106,* 751–758. doi:10.1002/cncr.21671

Bruera, E., Yennurajalingam, S., Palmer, J.L., Perez-Cruz, P.E., Frisbee-Hume, S., Allo, J.A., ... Cohen, M.Z. (2013). Methylphenidate and/or a nursing telephone intervention for fatigue in patients with advanced cancer: A randomized, placebo-controlled, phase II trial. *Journal of Clinical Oncology, 31,* 2421–2427. doi:10.1200/JCO.2012.45.3696

Butt, Z., Lai, J.S., Rao, A.V., Heinemann, A.W., Bill, A., & Cella, D. (2013). Measurement of fatigue in cancer, stroke, and HIV using the Functional Assessment of Chronic Illness Therapy–Fatigue (FACIT-F) scale. *Journal of Psychosomatic Research, 74,* 64–68. doi:10.1016/j.jpsychores.2012.10.011

Butt, Z., Rao, A.V., Lai, J.S., Abernethy, A.P., Rosenbloom, S.K., & Cella, D. (2010). Age-associated differences in fatigue among patients with cancer. *Journal of Pain and Symptom Management, 40,* 217–223. doi:10.1016/j.jpainsymman.2009.12.016

Carmack Taylor, C., Basen-Engquist, K., Shinn, E., & Bodurka, D. (2004). Predictors of sexual functioning in ovarian cancer patients. *Journal of Clinical Oncology, 22,* 881–889. doi:10.1200/JCO.2004.08.150

Cella, D., Kallich, J., McDermott, A., & Xu, X. (2004). The longitudinal relationship of hemoglobin, fatigue and quality of life in anemic cancer patients: Results from five randomized clinical trials. *Annals of Oncology, 15,* 979–986. doi:10.1093/annonc/mdh235

Chan, R.J., Yates, P., & McCarthy, A.L. (2016). Fatigue self-management behaviors in patients with advanced cancer: A prospective longitudinal survey. *Oncology Nursing Forum, 43,* 762–771. doi:10.1188/16.ONF.762-771

Cornelison, M., Jabbour, E.J., & Welch, M.A. (2012). Managing side effects of tyrosine kinase inhibitor therapy to optimize adherence in patients with chronic myeloid leukemia: The role of the midlevel practitioner. *Journal of Supportive Oncology, 10,* 14–24. doi:10.1016/j.suponc.2011.08.001

Duijts, S.F.A., van Egmond, M.P., Spelten, E., van Muijen, P., Anema, J.R., & van der Beek, A.J. (2014). Physical and psychosocial problems in cancer survivors beyond return to work: A systematic review. *Psycho-Oncology, 23,* 481–492. doi:10.1002/pon.3467

Erickson, M.M., Beck, S.L., Christian, B., Dudley, W.N., Hollen, P.J., Albritton, K., ... Godder, K. (2010) Patterns of fatigue in adolescents receiving chemotherapy. *Oncology Nursing Forum, 37,* 444–455. doi:10.1188/10.ONF.444-455

Fouladbakhsh, J.M., Balneaves, L., & Jenuwine, E. (2013). Understanding CAM natural health products: Implications of use among cancer patients and survivors. *Journal of the Advanced Practitioner in Oncology, 4,* 289–306. doi:10.6004/jadpro.2013.4.5.2

Gélinas, C., & Fillion, L. (2004). Factors related to persistent fatigue following completion of breast cancer treatment. *Oncology Nursing Forum, 31,* 269–278. doi:10.1188/04.ONF.269-278

Giacalone, A., Quitadamo, D., Zanet, E., Berretta, M., Spina, M., & Tirelli, U. (2013). Cancer-related fatigue in the elderly. *Supportive Care in Cancer, 21,* 2899–2911. doi:10.1007/s00520-013-1897-1

Greenberg, D.B. (1998). Fatigue. In J.C. Holland (Ed.), *Psycho-oncology* (pp. 485–493). New York, NY: Oxford University Press.

Griffie, J., & Godfroy, J. (2014). Improving cancer-related fatigue outcomes: Walking patients through treatment and beyond. *Clinical Journal of Oncology Nursing, 18*(Suppl. 5), 21–24. doi:10.1188/14.CJON.S2.21-24

Hauser, K., Rybicki, L., & Walsh, D. (2010). What's in a name? Word descriptors of cancer-related fatigue. *Palliative Medicine, 24,* 724–730. doi:10.1177/0269216310376557

Hofman, M., Ryan, J.L., Figueroa-Moseley, C.D., Jean-Pierre, P., & Morrow, G.R. (2007). Cancer-related fatigue: The scale of the problem. *Oncologist, 12*(Suppl. 1), S4–S10. doi:10.1634/theoncologist.12-S1-4

Horneber, M., Fischer, I., Dimeo, F., Rüffer, J.U., & Weis, J. (2012). Cancer-related fatigue. *Deutsches Ärzteblatt International, 109,* 161–172.

Hurter, B., & Bush, N.J. (2007). Cancer-related anemia: Clinical review and management update. *Clinical Journal of Oncology Nursing, 11,* 349–359. doi:10.1188/07.CJON.349-359

Jones, J.M., Olson, K.L., Catton, P., Catton, C.N., Fleshner, N.E., Krzyzanowska, M.J., ... Howell, D. (2016). Cancer-related fatigue and associated disability in post-treatment cancer survivors. *Journal of Cancer Survivorship, 10,* 51–61. doi:10.1007/s11764-015-0450-2

Keeney, C.E., & Head, B.A. (2011). Palliative nursing care of the patient with cancer-related fatigue. *Journal of Hospice and Palliative Nursing, 13,* 270–278. doi:10.1097/NJH.06013e318221aa36

Knight, K., Wade, S., & Balducci, L. (2004). Prevalence and outcomes of anemia in cancer. *American Journal of Medicine, 116*(Suppl. 7A), 11S–26S. doi:10.1016/j.amjmed.2003.12.008

Luciani, A., Jacobsen, P.B., Extermann, M., Foa, P., Marussin, D., Overcash, J.A., & Balducci, L. (2008). Fatigue and functional dependence in the older cancer patient. *American Journal of Clinical Oncology, 31,* 424–430. doi:10.1097/COC.0b013e31816d915f

Miller, E., Jacob, E., & Hockenberry, M.J. (2011). Nausea, pain, fatigue, and multiple symptoms in hospitalized children with cancer [Online exclusive]. *Oncology Nursing Forum, 38,* E382–E393. doi:10.1188/11.ONF.E382-E393

Mitchell, S.A. (2010). Cancer-related fatigue: State of the science. *PM&R, 2,* 364–383. doi:10.1016/j.pmrj.2010.03.024

Mitchell, S.A., Albrecht, T.A., Alkaiyat, M.O., Browne, K., Clark, J.C., DeGennaro, R.M., ... Weisbrod, B.M. (2016). Putting Evidence Into Practice: Fatigue. Retrieved from https://www.ons.org/practice-resources/pep/fatigue

Mitchell, S.A., Hoffman, A.J., Clark, J.C., DeGennaro, R.M., Poirier, P., Robinson, C.B., & Weisbrod, B.L. (2014). Putting evidence into practice: An update of evidence-based interventions for cancer-related fatigue during and following treatment. *Clinical Journal of Oncology Nursing, 18,* 38–58. doi:10.1188/14.CJON.S3.38-58

Mock, V. (2001). Fatigue management: Evidence and guidelines for practice. *Cancer, 92*(Suppl. 6), 1699–1707. doi:10.1002/1097-0142(20010915)92:6+<1699::AID-CNCR1500>3.0.CO;2-9

Morrow, G.R., Andrews, P.L.R., Hickok, J.T., Roscoe, J.A., & Matteson, S. (2002). Fatigue associated with cancer and its treatment. *Supportive Care in Cancer, 10,* 389–398. doi:10.1007/s005200100293

National Comprehensive Cancer Network. (2017a). *NCCN Clinical Practice Guidelines in Oncology (NCCN Guidelines®): Cancer- and chemotherapy-induced anemia* [v.2.2017]. Retrieved from http://www.nccn.org/professionals/physician_gls/pdf/anemia.pdf

National Comprehensive Cancer Network. (2017b). *NCCN Clinical Practice Guidelines in Oncology (NCCN Guidelines®): Cancer-related fatigue* [v.1.2017]. Retrieved from http://www.nccn.org/professionals/physician_gls/pdf/fatigue.pdf

Neefjes, E.C.W., van der Vorst, M.J.D.L., Blauwhoff-Buskermolen, S., & Verheul, H.M.W. (2013). Aiming for a better understanding and management of cancer-related fatigue. *Oncologist, 18,* 1135–1143. doi:10.1634/theoncologist.2013-0076

Nooner, A.K., Dwyer, K., DeShea, L., & Yeo, T.P. (2016). Using relaxation and guided imagery to address pain, fatigue, and sleep disturbances: A pilot study. *Clinical Journal of Oncology Nursing, 20,* 547–552. doi:10.1188/16.CJON.547-552

Nunes, M.D.R., Jacob, E., Adlard, K., Secola, R., & Nascimento, L.C. (2015). Fatigue and sleep experiences at home in children and adolescents with cancer. *Oncology Nursing Forum, 42,* 498–506. doi:10.1188/15.ONF.498-506

Piper, B.F. (1997). Measuring fatigue. In M. Frank-Stromborg & S.J. Olsen (Eds.), *Instruments for clinical health-care research* (pp. 482–496). Burlington, MA: Jones & Bartlett Learning.

Piper, B.F., Borneman, T., Sun, V.C., Koczywas, M., Uman, G., Ferrell, B., & James, R.L. (2008). Cancer-related fatigue: Role of oncology nurses in translating National Comprehensive Cancer Network assessment guidelines into practice. *Clinical Journal of Oncology Nursing, 12*(Suppl. 5), 37–47. doi:10.1188/08.CJON.S2.37-47

Piper, B.F., Dibble, S.L., Dodd, M.J., Weiss, M.C., Slaughter, R.E., & Paul, S.M. (1998). The revised Piper Fatigue Scale: Psychometric evaluation in women with breast cancer. *Oncology Nursing Forum, 25,* 677–684.

Puetz, T.W., & Herring, M.P. (2012). Differential effects of exercise on cancer-related fatigue during and following treatment: A meta-analysis [Online exclusive]. *American Journal of Preventive Medicine, 43*(2), E1–E24. doi:10.1016/j.amepre.2012.04.027

Ream, E., Gargaro, G., Barsevick, A., & Richardson, A. (2015). Management of cancer-related fatigue during chemotherapy through telephone motivational interviewing: Modeling and randomized exploratory trial. *Patient Education and Counseling, 98,* 199–206. doi:10.1016/j.pec.2014.10.012

Ream, E., & Richardson, A. (1999). From theory to practice: Designing interventions to reduce fatigue in patients with cancer. *Oncology Nursing Forum, 26,* 1295–1303.

Reeve, B.B., Stover, A.M., Alfano, C.M., Smith, A.W., Ballard-Barbash, R., Bernstein, L., ... Piper, B.F. (2012). The Piper Fatigue Scale-12 (PFS-12): Psychometric findings and item reduction in a cohort of breast cancer survivors. *Breast Cancer Research and Treatment, 136,* 9–20. doi:10.1007/s10549-012-2212-4

So, W.K.W., Marsh, G., Ling, W.M., Leung, F.Y., Lo, J.C.K., Yeung, M., & Li, G.K.H. (2009). The symptom cluster of fatigue, pain, anxiety, and depression and the effect on the quality of life of women receiving treatment for breast cancer: A multicenter study [Online exclusive]. *Oncology Nursing Forum, 36,* E205–E214. doi:10.1188/09.ONF.E205-E214

Stasi, R., Abriani, L., Beccaglia, P., Terzoli, E., & Amadori, S. (2003). Cancer-related fatigue: Evolving concepts in evaluation and treatment. *Cancer, 98,* 1786–1801. doi:10.1002/cncr.11742

Tariman, J.D., & Dhorajiwala, S. (2016). Genomic variants associated with cancer-related fatigue: A systematic review. *Clinical Journal of Oncology Nursing, 20,* 537–546. doi:10.1188/16.CJON.537-546

Tralongo, P., Respini, D., & Ferraù, F. (2003). Fatigue and aging. *Critical Reviews in Hematology, 48*(Suppl.), S57–S64. doi:10.1016/j.critrevonc.2003.07.003

Valdres, R., Escalante, C., & Manzullo, E. (2001). Fatigue: A debilitating symptom. *Nursing Clinics of North America, 36,* 685–694.

Weis, J. (2011). Cancer-related fatigue: Prevalence, assessment and treatment strategies. *Expert Review of Pharmacoeconomics and Outcomes Research, 11,* 441–446. doi:10.1586/erp.11.44

Whitehead, L. (2009). The measurement of fatigue in chronic illness: A systematic review of unidimensional and multidimensional fatigue measures. *Journal of Pain and Symptom Management, 37,* 107–128. doi:10.1016/j.jpainsymman.2007.08.019

Yilmaz, H.B., Taş, F., Muslu, G.K., Başbakkal, Z., & Kantar, M. (2010). Health professionals' estimation of cancer-related fatigue in children. *Journal of Pediatric Oncology, 27,* 330–337. doi:10.1177/1043454210377176

# CHAPTER 7

# Hope

*Tami Borneman, RN, MSN, CNS, FPCN*

> *We who lived in concentration camps can remember the men who walked through the huts comforting others, giving away their last piece of bread. They may have been few in number, but they offer sufficient proof that everything can be taken from a man but one thing: the last of the human freedoms—to choose one's attitude in any given set of circumstances, to choose one's own way.*
>
> —Viktor Frankl

The importance of hope cannot be overstated. Patients diagnosed with cancer may experience fear, uncertainty, denial, devastation, and a loss of self (Borneman, Irish, Sidhu, Koczywas, & Cristea, 2014; Lichwala, 2014; Weingarten, 2012). Patients often need help to recognize, foster, and sustain their hope as they experience a potentially life-threatening illness. Hope is described as being interrelated with coping in that the relationship between the two is dynamic and reciprocal.

As a multidimensional and complex construct, hope has been identified as an important element of a patient's existential needs. It is expressed as a behavior, feeling, and a way of thinking and is an important resource in influencing one's ability to cope with stressful events. Hope is derived from an inner power directed toward enhancement of self, giving life meaning and the patient direction and optimism. It is also associated with an increased energized mental state and an action-oriented positive outlook (Averill, Catlin, & Chon, 1990; Ballard, Green, McCaa, & Logsdon, 1997; Dufault & Martocchio, 1985; Duggleby et al., 2007; Folkman, 2010; Frankl, 1959; Herth, 1990a, 1990b, 1993, 1995; Herth & Cutcliffe, 2002; Irving, Snyder, & Crowson, 1998; Lillis & Prophit, 1991; McLean, 2011; Nowotny, 1989; Olsson, Östlund, Grassman, Friedrichsen, & Strang, 2010; Olver, 2012; Rustoen, Cooper, & Miaskowski, 2010; Saleh & Brockopp, 2001; Sand, Olsson, & Strang, 2009). Farran, Herth, and Popovich (1995) provided a seminal working definition of hope.

> Hope constitutes an essential experience of the human condition. It functions as a way of feeling, a way of thinking, a way of behaving, and a way of relating to oneself and one's world. Hope has the ability to be fluid in its expectations, and in the event that the desired object or outcome does not occur, hope can still be present. (p. 6)

## Hope and Hopelessness

When examining hope, it is also important to examine hopelessness. Initially, hopelessness came from the psychiatric literature as one of the symptoms of depression (Sachs, Kolva, Pessin, Rosenfeld, & Breitbart, 2013). Hopelessness is defined as a negative view and pessimistic attitude toward the future (Beck, Weissman, Lester, & Trexler, 1974; Stephenson, 1991). Physically, hopelessness is associated with illness, depression, and the desire to accelerate one's death (Rawdin, Evans, & Rabow, 2013). It can be expressed as despair, discouragement, or a de-energizing force. Farran et al. (1995) defined hopelessness as "an essential experience of the human condition. It functions as a feeling of despair and discouragement; a thought process that expects nothing; and a behavioral process in which the person attempts little or takes inappropriate action" (p. 25).

Sullivan (2003) suggested that hopelessness is not merely an outcome of a prognosis, but rather shaped by one's condition and characteristic psychological factors. Therefore, it is not just the absence of hope but an attachment to an aspect of hope that is lost. Sullivan noted that hopelessness for the dying patient (or those with a life-threatening illness) may be a form of anticipatory grief. This grief needs to be expressed and acknowledged. Otherwise, in an attempt to cling to any form of hope, patients may not make the best decisions about their care. When patients are able to experience the bereavement process, hope begins to emerge; however, if bereavement is complicated, hopelessness is prolonged. If the patient is attached to a hope for survival that is quickly becoming less likely, it will be difficult for the patient to see other forms of hope. Therefore, hope needs to be diversified and redirected in the patient (Sullivan, 2003).

Hope and hopelessness can coexist but represent opposite expectations and different outcomes. Particular to healthcare settings, hope and hopelessness are situationally determined by the patient's life stage; symptoms, stage, and duration of illness; and treatment setting (Herth, 1993). Hope and hopelessness are also interdependent, and each provides the potential for growth. Sachs et al. (2013) conducted semi-structured interviews with 22 terminally ill patients with cancer to identify definitions of hope and hopelessness and associated thoughts and emotions. From this analysis, the authors learned that hope became an adaptive coping tool when faced with the threat of hopelessness. Conversely, hopelessness occurred when attachments to a form of hope had been lost (Sachs et al., 2013).

## Theories and Conceptual Models of Hope

The literature provides various theories and models of hope. Dufault and Martocchio (1985) described hope as having two interrelated spheres: particularized and generalized.

Particularized hope is centered on specific goals or objects, with a critical component of doing. This is a hope that is more tangible or visible and is action oriented or goal focused. An example would be that of a grandmother who wants to live long enough to see the birth of a grandchild.

In contrast, generalized hope is broader and not related to goals. It represents the intangible inner experience, with a critical component of "being" that may not be easily expressed. Examples include statements such as "I feel hopeful" or "Things have worked out in the past. I'm not hoping for anything in particular; I just have hope." This is the aspect of one's self that gives rise to hope (Nekolaichuk & Bruera, 1998).

Using Dufault and Martocchio's six dimensions of hope (contextual, affective, cognitive, behavioral, affiliative, and temporal), Herth (1991) formed a framework based on the overlap of those six dimensions to create categorical items in the Herth Hope Scale: cognitive–temporal (perception that a positive outcome is probable in the near future), affective–behavioral (feeling of confidence to initiate plans to effect the desired outcome), and affiliative–contextual (recognition of both interdependence and interconnectedness between self and others and between self and spirit). Morse and Doberneck (1995) developed a conceptual framework comprising seven universal components involved in the process of developing hope in response to a threat: realistic assessment of the predicament or threat, envisioning alternatives and setting goals, bracing for negative outcomes, realistic assessment of personal resources and of external conditions and resources, solicitation of mutually supportive relationships, continuous evaluation for signs that reinforce the selected goals, and determination to endure.

Nekolaichuk and Bruera (1998) described hope as a holistic experience comprised of three dimensions: personal (personal spirit), situational (risk), and interpersonal (authentic caring). The first dimension of personal spirit is a dynamic process, interconnecting references of time and emphasizing the personal experience of hope based on the core theme of meaning. The second dimension of risk emphasizes the situational experience of hope, balancing predictability and uncertainty, and expanding one's object of hope beyond cure. Authentic caring, the third dimension, combines the components of credibility and comfort and seeks to balance maintaining hope and truth telling.

Others also have provided insight to hope through research. McGee (1984) conceptualized hope as having both a trait and state component. The trait component is one's disposition toward a hopeful or pessimistic approach to life. State components (e.g., perceived goal achievement, perceived internal–external support, importance of the goal) influence the level of demonstrated hope. Owen's (1989) conceptual model of hope included six subthemes, with the single unifying concept of energy. In each subtheme, energy was exchanged, transformed, or moved (i.e., revised goals), resulting in the preservation or loss of hope. The process of maintaining hope illustrated in Ersek's (1992) model outlined two components: "dealing with it" (confronting negative possibilities in the illness experience and allowing the resulting full range of emotions, behaviors, and thoughts) and "keeping it in its place" (managing the effect of illness by controlling one's response to the disease and treatment). In their model, Post-White et al. (1996) outlined five themes of hope: finding meaning, relying on inner resources, having affirming relationships, living in the present, and anticipating survival (see Figure 7-1). Although these five themes are viewed as central to all patients, many use different strategies to sustain their hope; some rely more on inner resources, while others choose to rely on external resources.

## Assessment of Hope in the Clinical Setting

The assessment of hope is important for effective strategies to help patients sustain their hope. Farran, Wilken, and Popovich (1992) created a framework for assessment that involved four central attributes of hope and hopelessness, applying the acronym HOPE as follows:
- **H**ealth—An experiential process: Looking at the relationship between the patient's health status and their present level of hope or hopelessness

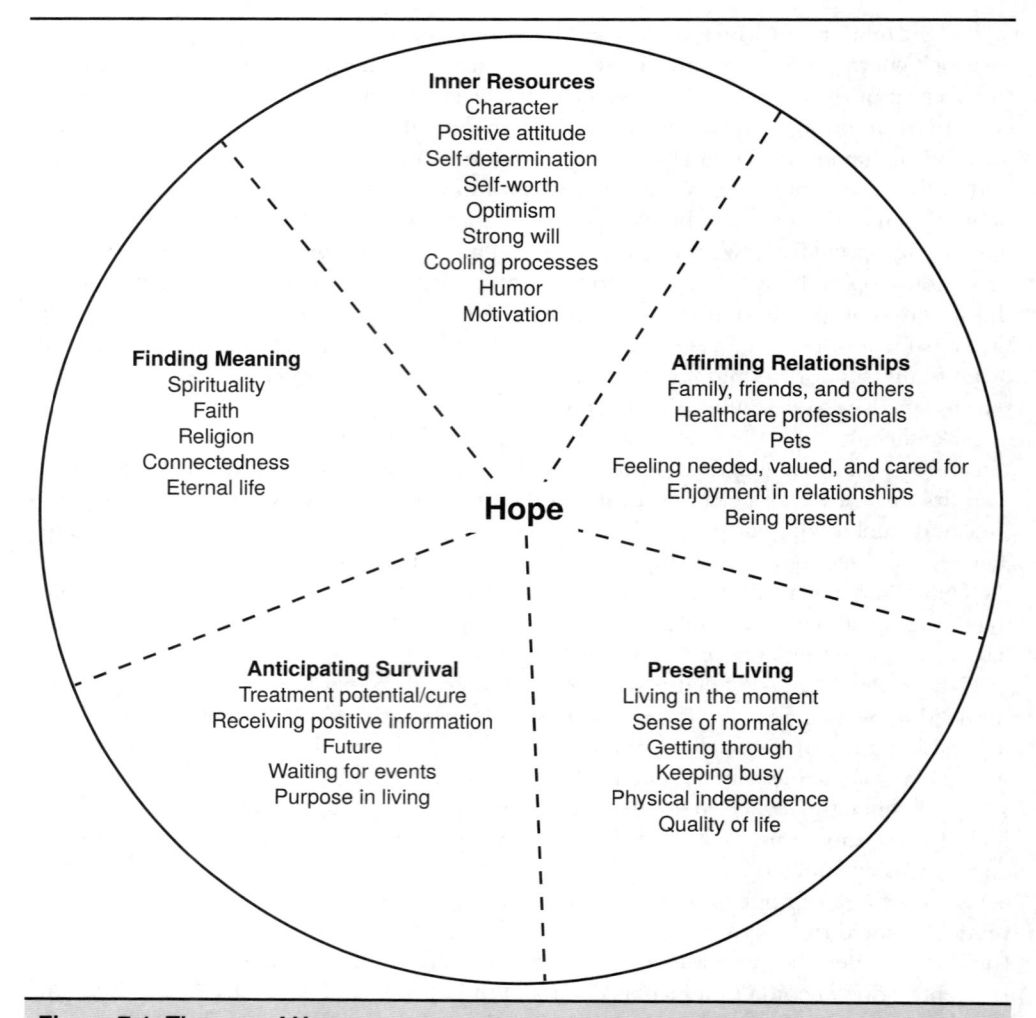

## Figure 7-1. Themes of Hope

**Inner Resources**
- Character
- Positive attitude
- Self-determination
- Self-worth
- Optimism
- Strong will
- Cooling processes
- Humor
- Motivation

**Finding Meaning**
- Spirituality
- Faith
- Religion
- Connectedness
- Eternal life

**Affirming Relationships**
- Family, friends, and others
- Healthcare professionals
- Pets
- Feeling needed, valued, and cared for
- Enjoyment in relationships
- Being present

**Hope**

**Anticipating Survival**
- Treatment potential/cure
- Receiving positive information
- Future
- Waiting for events
- Purpose in living

**Present Living**
- Living in the moment
- Sense of normalcy
- Getting through
- Keeping busy
- Physical independence
- Quality of life

*Note.* From "Hope, Spirituality, Sense of Coherence, and Quality of Life in Patients With Cancer," by J. Post-White, C. Ceronsky, M.J. Kreitzer, K. Nickelson, D. Drew, K.W. Mackey, ... S. Gutknecht, 1996, *Oncology Nursing Forum, 23*, p. 1576. Copyright 1996 by Oncology Nursing Society. Reprinted with permission.

- **O**ther—A relational process: Assessing the importance the patient places on others in restoring or maintaining hope and preventing hopelessness
- **P**urpose—A spiritual/transcendent process: Assessing the patient's source of hope
- **E**ngaging—A rational thought process: Assessing the patient's use of setting goals, refining goals, and refocusing goals when needed. If the patient's hope is based on God or a higher power, then a more in-depth spiritual assessment should be completed.

Several quantitative measures with acceptable psychometrics for assessing hope exist. The Time Opinion Survey identifies attributes of hope and how those factors influence hope in the ill adult (Raleigh, 1992). The Stoner Hope Scale assesses the intrapersonal, interpersonal, and global domains of hope (Stoner, 2004; Stoner & Keampfer, 1985). The Nowotny Hope Scale assesses six dimensions of hope: confidence, relating to others, feeling that the future is possible, religious faith, active involvement, and feeling that hope comes from within (Nowotny, 1989). The Herth Hope Index (HHI), an abbreviated version of the Herth Hope Scale, is used to assess the cognitive-temporal, affective-behavioral, and interconnectedness dimensions of hope (Herth, 1992). HHI is intended for clinical use as well as for research. Another well-known instrument, the Miller Hope Scale, assesses three factors: satisfaction with self, others, and life; avoidance of hope threats; and anticipation of the future (Miller & Powers, 1988). Further information on validated assessment tools can be found in Table 7-1.

An important consideration for assessing hope is culture. Unfortunately, a tremendous gap still exists in the research literature regarding the influence of culture on hope (Cotter & Foxwell, 2015; Farran et al., 1995). The aforementioned studies were con-

### Table 7-1. Sample Hope Assessment Tools

| Instrument | Description |
| --- | --- |
| Beck Hopelessness Scale | Assesses pessimism and quantifies hopelessness in psychopathological conditions<br>20-item scale<br>True or false |
| Herth Hope Index | Assesses hope in adults who have an altered health status<br>12-item scale across 3 subscales<br>4-point Likert scale (strongly agree, agree, disagree, strongly disagree) |
| Herth Hope Scale | Assesses the multidimensionality of hope in well adults, older adults, and adults with cancer<br>30-item scale<br>4-point Likert scale (rating scale of 0 [never applies] to 3 [often applies]) |
| Hinds Hopefulness Scale | Assesses relational and rational thought processes of hope and the degree of positive future orientation<br>24-item scale<br>Uses a line with phrase anchors on both ends |
| Miller Hope Scale | Assesses hope in adults in three subscales: satisfaction with self, others, and life; avoidance of hope threats; and anticipation of a future<br>40-item scale<br>5-point Likert scale |
| Nowotny Hope Scale | Assesses hope following a stressful event<br>29-item scale within 6 factors<br>4-point Likert scale (strongly agree, agree, disagree, strongly disagree) |
| Snyder Hope Scale | Assesses hope in adults and is goal and control oriented<br>12-item scale<br>4-point Likert scale |
| Stoner Hope Scale | Assesses intrapersonal, interpersonal, and global hope<br>30-item scale<br>4-point Likert scale |

*Note.* Based on information from Beck et al., 1974; Herth, 1990a, 1990b, 1991, 1992; Hinds & Gattuso, 1991; Miller, 1989; Miller & Powers, 1988; Nowotny, 1989; Snyder et al., 1991; Stoner, 2004; Stoner & Keampfer, 1985.

ducted with homogenous groups of patients. European studies have contributed to further understanding hope but were conducted using existing tools or frameworks created in the United States (Kylmä, Vehviläinen-Julkunen, & Lähdevirta, 2001; Olsson et al., 2010; Rustoen, Cooper, & Miaskowski, 2011). HHI has been translated into Portuguese with good results, but cultural and conceptual equivalence was not conducted in Brazil because of a lack of experts in the field (Balsanelli, Grossi, & Herth, 2010; Orlandi & Praca, 2013). Cultural factors that could affect a patient's hope are time orientation (future oriented or present focused), truth telling (disclosure or nondisclosure of information), and feeling in control (personal control or more passive role) (Cotter & Foxwell, 2015; McLean, 2011). It is important for nurses to consider cultural influences on hope during assessment.

## Hope-Fostering Strategies

Being diagnosed with cancer suddenly puts the patient's life in a whole different perspective. How can nurses help them to foster or maintain their hope? Recent literature does not reveal any new nursing interventions but reinforces existing ones. Figure 7-2 reviews common nursing strategies to help patients with cancer foster and maintain hope.

The following strategies are organized using the framework by Farran et al. (1992, 1995), which includes the following four central attributes of hope discussed previously: experiential (health), relational (others), spiritual/transcendent (purpose), and rational thought (encourage). These strategies, however, are not mutually exclusive to each process.

**Suggestions for Assessing Hope**
- What is your understanding of your cancer?
- What does that mean to you?
- What gives you hope?
- Has your cancer affected your hope?
- Will your hope help you through this journey?
- How might I, as your nurse, help you to maintain hope?

**Suggestions for Supporting Hope**
- Affirm the patient's values (not necessarily the goal of hope).
- Use humor when appropriate.
- Practice focused listening.
- Control physical symptoms.
- Set short-term goals.
- Encourage the patient to engage in activities of choice.
- Help identify tasks that are challenging but realistic.
- Encourage visitation of supportive relationships.
- Help identify strengths and resources.
- Encourage attributes of determination.
- Normalize the patient's feelings.
- Facilitate leaving a legacy.
- Support the patient's goals as appropriate.
- Clarify information.

**Figure 7-2. Suggestions for Assessing and Supporting Hope**

*Note.* Based on information from Borneman et al., 2014; Duggleby, 2001; Penrod & Morse, 1997; Saleh & Brockopp, 2001.

## Experiential Process/Health

The experiential process can be translated as the "pain" of hope (Farran et al., 1995). It involves the process of accepting what is happening physically (symptoms and physical changes), psychologically (effect on one's life), socially (how others respond), and spiritually (questioning why).

### *Physically*

Poorly or uncontrolled symptoms, especially pain, affect one's ability to hope because they serve as a reminder of disease and the possibility of death (Benzein, Norberg, & Saveman, 2001; Buckley & Herth, 2004; Herth, 1990a; Hsu, Lu, Tsou, & Lin, 2003). Research has shown that lower levels of pain are associated with higher levels of hope. Laboratory research has indicated that patients with higher levels of hope demonstrate greater tolerance to pain (Berendes et al., 2010; Hsu et al., 2003; Snyder et al., 2005). Patients may use hope as a way to obtain realistic goals about their health; therefore, it is important for symptoms and side effects of treatment to be effectively controlled (Lacasse & Beck, 2007; Lichwala, 2014).

### *Psychologically*

The use of humor or lightheartedness has been shown to help patients maintain hope (Buckley & Herth, 2004; Duggleby, 2001; Herth, 1990a, 1993). Humor can be used to counter or moderate the effects of stressful events as well as reduce psychological symptoms (Bennett & Lengacher, 2006). Being able to maintain a self-enhancing humorous perspective about one's situation has been positively related to resilience and improved psychological health (Cann & Collette, 2014). The ability to laugh with other patients helps to maintain hope and has been referred to as an important inner resource (Buckley & Herth, 2004). Lightheartedness, sometimes used interchangeably with humor, is described as a feeling of delight and sense of playfulness of the inner spirit (Herth, 1990a, 1993). By being lighthearted and using humor, patients have reported having a better perspective of their situation, feeling a sense of control, experiencing a temporary escape, and viewing humor as a necessity for coping with multiple changes (Herth, 1990a, 1993). Engaging patients with humor must always be done with sensitivity.

### *Socially*

How others respond to the patient can be detrimental to their hope; feeling that no one cares or feeling abandoned and isolated threatens a patient's hope (Buckley & Herth, 2004; Haugan, 2014; Herth, 1990a; Miller, 1989). When friends and relatives distance themselves physically or emotionally for various reasons, the patient can feel even more isolated. Experiencing physical presence with emotional withdrawal of family and friends is worse than being totally absent because it constantly reminds the patient of losses, making it extremely hard to maintain any hope (Buckley & Herth, 2004; Haugan, 2014; Herth, 1990a). Additionally, when family or friends talk as if the patient is not there, it devalues the patient, leaving a feeling of being a nonperson with little ability to maintain hope (Herth, 1990a). It is important that nurses affirm patients by role modeling to family and friends, talking directly to the patient, and affirming the patient's worth and value by active listening and interacting. When patients feel understood, validated, and treated with respect, their hope increases (Buckley & Herth, 2004; Haugan, 2014; Herth, 1990a). Engaging patients in conversation about happy memories or stories was found to increase and renew hope, especially memories from early life with family (Buckley & Herth, 2004; Duggleby, 2001; Haugan, 2014; Herth, 1990a, 1993). Helping patients to maintain a positive attitude also enables hope (Salander, Bergknut, & Henriksson, 2014).

### *Spiritually*

Having active spiritual beliefs and practices fosters hope (Herth, 1990a). Although the concept of spiritual pain has no formal definition, one commonly used description is "a pain deep in your being that is not physical" (Mako, Galek, & Poppito, 2006, p. 1108). Spiritual pain can lead to questions of "Why?" or "Why me?" These questions come from a place of personal experience; they are not mere words used to convey a theoretical sense of suffering. Spiritual pain stemming from a cancer diagnosis can lead to feelings of isolation in that the patient is now different from others. This sense of isolation, whether perceived or real, can rob the patient of hope. Existential questions are common for those facing a life-threatening illness, and interventions that support a patient's dignity, hope, and meaning may reduce spiritual distress (Chochinov & Cann, 2005; Chochinov et al., 2008).

## Relational Process/Others

The relational process is translated as the "heart" of hope (Farran et al., 1995). Relationships with others are paramount for sustaining hope and include not only family and friends but healthcare professionals as well (Benzein et al., 2001; Buckley & Herth, 2004; Duggleby, 2001; Sachs et al., 2013; Saleh & Brockopp, 2001). Families can serve as encouragers, cheerleading for the patient when hope becomes difficult. The presence of family was demonstrated to reflect acceptance, which enabled some patients to hope for more short-term events, especially those involving children (Sachs et al., 2013). The presence of children can provide a sense of future; patients' hopes have been shown to increase when feeling needed by their families (Miller, 1989). Another important relationship that fosters hope is the patient's pet (Benzein et al., 2001).

Nurses can encourage the patient to have friends and family around them who have been a major support over the years. Olsson et al. (2010) referred to this as "fellow travelers," those who help in the process of bringing hope. Nurses can support the patient's hope by educating family and friends about the importance of maintaining a caring relationship (Duggleby, 2001). If feasible, nurses should enable patients to actively engage with others online and provide information on support groups (Hansen et al., 2012). Encouraging a patient to leave a legacy is a tangible expression of maintaining hope, as it provides affirmation of the patient's presence and value in life (Borneman & Brown-Saltzman, 2015). Social media provides a way for patients and families with similar experiences to engage in mutual support. Gage-Bouchard, LaValley, Mollica, and Beaupin (2017) conducted a content analysis of 12 months' worth of data from 18 public Facebook pages hosted by parents of children with leukemia. Support exchange content included specialized health-related information, such as health services, recognizing symptoms, compliance, medication use, treatments, and procedures. Emotional support was exchanged through comparison, encouragement, empathy, and hope.

Hope can also be fostered through the nurse–patient relationship. Treating the patient with dignity, being willing to answer questions, having a positive attitude, taking the time to talk without interruptions, being encouraging, sincerely pushing for positive accomplishments, and verbally acknowledging fears without judgment are all interventions nurses can provide that have shown to help sustain patient hope (Benzein et al., 2001; Buckley & Herth, 2004; Cotter & Foxwell, 2015; Duggleby, 2001; Haugan, 2014; Lichwala, 2014; Saleh & Brockopp, 2001).

## Spiritual/Transcendent Process/Purpose

The spiritual/transcendent process can be translated as the "soul" of hope (Farran et al., 1995). For some patients, hope is inseparable from one's religion, spiritual life, or faith (Farran, Wilken, & Popovich, 1992; Pattison & Lee, 2011). Whatever a patient's faith, beliefs, or spirituality, nurses do not have to agree with whatever the patient is hoping. Rather, nurses can support their patients by affirming their values (Borneman et al., 2014). Many patients strive for normalcy and significance as they face a life-threatening illness or death, and being able to express their beliefs and engage in spiritual activities helps to maintain hope (Herth, 1990a, 1993; Olsson et al., 2010). Activities may include reading the Bible or inspirational books, watching or listening to religious programs, attending religious services, listening to spiritual music, praying, and engaging in hobbies (Herth, 1990a, 1993; Olsson et al., 2010). Spiritual faith and practices can provide a sense of meaning that enables patients to transcend their suffering and foster hope. This is evidenced in patient statements such as "God has a reason" and "He is with me" (Herth, 1990a; Miller, 1989). Nurses can help patients to identify meanings that help sustain them beyond just being emotionally happy (Weingarten, 2007). Nurses can also help patients identify sources of strength through using creative expressions of hope as they think about life and death (Herth, 2000). If comfortable, the nurse can pray with the patient. Assess for spiritual distress so that an appropriate referral can be made, along with community resources if warranted. Perhaps most important to providing spiritual interventions to foster hope is knowing and being comfortable with one's own spirituality.

## Rational Thought Process/Encouragement

The process of rational thought is also known as the "mind" of hope and involves setting goals, using resources, taking action, gaining control, and placing this process within a time frame (Farran et al., 1992, 1995).

Hope normally involves setting goals that are flexible, nonspecific, and realistic (Farran et al., 1992). In general, people are more motivated when faced with a high probability of achieving their goal. Nurses need to assess whether the patient's goals are consistent with physical capabilities, thoughts, and actions. Can the goal realistically be achieved?

The second element includes resources, which are both internal (courage, cognitive strategies, and energy level) and external (community support and family). Without resources, the patient may have difficulty attaining hope.

The next element of hope is action. This element involves assessing how active the patient is in planning, creating, visualizing, and participating in hopeful behavior or whether anything may prevent the patient from being actively engaged.

The fourth element of hope is control. Sometimes when life events become so uncontrollable, interpersonal control may become impotent. Assessing for functional control is important and focuses on things being under control instead of one's self being in control.

The final element is time. Past experiences help one deal with present situations (Farran et al., 1992, 1995). Nurses need to assess whether the patient's hope is based in the past, present, or future and how past experiences influence the present situation.

## Reframing

Another way patients can maintain hope is through reframing. Meaning exists within a historical context (Breitbart, 2003). What has given life meaning in the past and provided hope still can. Hope and meaning must be reframed to fit the new context of illness. One way of accomplishing this is by having short-term hopes, such as living day by day instead of worrying about the long-term future, or focusing on the smaller things in life (Eustache, Jibb, & Grossman, 2014). Reframing can be operationalized by placing oneself on the same level with healthy people and comparing statistical risks of dying (Salander, Bergenheim, & Henriksson, 1996). Shifting one's mental focus can also maintain hope. For example, instead of focusing on their failing physical body, patients may shift their focus to their intellect or escape in dreams (Olsson et al., 2010). Another example of reframing is looking at one's declining physical abilities as an opportunity for others to return the favor of helping. These positive thought processes help to foster hope (Miller, 1989). Refocusing time is a way to reframe hope. Rather than measuring time with a calendar or clock, time may become associated with anticipated events, such as birthday parties, weddings, or even changes in the seasons (Herth, 1993). By finding out what is important to patients, nurses can assist them in reframing their hope.

## Conclusion

Hope is an essential part of the human experience and especially so for patients with cancer. It is affected by the patient's physical, psychological, social, and spiritual well-being. Nurses play a vital role in facilitating hope by controlling symptoms, encouraging the presence of supportive relationships, affirming the patient's religious or spiritual beliefs, and facilitating the engagement of activities. Reframing hope within the context of illness helps to bring meaning to the present. Affirming what the patient values can foster hope, as it validates life for the patient. Nurses can enable hope by providing an opportunity to make something possible—whether by facilitating a mental shift in the patient's object of hope or in setting or achieving goals. Nursing interventions chosen to foster hope should be tailored to individual patient and family needs.

*The author would like to acknowledge Phyllis Gorney Cooper, RN, MN, for her contribution to this chapter from the previous edition of this book.*

## References

Averill, J.R., Catlin, G., & Chon, K.K. (1990). *Rules of hope.* New York, NY: Springer.

Ballard, A., Green, T., McCaa, A., & Logsdon, M.C. (1997). A comparison of the level of hope in patients with newly diagnosed and recurrent cancer. *Oncology Nursing Forum, 24,* 899–904.

Balsanelli, A., Grossi, S., & Herth, K. (2010). Cultural adaptation and validation of the Herth Hope Index for Portuguese language: Study in patients with chronic illness. *Texto Contexto-Enferm, 19,* 754–761. doi:10.1590/S0104-07072010000400019

Beck, A.T., Weissman, A., Lester, D., & Trexler, L. (1974). The measurement of pessimism: The hopelessness scale. *Journal of Consulting and Clinical Psychology, 42,* 861–865. doi:10.1037/h0037562

Bennett, M.P., & Lengacher, C. (2006). Humor and laughter may influence health: II. Complementary therapies and humor in a clinical population. *Evidence-Based Complementary and Alternative Medicine, 3,* 187–190. doi:10.1093/ecam/nel014

Benzein, E., Norberg, A., & Saveman, B.I. (2001). The meaning of the lived experience of hope in patients with cancer in palliative home care. *Palliative Medicine, 15,* 117–126. doi:10.1191/026921601675617254

Berendes, D., Keefe, F.J., Somers, T.J., Kothadia, S.M., Porter, L.S., & Cheavens, J.S. (2010). Hope in the context of lung cancer: Relationships of hope to symptoms and psychological distress. *Journal of Pain and Symptom Management, 40,* 174–182. doi:10.1016/j.jpainsymman.2010.01.014

Borneman, T., & Brown-Saltzman, K. (2015). Meaning in illness. In B. Ferrell, N. Coyle, & J.A. Paice (Eds.), *Oxford textbook of palliative nursing* (4th ed., pp. 554–566). New York, NY: Oxford University Press.

Borneman, T., Irish, T., Sidhu, R., Koczywas, M., & Cristea, M. (2014). Death awareness, feelings of uncertainty, and hope in advanced lung cancer patients: Can they coexist? *International Journal of Palliative Nursing, 20,* 271–277. doi:10.12968/ijpn.2014.20.6.271

Breitbart, W. (2003). Reframing hope: Meaning-centered care for patients near the end of life. Interview by Karen S. Heller. *Journal of Palliative Medicine, 6,* 979–988. doi:10.1089/109662103322654901

Buckley, J., & Herth, K. (2004). Fostering hope in terminally ill patients. *Nursing Standard, 19*(10), 33–41. doi:10.7748/ns2004.11.19.10.33.c3759

Cann, A., & Collette, C. (2014). Sense of humor, stable affect, and psychological well-being. *Europe's Journal of Psychology, 10.* doi:10.5964/ejop.v10i3.746

Chochinov, H.M., & Cann, B.J. (2005). Interventions to enhance the spiritual aspects of dying. *Journal of Palliative Medicine, 8*(Suppl. 1), S103–S115. doi:10.1089/jpm.2005.8.s-103

Chochinov, H.M., Hassard, T., McClement, S., Hack, T., Kristjanson, L.J., Harlos, M., ... Murray, A. (2008). The patient dignity inventory: A novel way of measuring dignity-related distress in palliative care. *Journal of Pain and Symptom Management, 36,* 559–571. doi:10.1016/j.jpainsymman.2007.12.018

Cotter, V., & Foxwell, A. (2015). The meaning of hope in the dying. In B. Ferrell, N. Coyle, & J.A. Paice (Eds.), *Oxford textbook of palliative nursing* (4th ed., pp. 475–486). New York, NY: Oxford University Press.

Dufault, K., & Martocchio, B.C. (1985). Symposium on compassionate care and the dying experience. Hope: Its spheres and dimensions. *Nursing Clinics of North America, 20,* 379–391.

Duggleby, W.D. (2001). Hope at the end of life. *Journal of Hospice and Palliative Nursing, 3,* 51–57. doi:10.1097/00129191-200103020-00003

Duggleby, W.D., Degner, L., Williams, A., Wright, K., Cooper, D., Popkin, D., & Holtslander, L. (2007). Living with hope: Initial evaluation of a psychosocial hope intervention for older palliative home care patients. *Journal of Pain and Symptom Management, 33,* 247–257. doi:10.1016/j.jpainsymman.2006.09.013

Ersek, M. (1992). The process of maintaining hope in adults undergoing bone marrow transplantation for leukemia. *Oncology Nursing Forum, 19,* 883–889.

Eustache, C., Jibb, E., & Grossman, M. (2014). Exploring hope and healing in patients living with advanced non-small cell lung cancer. *Oncology Nursing Forum, 41,* 497–508. doi:10.1188/14.ONF.497-508

Farran, C.J., Herth, K., & Popovich, J. (1995). *Hope and hopelessness: Critical clinical constructs.* Thousand Oaks, CA: Sage Publications.

Farran, C.J., Wilken, C., & Popovich, J.M. (1992). Clinical assessment of hope. *Issues in Mental Health Nursing, 13,* 129–138. doi:10.3109/01612849209040528

Folkman, S. (2010). Stress, coping, and hope. *Psycho-Oncology, 19,* 901–908. doi:10.1002/pon.1836

Frankl, V.E. (1959). *Man's search for meaning: An introduction to logotherapy.* Boston, MA: Beacon Press.

Gage-Bouchard, E.A., LaValley, S., Mollica, M., & Beaupin, L.K. (2017). Communication and exchange of specialized health-related support among people with experiential similarity on Facebook. *Health Communication, 32,* 1233–1240. doi:10.1080/10410236.2016.1196518

Hansen, B.S., Rørtveit, K., Leiknes, I., Morken, I., Testad, I., Joa, I., & Severinsson, E. (2012). Patient experiences of uncertainty—A synthesis to guide nursing practice and research. *Journal of Nursing Management, 20,* 266–277. doi:10.1111/j.1365-2834.2011.01369.x

Haugan, G. (2014). Meaning-in-life in nursing-home patients: A valuable approach for enhancing psychological and physical well-being? *Journal of Clinical Nursing, 23,* 1830–1844. doi:10.1111/jocn.12402

Herth, K.A. (1990a). Fostering hope in terminally-ill people. *Journal of Advanced Nursing, 15,* 1250–1259. doi:10.1111/j.1365-2648.1990.tb01740.x

Herth, K.A. (1990b). Relationship of hope, coping styles, concurrent losses, and setting to grief resolution in the elderly widow(er). *Research in Nursing and Health, 13,* 109–117. doi:10.1002/nur.4770130207

Herth, K.A. (1991). Development and refinement of an instrument to measure hope. *Scholarly Inquiry for Nursing Practice, 5,* 39–56.

Herth, K.A. (1992). Abbreviated instrument to measure hope: Development and psychometric evaluation. *Journal of Advanced Nursing, 17,* 1251–1259. doi:10.1111/j.1365-2648.1992.tb01843.x

Herth, K.A. (1993). Hope in older adults in community and institutional settings. *Issues in Mental Health Nursing, 14,* 139–156. doi:10.3109/01612849309031613

Herth, K.A. (1995). Engendering hope in the chronically and terminally ill: Nursing interventions. *American Journal of Hospice and Palliative Care, 12*(5), 31–39. doi:10.1177/104990919501200510

Herth, K.A. (2000). Enhancing hope in people with a first recurrence of cancer. *Journal of Advanced Nursing, 32,* 1431–1441. doi:10.1046/j.1365-2648.2000.01619.x

Herth, K.A., & Cutcliffe, J.R. (2002). The concept of hope in nursing. 6: Research/education/policy/practice. *British Journal of Nursing, 11,* 1404–1411. doi:10.12968/bjon.2002.11.21.12277

Hinds, P.S., & Gattuso, J.S. (1991). Measuring hopefulness in adolescents. *Journal of Pediatric Oncology Nursing, 8,* 92–94. doi:10.1177/104345429100800241

Hsu, T.H., Lu, M.S., Tsou, T.S., & Lin, C.C. (2003). The relationship of pain, uncertainty, and hope in Taiwanese lung cancer patients. *Journal of Pain and Symptom Management, 26,* 835–842. doi:10.1016/S0885-3924(03)00257-4

Irving, L.M., Snyder, C.R., & Crowson, J.J., Jr. (1998). Hope and coping with cancer by college women. *Journal of Personality, 66,* 195–214. doi:10.1111/1467-6494.00009

Kylmä, J., Vehviläinen-Julkunen, K., & Lähdevirta, J. (2001). Hope, despair and hopelessness in living with HIV/AIDS: A grounded theory study. *Journal of Advanced Nursing, 33,* 764–775. doi:10.1046/j.1365-2648.2001.01712.x

Lacasse, C., & Beck, S.L. (2007). Clinical assessment of symptom clusters. *Seminars in Oncology Nursing, 23,* 106–112. doi:10.1016/j.soncn.2007.01.007

Lichwala, R. (2014). Fostering hope in the patient with cancer. *Clinical Journal of Oncology Nursing, 18,* 267–269. doi:10.1188/14.CJON.267-269

Lillis, P.P., & Prophit, P. (1991). Keeping hope alive. *Nursing, 21*(12), 65–66. doi:10.1097/00152193-199112000-00021

Mako, C., Galek, K., & Poppito, S. (2006). Spiritual pain among patients with advanced cancer in palliative care. *Journal of Palliative Medicine, 9,* 1106–1113. doi:10.1089/jpm.2006.9.1106

McGee, R.F. (1984). Hope: A factor influencing crisis resolution. *Advances in Nursing Science, 6,* 34–44. doi:10.1097/00012272-198406040-00006

McLean, P. (2011). Balancing hope and hopelessness in family therapy for people affected by cancer. *Australian and New Zealand Journal of Family Therapy, 32,* 329–342. doi:doi:10.1375/S0814723X00001923

Miller, J.F. (1989). Hope-inspiring strategies of the critically ill. *Applied Nursing Research, 2,* 23–29. doi:10.1016/S0897-1897(89)80021-7

Miller, J.F., & Powers, M.J. (1988). Development of an instrument to measure hope. *Nursing Research, 37,* 6–10. doi:10.1097/00006199-198801000-00002

Morse, J.M., & Doberneck, B. (1995). Delineating the concept of hope. *Image: The Journal of Nursing Scholarship, 27,* 277–285. doi:10.1111/j.1547-5069.1995.tb00888.x

Nekolaichuk, C.L., & Bruera, E. (1998). On the nature of hope in palliative care. *Journal of Palliative Care, 14,* 36–42.

Nowotny, M.L. (1989). Assessment of hope in patients with cancer: Development of an instrument. *Oncology Nursing Forum, 16,* 57–61.

Olsson, L., Östlund, G., Grassman, E.J., Friedrichsen, M., & Strang, P. (2010). Maintaining hope when close to death: Insight from cancer patients in palliative home care. *International Journal of Palliative Nursing, 16,* 607–612. doi:10.12968/ijpn.2010.16.12.607

Olver, I. (2012). Evolving definitions of hope in oncology. *Current Opinion in Supportive and Palliative Care, 6,* 236–241. doi:10.1097/SPC.0b013e3283528d0c

Orlandi, F., & Praca, N. (2013). The hope of women with HIV/AIDS: Evaluation using the Herth Scale. *Texto y Contexto Enfermagem, 22,* 141–148. doi:10.1590/S0104-07072013000100017

Owen, D.C. (1989). Nurses' perspectives on the meaning of hope in patients with cancer: A qualitative study. *Oncology Nursing Forum, 16,* 75–79.

Pattison, N.A., & Lee, C. (2011). Hope against hope in cancer at the end of life. *Journal of Religious Health, 50,* 731–742. doi:10.1007/s10943-009-9265-7

Penrod, J., & Morse, J.M. (1997). Strategies for assessing and fostering hope: The hope assessment guide. *Oncology Nursing Forum, 24,* 1055–1063.

Post-White, J., Ceronsky, C., Kreitzer, M.J., Nickelson, K., Drew, D., Mackey, K.W., … Gutknecht, S. (1996). Hope, spirituality, sense of coherence, and quality of life in patients with cancer. *Oncology Nursing Forum, 23,* 1571–1579.

Raleigh, E.D. (1992). Sources of hope in chronic illness. *Oncology Nursing Forum, 19,* 443–448.

Rawdin, B., Evans, C., & Rabow, M.W. (2013). The relationships among hope, pain, psychological distress, and spiritual well-being in oncology outpatients. *Journal of Palliative Medicine, 16,* 167–172. doi:10.1089/jpm.2012.0223

Rustoen, T., Cooper, B.A., & Miaskowski, C. (2010). The importance of hope as a mediator of psychological distress and life satisfaction in a community sample of cancer patients. *Cancer Nursing, 33,* 258–267. doi:10.1097/NCC.0b013e3181d6fb61

Rustoen, T., Cooper, B.A., & Miaskowski, C. (2011). A longitudinal study of the effects of a hope intervention on levels of hope and psychological distress in a community-based sample of oncology patients. *European Journal of Oncology Nursing, 15,* 351–357. doi:10.1016/j.ejon.2010.09.001

Sachs, E., Kolva, E., Pessin, H., Rosenfeld, B., & Breitbart, W. (2013). On sinking and swimming: The dialectic of hope, hopelessness, and acceptance in terminal cancer. *American Journal of Hospice and Palliative Care, 30,* 121–127. doi:10.1177/1049909112445371

Salander, P., Bergenheim, T., & Henriksson, R. (1996). The creation of protection and hope in patients with malignant brain tumours. *Social Science and Medicine, 42,* 985–996. doi:10.1016/0277-9536(95)00204-9

Salander, P., Bergknut, M., & Henriksson, R. (2014). The creation of hope in patients with lung cancer. *Acta Oncologica, 53,* 1205–1211. doi:10.3109/0284186X.2014.921725

Saleh, U.S., & Brockopp, D.Y. (2001). Hope among patients with cancer hospitalized for bone marrow transplantation: A phenomenologic study. *Cancer Nursing, 24,* 308–314. doi:10.1097/00002820-200108000-00012

Sand, L., Olsson, M., & Strang, P. (2009). Coping strategies in the presence of one's own impending death from cancer. *Journal of Pain and Symptom Management, 37,* 13–22. doi:10.1016/j.jpainsymman.2008.01.013

Snyder, C.R., Berg, C., Woodward, J.T., Gum, A., Rand, K.L., Wrobleski, K.K., ... Hackman, A. (2005). Hope against the cold: Individual differences in trait hope and acute pain tolerance on the cold pressor task. *Journal of Personality, 73,* 287–312. doi:10.1111/j.1467-6494.2005.00318.x

Snyder, C.R., Harris, C., Anderson, J.R., Holleran, S.A., Irving, L.M., Sigmon, S.T., ... Harney, P. (1991). The will and the ways: Development and validation of an individual-differences measure of hope. *Journal of Personality and Social Psychology, 60,* 570–585. doi:10.1037/0022-3514.60.4.570

Stephenson, C. (1991). The concept of hope revisited for nursing. *Journal of Advanced Nursing, 16,* 1456–1461. doi:10.1111/j.1365-2648.1991.tb01593.x

Stoner, M.H. (2004). Measuring hope. In M. Frank-Stromborg & S.J. Olsen (Eds.), *Instruments for clinical healthcare research* (3rd ed., pp. 215–238). Burlington, MA: Jones & Bartlett Learning.

Stoner, M.H., & Keampfer, S.H. (1985). Recalled life expectancy information, phase of illness and hope in cancer patients. *Research in Nursing and Health, 8,* 269–274. doi:10.1002/nur.4770080309

Sullivan, M.D. (2003). Hope and hopelessness at the end of life. *American Journal of Geriatric Psychiatry, 11,* 393–405. doi:10.1097/00019442-200307000-00002

Weingarten, K. (2007). Hope in a time of global despair. In C. Flaskas, I. McCarthy, & J. Sheehan (Eds.), *Hope and despair in narrative therapy: Adversity, forgiveness and reconciliation* (pp. 13–23). New York, NY: Routledge.

Weingarten, K. (2012). Sorrow: A therapist's reflection on the inevitable and the unknowable. *Family Process, 51,* 440–455. doi:10.1111/j.1545-5300.2012.01412.x

# CHAPTER 8

# Pain

*Carol P. Curtiss, MSN, RN-BC*

> *Pain is the common companion of birth and growth, disease and death, and is a phenomenon deeply intertwined with the very question of human existence. It is among the most salient of human experiences, and it precipitates questioning the meaning of life itself.*
>
> —David Bakan

Pain is one of the most distressing and feared symptoms associated with cancer (Gorin et al., 2012; National Comprehensive Cancer Network® [NCCN®], 2017a; Paice & Ferrell, 2011; van den Beuken-van Everdingen et al., 2007). Pain is a significant threat to every aspect of quality of life in adults and children (Hui & Bruera, 2014; Paice & Ferrell, 2011). Saunders (1978) first described the concept of total pain to illustrate the complex interplay among physical, existential, and emotional suffering. The multidimensional biopsychosocial nature of pain affects the whole person and their loved ones. Unrelieved pain increases suffering, influences the patient's ability to complete treatment, compromises return to health, and interferes with a peaceful death (Fishman et al., 2013; Kopf & Patel, 2010; Paice & Ferrell, 2011). Increasing evidence also shows that survival from cancer is linked to symptom control, including pain management (NCCN, 2017a; Temel et al., 2010). Epidemiologic evidence indicates that cancer pain substantially adds to the already considerable national disease burden of cancer (NCCN, 2017a). Although pain is one of the most common symptoms reported by people with cancer, published studies are virtually restricted to prevalence data; no reliable incidence studies currently exist. However, pain may occur anywhere in the illness trajectory, from prediagnosis through end of life, and in cancer survivors of all ages who may experience persistent pain as a long-term complication of otherwise curative therapy. Estimates of prevalence range from 25% in newly diagnosed individuals, 33% for people undergoing active treatment, and up to 85% of people with advanced disease (Green, Hart-Johnson, & Loeffler, 2011; Paice & Ferrell, 2011). For many long-term cancer survivors, persistent pain lingers long after treatment (Glare et al., 2014; Meretoja, Leidenius, Tasmuth, Sipilä, & Kalso, 2014). Between 5% and 33% of cancer survivors have chronic pain that interferes with quality of life (Glare et al., 2014; Green et al., 2011; National Cancer Institute [NCI], 2016).

Cancer pain can be relieved or controlled for nearly everyone (NCI, 2016; NCCN, 2017a). However, unrelieved cancer pain continues to be a significant public health problem, causing needless suffering for patients and their families (Greco et al., 2014; Institute of Medicine [IOM], 2011; NCI, 2016; Paice & Ferrell, 2011; Zhao et al., 2014). IOM calls effective pain management a "moral imperative, professional responsibility, and duty of all healthcare providers" and stresses the need for a biopsychosocial approach to care (IOM, 2011, p. 3). The Joint Commission (2014) accreditation standards identify a patient's right to pain assessment and management as a key component of patient-centered care. See Figure 8-1 for a list of best practices for effectively managing pain.

Pain is a subjective, complex, unique, individual experience. The International Association for the Study of Pain (2012) defined it as "an unpleasant sensory and emotional experience associated with actual or potential tissue damage or described in terms of such damage" (para. 1). McCaffery (1968) defined pain as whatever the person says it is, occurring whenever the person says it occurs. However pain is defined, the best indicator of pain and pain relief is self-report of the individual (American Cancer Society [ACS], 2014; NCCN, 2017a). People with persistent pain from cancer may not exhibit acute pain physiologic indicators, such as increased blood pressure and heart rate, because of sympathetic nervous system adaptation to long-term pain, leading clinicians to wrongly conclude that the person is not in pain (American Pain Society [APS], 2008; Pasero & McCaffery, 2011). Clinicians must accept verbal reports from the person in pain as the gold standard for understanding pain and pain relief (ACS, 2014; APS, 2016; NCCN, 2017a). Pain, pain perception, and pain expression are uniquely different for each person, even when the source of the pain is similar. Interventions that work for one person, including medications, may be ineffective for another

---

- Encourage patients to be active participants in their care.
- Systematically screen all patients for pain—ask routinely and accept self-report.
- Complete a thorough history and physical examination.
- Assess pain, pain relief, the effects of pain on the person, function, and side effects of pain relief measures.
- Establish mutually agreeable, written, and measurable goals for pain care.
- Consider the patient's ability to sleep, mood, energy, emotional state, and quality of life when planning care.
- Develop an individualized, multimodal plan of care that includes nonpharmacologic interventions, medications as needed, and lifestyle changes when appropriate.
- Use medications in a systematic way and adjust doses based on individual responses, pain intensity, responses to previous treatment, and safety. Use the oral route unless contraindicated.
- If opioids are part of the treatment plan, assess all patients with reliable and valid tools for risks of misuse and abuse.
- Reassess for analgesia, adverse events, activities of daily living, and aberrant behavior at each visit.
- Reassess for new pain, pain that changes, and unrelieved pain at transitions in health care and before, during, and after procedures that cause pain.
- Anticipate, prevent, and manage side effects aggressively.
- Begin a prophylactic bowel management program to prevent constipation for all patients taking opioids.
- Educate patients and families about pain, pain interventions, and the use, safe handling, storage, and disposal of medications.
- Evaluate the effectiveness of the plan regularly.
- Keep the plan simple.
- Communicate the plan to other healthcare providers.
- Identify strategies to continuously improve.

**Figure 8-1. Best Practices for Effectively Managing Pain**

*Note.* Based on information from Curtiss, 2010; Paice & Ferrell, 2011; Pasero & McCaffery, 2011.

person with similar pain. Therefore, all pain management plans are developed based on each individual's systematic screening and comprehensive assessment, using self-report as a guide whenever possible (ACS, 2014; APS, 2016; Hui & Bruera, 2014; NCCN, 2017a).

# Pain and Quality of Life

Unrelieved pain is all-consuming and threatens every aspect of quality of life. Pain is complex; multidimensional; and influences physical, psychological, social, and spiritual or existential well-being (Ferrell, 1995; Gorin et al., 2012; Syrjala et al., 2014). Imaging studies confirm that pain activates sensory, affective, and cognitive areas of the brain (Kopf & Patel, 2010). Pain causes multiple losses for individuals and families and increases caregiver burden (Adler & Page, 2008; Paice & Ferrell, 2011; Syrjala et al., 2014). Overall, people with cancer pain report significantly worse quality of life than those without pain throughout the illness trajectory, including long-term survival (Gold et al., 2012; IOM, 2011; NCCN, 2017a). Figure 8-2 presents a framework for examining the effect of pain on quality of life.

## Physical Effects of Unrelieved Pain

Pain negatively affects every body system, including immune response, and results in multiple physical problems for people with cancer (Pasero & McCaffery, 2011). Pain interrupts sleep, diminishes appetite, and decreases mobility, endurance, and energy. Pain-related symptoms, such as fatigue, depression, constipation, anorexia, and decreased functional ability, further strain individual resources. Persistent pain causes irreversible peripheral and

**Physical Well-Being and Symptoms**
Functional ability
Strength/fatigue
Sleep and rest
Nausea
Appetite
Constipation

**Psychological Well-Being**
Anxiety
Depression
Enjoyment/leisure
Pain distress
Happiness
Fear
Cognition/attention

**Pain**

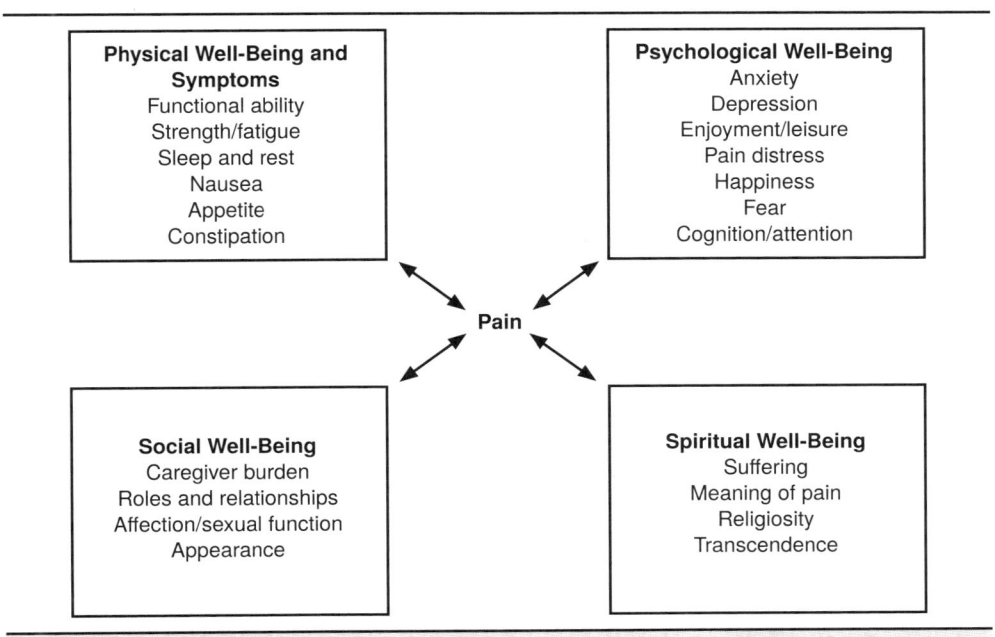

**Social Well-Being**
Caregiver burden
Roles and relationships
Affection/sexual function
Appearance

**Spiritual Well-Being**
Suffering
Meaning of pain
Religiosity
Transcendence

**Figure 8-2. The Impact of Pain on the Dimensions of Quality of Life**

*Note.* Copyright 2003 by Betty Ferrell. Used with permission.

central nervous system changes leading to the development of chronic pain, hypersensitivity (hyperalgesia), and over-responsiveness to stimuli that ordinarily would not be painful (allodynia) (IOM, 2011; Starkweather & Pair, 2013; Tennant, 2009). Pain signals from persistent pain are permanently embedded in the central nervous system, causing hypersensitivity to additional painful stimuli and a decrease in antinociceptive mechanisms. Pain impulses may continue long after healing occurs (APS, 2016; IOM, 2011; Starkweather & Pair, 2013; Tennant, 2009).

## Psychological Effects of Unrelieved Pain

Distress management is a core component of quality cancer care (Adler & Page, 2008; Andersen et al., 2014; NCCN, 2017b). Pain, fatigue, and emotional distress are the three most commonly co-occurring symptoms in people with cancer (Syrjala et al., 2014). Dealing with persistent pain is an emotional challenge and a major cause of distress for patients, their loved ones, and caregivers (Adler & Page, 2008; NCCN, 2017b). Unrelieved cancer pain is associated with higher levels of depression, fatigue, anxiety, distress, mood disturbance, and post-traumatic stress disorder (Adler & Page, 2008; Gold et al., 2012; Hui & Bruera, 2014; NCCN, 2017a). Individuals with persistent pain describe diminished self-worth, loss of control, guilt, anger, helplessness, a negative effect on overall coping, and decreased ability to participate in leisure and work activities (IOM, 2011). Coping style also influences pain perception. Catastrophizing, a set of exaggerated, negative cognitive and emotional responses to actual or anticipated pain, results in worse pain, more disability, and slower recovery (Quartana, Campbell, & Edwards, 2009). Self-efficacy regarding pain increases pain tolerance and improves physical and psychological functioning (IOM, 2011).

Unrelieved cancer pain is a primary risk factor for developing depressive disorders (IOM, 2011; Syrjala et al., 2014). The prevalence of depression and anxiety is higher in patients with cancer than in the general population. Prevalence of depression in people with cancer ranges from 1%–69% (Mitchell et al., 2011). As pain worsens, depressive symptoms and emotional distress increase (O'Connor et al., 2012). Although the incidence of suicide in people with cancer is poorly understood, depression, hopelessness, and uncontrolled pain are among the risk factors for suicidal ideation (Carlson, 2010; NCI, 2016). Some people consider suicide as an option when severe pain is unrelieved but often reconsider when pain is treated effectively (see Chapter 17 for more information on depression and suicide).

Poorly managed pain may distort mood and personality (Adler & Page, 2008; O'Connor et al., 2012). Family members often describe changes in the patients' personality (e.g., "He's not the same person I knew because of the pain."). Unrelieved pain affects the patient's enjoyment, lifestyle, and relationships with others. In addition, if pain is poorly managed, personal control is undermined, taxing coping skills and emotional well-being. The sense of hopelessness, vulnerability, and fear that accompanies unrelieved pain may add to and exaggerate pain and contribute to the overall suffering (Adler & Page, 2008).

Anxiety, like depression, may increase pain (Adler & Page, 2008; IOM, 2011; O'Connor et al., 2012). Conversely, poorly managed pain may precipitate, exacerbate, or intensify anxiety and depression (Hui & Bruera, 2014). Muscle tension caused by anxiety or fear further aggravates the problem. Treatment for anxiety disorders can augment pain management, and conversely, managing pain can reduce anxiety. Patient anxiety also influences family distress about pain (see Chapter 14). Fear is a powerful emotion that increases pain perception. Patients with cancer and their families are frightened by pain and concerned that pain will worsen with time. They worry that treatments will be ineffective. Families sometimes see pain as the indicator of overall health status, a signal that the cancer is getting worse, or a metaphor for death. Fear of addiction to opioid medications is one of the primary reasons people abandon therapy and do not obtain adequate pain control.

Physicians, nurses, and other healthcare providers are often reluctant to prescribe or recommend adequate doses of opioids, and patients experiencing pain may be afraid to take medicines for comfort (American Geriatrics Society [AGS] Panel on the Pharmacological Management of Persistent Pain in Older Persons, 2009; NCCN, 2017a). Patients commonly stop taking opioids because providers fail to anticipate and manage opioid-induced constipation. The current public health problems of prescription drug misuse and abuse, with extensive and sometimes sensational media coverage, further increase fears of taking opioid analgesics for cancer pain (Paice & Von Roenn, 2014). Failure to understand that the symptoms of tolerance and physical dependence are different syndromes from psychological addiction continues to compromise adequate pain relief (American Academy of Pain Medicine [AAPM], APS, & American Society of Addiction Medicine [ASAM], 2001; ASAM, 2011; Federation of State Medical Boards [FSMB], 2013). AAPM, APS, ASAM, and FSMB provide recommendations for differentiating, understanding, and managing each of these syndromes. It is essential to educate providers about risk assessment and stratification of patients for misuse of opioids and other safe prescribing strategies (Denenberg & Curtiss, 2016; NCCN, 2017a). Patients at high risk for misuse or abuse need effective pain management that may include opioids, but when opioids are part of the plan, these patients require more frequent and careful monitoring (Denenberg & Curtiss, 2016). Teaching patients and families about safe storage and disposal of medications is also essential (NCCN, 2017a). Despite the multitude of published guidelines for pain management and recommendations for the safe use of opioids for pain, undertreatment of cancer pain persists in all clinical settings.

Although national certification in pain management is available for nurses and physicians, the number of people needing expert care for pain control far exceeds the number of pain specialists in the United States. Many nonpain specialists are uncomfortable treating chronic pain, are reluctant to prescribe opioids for pain, and fear regulatory scrutiny and oversight (IOM, 2011). In addition, some pharmacies do not routinely stock opioids. Patients wait in pain for medications to arrive. In response to concerns about the opioid epidemic in the United States and fear of oversight, many providers refuse to prescribe opioids for pain, even if it is harmful to patients (Freyer, 2017).

A person's understanding of pain, pain relief, and the meaning attributed to pain influence the experience of pain. For some, pain is a constant reminder of illness and death. For others, pain is seen as a punishment, an enemy, a challenge, or a sense of purpose. People who have had poor experiences with pain relief are more likely to be anxious and fearful with new pain. Comprehensive interprofessional assessment, a team approach, and individualized plans for pain management help to address these individual differences (APS, 2016; IOM, 2011; NCCN, 2017a).

## Social Effects of Unrelieved Pain

Unrelieved pain causes many social losses, including changes in lifestyle, roles and relationships, and the ability to work, play, and socialize. Pain influences sexuality, intimacy, and the ability to give and receive affection (Adler & Page, 2008; NCCN, 2017a; Paice & Ferrell, 2011). Chronic pain may cause changes in appearance and diminished self-esteem. Persistent pain forces some people to be socially isolated and unable to resume work or education. For long-term cancer survivors, the consequences of persistent pain from cancer or cancer treatment may last a lifetime.

Pain is a family experience, and patient comfort is a high priority for family members. Family caregivers feel helpless, frustrated, heartbroken, frightened, and overwhelmed when a loved one has pain (Adler & Page, 2008). Loved ones share the suffering, loss of control, and impaired quality of life caused by pain and also experience psychological and social distress (Adler & Page, 2008). Family caregivers have the additional burden of experiencing interrupted sleep, learning to make decisions about pain assessment and management, and dealing with medicines and technology at home. Other issues include financial burdens from costs of therapy, loss of employment, and lost time from work for the patient or family members.

## Spiritual Effects of Unrelieved Pain

Unrelieved pain causes suffering for individuals and families and often results in a reevaluation of spiritual values and beliefs. For many people, spiritual beliefs shape their views of pain (Weinstein, Bernstein, Kapenstein, & Penn, 2014). Some people derive existential meaning from pain and suffering, describing positive life changes, opportunities for transcendence, increased control or power, and an enhanced sense of purpose. Others experience pain as punishment, a test, or an existential crisis that adds to additional pain and suffering. Spiritual support serves as a powerful intervention that may decrease pain intensity and enhance coping (Weinstein et al., 2014). Although often interrelated, pain and suffering are not the same concepts. Pain is managed with relative ease for most people by using medications and nondrug interventions. Suffering, however, is far more complex and requires a more in-depth interprofessional approach (see Chapters 9 and 10 for information on spiritual support and suffering).

## Developmental Issues Related to Pain Control

### Infants and Children

Children are at risk for poorly managed pain throughout the cancer experience (Mercadante & Giarratano, 2014; Sharek, Powers, Koehn, & Anand, 2006). Pain in children with cancer occurs most often from diagnostic procedures and treatments but may also be caused by cancer itself (World Health Organization [WHO], 2012). As with adults, non–cancer-related sources also can cause pain. Prevention of pain is vital in order to prevent fear, anxiety, depression, and additional suffering in children (Mercadante & Giarratano, 2014). Severe pain in children with cancer is an emergency and should be handled expeditiously. Pain sensation, perception, and management are similar in children and adults, but children may experience increased physiologic and psychological trauma from cancer, diagnostic procedures, unfamiliar settings, and separation from family. Pain affects cognitive, affective, and behavioral domains and influences concentration, social development, and the ability to learn and play (WHO, 2012). Neonates feel pain, and infants can remember painful experiences by six months of age. Most four-year-old children can provide a self-report of pain using age-appropriate assessment tools. The child's developmental level, emotional and cognitive state, physical condition, family attitudes and beliefs, and previous pain experiences influence responses to pain. A child's pain has a profound effect on the entire family, with parents or caregivers experiencing an overwhelming sense of devastation and helplessness (WHO, 2012).

Children's cancer pain can be relieved using strategies similar to those used with adults. Appropriate preparation for and adequate prevention of pain are critical. When healthcare providers anticipate and prevent pain from occurring, children are less fearful, tense, and anxious and feel more in control. Information about the child's, parent's, and family's beliefs and expectations; the illness; and the child's environment are needed to prevent and control pain adequately. Self-report is the primary source of information for verbal children, whereas keen observational skills and developmentally appropriate assessment tools are required to assess children who are preverbal or nonverbal (APS, 2008; Herr, Coyne, McCaffery, Manworren, & Merkel, 2011; WHO, 2012). Initially, acute pain in nonverbal or preverbal children elicits crying with physical withdrawal from the stimuli, but children with long-term pain may instead appear depressed and withdrawn (Herr et al., 2011). As pain continues, responses are further blunted, increasing the risk of undertreatment.

Parents or caregivers can provide information and help children to feel comforted and more secure. A child's hospital room should be a safe haven, with treatments and painful tests done elsewhere. A child-centered environment with familiar people, objects, and toys provides comfort during stressful periods. Family support throughout the experience is critical. Accurate and ongoing assessment and a comprehensive plan that integrates nondrug interventions, emotional support, and appropriately selected medications titrated to each child's needs are vital.

## Older Adults

Older adults are vulnerable to undertreatment of pain (Abdulla et al., 2013; AGS, 2009; Curtiss, 2010; Herr et al., 2011). Consequences of untreated pain among older people include depression, anxiety, decreased socialization, sleep disturbances, impaired mobility, and increased healthcare utilization. Common myths leading to poor management in older adults are that pain is a normal process of aging, that tolerance to pain sensations increases with aging, and that opioids cannot be used safely with older adults. Clinical experience, guidelines, and research do not support these misconceptions (AGS, 2009; Curtiss, 2010; Herr et al., 2011; NCCN, 2017a). Effective pain control improves mood, physical function, and quality of life for older people.

Principles for assessing and managing pain in older adults are similar to those in younger adults but more complex and multifactorial. Older adults often underreport pain, have multiple comorbidities, and experience changes in metabolism from aging that affect medication titration. Multiple drug–drug interactions are common (AGS, 2009). A comprehensive assessment includes a medical evaluation and physical examination, thorough pain history, evaluation of the effects of pain on functional ability, evaluation of the effects of pain on the primary caregiver and family, psychosocial and financial issues, history of trauma or falls, and a complete evaluation of current medications, herbs, and dietary supplements. Accommodations should be made for visual, auditory, and cognitive deficits.

Many cognitively impaired people with cancer can self-report pain, and some can use intensity rating scales to report current pain (Ferrell, Ferrell, & Rivera, 1995; Herr et al., 2011), but even those able to self-report pain require consistent, keen evaluation and observation. Subtle changes in normal behaviors in a cognitively impaired person increases suspicion that pain may be a problem. Pain behavior is more difficult to identify in the cognitively impaired and may include belligerence, withdrawal, restlessness, and a variety of other symptoms not commonly associated with pain. Some cognitive changes can be caused by unrelieved pain and may improve with adequate pain control. A useful hierarchy for assessing pain in nonverbal patients who are unable to self-report recommends the following assessment strategies (in the order listed) (Herr et al., 2011):
1. Attempt to obtain self-report.

2. If unable to obtain self-report, consider whether the patient's diagnoses and treatments would ordinarily cause pain in someone who could self-report.
3. Use a valid and reliable pain assessment tool to observe individual patient behaviors.
4. Ask family members or staff who know the patient (surrogate reporting).
5. Attempt an analgesic trial.

If the possibility of pain exists at any point in the hierarchy, treat pain and observe for improvements in behavior, mood, function, or cognition. When using medications as part of a comprehensive pain management plan, WHO's analgesic ladder for treating cancer pain needs only minor adaptation for use with older adults (AGS, 2009; WHO, 1990). Older adults may be more sensitive to the peak effects and duration of analgesics because of changes in pharmacokinetics, including slower excretion of medicines. "Start low and go slow" when titrating analgesics in the older adult. Begin dose escalation at the lower end of the spectrum and raise doses slowly and carefully. Monitor and assess for pain relief and aggressively anticipate and manage side effects (AGS, 2009).

As the population ages, as more people live longer, and as society becomes more mobile, older adults often are the primary caregivers for other older adults. Fatigue, lack of energy, sleep deprivation, worry, hopelessness, and frustration are common problems of both patients with unrelieved pain and caregivers. Attentive pain management can ease the burden and promote physical and psychosocial well-being.

# The Effects of Culture on Pain and Pain Relief

People from minority cultures are at increased risk for inadequate cancer pain management (Cleeland et al., 1994; IOM, 2011). Multiple studies report racial and gender disparities related to cancer pain incidence and pain's effect on quality of life (Clyde & Kwiatkowski, 2010; Green et al., 2011; Kopf & Patel, 2010). Causes of disparities leading to inadequate treatment of pain include negative stereotyping; difficulty in obtaining accurate assessment, especially when language is a barrier; poor quality of patient–provider interactions; and physiologic and sociocultural differences among various racial and ethnic groups (Tait & Chibnall, 2014). Healthcare providers must examine personal values, beliefs, communication skills, and negotiating skills to provide competent, culturally sensitive care (see Chapter 5).

People universally perceive pain but react to it with individual emotions and behaviors. Studies show racial and ethnic differences in both experimental and clinical pain, with African Americans showing greater pain severity and higher levels of disability than Hispanics and Whites (Rahim-Williams, Riley, Williams, & Fillingim, 2012). Genetic polymorphisms that affect medication metabolism also differ among races (IOM, 2011). The genetic makeup of each person influences how that individual responds to different medications. The results of genetic variations on medication efficacy are wide, variable, and unpredictable. The selection of one opioid over another essentially is by trial and error. Genetic testing to predict whether a person will have a good or bad response to an individual pain medication is available but often not used in practice, largely because of cost (Trescot & Faynboym, 2014). Factors such as culture, family beliefs, and religion contribute significantly to the expression of pain. The experience of pain, reactions to pain, and the willingness to try different methods to control pain are each learned experiences influenced by cultural expectations, values, and beliefs. These influences determine whether pain is reported, how it is reported, how it is expressed, and the ability to accept or reject a treatment plan. The way in which a culture treats and regards cancer can influence the quality and tolerance of cancer-related pain (IOM, 2011). When cancer is viewed as a punishment, pain may be seen as a necessary problem to endure. If cancer is a taboo subject in a culture, cancer pain may not be acknowledged at all. Some cultural variables that influence pain and pain control include the meaning of pain; religious beliefs, rituals, and values; methods of acceptable pain expression and pain tolerance; comfort with the use of medications (e.g., some cultures prefer externally applied medicines, such as salves and ointments, versus internally applied medicines, such as pills or injections); culturally acceptable coping styles and levels of anxiety in the presence of pain; significance of pain to the person; the body part involved; use of folk or non-Western medicine; concepts of illness and health; age; sex; and degree of acculturation (Clyde & Kwiatkowski, 2010; IOM, 2011). Understanding individual values, beliefs, and cultural influences is essential for caregivers to provide patient-centered care.

The patient–provider relationship is a significant factor in adequate assessment and adherence to treatment plans (IOM, 2011; Tait & Chibnall, 2014). Healthcare providers must honor personal preferences, embrace diversity, and consider health literacy to effectively care for people with pain (IOM, 2011). For example, a focus on individual autonomy in health care is a Western value that does not transcend to cultures in which decisions are determined based on the needs and ideas of the group. In some cultures, the individual's wants and desires are secondary to group needs, making it inappropriate for an individual to make any decisions about health care without including other significant people in the process. Eye contact also is a Western value. Some cultures see direct eye contact as disrespectful or threatening. Specific words used to describe pain differ from culture to culture, and some languages do not have a word for "pain." A pause or silence before responding to a question can be a cultural expectation. Healthcare providers lose valuable information and respect by failing to wait a sufficient amount of time for a response.

Some cultures find it rude and disrespectful to question someone in authority, even when disagreement exists. In this case, the person may respond "yes," "no," or "all right" or simply nod but not adhere to recommendations if they are inconsistent with personal values and beliefs. The person's definition of pain may determine the amount of pain tolerated or reported. If an individual believes pain should be endured, the patient may not express pain even when asked about it. Remembering that each person responds to pain as an individual is important, even in the presence of strong cultural ties. Accurate and complete assessment and frequent reassessment of pain, including the person's beliefs, understanding, values, experiences with pain and pain relief, and the actual words used to describe pain, will assist healthcare providers in delivering comprehensive pain management to individuals of many cultures (IOM, 2011).

## Promoting Evidence-Based Pain Care

Scheduled routine screening for the presence of pain, comprehensive assessment when pain is reported, development and implementation of multimodal plans of care, and pain management outcomes are core competencies for all clinicians, regardless of their discipline or clinical specialty (Herr et al., 2015). At least 15 organizations have published consistent guidelines for evidence-based practices (EBP) in pain assessment and management over many years, including a frequently updated guideline for cancer pain management in adults (NCCN, 2016a). The Oncology Nursing Society (ONS) publishes recommendations for evidence-based interventions for acute pain, breakthrough pain, chronic pain, and refractory/intractable pain (ONS, 2016). These publications form the research base for clinical decisions regarding evidence-based pain control. Nursing expertise and patient preferences complete the EBP process. According to Eaton, Meins, Mitchell, Voss, and Doorenbos (2015), although nurses value EBP, they rely on physicians, advanced practice nurses, and policies and procedures to guide best practices for pain management and do not often implement best practices in pain management. Lack of prelicensure and continuing education in pain assessment and management place nurses and other clinicians at a disadvantage when implementing EBP. Finding time to appraise and interpret the literature and develop best practices is another barrier. Symptom distress from pain and other symptoms challenge quality of life for people with cancer (McMillan & Small, 2002; McMillan, Tofthagen, Choe, & Rheingans, 2015). A consistent evidence-based approach to assessing pain and other distressing symptoms provides quality care that can influence pain intensity, symptom distress, overall quality of life, and patient and family satisfaction. Nurses advocate for people with cancer every day. Implementing EBP ensures that all patients receive the quality care they deserve.

## Conclusion

Most pain can be relieved using principles in published guidelines. Despite these and other resources, however, unrelieved pain continues to burden people with cancer and their families throughout the cancer continuum. The unnecessary burden of unrelieved pain in people with cancer adds needless distress, discomfort, and suffering to an already difficult situation and profoundly diminishes quality of life. In the United States, healthcare professionals have the knowledge, skills, medications, and, when needed, technology to manage most cancer pain. Nurses have a professional responsibility to relieve suffering, aggressively identify pain, and attentively control it. Spross (1985) noted, "Pain is an emergency for the person experiencing it regardless of the underlying pathology. We must apply the science and art of pain relief as though a life depended on it. Certainly, the quality of life does" (p. 31).

## References

Abdulla, A., Adams, N., Bone, M., Elliott, A.M., Gaffin, J., Jones, D., ... Schofield, P. (2013). Guidance on the management of pain in older people. *Age and Ageing, 42*(Suppl. 1), i1–i57. doi:10.1093/ageing/afs200

Adler, N.E., & Page, A.E.K. (Eds.). (2008). *Cancer care for the whole patient: Meeting psychosocial health needs*. Washington, DC: National Academies Press.

American Academy of Pain Medicine, American Pain Society, & American Society of Addiction Medicine. (2001). *Definitions related to the use of opioids for the treatment of pain: A consensus document*. Retrieved from https://www.naabt.org/documents/APS_consensus_document.pdf

American Cancer Society. (2014). Guide to controlling cancer pain. Retrieved from http://www.cancer.org/content/dam/cancer-org/cancer-control/en/booklets-flyers/guide-to-controlling-cancer-pain.pdf

American Geriatrics Society Panel on Pharmacological Management of Persistent Pain in Older Persons. (2009). Pharmacological management of persistent pain in older persons. *Journal of the American Geriatrics Society, 57*, 1331–1346. doi:10.1111/j.1532-5415.2009.02376.x

American Pain Society. (2016). *Principles of analgesic use* (7th ed.). Chicago, IL: Author.

American Society of Addiction Medicine. (2011). Definition of addiction. Retrieved from http://www.asam.org/for-the-public/definition-of-addiction

Andersen, B.L., DeRubeis, R.J., Berman, B.S., Gruman, J., Champion, V.L., Massie, M.J., ... Rowland, J.H. (2014). Screening, assessment, and care of anxiety and depressive symptoms in adults with cancer: An American Society of Clinical Oncology guideline adaptation. *Journal of Clinical Oncology, 32,* 1605–1619. doi:10.1200/JCO.2013.52.4611

Carlson, R. (2010). Helping prevent suicide in cancer patients. *Oncology Times, 32*(18), 15–19. doi:10.1097/01.COT.0000389877.67594.b8

Cleeland, C.S., Gonin, R., Hatfield, A.K., Edmonson, J.H., Blum, R.H., Stewart, J.A., & Pandya, K.J. (1994). Pain and pain treatment in outpatients with metastatic cancer. *New England Journal of Medicine, 330,* 592–596. doi:10.1056/NEJM199403033300902

Clyde, C.L., & Kwiatkowski, K.A. (2010). Historical and cultural influences on pain perceptions and barriers to treatment. In B. St. Marie (Ed.), *Core curriculum for pain management nursing* (2nd ed., pp. 123–149). Dubuque, IA: Kendall Hunt Professional.

Curtiss, C.P. (2010). Challenges in pain assessment in cognitively intact and cognitively impaired older adults with cancer. *Oncology Nursing Forum, 37*(Suppl. 5), S7–S16. doi:10.1188/10.ONF.S1.7-16

Denenberg, R., & Curtiss, C.P. (2016). Appropriate use of opioids in the management of chronic pain. *American Journal of Nursing, 116*(7), 26–38. doi:10.1097/01.NAJ.0000484931.50778.6f

Eaton, L.H., Meins, A.R., Mitchell, P.H., Voss, J., & Doorenbos, A.Z. (2015). Evidence-based practice beliefs and behaviors of nurses providing cancer pain management: A mixed-methods approach. *Oncology Nursing Forum, 42,* 165–173. doi:10.1188/15.ONF.165-173

Federation of State Medical Boards. (2013). *Model policy on the use of opioid analgesics in the treatment of chronic pain.* Washington, DC: Author.

Ferrell, B.A., Ferrell, B.R., & Rivera, L. (1995). Pain in cognitively impaired nursing home patients. *Journal of Pain and Symptom Management, 10,* 591–595. doi:10.1016/0885-3924(95)00121-2

Ferrell, B.R. (1995). The impact of pain on quality of life: A decade of research. *Nursing Clinics of North America, 30,* 609–624.

Fishman, S.M., Young, H.M., Arwood, E.L., Chou, R., Herr, K., Murinson, B.B., ... Strassels, S.A. (2013). Core competencies for pain management: Results of an interprofessional consensus summit. *Pain Medicine, 14,* 971–981. doi:10.1111/pme.12107

Freyer, F.J. (2017, January 3). Doctors are cutting opioids, even if it harms patients. *Boston Globe.* Retrieved from http://www.bostonglobe.com/metro/2017/01/02/doctors-curtail-opioids-but-many-see-harm-pain-patients/z4Ci68TePafcD9AcORs04J/story.html

Glare, P.A., Davies, P.S., Finlay, E., Gulati, A., Lemanne, D., Moryl, N., ... Syrjala, K.L. (2014). Pain in cancer survivors. *Journal of Clinical Oncology, 32,* 1739–1747. doi:10.1200/JCO.2013.52.4629

Gold, J.I., Douglas, M.K., Thomas, M.L., Elliott, J.E., Rao, S.M., & Miaskowski, C. (2012). The relationship between post-traumatic stress disorder, mood states, functional status, and quality of life in oncology outpatients. *Journal of Pain and Symptom Management, 44,* 520–531. doi:10.1016/j.jpainsymman.2011.10.014

Gorin, S.S., Krebs, P., Badr, H., Janke, E.A., Jim, H.S.L., Spring, B., ... Jacobson, P.B. (2012). Meta-analysis of psychosocial interventions to reduce pain in patients with cancer. *Journal of Clinical Oncology, 30,* 539–547. doi:10.1200/JCO.2011.37.0437

Greco, M.T., Roberto, A., Corli, O., Deandrea, S., Bandieri, E., Cavuto, S., & Apolone, G. (2014). Quality of cancer pain management: An update of a systematic review of undertreatment of patients with cancer. *Journal of Clinical Oncology, 32,* 4149–4154. doi:10.1200/JCO.2014.56.0383

Green, C.R., Hart-Johnson, T., & Loeffler, D.R. (2011). Cancer-related chronic pain. *Cancer, 117,* 1994–2003. doi:10.1002/cncr.25761

Herr, K., Coyne, P.J., McCaffery, M., Manworren, R., & Merkel, S. (2011). Pain assessment in the patient unable to self-report: Position statement with clinical practice recommendations. *Pain Management Nursing, 12,* 230–250. doi:10.1016/j.pmn.2011.10.002

Herr, K., St. Marie, B., Gordon, D.B., Paice, J.A., Watt-Watson, J., Stevens, B.J., ... Young, H.M. (2015). An interprofessional consensus of core competencies for prelicensure education in pain management: Curriculum application for nursing. *Journal of Nursing Education, 54,* 317–328. doi:10.3928/01484834-20150515-02

Hui, D., & Bruera, E. (2014). A personalized approach to assessing and managing pain in patients with cancer. *Journal of Clinical Oncology, 32,* 1640–1646. doi:10.1200/JCO.2013.52.2508

Institute of Medicine. (2011). *Relieving pain in America: A blueprint for transforming prevention, care, education, and research.* Washington, DC: Author.

International Association for the Study of Pain. (2012). IASP taxonomy. Retrieved from http://www.iasp-pain.org/Taxonomy

Joint Commission. (2014). Pain management. Retrieved from http://www.jointcommission.org/topics/pain_management.aspx

Kopf, A., & Patel, N. (2010). *Guide to pain management in low-resource settings.* Seattle, WA: International Association for the Study of Pain.

McCaffery, M. (1968). *Nursing practice theories related to cognition, bodily pain, and man-environment interactions.* Los Angeles, CA: UCLA Students' Store.

McMillan, S.C., & Small, B.J. (2002). Symptom distress and quality of life in patients with cancer and newly admitted to hospice home care. *Oncology Nursing Forum, 29,* 1421–1428. doi:10.1188/02.ONF.1421-1428

McMillan, S.C., Tofthagen, C., Choe, R., & Rheingans, J. (2015). Assessing symptoms experienced by patients with cancer. *Journal of Hospice and Palliative Nursing, 17,* 56–65. doi:10.1097/NJH.0000000000000123

Mercadante, S., & Giarratano, A. (2014). Pharmacological management of cancer pain in children. *Critical Reviews in Oncology/Hematology, 91,* 93–97. doi:10.1016/j.critrevonc.2014.01.005

Meretoja, T.J., Leidenius, M.H.K., Tasmuth, T., Sipilä, R., & Kalso, E. (2014). Pain at 12 months after surgery for breast cancer. *JAMA, 311,* 90–92. doi:10.1001/jama.2013.278795

Mitchell, A.J., Chan, M., Bhatti, H., Halton, M., Grassi, L., Johansen, C., & Meader, N. (2011). Prevalence of depression, anxiety, and adjustment disorder in oncological, haematological, and palliative-care settings: A meta-analysis of 94 interview-based studies. *Lancet Oncology, 12,* 160–174. doi:10.1016/S1470-2045(11)70002-X

National Cancer Institute. (2016). Cancer pain (PDQ®)–Health professional version. Retrieved from http://www.cancer.gov/cancertopics/pdq/supportivecare/pain/HealthProfessional/page1

National Comprehensive Cancer Network. (2017a). *NCCN Clinical Practice Guidelines in Oncology (NCCN Guidelines®): Adult cancer pain* [v.2.2017]. Retrieved from https://www.nccn.org/professionals/physician_gls/pdf/pain.pdf

National Comprehensive Cancer Network. (2017b). *NCCN Clinical Practice Guidelines in Oncology (NCCN Guidelines®): Distress management* [v.2.2017]. Retrieved from https://www.nccn.org/professionals/physician_gls/pdf/distress.pdf

O'Connor, M., Weir, J., Butcher, I., Kleiboer, A., Murray, G., Sharma, N., ... Sharpe, M. (2012). Pain in patients attending a specialist cancer service: Prevalence and association with emotional distress. *Journal of Pain and Symptom Management, 43,* 29–38. doi:10.1016/j.jpainsymman.2011.03.010

Oncology Nursing Society. (2016). PEP rating system overview. Retrieved from https://www.ons.org/practice-resources/pep

Paice, J.A., & Ferrell, B. (2011). The management of cancer pain. *CA: A Cancer Journal for Clinicians, 61,* 157–182. doi:10.3322/caac.20112

Paice, J.A., & Von Roenn, J.H. (2014). Under- or overtreatment of pain in the patient with cancer: How to achieve proper balance. *Journal of Clinical Oncology, 32,* 1721–1726. doi:10.1200/JCO.2013.52.5196

Pasero, C., & McCaffery, M. (2011). *Pain assessment and pharmacological management.* St. Louis, MO: Elsevier Mosby.

Quartana, P.J., Campbell, C.M., & Edwards, R.R. (2009). Pain catastrophizing: A critical review. *Expert Review of Neurotherapeutics, 9,* 745–758. doi:10.1586/ern.09.34

Rahim-Williams, B., Riley, J.L., Williams, A.K.K., & Fillingim, R.B. (2012). A quantitative review of ethnic group differences in experimental pain response: Do biology, psychology, and culture matter? *Pain Medicine, 13,* 522–540. doi:10.1111/j.1526-4637.2012.01336.x

Saunders, C.M. (1978). *The management of terminal malignant disease.* London, England: Edward Arnold.

Sharek, P.J., Powers, R., Koehn, A., & Anand, K.J.S. (2006). Evaluation and development of potentially better practices to improve pain management of neonates. *Pediatrics, 118*(Suppl. 2), S78–S86. doi:10.1542/peds.2006-0913D

Spross, J.A. (1985). Cancer pain and suffering: Clinical lessons from life, literature, and legend. *Oncology Nursing Forum, 12*(4), 23–31.

Starkweather, A.R., & Pair, V.E. (2013). Decoding the role of epigenetics and genomics in pain management. *Pain Management Nursing, 14,* 358–367. doi:10.1016/j.pmn.2011.05.006

Syrjala, K.L., Jensen, M.P., Mendoza, M.E., Yi, J.C., Fisher, H.M., & Keefe, F.J. (2014). Psychological and behavioral approaches to cancer pain management. *Journal of Clinical Oncology, 32,* 1703–1711. doi:10.1200/JCO.2013.54.4825

Tait, R.C., & Chibnall, J.T. (2014). Racial/ethnic disparities in the assessment and treatment of pain: Psychosocial perspectives. *American Psychologist, 69,* 131–141. doi:10.1037/a0035204

Temel, J.S., Greer, J.A., Muzikansky, A., Gallagher, E.R., Admane, N.S., Jackson, V.A., ... Lynch, T.J. (2010). Early palliative care for patients with metastatic non–small-cell lung cancer. *New England Journal of Medicine, 363,* 733–742. doi:10.1056/NEJMoa1000678

Tennant, F. (2009). Brain atrophy with chronic pain: A call for enhanced treatment. *Practical Pain Management, 9*(2). Retrieved from https://www.practicalpainmanagement.com/pain/other/brain-injury/brain-atrophy-chronic-pain-call-enhanced-treatment

Trescot, A.M., & Faynboym, S. (2014). A review of the role of genetic testing in pain medicine. *Pain Physician, 17,* 425–445. doi:10.1093/annonc/mdm056 van den Beuken-van Everdingen, M.H.J., de Rijke, J.M., Kessels, A.G., Schouten, H.C., van Kleef, M., & Patijn, J. (2007). Prevalence of pain in patients with cancer: A systematic review of the past 40 years. *Annals of Oncology, 18,* 1437–1449. doi:10.1093/annonc/mdm056

Weinstein, F., Bernstein, A., Kapenstein, T., & Penn, E. (2014). Spirituality assessments and interventions in pain medicine. *Practical Pain Management, 14*(5), 1–11. Retrieved from http://www.practicalpainmanagement.com/treatments/psychological/spirituality-assessments-interventions-pain-medicine

World Health Organization. (1990). *Cancer pain relief and palliative care: Report of a WHO Expert Committee.* Technical Report Series 804. Retrieved from http://apps.who.int/iris/bitstream/10665/39524/1/WHO_TRS_804.pdf

World Health Organization. (2012). WHO guidelines on the pharmacological treatment of persisting pain in children with medical illnesses. Retrieved from http://apps.who.int/iris/bitstream/10665/44540/1/9789241548120_Guidelines.pdf

Zhao, F., Chang, V.T., Cleeland, C., Cleary, J.F., Mitchell, E.P., Wagner, L.I., & Fisch, M.J. (2014). Determinants of pain severity changes in ambulatory patients with cancer: An analysis from Eastern Cooperative Oncology Group Trial E2Z02. *Journal of Clinical Oncology, 32,* 312–319. doi:10.1200/JCO.2013.50.6071

# CHAPTER 9

# Spiritual and Religious Support

*Elizabeth Johnston Taylor, PhD, RN*

> *And almost everyone when age,*
> *Disease, or sorrows strike him,*
> *Inclines to think there is a God,*
> *Or something very like Him.*
>
> —Arthur Hugh Clough

Spirituality and religion often influence patients' responses to the psychosocial and physical experiences of living with cancer. Likewise, the psychosocial and physical sequelae of cancer can influence patients' spirituality or religiosity. This interplay between spirituality and religion and living with cancer can contribute to the transformation and enhancement of spiritual and general well-being or to doubts and struggles (Bulkley et al., 2013). It is beneficial for oncology nurses to understand the spirituality and religion of their patients and family caregivers to provide appropriate support.

## Concept Descriptions

Although most Americans identify themselves as spiritual and religious, a substantial minority self-define as only spiritual—and very few self-define as neither (Chatters, Taylor, Bullard, & Jackson, 2008). In a study of more than 5,000 Americans, 63% of Caucasians and 81% of African Americans considered themselves both religious and spiritual, while 8% of African Americans and 15% of Caucasians labeled themselves as neither. Of these participants, 8% of African Americans and 19% of Caucasians considered themselves as "spiritual only." A Gallup poll indicated that 78% of Americans view religion as either "fairly" or "very important" in their life. However, only 54% of Americans were members of a religious congregation (Gallup, 2016).

A qualitative study of underserved and ethnically diverse patients with cancer found that some patients viewed spirituality and religion as "intertwined," whereas others viewed religion as an expression of spirituality, and others perceived them as different concepts, with spirituality being less desirable than religion (Stein, Kolidas, & Moadel, 2015). This postmodern view of spirituality and religion is likely reflected in the thinking of nurses.

## Comparison

Nursing literature consistently differentiates religion from spirituality (Nardi & Rooda, 2011; White, Peters, & Schim, 2011). Murray and Zentner (1989) provided a classic definition of spirituality that is often quoted in nursing literature:

> A quality that goes beyond religious affiliation, that strives for inspirations, reverence, awe, meaning and purpose, even in those who do not believe in any god. The spiritual dimension tries to be in harmony with the universe, and strives for answers about the infinite, and comes into focus when the person faces emotional stress, physical illness or death. (p. 259)

Religion, on the other hand, is typically described in the nursing literature as an expression of spirituality. Religion offers people beliefs that provide answers to the questions of ultimate meaning. Religion also recommends how one is to live harmoniously with oneself, others, nature, and God. Such explanations and recommendations are presented in a religion's belief system (e.g., myths/stories, doctrines, dogmas) and are remembered and appreciated through rituals and other religious practices or observances (Taylor, 2012).

Spirituality is often misconstrued as subjective and individual, whereas religion is thought to be objective and institutional (Hill et al., 2000). However, those who study spirituality and religion scientifically debate that this concept belittles religion. Religionists see the two concepts as similar or overlapping. For example, psychologists of religion Hill et al. (2000) defined spirituality as the following:

> The feelings, thoughts, experiences, and behaviors that arise from a search for the sacred. The term "search" refers to attempts to identify, articulate, maintain, or transform. The term "sacred" refers to a divine being, divine object, Ultimate Reality, or Ultimate Truth as perceived by the individual. (p. 66)

Hill et al. (2000) then defined religion by extending the definition of spirituality to include "a search for non-sacred goals (such as identity, belongingness, meaning, health, or wellness) in a context that has as its primary goal the facilitation" of the criterion for spirituality and "the means and methods (e.g., rituals or prescribed behaviors) of the search that receive validation and support from within an identifiable group of people" (p. 66). This definition indicates that religion is characterized by group-endorsed beliefs and behaviors that enable a search for what is sacred. Although religion is within the context of "an identifiable group," this does not mean that the group is institutionalized; it also does not mean that the religious beliefs or practices are codified or formalized.

The Association of Religion Data Archives (ARDA, n.d.) defines religiosity as the "degree to which a person is religious or spiritual," suggesting that no difference exists between the two concepts. However, Reinert and Koenig (2013) proposed that both concepts are helpful in nursing. Although religion is a more objective and measurable concept that can be used for research purposes, the term *spiritual* can be useful in clinical practice as a colloquial word that implies a broad concept with which most patients can identify.

## Spiritual Support

Spiritual and religious support (also known as spiritual care or spiritually sensitive nursing care) is rarely defined in the nursing literature. Barss (2012) described spiritual care as "relevant, nonintrusive care, which tends to the spiritual dimension of health by addressing universal spiritual needs, honoring unique spiritual worldviews, and helping individuals explore and mobilize factors that can help them gain/regain a sense of trust to promote optimum healing" (p. 24). Another definition for spiritual care describes it as an expression of self that is founded in a compassionating love (Sawatzky & Pesut, 2005). After qualitative interviews with 10 dialysis nurses about their experiences of providing spiritual care, Deal and Grassley (2012) portrayed spiritual care as an aspect of nursing care that is deeper and more intimate than psychosocial care, suggesting that spiritual care requires nurses to "reach deep within to respond to the patient" (p. 476). These examples suggest that it is not only an aspect of care that addresses another's spirituality and religion; it also involves drawing on the nurse's own spirituality and religion. Perhaps it is a type of "holistic empathy" where the nurse's own spirituality allows him or her to deeply listen to the patient's spirituality, thoughts, feelings, and body messages (Taylor, 2007).

## Spirituality and Religiosity in Cancer Care: Rationale

Several arguments verify the importance of supporting patient and family caregiver spirituality and religion in oncology nursing care.

### Spirituality as Part of the Whole

Nursing prides itself on being a profession that cares for the whole person. Many nursing theories implicitly or explicitly include spirituality as a dimension of nursing care (Martsolf & Mickley, 1998; Taylor, 2002). The International Council of Nurses (ICN) stated that nurses should create "an environment in which the human rights, values, customs, and spiritual beliefs of the individual, family and community are respected" (ICN, 2012, p. 2). Since 1978, NANDA International has supported this notion by including the diagnosis of "spiritual distress" in its formulary. Subsequently, NANDA International has added related diagnoses, such as "impaired religiosity" (Gordon, 2007). Several organizations that provide accreditation to nursing programs (e.g., American Association of Colleges of Nursing) identify spiritual assessment and care as content that baccalaureate-prepared nurses should receive (Taylor, Testerman, & Hart, 2014). These positions and practices indicate a commitment to holistic care that includes supporting spirituality and religion.

### Pragmatic Reasons

Pragmatic reasons exist for including spiritual care in nursing. The Joint Commission (2009) requires that patients' rights be respected, protected, and promoted. The Joint Commission stipulates that a patient's right to religious and other spiritual services be accommodated. To accommodate such rights, nurses are often involved in inquiring patients about their spirituality and religion during admission assessments. The Joint Commission particularly emphasizes the need for spiritual assessment for patients at the end of life.

Although little evidence currently exists, spiritual care may save healthcare dollars. A multisite study (N = 343) investigating the effects of team (i.e., doctors, nurses, and chaplains) approaches to spiritual care among patients with advanced cancer observed lower healthcare costs among those who believed they received spiritual care (Balboni et al., 2010, 2011). Furthermore, spiritual support was found to be associated with receipt of hospice care. In contrast, those who perceived their spiritual needs were unmet were more apt to receive aggressive therapies and die in an intensive care unit. Of note for nurses is the fact that these patients' perceptions of having received spiritual care were not related to having a chaplain visit but rather to any clinician's provision of spiritual support.

Nurturing the spirit also has marketing value. Those who market healthcare institutions often understand that consumers are interested in health care that cares for the body, mind, and spirit. It is not unusual to find advertisements for healthcare institutions that proclaim they care holistically. Providing spiritual support may be one way an institution can set itself apart from others.

## Spiritual and Religious Responses to Cancer: Evidence

Nursing and healthcare philosophies and policies encourage the provision of spiritual and/or religious support for those living with cancer. The most significant argument for provision of spiritual and religious support, however, comes from the hundreds of studies that document how spirituality and religion are associated with, or contribute to, positive health-related outcomes (Koenig, King, & Carson, 2012).

### Patients' Spirituality and Religiosity

Although little evidence quantifies the spirituality and religion of people living with cancer, the baseline presumably reflects that of the American population. In a 2014 survey of more than 35,000 Americans, 77% reported that religion was important in their lives; conversely, 22% indicated that it was either not too important or not at all important (Pew Research Center, 2017). Similarly, 83% held a belief in the existence of God (or were at least fairly certain). However, strong evidence from a large national survey (N = 3,443) and a metasynthesis of 22 studies indicate that religiosity increases once a person is diagnosed with cancer (McFarland, Pudrovska, Schieman, Ellison, & Bierman, 2013; Moreno & Stanton, 2013).

Whereas the focus of this chapter is about adult persons living with cancer, many of the themes and spiritual care therapeutics can be adapted for children, adolescents, and young adults. Younger children's spirituality and religion typically will mirror that of their parents or authority figures. Reflecting their psychological development involving individuation, adolescents and young adults (AYA) will likely test or begin to reappraise their spirituality and religion. Indeed, considerable evidence indicates that AYA tend to become less religious in their late teens while maintaining a spiritual awareness (Taylor, Petersen, Oyedele, & Haase, 2015).

## Prevalence and Types of Spiritual Needs

To describe that a patient may need spiritual support, clinicians often use the term *spiritual need*. Over the past few decades, several health researchers have identified the prevalence and types of spiritual needs among patients with cancer (Maguire et al., 2013; Nixon, Narayanasamy, & Penny, 2013; Paterson, Robertson, Smith, & Nabi, 2015). Observed prevalence rates of spiritual needs among patients with cancer vary by study. For example, in a study of cancer survivors in Vermont (an area known for low religious affiliation), 30% admitted that they had at least one unmet psychosocial or spiritual need (Geller, Vacek, Flynn, Lord, & Cranmer, 2014). A Northern European study, on the other hand, found that 94% of

285 patients with cancer had one or more spiritual needs (Hocker, Krull, Koch, & Mehnert, 2014). When categorizing spirituality and religion as conducive to positive or negative coping, studies consistently show a minority (roughly 20%–30%) of patients experience significant spiritual distress (Bulkley et al., 2013; Frost et al., 2013; King, Fitchett, & Berry, 2013).

Types of spiritual needs vary. How researchers and clinicians categorize needs as spiritual also varies. This contributes to lists of spiritual needs that may overlap with other psychosocial needs. The National Comprehensive Cancer Network® (2017) guidelines on distress provide a list of spiritual needs identified as requiring spiritual support:
- Grief
- Concerns about death and an afterlife
- Guilt
- Conflicted or challenged belief systems
- Conflicts between religious beliefs and recommended treatment
- Loss of faith
- Concerns about a relationship with a deity
- Concerns about meaning and purpose in life
- Isolation from a religious community
- Hopelessness

These spiritual needs can be manifested in a myriad of ways (see Table 9-1).

## Factors Related to Spirituality and Religiosity

Several longitudinal studies provide evidence about how spirituality and religion changes over the trajectory of the cancer experience. When considered together to make a broad generalization, these studies suggest that spirituality and religion, especially if it is of a positive and nonorganizational nature prior to diagnosis, tends to continue over the span of the illness and increase (Leeson et al., 2015; McFarland et al., 2013; Moreno & Stanton, 2013) or remain high (Bai, Lazenby, Jeon, Dixon, & McCorkle, 2015; Bulkley et al., 2013; Caplan, Sawyer, Holt, & Brown, 2014; Frost et al., 2013). Two time points in the illness trajectory when spirituality and religion may substantially shift include the initial phase (i.e., "existential plight"), when it may decrease or increase (Danhauer et al., 2013; Leeson et al., 2015), and at the end of life, when it may increase slightly (King et al., 2013). Although spiritual well-being was observed to be relatively stable over time in a sample of nearly 1,600 patients with lung cancer, Frost et al. (2013) noted that individual spiritual and religious trajectories were often highly variable. This evidence led the research team to conclude that it is important to continually monitor for shifts in a patient's spiritual well-being as well as during the initial and final phases of cancer.

Four demographic factors appear to be linked with spirituality and religion: gender, age, social support, and ethnicity. As found in other research about spirituality and religion in the general adult population, some evidence suggests that women with cancer self-report greater spirituality and religion than men (Hocker et al., 2014; Munoz, Salsman, Stein, & Cella, 2015). Two strong studies suggest that younger adult patients are more likely to experience spiritual and religious growth than older adult patients (McFarland et al., 2013; Moreno & Stanton, 2013). Another large national study of 8,864 cancer survivors showed that survivors between the ages of 60 and 80 reported higher spiritual well-being than those between the ages of 18 and 39 (Munoz et al., 2015). This may be because, although older adults generally have higher spiritual well-being, the cancer experience is more spiritually catapulting for young adults.

## Table 9-1. Spiritual Needs Illustrated

| Spiritual Dimensions Conceptualized* | How Dimensions May Be Manifested With Spiritual Needs |
|---|---|
| Beliefs and meaning (i.e., mission, purpose, religious and nonreligious meaning in life) | "My cancer was a wake-up call for me to get my house in order."<br>"I am now more sympathetic toward others who are also suffering."<br>"There has to be a reason for this; there just has to be."<br>"I've been making a scrapbook about my life so that when I'm gone, others will know I've lived a good life." |
| Authority and guidance (i.e., exploring where or with whom one places trusts, seeking guidance) | "I pray that God will guide my surgeon's hands."<br>"I've learned that I am stronger than I thought, and I'm using that inner strength to get me through this."<br>"I just keep telling myself to live in the power of the present moment and not worry about the future." |
| Experience (i.e., of the divine or demonic) and emotion (i.e., the tone emerging from one's spiritual experience) | "Having cancer makes me feel closer to God."<br>"I'm just more grateful now. I have so many blessings!"<br>"I now stop and smell the roses." |
| Fellowship (i.e., involvement in any formal or informal community that shares spiritual beliefs and practices) | "My support group is my church family now."<br>"Now that I am too sick to go to services, I feel it's hard to stay connected to God."<br>"It seems like the people at church have forgotten me." |
| Ritual and practice (i.e., activities that make life meaningful) | "Every night I list three things that made the day satisfying."<br>"I try to keep doing my hobbies."<br>"Seems my prayers now are not being answered. Am I doing it the wrong way?" |
| Courage and growth (i.e., the ability to encounter doubt and inner change) | "I grew up believing there was a God, but now that I have cancer, I wonder where that God is."<br>"It's scary facing the fact that I might die, so I try not to think about it." |
| Vocation and consequences (i.e., what people believe they should do, what is their calling) | "I think I need to fight this cancer with all my might so that I can be there for my kids."<br>"I've lived a good life; I'm going to let nature take its course because it is not right to use up so many healthcare resources just to make me live a couple years longer." |

*These spiritual needs can be expressed along a continuum from healthy or positive spirituality and religion to unhealthy and negative spirituality and religion.

Note. Based on information from Fitchett, 1993.

A number of studies document that African Americans report higher spirituality and religion than Caucasians (Best et al., 2014; Canada et al., 2013). A few studies suggested that patients with cancer who are in partnered relationships and have social support have higher spiritual well-being (Hocker et al., 2014; Moreno & Stanton, 2013). These demographic factors can provide clues as to which patients may be at risk for spiritual distress and which may be more welcoming of spiritual support.

Most importantly, however, are the research findings that spirituality and religion are associated with, or predictive of, other pertinent aspects of adaptation to cancer. Numerous studies have shown spirituality and religion to be related to quality of life (Frost et al., 2013; Rabow & Knish, 2015; Sirilla & Overcash, 2013; Taylor & Davenport, 2012). Bai et al. (2015) found that spiritual well-being predicted quality of life more so than physical or emotional well-being in a sample of 52 patients with advanced cancers. Other important factors found to be inversely related to spirituality and religion included anxiety, depression, pain, and fatigue (Leeson et al., 2015; Lewis, Salins, Rao, & Kadam, 2014; Rabow & Knish, 2015). Especially significant are the findings from Leeson et al. (2015) that patients undergoing stem cell transplant (N = 220) who had higher levels of meaning and peace predicted lower anxiety, depression, and fatigue, and better physical well-being a year after the transplant.

A few studies provide evidence that spirituality and religion appear to contribute to well-being for people living with cancer. These linkages are typically illuminated when specific psychological facets of spirituality and religion are studied. For instance, it is high intrinsic religiosity, or internalized religion, (versus a religion used for personal gain) that is associated with low depression (Caplan et al., 2013; Pérez & Smith, 2015). In a study of 179 outpatients with cancer, Pérez and Smith (2015) further identified how intrinsic religiosity and well-being were associated with the active process of spiritual and religious surrender.

Another significant facet to spirituality and religion that provides clear distinctions in how well a patient with cancer adapts to living with illness is the patient's religious coping. Negative religious coping includes spiritual and religious doubts and disturbing beliefs such as "cancer is a punishment from God" or "God has abandoned me." Thune-Boyle, Stygall, Keshtgar, Davidson, and Newman (2013) studied 155 women in their first year of living with breast cancer and learned that "feeling punished and abandoned by God" explained 4%–5% of their anxiety and depressed mood. Pérez and Smith (2015) found that negative religious coping that involved pleading for God's intervening or passively deferring decisions to God were inversely related to various types of well-being. Similarly, McLaughlin et al. (2013) noted that passively deferring control to God contributed to decreased quality of life. This finding led them to advise that religious patients be encouraged to "keep their end of the bargain and maintain an active coping style" (p. 2747). Trevino, Balboni, Zollfrank, Balboni, and Prigerson (2014) observed that suicidal ideation was 2–3 times more frequent among patients with negative religious coping. Although positive religious coping is generally associated with adaptation to illness, health research in this area intimates that negative religious coping is most predictive of maladaptation to illness.

Spiritual and religious beliefs also often provide comfort (e.g., reasons and solutions for the problem of suffering). One large study observed that it was whether or not a patient experienced comfort from spirituality and religion that linked them with high quality of life (Préau, Bouhnik, & Le Coroller Soriano, 2013). Numerous studies described how spiritual and religious beliefs and practices provided patients with cancer with comfort and a general means of coping (Asiedu, Eustace, Eton, & Radecki Breitkopf, 2014; Lynn, Yoo, & Levine, 2014; Seibaek, Hounsgaard, & Hvidt, 2013). For example, in a qualitative study of African American patients with cancer, Hamilton, Galbraith, Best, Worthy, and Moore (2015) noted that the participants found comfort in beliefs about God; they believed that good things were promised by God to those who believed in Him. These patients also noted that prayer and worshipful experiences provided comfort and courage.

Patients' spirituality and religion also typically provides them with beliefs about health. Thus, health-related decisions (e.g., about surgery or treatment options) are often influenced by spiritual and religious beliefs or one's faith in God (Rubin, Chavez, Alderman, & Pusic, 2013; Silvestri, Knittig, Zoller, & Nietert, 2003). For this reason, numerous studies examine how spirituality and religion affect cancer-screening behavior and how conducting cancer screening in a religious context may improve participation (Daverio-Zanetti et al., 2014; Leyva, Nguyen, Allen, Taplin, & Moser, 2014). Padela, Peek, Johnson-Agbakwu, Hosseinian, and Curlin (2014) observed that Muslim American women who believed that a disease was punishment from God were significantly less likely to have a Pap smear. Participants from a Latino Roman Catholic focus group discussed how their spiritual and religious beliefs contributed to their seeking health care and practicing a healthful lifestyle (Allen et al., 2014). A focus group study with Orthodox Jewish women identified how spiritual and religious beliefs about the possibility of a miracle and fate could be barriers to cancer screening (Tkatch et al., 2014). Best, Spencer, Hall, Friedman, and Billings (2015) asked African American women not how spiritual and religious beliefs could become a barrier to screening, but rather how they could be framed so as to promote cancer screening. They concluded that African American women could be encouraged to get screened by messages such as "The human body is the temple for God—so keep it fit so that God can reside therein"; "Seeking medical care does not reflect a lack of faith"; and "God's spirit gives one courage to face physical challenges."

## Family Caregivers' Spirituality and Religiosity

Although most of the research on spirituality and religion among people living with cancer focuses on the patient, evidence exists on the spiritual and religious experiences and needs of family caregivers. Findings generally mirror that of studies on patients. A phenomenological study of 135 family caregivers (Williams & Bakitas, 2012) identified spiritual and meaning-making responses to being a caregiver; these included positive and challenging experiences. Negative spiritual aspects of caring for a family member with cancer included struggling to ascribe satisfying meaning, experiencing uncertainty, facing death, having difficulty enjoying living in the present, and asking questions about the purpose of suffering and dying. In contrast, caregivers also identified positive aspects of caring, which included being prompted to reflect on and celebrate life, prioritizing and living more congruently with values, becoming kinder and more communicative, and collaborating with and getting to know other family members better. For these caregivers, comfort was found in rituals, such as prayer, that afforded solace, as well as in spiritual and religious beliefs that provided caregivers with "the bigger picture." These spiritual and religious responses to family caregiving, however, are similar to those identified in qualitative studies of patients describing their responses to living with a life-threatening illness.

A few studies of family caregivers provide insight about factors that may precipitate and result from spiritual distress. Williams, Dixon, Feinn, and McCorkle (2014) found that, although use of prayer was not associated with depression, religious service attendance was inversely related to depression. This finding may be explained by the social support provided by attending services. Another study of 70 family caregivers indicated that social support provided by fellow family members was directly related to a sense of meaning and peace (Adams, Mosher, Cannady, Lucette, & Kim, 2014). A small study (N = 43) of family caregivers of patients receiving palliative care found that over half of the patients experienced spiritual pain (Delgado-Guay et al., 2013). These caregivers with spiritual pain were found to also have increased depression and anxiety and other indications of dysfunctional coping. Studies such as these portrayed the family caring experience as involving spiritual and religious benefits and challenges. Social support from family or a religious congregation, spirituality and religion beliefs that provide meaning, and spirituality and religion rituals that provide comfort can all aid family caregivers during the arduous experience of caring for a loved one with cancer.

# Spiritual Support: Evidence-Based Approaches

Individuals with or without a life-threatening illness seek spiritual nurture in myriad ways. Some may find spiritual solace by being in nature (e.g., going to the beach, watching a sunset, watching a seedling grow). Some may seek an informal or formal spiritual mentor (e.g., spiritual director, shaman, clergy, friend, family). Some may purposefully pursue activities that enhance spiritual awareness (e.g., meditation, journal writing, listening to music, viewing or creating artistic expressions, reading an inspirational book or sacred text). The spiritual experience and what supports its nurture vary.

For people living with cancer, sources of spiritual nurture that provided support prior to the diagnosis often continue to provide support after the diagnosis. It is not uncommon, however, that the diagnosis challenges previously accepted spirituality and religion beliefs or forces examination of spirituality and religion beliefs and practices that never were completely accepted. For example, a patient or family caregiver may have wondered for years how there could be a loving, personal, and powerful God when people are suffering. If such a concern simmered preconsciously prior to the diagnosis, it would likely become a pressing concern after it. Thus, the cancer experience often prompts a spiritual revolution, one that seeks meaning for suffering, purpose for life, forgiveness, love, and so forth. The following approaches can help nurses to support patients on this spiritual journey.

## Screening and Assessment

To determine if patients have spiritual concerns and if they want spiritual support, a spiritual screening is necessary (Taylor, 2015). If findings from the screening indicate a spiritual concern with health implications, a more in-depth and focused assessment is in order. If an immediate referral to an expert is not made, the nurse may need to provide the spiritual support. Appropriate questions for spiritual screening and assessment are provided in Figure 9-1.

## Mindfulness-Based Stress Reduction Therapies

Several clinical trials have provided evidence for the effectiveness of mindfulness-based stress reduction (MBSR) therapies (Cramer, Lauche, Paul, & Dobos, 2012). MBSR is known to decrease anxiety, depression, distress, and mood disturbance, as well as improve spiritual well-being (Charlson et al., 2014; Dobos et al., 2015; Fish, Ettridge, Sharplin, Hancock, & Knott, 2014; Zernicke et al., 2014). Mindfulness is the core feature of meditation and involves bringing one's awareness to the present moment. This attention to the present is nonjudgmental; by not letting the past or future judge the present, one becomes accepting and joyful in the "power of now" (Tolle, 1997). When practiced regularly, the beneficial experience of the meditative state seeps into daily life. Thus, it is probably no surprise to Buddhists and others who have practiced meditation that people living with cancer now find spiritual, emotional, and physical benefits from MBSR.

Trials that assessed the efficacy of MBSR among people living with cancer generally teach meditation to participants over a period of at least eight weeks. The MBSR sessions are usually about two hours long, and participants are then given homework that includes daily meditation practice for approximately 45 minutes. The tested intervention in studies often also includes hatha yoga (movement or positioning the body so as to develop greater balance) and cognitive behavioral instruction about coping with illness (Charlson et al., 2014; Dobos et al., 2015; Zernicke et al., 2014). Zernicke et al. (2014) demonstrated feasibility and positive

**Step 1: Spiritual Screening**
Purpose:
- To identify spiritual distress that could have health-related implications
- To understand any spirituality and religion beliefs or practices requiring healthcare team support
- To determine from whom the patient would like to receive spiritual support

Preferred timing:
- When the patient enters the healthcare organization
- When a significant change in health status has occurred

Examples of screening questions:
- How important is spirituality and religion to you as you live with cancer?
- If 0 = not at all at peace and 10 = completely at peace, how would you rate yourself?
- Please tell us about any religious or spiritual beliefs or practices that are especially important to you now. How would you like for your healthcare team to support these?

**Step 2: Spiritual Assessment**
Purpose:
- To further understand any spiritual needs or distress identified during the screening
- If a primary care provider, to gather more complete data about how spirituality and religion affects health care

Preferred timing:
- Prior to episodes of care that would benefit from spiritual support (e.g., major surgery, bone marrow transplant)
- If beginning to serve the patient in a long-term significant or primary capacity

Examples of assessment questions:
- What beliefs or practices help you to face tough challenges like this? From where do you get your courage to keep going? Comfort? Strength? What helps you to cope?
- What kind of person do you see yourself as? What are you famous for?
- What do you see as the purpose for your life now?
- Follow-up questions that reflect specific spirituality and religion concerns raised during the screening

**Figure 9-1. Spiritual Screening and Assessment Questions**

*Note.* Based on information from Taylor, 2015.

outcomes from an online MBSR course that allowed participants to synchronously learn, practice, and discuss. Given that many patients are unable to attend so many MBSR classes away from home, this is especially useful.

The MBSR intervention in the aforementioned clinical trials was taught by psychologists or others with training in meditation. Although nurses may not be trained to provide MBSR, they can provide encouragement or supportive environments for patients who do want to meditate. Nurses can also incorporate elements of MBSR in clinical practice when appropriate (e.g., focused and deep breathing, assisting patients to identify a comforting visual image on which to focus attention, encouraging a "body scan," or focusing awareness on how areas of the body feel).

## Dignity Therapy and Life Storytelling

Telling the story of one's life gives it meaning; it also helps one to weave together its disparate pieces and to pass one's values to the next generation (Taylor, 1997). Being able to tell one's story can diminish anxiety and depression, and improve spiritual well-being (Fitchett, Emanuel, Handzo, Boyken, & Wilkie, 2015; Lloyd-Williams, Cobb, O'Connor, Dunn, & Shiels, 2013). Although reminiscence therapy and life storytelling are not new therapeutics, an interprofessional team, led by Dr. Chochinov, provided structure, evidence, and a label for such therapy: dignity therapy (Fitchett et al., 2015).

Dignity therapy involves a trained interviewer spending several hours with a patient to audio-record responses to a set of 10 questions (Fitchett et al., 2015). These responses are then transcribed, edited, and placed in a document that is given to the patient. The patient can then share the document as desired; it may be left to family as a legacy. Prompts cover the following topics: important parts of their life story, what they wish the family would remember of themselves, important roles they have played in life, accomplishments, what they wish to say to others, what life lessons they wish to pass on, and instructions they would like to give to prepare others for when they pass away (Chochinov et al., 2005). Although these questions were designed for use with patients near the end of life, the ones that prompt reflection on life could be useful to other patients. Patients could also adapt the therapy by keeping a personal journal or scrapbook.

## Religious Rituals and Community Support

Religious traditions offer beliefs and practices that support spiritual well-being (Taylor, 2012). These beliefs and practices are often deeply rooted, having been developed and used over centuries. Beliefs differ between religions but generally offer the adherent explanations about how the world and humanity came into existence, why suffering exists, what the purpose of life is, what happens after death, and so forth. Understanding such topics is typically important for patients with cancer who sense their lives are threatened. For the nurse caring for a patient with a stated religious affiliation, it is important to remember that even among members of the same religious tradition, considerable variation can exist in how doctrines are interpreted. In today's pluralistic societies, an individual's religiosity often is "hyphenated"—that is, more than one religious belief system influences the person (e.g., a Baptist-Buddhist who attends an interdenominational congregation). Therefore, it is important for a nurse to not pigeonhole patients by their religious affiliations. Whenever necessary, it is important to assess each patient's unique beliefs and practices as they pertain to the healthcare circumstance (Taylor, 2012).

Religious practices will reflect the basic assumptions espoused by a religious tradition and typically aim to facilitate relationship or connection between the believer and the divine (Taylor, 2012). For example, prayer, meditation, worship experiences, and even prescribed diet, dress, holy days, and other religious practices allow the believer to more fully experience sacredness. They also afford a communal experience that typically provides social support (e.g., "It is nice to know that church members are praying for me," or "I feel connected when I am singing with a hundred other believers during services."). Thus, patients benefit socially and spiritually when nurses assist them to continue their religious practices as needed. Such support can vary, from assisting a patient to connect with a local faith community, to practicing worshipful rituals or observing religious prescriptions related to diet, modesty, or holy days. However, such support should only be given if the patient has requested or consented to it (Taylor, 2012).

## Prayer

One religious practice commonly used by Americans, whether religious or not, is prayer (Jors, Büssing, Hvidt, & Baumann, 2015). In 2010, the General Social Survey of Americans showed that only 13% reported not praying, whereas 57% prayed at least once a day (ARDA, n.d.). In a survey about prayer habits by the National Health Interview Survey, 49% of more than 22,000 Americans reported praying about their health during the previous year (Wachholtz & Sambamoorthi, 2011).

In several studies about complementary and alternative medicine (CAM) therapies use among patients with cancer, prayer is often identified as a frequently used CAM (Huebner et al., 2014; Kang, McArdle, & Suh, 2014; Taylor, 2005).

Although many styles of prayer exist, and these styles vary across religious traditions, Smith et al. (2012) found in a focus group study with 13 Christian women with cancer that the most common types of prayer included those that prayed for others, conversed colloquially with God, petitioned God for something, expressed thankfulness, or used a ritual prayer (e.g., memorized prayer). Whether a patient requests the nurse pray with him or her, or whether the nurse is listening to a patient talk about praying, the evidence and clinical guidelines offered in Figure 9-2 will be helpful.

## Empathic Listening and Presence

When persons living with cancer express their spiritual doubts, struggles, and pain, it is instinctive for most nurses to avoid being present to that spiritual suffering (Taylor, 2007). Nurses' avoidance strategies include making comments that will cause all but the most desperate of patients to stop talking and finding legitimate reasons for physically leaving the patient. For example, a nurse can minimize the patient's suffering (e.g., "Do not worry; I've seen worse.") or impose a positive spin when the patient is not ready to hear it (e.g., "This is going to make you strong."). A nurse can also simply avoid being at the patient's bedside or give nonverbal messages to the patient to indicate they are discomforted by verbalized spiritual pain. Although patient expressions of spiritual suffering are upsetting to most anyone, the nurse who cares to ease this distress can do so, even if in an incremental way. This is generally done by actively and nonjudgmentally listening to the patient's thoughts and feelings with intellect, emotions, and awareness of physical responses. Communication skills, such as restating open-ended questions and

---

- Ethical considerations prior to offering to pray with a patient
  – Understand spiritual needs, resources, and preferences.
  – Follow expressed wishes.
  – Do not prescribe your own spiritual beliefs or practices, or pressure client to relinquish theirs.
  – Strive to know your own spirituality.
  – Provide care that is consonant with your own integrity.
- Positive prayer content is associated with positive mood. That is, if a patient's prayers include thanksgiving, adoration, and/or reception (i.e., passively waiting for divine insight), this likely will accompany positive mood and emotional well-being.
- Prayer with trust-based beliefs contributes to positive psychological outcomes (e.g., self-esteem). Trusting prayers include recognition that God will respond.
  – When is best (e.g., "I'll wait patiently for the answer because God's timing is best.")
  – How is best (e.g., "I pray with my hands and heart open to whatever God gives me.")
- Prayer that allows self-disclosure is associated with positive mental health outcomes. Writing a prayer as a letter or diary entry can allow such self-disclosure.
- Telling a patient or family caregiver that you are praying for them can contribute to increasing their optimism.
- "Making God real and making God good" may be mechanisms that explain the positive health outcomes of prayer. Thus, prayer experiences that vividly imagine God and experiences of others who portray a loving God (e.g., a compassionate nurse) likely foster positive outcomes of prayer.

**Figure 9-2. Prayer: Ethical and Evidence-Based Guidelines**

*Note.* Based on information from Krause, 2011; Krause & Hayward, 2013; Luhrmann, 2013; Pérez et al., 2011; Pössel et al., 2014; Schafer, 2013; Whittington & Scher, 2010; Winslow & Winslow, 2003.

reflecting feelings, can be used to formulate therapeutic responses to expressions of spiritual pain (Taylor, 2007).

## Other Potential Approaches to Spiritual Support

Numerous other approaches support patient spiritual well-being. For example, limited evidence suggests yoga (Cramer, Lange, Klose, Paul, & Dobos, 2012), relaxation and guided imagery (Elias et al., 2015), self-forgiveness therapy (Toussaint, Barry, Bornfriend, & Markman, 2014), being with nature (Nakau et al., 2013), and advance care planning (Lyon, Jacobs, Briggs, Cheng, & Wang, 2014) all may support spiritual well-being among patients with cancer. Strong evidence indicates that meaning-centered psychotherapy is also effective (Breitbart et al., 2015) (see Chapter 25).

## Role of the Nurse in Providing Spiritual Support

Although healthcare facilities typically have relegated spiritual care to chaplains, this compartmentalization of services is inadequate for several reasons. First, spiritual needs can surface at any time and often are best cared for if immediately addressed. Second, spiritual needs do not occur in isolation or only during a pastoral visit. Third, many people are unable to benefit from spiritual care from a chaplain because of negative associations with organized religion. Fourth, much of spiritual caregiving requires rapport and a good relationship, which can be difficult to achieve when patients are isolated or receive only brief chaplain visits.

Nursing, however, lends itself to at least an initial level of spiritual support. Nurses can develop rapport, and nurses' constant presence allows them to witness spiritual needs if they are observant and deeply listening.

Although nurses are expected to provide holistic care that includes spiritual support, it is important for nurses to recognize the limitations of their generalist role in this regard. It is the chaplain who is the spiritual care expert. Thus, when a nurse screens or assesses that a patient or family caregiver is experiencing spiritual and religious distress, a referral should be made. Even nurses with rich and positive spiritual and religious backgrounds who are eager to support client spirituality and religion should be mindful that this is not their primary role or a role for which they have training and expertise. Reflection questions posed in Figure 9-3 can also prompt nurses to consider their motivations for initiating spirituality and religion discourse with patients, as any coercive proselytization is unethical (Taylor, 2012).

---

What prompts my actions and reactions related to patient spirituality and religiosity?
- Am I simply curious? Or is there clearly a healthcare-related reason to introduce a spirituality and religion topic with a patient?
- Do I believe my spiritual and religious beliefs are better than most patients' beliefs and therefore need to gently persuade them of that?
- How much do I accept and even value diverse spiritual and religious experiences?
- What guides me as I inquire about or listen to a patient discuss spirituality and religion? Is it my intuition, gut, divine influence, or personal need?
- Is my desire to talk about spirituality and religion with a patient self-centered or patient centered?

**Figure 9-3. Questions for Reflection**

*Note.* Based on information from Taylor, 2010.

## Conclusion

This chapter identifies the growing body of evidence that describes and begins to explain the spiritual and religious experience among people living with cancer, patients and family caregivers alike. Because cancer can undermine one's spiritual and religious beliefs and/or be a catalyst for spirituality and religion growth—and because this interplay between illness and spirituality and religion often affects health-related outcomes—it is important that nurses understand how spiritual and religious beliefs and practices affect patient well-being and strive to provide spirituality and religion support. Although several evidence-informed approaches to spirituality and religion support are introduced, what may be most effective is the nurse's expert use of self when fully present and deeply listening. It is imperative, however, that nurses practice spiritual care within their scope of practice.

## References

Adams, R.N., Mosher, C.E., Cannady, R.S., Lucette, A., & Kim, Y. (2014). Caregiving experiences predict changes in spiritual well-being among family caregivers of cancer patients. *Psycho-Oncology, 23,* 1178–1184. doi:10.1002/pon.3558

Allen, J.D., Leyva, B., Torres, A.I., Ospino, H., Tom, L., Rustan, S., & Bartholomew, A. (2014). Religious beliefs and cancer screening behaviors among Catholic Latinos: Implications for faith-based interventions. *Journal of Health Care for the Poor and Underserved, 25,* 503–526. doi:10.1353/hpu.2014.0080

Asiedu, G.B., Eustace, R.W., Eton, D.T., & Radecki Breitkopf, C. (2014). Coping with colorectal cancer: A qualitative exploration with patients and their family members. *Family Practice, 31,* 598–606. doi:10.1093/fampra/cmu040

Association of Religion Data Archives. (n.d.). Religion dictionary. Retrieved from http://www.thearda.com/learningcenter/religiondictionary.asp

Bai, M., Lazenby, M., Jeon, S., Dixon, J., & McCorkle, R. (2015). Exploring the relationship between spiritual well-being and quality of life among patients newly diagnosed with advanced cancer. *Palliative and Supportive Care, 13,* 927–935. doi:10.1017/S1478951514000820

Balboni, T.A., Balboni, M., Paulk, M.E., Phelps, A., Wright, A., Peteet, J., ... Prigerson, H. (2011). Support of cancer patients' spiritual needs and associations with medical care costs at the end of life. *Cancer, 117,* 5383–5391. doi:10.1002/cncr.26221

Balboni, T.A., Paulk, M.E., Balboni, M.J., Phelps, A.C., Loggers, E.T., Wright, A.A., ... Prigerson, H.G. (2010). Provision of spiritual care to patients with advanced cancer: Associations with medical care and quality of life near death. *Journal of Clinical Oncology, 28,* 445–452. doi:10.1200/JCO.2009.24.8005

Barss, K.S. (2012). T.R.U.S.T.: An affirming model for inclusive spiritual care. *Journal of Holistic Nursing, 30,* 24–34. doi:10.1177/0898010111418118

Best, A.L., Alcaraz, K.I., McQueen, A., Cooper, D.L., Warren, R.C., & Stein, K. (2014). Examining the mediating role of cancer-related problems on spirituality and self-rated health among African American cancer survivors: A report from the American Cancer Society's Studies of Cancer Survivors-II. *Psycho-Oncology, 24,* 1051–1059, doi:10.1002/pon.3720

Best, A.L., Spencer, M., Hall, I.J., Friedman, D.B., & Billings, D. (2015). Developing spiritually framed breast cancer screening messages in consultation with African American women. *Health Communication, 30,* 290–300. doi:10.1080/10410236.2013.845063

Breitbart, W., Rosenfeld, B., Pessin, H., Applebaum, A., Kulikowski, J., & Lichtenthal, W.G. (2015). Meaning-centered group psychotherapy: An effective intervention for improving psychological well-being in patients with advanced cancer. *Journal of Clinical Oncology, 33,* 749–754. doi:10.1200/JCO.2014.57.2198

Bulkley, J., McMullen, C.K., Hornbrook, M.C., Grant, M., Altschuler, A., Wendel, C.S., & Krouse, R.S. (2013). Spiritual well-being in long-term colorectal cancer survivors with ostomies. *Psycho-Oncology, 22,* 2513–2521. doi:10.1002/pon.3318

Canada, A.L., Fitchett, G., Murphy, P.E., Stein, K., Portier, K., Crammer, C., & Peterman, A.H. (2013). Racial/ethnic differences in spiritual well-being among cancer survivors. *Journal of Behavioral Medicine, 36,* 441–453. doi:10.1007/s10865-012-9439-8

Caplan, L., Sawyer, P., Holt, C., & Brown, C.J. (2014). Religiosity after a diagnosis of cancer among older adults. *Journal of Religion, Spirituality, and Aging, 26,* 357–369. doi:10.1080/15528030.2014.928922

Charlson, M.E., Loizzo, J., Moadel, A., Neale, M., Newman, C., Olivo, E., ... Peterson, J.C. (2014). Contemplative self healing in women breast cancer survivors: A pilot study in underserved minority women shows improvement in quality of life and reduced stress. *BMC Complementary and Alternative Medicine, 14,* 349. doi:10.1186/1472-6882-14-349

Chatters, L.M., Taylor, R.J., Bullard, K.M., & Jackson, J.S. (2008). Spirituality and subjective religiosity among African Americans, Caribbean Blacks and non-Hispanic Whites. *Journal for the Scientific Study of Religion, 47,* 725–737. doi:10.1111/j.1468-5906.2008.00437.x

Chochinov, H.M., Hack, T., Hassard, T., Kristjanson, L.J., McClement, S., & Harlos, M. (2005). Dignity therapy: A novel psychotherapeutic intervention for patients near the end of life. *Journal of Clinical Oncology, 23,* 5520–5525. doi:10.1200/JCO.2005.08.391

Cramer, H., Lange, S., Klose, P., Paul, A., & Dobos, G. (2012). Yoga for breast cancer patients and survivors: A systematic review and meta-analysis. *BMC Cancer, 12,* 412. doi:10.1186/1471-2407-12-412

Cramer, H., Lauche, R., Paul, A., & Dobos, G. (2012). Mindfulness-based stress reduction for breast cancer: A systematic review and meta-analysis. *Current Oncology, 19,* E343–E352. doi:10.3747/co.19.1016

Danhauer, S.C., Case, L.D., Tedeschi, R., Russell, G., Vishnevsky, T., Triplett, K., ... Avis, N.E. (2013). Predictors of posttraumatic growth in women with breast cancer. *Psycho-Oncology, 22,* 2676–2683. doi:10.1002/pon.3298

Daverio-Zanetti, S., Schultz, K., Del Campo, M.A., Malcarne, V., Riley, N., & Sadler, G.R. (2014). Is religiosity related to attitudes toward clinical trials participation? *Journal of Cancer Education, 30,* 220–224. doi:10.1007/s13187-014-0696-9

Deal, B., & Grassley, J.S. (2012). The lived experience of giving spiritual care: A phenomenological study of nephrology nurses working in acute and chronic hemodialysis settings. *Nephrology Nursing Journal, 39,* 471–481, 496.

Delgado-Guay, M.O., Parsons, H.A., Hui, D., De la Cruz, M.G., Thorney, S., & Bruera, E. (2013). Spirituality, religiosity, and spiritual pain among caregivers of patients with advanced cancer. *American Journal of Hospice and Palliative Care, 30,* 455–461. doi:10.1177/1049909112458030

Dobos, G., Overhamm, T., Büssing, A., Ostermann, T., Langhorst, J., Kümmel, S., ... Cramer, H. (2015). Integrating mindfulness in supportive cancer care: A cohort study on a mindfulness-based day care clinic for cancer survivors. *Supportive Care in Cancer, 23,* 2945–2955. doi:10.1007/s00520-015-2660-6

Elias, A.C., Ricci, M.D., Rodriguez, L.H., Pinto, S.D., Giglio, J.S., & Baracat, E.C. (2015). The biopsychosocial spiritual model applied to the treatment of women with breast cancer, through RIME intervention (relaxation, mental images, spirituality). *Complementary Therapies in Clinical Practice, 21,* 1–6. doi:10.1016/j.ctcp.2015.01.007

Fish, J.A., Ettridge, K., Sharplin, G.R., Hancock, B., & Knott, V.E. (2014). Mindfulness-based cancer stress management: Impact of a mindfulness-based programme on psychological distress and quality of life. *European Journal of Cancer Care, 23,* 413–421. doi:10.1111/ecc.12136

Fitchett, G. (1993). *Assessing spiritual needs: A guide for caregivers.* Minneapolis, MN: Augsberg Publishing House.

Fitchett, G., Emanuel, L., Handzo, G., Boyken, L., & Wilkie, D.J. (2015). Care of the human spirit and the role of dignity therapy: A systematic review of dignity therapy research. *BMC Palliative Care, 14,* 8. doi:10.1186/s12904-015-0007-1

Frost, M.H., Novotny, P.J., Johnson, M.E., Clark, M.M., Sloan, J.A., & Yang, P. (2013). Spiritual well-being in lung cancer survivors. *Supportive Care in Cancer, 21,* 1939–1946. doi:10.1007/s00520-013-1757-z

Gallup. (2016). Religion. Retrieved from http://www.gallup.com/poll/1690/religion.aspx

Geller, B.M., Vacek, P.M., Flynn, B.S., Lord, K., & Cranmer, D. (2014). What are cancer survivors' needs and how well are they being met? *Journal of Family Practice, 63,* E7–E16.

Gordon, M. (2007). *Manual of nursing diagnosis.* Burlington, MA: Jones & Bartlett Learning.

Hamilton, J.B., Galbraith, K.V., Best, N.C., Worthy, V.C., & Moore, L.T. (2015). African American cancer survivors' use of religious beliefs to positively influence the utilization of cancer care. *Journal of Religion and Health, 54,* 1856–1869. doi:10.1007/s10943-014-9948-6

Hill, P.C., Pargament, K., Hood, R.W., McCullough, M.E., Swyers, J.P., Larson, D.B., & Zinnbauer, B.J. (2000). Conceptualizing religion and spirituality: Points of commonality, points of departure. *Journal for the Theory of Social Behaviour, 30,* 51–77. doi:10.1111/1468-5914.00119

Hocker, A., Krull, A., Koch, U., & Mehnert, A. (2014). Exploring spiritual needs and their associated factors in an urban sample of early and advanced cancer patients. *European Journal of Cancer Care, 23,* 786–794. doi:10.1111/ecc.12200

Huebner, J., Prott, F.J., Micke, O., Muecke, R., Senf, B., Dennert, G., & Muenstedt, K. (2014). Online survey of cancer patients on complementary and alternative medicine. *Oncology Research and Treatment, 37,* 304–308. doi:10.1159/000362616

International Council of Nurses. (2012). *The ICN Code for Nurses.* Retrieved from http://www.icn.ch/images/stories/documents/about/icncode_english.pdf

Joint Commission. (2009). *The Joint Commission 2009 requirements related to the provision of culturally competent patient-centered care Hospital Accreditation Program (HAP).* Retrieved from http://www.jointcommission.org/assets/1/6/2009_CLASRelatedStandardsHAP.pdf

Jors, K., Büssing, A., Hvidt, N.C., & Baumann, K. (2015). Personal prayer in patients dealing with chronic illness: A review of the research literature. *Evidence-Based Complementary and Alternative Medicine, 2015,* Article ID 927973. doi:10.1155/2015/927973

Kang, D.H., McArdle, T., & Suh, Y. (2014). Changes in complementary and alternative medicine use across cancer treatment and relationship to stress, mood, and quality of life. *Journal of Alternative and Complementary Medicine, 20,* 853–859. doi:10.1089/acm.2014.0216

King, M., Llewellyn, H., Leurent, B., Owen, F., Leavey, G., Tookman, A., & Jones, L. (2013). Spiritual beliefs near the end of life: A prospective cohort study of people with cancer receiving palliative care. *Psycho-Oncology, 22,* 2505–2512. doi:10.1002/pon.3313

King, S.D., Fitchett, G., & Berry, D.L. (2013). Screening for religious/spiritual struggle in blood and marrow transplant patients. *Supportive Care in Cancer, 21,* 993–1001. doi:10.1007/s00520-012-1618-1

Koenig, H.G., King, D.E., & Carson, V.B. (2012). Handbook of religion and health (2nd ed.). New York, NY: Oxford University Press.

Krause, N. (2011). Assessing the prayer lives of older whites, older blacks and older Mexican Americans: A descriptive analysis. *International Journal for the Psychology of Religion, 22,* 60–78. doi:10.1080/10508619.2012.635060

Krause, N., & Hayward, R.D. (2013). Prayer beliefs and change in life satisfaction over time. *Journal of Religion and Health, 52,* 674–694. doi:10.1007/s10943-012-9638-1

Leeson, L.A., Nelson, A.M., Rathouz, P.J., Juckett, M.B., Coe, C.L., Caes, E.W., & Costanzo, E.S. (2015). Spirituality and the recovery of quality of life following hematopoietic stem cell transplantation. *Health Psychology, 34,* 920–928. doi:10.1037/hea0000196

Lewis, S., Salins, N., Rao, M.R., & Kadam, A. (2014). Spiritual well-being and its influence on fatigue in patients undergoing active cancer directed treatment: A correlational study. *Journal of Cancer Research and Therapy, 10,* 676–680. doi:10.4103/0973-1482.138125

Leyva, B., Nguyen, A.B., Allen, J.D., Taplin, S.H., & Moser, R.P. (2014). Is religiosity associated with cancer screening? Results from a national survey. *Journal of Religion and Health, 54,* 998–1013. doi:10.1007/s10943-014-9843-1

Lloyd-Williams, M., Cobb, M., O'Connor, C., Dunn, L., & Shiels, C. (2013). A pilot randomised controlled trial to reduce suffering and emotional distress in patients with advanced cancer. *Journal of Affective Disorders, 148,* 141–145. doi:10.1016/j.jad.2012.11.013

Luhrmann, T.M. (2013). Making God real and making God good: Some mechanisms through which prayer may contribute to healing. *Transcultural Psychiatry, 50,* 707–725. doi:10.1177/1363461513487670

Lynn, B., Yoo, G.J., & Levine, E.G. (2014). "Trust in the Lord": Religious and spiritual practices of African American breast cancer survivors. *Journal of Religion and Health, 53,* 1706–1716. doi:10.1007/s10943-013-9750-x

Lyon, M.E., Jacobs, S., Briggs, L., Cheng, Y.I., & Wang, J. (2014). A longitudinal, randomized, controlled trial of advance care planning for teens with cancer: Anxiety, depression, quality of life, advance directives, spirituality. *Journal of Adolescent Health, 54,* 710–717. doi:10.1016/j.jadohealth.2013.10.206

Maguire, R., Papadopoulou, C., Kotronoulas, G., Simpson, M.F., McPhelim, J., & Irvine, L. (2013). A systematic review of supportive care needs of people living with lung cancer. *European Journal of Oncology Nursing, 17,* 449–464. doi:10.1016/j.ejon.2012.10.013

Martsolf, D.S., & Mickley, J.R. (1998). The concept of spirituality in nursing theories: Differing world-views and extent of focus. *Journal of Advanced Nursing, 27,* 294–303. doi:10.1046/j.1365-2648.1998.00519.x

McFarland, M.J., Pudrovska, T., Schieman, S., Ellison, C.G., & Bierman, A. (2013). Does a cancer diagnosis influence religiosity? Integrating a life course perspective. *Social Science Research, 42,* 311–320. doi:10.1016/j.ssresearch.2012.10.006

McLaughlin, B., Yoo, W., D'Angelo, J., Tsang, S., Shaw, B., Shah, D., … Gustafson, D. (2013). It is out of my hands: How deferring control to God can decrease quality of life for breast cancer patients. *Psycho-Oncology, 22,* 2747–2754. doi:10.1002/pon.3356

Moreno, P.I., & Stanton, A.L. (2013). Personal growth during the experience of advanced cancer: A systematic review. *Cancer Journal, 19,* 421–430. doi:10.1097/PPO.0b013e3182a5bbe7

Munoz, A.R., Salsman, J.M., Stein, K.D., & Cella, D. (2015). Reference values of the Functional Assessment of Chronic Illness Therapy–spiritual well-being: A report from the American Cancer Society's studies of cancer survivors. *Cancer, 121,* 1838–1844. doi:10.1002/cncr.29286

Murray, R.B., & Zentner, J.P. (1989). *Nursing concepts for health promotion*. Englewood Cliffs, NJ: Prentice Hall.

Nakau, M., Imanishi, J., Imanishi, J., Watanabe, S., Imanishi, A., Baba, T., ... Morimoto, Y. (2013). Spiritual care of cancer patients by integrated medicine in urban green space: A pilot study. *Explore, 9,* 87–90. doi:10.1016/j.explore.2012.12.002

Nardi, D., & Rooda, L. (2011). Spirituality-based nursing practice by nursing students: An exploratory study. *Journal of Professional Nursing, 27,* 255–263. doi:10.1016/j.profnurs.2011.03.006

National Comprehensive Cancer Network. (2017). *NCCN Clinical Practice Guidelines in Oncology (NCCN Guidelines®): Distress management* [v.2.2017]. Retrieved from http://www.nccn.org/professionals/physician_gls/pdf/distress.pdf

Nixon, A.V., Narayanasamy, A., & Penny, V. (2013). An investigation into the spiritual needs of neuro-oncology patients from a nurse perspective. *BMC Nursing, 12,* 2. doi:10.1186/1472-6955-12-2

Padela, A.I., Peek, M., Johnson-Agbakwu, C.E., Hosseinian, Z., & Curlin, F. (2014). Associations between religion-related factors and cervical cancer screening among Muslims in greater Chicago. *Journal of Lower Genital Tract Disease, 18,* 326–332. doi:10.1097/LGT.0000000000000026

Paterson, C., Robertson, A., Smith, A., & Nabi, G. (2015). Identifying the unmet supportive care needs of men living with and beyond prostate cancer: A systematic review. *European Journal of Oncology Nursing, 19,* 405–418. doi:10.1016/j.ejon.2014.12.007

Pérez, J.E., & Smith, A.R. (2015). Intrinsic religiousness and well-being among cancer patients: The mediating role of control-related religious coping and self-efficacy for coping with cancer. *Journal of Behavioral Medicine, 38,* 183–193. doi:10.1007/s10865-014-9593-2

Pérez, J.E., Smith, A.R., Norris, R.L., Canenguez, K.M., Tracey, E.F., & Decristofaro, S.B. (2011). Types of prayer and depressive symptoms among cancer patients: The mediating role of rumination and social support. *Journal of Behavioral Medicine, 34,* 519–530. doi:10.1007/s10865-011-9333-9

Pew Research Center. (2017). Religious landscape survey. Available from http://www.pewforum.org/religious-landscape-study/

Pössel, P., Black, S.W., Bjerg, A., Jeppsen, B., & Wooldridge, D. (2014). Do trust-based beliefs mediate the associations of frequency of private prayer with mental health? A cross-sectional study. *Journal of Religion and Health, 53,* 904–916. doi:10.1007/s10943-013-9688-z

Préau, M., Bouhnik, A.D., & Le Coroller Soriano, A.G. (2013). Two years after cancer diagnosis, what is the relationship between health-related quality of life, coping strategies and spirituality? *Psychology, Health, and Medicine, 18,* 375–386. doi:10.1080/13548506.2012.736622

Rabow, M.W., & Knish, S.J. (2015). Spiritual well-being among outpatients with cancer receiving concurrent oncologic and palliative care. *Supportive Care in Cancer, 23,* 919–923. doi:10.1007/s00520-014-2428-4

Reinert, K.G., & Koenig, H.G. (2013). Re-examining definitions of spirituality in nursing research. *Journal of Advanced Nursing, 69,* 2622–2634. doi:10.1111/jan.12152

Rubin, L.R., Chavez, J., Alderman, A., & Pusic, A.L. (2013). 'Use what God has given me': Difference and disparity in breast reconstruction. *Psychology and Health, 28,* 1099–1120. doi:10.1080/08870446.2013.782404

Sawatzky, R., & Pesut, B. (2005). Attributes of spiritual care in nursing practice. *Journal of Holistic Nursing, 23,* 19–33. doi:10.1177/0898010104272010

Schafer, M.H. (2013). Close ties, intercessory prayer, and optimism among American adults: Locating God in the social support network. *Journal for the Scientific Study of Religion, 52,* 35–56. doi:10.1111/jssr.12010

Seibaek, L., Hounsgaard, L., & Hvidt, N.C. (2013). Secular, spiritual, and religious existential concerns of women with ovarian cancer during final diagnostics and start of treatment. *Evidence-Based Complementary and Alternative Medicine, 2013,* Article ID 765419. doi:10.1155/2013/765419

Silvestri, G.A., Knittig, S., Zoller, J.S., & Nietert, P.J. (2003). Importance of faith on medical decisions regarding cancer care. *Journal of Clinical Oncology, 21,* 1379–1382. doi:10.1200/JCO.2003.08.036

Sirilla, J., & Overcash, J. (2013). Quality of life, supportive care, and spirituality in hematopoietic stem cell transplant patients. *Supportive Care in Cancer, 21,* 1137–1144. doi:10.1007/s00520-012-1637-y

Smith, A.R., DeSanto-Madeya, S., Pérez, J.E., Tracey, E.F., DeCristofaro, S., Norris, R.L., & Mukkamala, S.L. (2012). How women with advanced cancer pray: A report from two focus groups [Online exclusive]. *Oncology Nursing Forum, 39,* E310–E316. doi:10.1188/12.ONF.E310-E316

Stein, E.M., Kolidas, E., & Moadel, A. (2015). Do spiritual patients want spiritual interventions?: A qualitative exploration of underserved cancer patients' perspectives on religion and spirituality. *Palliative and Supportive Care, 13,* 19–25. doi:10.1017/S1478951513000217

Taylor, E.J. (1997). The story behind the story: The use of storytelling in spiritual caregiving. *Seminars in Oncology Nursing, 13,* 252–254. doi:10.1016/S0749-2081(97)80020-4

Taylor, E.J. (2002). *Spiritual care: Nursing theory, research, and practice*. Upper Saddle River, NJ: Prentice Hall.

Taylor, E.J. (2007). *What do I say? Talking with patients about spirituality*. West Conshohocken, PA: Templeton Press.

Taylor, E.J. (2012). *Religion: A clinical guide for nurses*. New York, NY: Springer.

Taylor, E.J. (2015). Spiritual assessment. In B.R. Ferrell, N. Coyle, & J.A. Paice (Eds.), *Oxford textbook of palliative nursing care* (4th ed., pp. 531–545). New York, NY: Oxford University Press.

Taylor, E.J., & Davenport, F. (2012). Spiritual quality of life. In C. King & P. Hinds (Eds.), *Quality of life: From nursing and patient perspective* (3rd ed., pp. 83–104). Burlington, MA: Jones & Bartlett Learning.

Taylor, E.J., Petersen, C., Oyedele, O., & Haase, J. (2015). Spirituality and spiritual care of adolescents and young adults with cancer. *Seminars in Oncology Nursing, 31,* 227–241. doi:10.1016/j.soncn.2015.06.002

Taylor, E.J., Testerman, N., & Hart, D. (2014). Teaching spiritual care to nursing students: An integrated model. *Journal of Christian Nursing, 31,* 94–99. doi:10.1097/CNJ.0000000000000058

Thune-Boyle, I.C., Stygall, J., Keshtgar, M.R., Davidson, T.I., & Newman, S.P. (2013). Religious/spiritual coping resources and their relationship with adjustment in patients newly diagnosed with breast cancer in the UK. *Psycho-Oncology, 22,* 646–658. doi:10.1002/pon.3048

Tkatch, R., Hudson, J., Katz, A., Berry-Bobovski, L., Vichich, J., Eggly, S., … Albrecht, T.L. (2014). Barriers to cancer screening among orthodox Jewish women. *Journal of Community Health, 39,* 1200–1208. doi:10.1007/s10900-014-9879-x

Tolle, E. (1997). *The power of now: A guide to spiritual enlightenment.* Novato, CA: New World Library.

Toussaint, L., Barry, M., Bornfriend, L., & Markman, M. (2014). Restore: The journey toward self-forgiveness: A randomized trial of patient education on self-forgiveness in cancer patients and caregivers. *Journal of Health Care Chaplaincy, 20,* 54–74. doi:10.1080/08854726.2014.902714

Trevino, K.M., Balboni, M., Zollfrank, A., Balboni, T., & Prigerson, H.G. (2014). Negative religious coping as a correlate of suicidal ideation in patients with advanced cancer. *Psycho-Oncology, 23,* 936–945. doi:10.1002/pon.3505

Wachholtz, A., & Sambamoorthi, U. (2011). National trends in prayer use as a coping mechanism for health concerns: Changes from 2002 to 2007. *Psychology of Religion and Spirituality, 3,* 67–77. doi:10.1037/a0021598

White, M.L., Peters, R., & Schim, S.M. (2011). Spirituality and spiritual self-care: Expanding self-care deficit nursing theory. *Nursing Science Quarterly, 24,* 48–56. doi:10.1177/0894318410389059

Whittington, B.L., & Scher, S.J. (2010). Prayer and subjective well-being: An examination of six different types of prayer. *International Journal for the Psychology of Religion, 20,* 59–68. doi:10.1080/10508610903146316

Williams, A.-L., & Bakitas, M. (2012). Cancer family caregivers: A new direction for interventions. *Journal of Palliative Medicine, 15,* 775–783. doi:10.1089/jpm.2012.0046

Williams, A.-L., Dixon, J., Feinn, R., & McCorkle, R. (2014). Cancer family caregiver depression: Are religion-related variables important? *Psycho-Oncology, 24,* 825–831. doi:10.1002/pon.3647

Winslow, G.R., & Winslow, B.W. (2003). Examining the ethics of praying with patients. *Holistic Nursing Practice, 17,* 170–177. doi:10.1097/00004650-200307000-00002

Zernicke, K.A., Campbell, T.S., Speca, M., McCabe-Ruff, K., Flowers, S., & Carlson, L.E. (2014). A randomized wait-list controlled trial of feasibility and efficacy of an online mindfulness-based cancer recovery program: The eTherapy for cancer applying mindfulness trial. *Psychosomatic Medicine, 76,* 257–267. doi:10.1097/PSY.0000000000000053

# CHAPTER 10

# Suffering

*Betty R. Ferrell, PhD, FAAN, and Virginia Sun, PhD, RN*

> *Out of suffering have emerged the strongest souls.*
> —E.H. Chapin

In 1982, Cassell challenged the separation of illness into physical and psychological states in his classic paper "The Nature of Suffering and the Goals of Medicine." He asserted that "suffering is experienced by persons, not merely by bodies" (p. 639) and suggested that understanding the place of the person in human illness requires a rejection of the historical dualism of mind and body. According to Cassell (1999), suffering occurs when the intactness or integrity of an individual is threatened or disrupted. It involves some symptom or process (physical or otherwise) that poses a threat, the meaning of that threat, fear, and concerns about the future.

Cassell's classic work has challenged the medical profession to examine its goals and recognize the moral mandate to attend not only to physical illness but also to the suffering that accompanies it. Nurses, perhaps, have been less inclined to consider the mind and the body as separate, because professionally, they recognize and embrace the whole person. The vision and standards of oncology nursing are embedded in the view that cancer is a life-threatening illness with physical, psychological, social, and spiritual dimensions (Ferrell, 1996). Oncology nurses view their profession as family centered, with cancer affecting the entire family and the patient's significant others, not just the individual with cancer.

Thus, for oncology nurses, recognition of suffering is not a novel notion but rather the reaffirmation of the importance of holistic care amid a rapidly changing healthcare environment. Nurses are confronted with the challenges posed by increasingly depersonalized cancer care that is characterized by high-tech treatments, more invasive and aggressive care, and a new frontier of scientific strides, including gene therapy, transplantation, and surgical approaches to eradicate disease. At the same time, nursing as a profession is rapidly moving toward a managed-care environment with many potentially threatening components, including decreased staffing, increased reliance on assistive personnel, and transfer of even the most intensive patient care to family caregivers in the home. The need to explore the basis of suffering is rooted in a reaffirmation of nursing's commitment to the wholeness of the patient and the existential crisis caused by a cancer diagnosis.

# The Nature of Suffering in Patients With Cancer

Suffering is discussed in oncology literature as a component of quality of life (QOL). A cancer diagnosis and subsequent treatment profoundly influence QOL. Patients with cancer have described seeing their image in a mirror and reflecting on the physical devastation of disease and treatment and the insult to the spirit. This recognition of decreased QOL makes the patient aware of the disease's devastation and of an altered life with diminished meaning. As many previous theorists (Copp, 1974; Frankl, 1963) have described, this decreased meaning leads to suffering. Therefore, relief of suffering is seen as a critical QOL intervention, particularly when the patient has advanced disease and the goals of care shift from cure to comfort. Suffering is included in the domain of spiritual well-being as an aspect of QOL, but it is also a component that transcends the other domains of physical, psychological, and social well-being (Ferrell, 1996). This model has been applied to patients with advanced cancer who are experiencing pain (Borneman et al., 2011); survivors of bone marrow transplant (Cooke, Chung, & Grant, 2011; Wong et al., 1992), breast cancer (Dow, Ferrell, Leigh, Ly, & Gulasekaram, 1996), ovarian cancer (O'Sullivan, Bowles, Jeon, Ercolano, & McCorkle, 2011; Pinar, Ayhan, & Pinar, 2013); and other long-term survivors of cancer (Koch, Jansen, Brenner, & Arndt, 2013). These QOL studies have included varying populations across the cancer trajectory, and suffering is evident as a component in each. Suffering begins not at the transition from chronic illness to terminal illness but rather at the moment of diagnosis.

As an elusive and abstract concept, suffering often has been confused with other psychological constructs. Morse and Carter (1996) studied the concept of enduring and expressions of suffering and used narratives of illness experiences to analyze them. They defined three types of enduring: enduring to survive, enduring to live, and enduring to die. Suffering was defined as an emotional response to that which was endured, to the changed present, or to anticipating a changed future.

In another study, Morse, Bottorff, and Hutchinson (1995) examined the paradox of comfort. This conceptualization is applicable to cancer because cancer causes significant physical deterioration, symptoms, and resulting discomfort. Eight themes of discomfort emerged in this study: the diseased body, the disobedient body, the deceiving body, the vulnerable body, the violated body, the resigned body, the enduring body, and the betraying body. The authors concluded that illness places patients' bodies in the foreground, thus dominating their lives.

Frankl (1963), another classic contributor to the field of suffering, developed a psychotherapy modality known as logotherapy. Logotherapy attempted to help individuals find meaning in their experiences. Having been a concentration camp prisoner and survivor, Frankl applied his personal observations and experiences to individuals who survive life-threatening illnesses. Frankl observed that prisoners like himself, who had a will to live or a purpose to sustain themselves, were able to find meaning in their suffering and, thus, survive. In applying these lessons to therapeutic relationships, Frankl contended that the clinician's role was to assist the patient in finding meaning in suffering. Studies have built on Frankl's work, making significant contributions to the area of meaning in oncology (Breitbart & Applebaum, 2011; Chochinov, 2012).

Just as nursing plays a key role in cancer care, it also has a pivotal role in relieving suffering. Copp (1974, 1990a, 1990b), a pioneer in making the relief of suffering a goal in the nursing profession, defined *suffering* as a state of anguish in one who bears pain, injury, or loss. Her classic work challenged nurses to assess and intervene in suffering.

Oncology nurses are intimately involved in the cancer journey, traversing the phases of cancer survivorship. Nurses are present during the shock and suffering associated with a new diagnosis, through the trials of aggressive treatment, the uncertainty and apprehension of remission, the devastation of recurrence, and the suffering associated with facing death from advanced disease. Nurses are instrumental in moving patients from the anguish of suffering to finding meaning from suffering.

Recognizing the trajectory of cancer, Reich (1987, 1989) described the experience of suffering through the metaphor of language. He described the sufferers' struggle to discover a voice that would express the search for suffering's meaning in three phases: mute suffering, expressive suffering, and new identity. In mute suffering, patients are so affected by their circumstances that they cannot verbally express their needs. This is not suffering in silence, however, because these individuals may be screaming in pain. The scream of pain may be the expression of mute suffering. In expressive suffering, the sufferer seeks a language to express the suffering. The language may be one of lament (complaint), story (in telling their story they gain voice, transform the suffering, or gain distance), or interpretation (often through metaphor). The third phase is new identity or having a voice of one's own. This occurs through experiencing solidarity with compassionate others and by taking on a language of suffering through reforming one's story, which then identifies the new self.

## Sources of Suffering

In oncology, uncontrolled symptoms have been recognized as a major source of suffering. The side effects of cancer treatment often are reported to be more debilitating than the disease itself. Patients with ovarian cancer have described the suffering from uncontrolled pain, such as peripheral neuropathy, as both severe and lingering (Borneman et al., 2011). Research on fatigue has revealed that symptoms previously viewed as only physical problems also are associated with suffering. The experience of fatigue is a reminder of patients' many losses and results in their inability to participate in life activities. Patients often suffer from guilt and frustration because fatigue affects their ability to take care of their families (Borneman et al., 2010).

Fatigue, pain, dyspnea, and poor appetite are commonly reported symptoms in pediatric palliative care (Montoya-Juárez et al., 2013). Children who die of a treatment-related complication suffer more symptoms than those who die of progressive disease.

Literature in palliative care is extensive and growing, and studies have documented the numerous factors contributing to suffering and psychological distress. Uncontrolled physical symptoms, including pain, dyspnea, and nausea, can make life seem unbearable for patients. Family caregivers who observe patients with uncontrolled symptoms also have increased suffering. Psychological factors can evoke suffering, such as anxiety, depression, fears regarding the future, or living with uncertainty. Social factors, such as sexual concerns or loss of intimacy, can create suffering. Spiritual factors, such as unresolved regrets, the need for forgiveness, spiritual longing, or a loss of meaning in life, can contribute greatly to suffering (Ferrell et al., 2015; Sun, Grant, et al., 2015; Sun, Kim, et al., 2015). Throughout the literature, when the terms *pain* and *suffering* appear, it often is implied that these terms are synonymous or always experienced together. Although these experiences are closely akin, they are quite separate. Many patients endure significant pain with little suffering, whereas others experience extreme suffering, even in the absence of pain.

Beyond physical symptoms, psychological aspects of the cancer diagnosis are also sources of suffering. Suffering is intensified as patients recognize that their cancer will not be cured and, thus, serves no meaning. As Frankl (1963) stated, "Suffering ceases to be suffering . . . at the moment it finds meaning" (p. 113). Suffering creates one of the greatest challenges to uncovering meaning. This search for meaning is not a stagnant process but changes as each day unfolds and occurrences are interpreted (Borneman & Brown-Saltzman, 2015).

Specific events related to cancer are recognized as sources of suffering. One of the hallmarks of the cancer experience is that of loss. Patients with cancer experience phenomenal sacrifice, beginning with the physical losses associated with cancer treatment such as breast or hair loss. Continued illness involves losses of relationships and responsibilities, autonomy, and the threat of loss of life itself. Many patients have described their experiences as a gradual unraveling in which one layer of their lives is removed at a time. Patients have described losing their sense of health once hearing the devastating diagnosis. Many cancer survivors experiencing long-term remission have discussed the loss of their future because the physical effects of illness and treatment, despite a good prognosis, cause them to believe they will not live a long life. Suffering is intensified when patients face the dilemma of limited time to enjoy altered life goals and priorities after discovering what is truly important to them.

## Suffering Across the Cancer Trajectory

Suffering is evident in all phases of cancer, and the needs for nursing care vary across phases. At the time of initial diagnosis, psychological needs are profound as patients confront what is often the worst experience of their lives. Many patients equate their diagnosis with an inevitable death sentence (Ferrell, Smith, Cullinane, & Melancon, 2003). During cancer treatment, patients' physical needs intensify as they experience the effects of surgery, chemotherapy, or radiation. The degree of physical symptoms caused by cancer treatments tremendously affects suffering at this stage of the cancer trajectory. Patients describe the suffering associated with remission as they regain physical strength and health, yet they often have intense psychological distress as they adjust to living beyond the cancer diagnosis. Suffering often accompanies the completion of active treatment, arising from the uncertainty of the future and the distress that nothing is being actively done to fight the disease (Ferrell et al., 2003). The phase of recurrence has been described as one of the most intense times of suffering (Koch et al., 2013). For many, recurrence creates awareness that, in fact, the treatment did not cure, and the patient is thus living with a terminal illness rather than only a chronic one. For those who are still struggling with the effects of initial treatment, recurrence means having to cope with renewed physical and psychological distress. During the final phase of advanced disease or terminal illness, spiritual needs may become more intense, as patients question the meaning of their lives and transcendence beyond death (Boston, Bruce, & Schreiber, 2011; Ferrell, 1993; Ferrell & Dean, 1995).

## Suffering Across the Life Span

The experience of a cancer diagnosis is similar, but also profoundly different, across various age groups. A child with leukemia may struggle less with life's meaning but may be more overwhelmed by the unknown and uncertainty of illness and the disruption of all that has created the child's feeling of security. Narratives of nurses caring for pediatric hospice patients demonstrated the child's need to discuss death. Children also sought to discuss questions about spirituality. Parents' suffering was expressed as they struggled to understand why their child would die or the unfairness of this unreal circumstance (Ferrell, Wittenberg, Battista, & Walker, 2016a, 2016b). Research has shown that children might suffer more because they frequently are treated with highly aggressive regimens (Montoya-Juárez et al., 2013; Wolfe et al., 2000). The diagnosis of an illness often perceived as reserved for the old complicates the developmental tasks of adolescents and their normal struggles to gain identity and autonomy. Young adults' cancer experiences cause suffering and impede the development of autonomy and the pursuit of life goals. Patients may perceive cancer at this period of life as an ultimate punishment as one is robbed of life goals and dreams before they even begin. Suffering associated with cancer for middle-aged adults may involve the struggle to maintain the roles and relationships of spouse, parent, and productive adult. Cancer in older adults and its associated suffering have widely diverse meanings. In many studies, older adults have been identified as a population for whom cancer caused less suffering, because these patients perceived the disease as a normal occurrence and end to life as inevitable in the near future (Boston et al., 2011).

Across the life span, cancer suffering can be related to the losses associated with that phase of life and one's current roles and relationships. A young mother's anguish and suffering at a breast cancer diagnosis may primarily focus on the reality that this will disrupt her role as a mother. The suffering associated with breast cancer in a middle-aged woman may center on the unfairness of receiving the diagnosis just as she has completed the responsibilities of raising her children; she feels robbed of the much-anticipated time in her life when she could focus on her own needs.

Although the patient's chronologic age provides valuable information, one's psychological place in life also provides insight into suffering. Understanding what gives life meaning for an individual at any age is an important aspect of assessment. Ferrell (1996) interviewed an older woman with breast cancer whose entire life had centered on caring for her family and mentally disabled daughter. Providing physical care to her daughter had consumed this mother's life since age 40 to her current age of 75. The woman found a breast lump and, although she was aware that it was cancer, she chose not to seek any health care. To do so, she felt, would put her ability to continue her caregiving responsibilities in jeopardy. The physical pain and deterioration she endured from an untreated cancer was less important than the loss of meaning she would have experienced in "abandoning" her daughter and her caregiver role. For this woman, continuing to do what was meaningful lessened the severe physical pain and fear of her own approaching death.

Similar to other aspects of oncology nursing, a need exists for heightened sensitivity and intervention when caring for those in vulnerable populations. Young children and frail older adults are less able to express their needs and are most vulnerable to suffering, just as they are most vulnerable to other untreated physical symptoms (Shapiro, 1996).

The cancer experience varies greatly among a mother observing her adult daughter with breast cancer, a preschool-aged child confused by the changes in his father who has been diagnosed with leukemia, the husband caring for his wife of 50 years, and a teenager accompanying her younger sibling to radiation therapy for a brain tumor. Reich's (1989) metaphor of "giving voice" applies to recognition of suffering across the age continuum because those most vulnerable to unrelieved suffering may be least able to articulate their needs.

## Cultural Considerations

Culture significantly influences one's reaction to a diagnosis of cancer or any illness. It provides the foundation for all life experiences and profoundly influences the response to illness. Cultures hold strong beliefs about cancer as an illness and can influence how one responds to the cancer diagnosis as well as to all aspects of treatment and the cancer trajectory. Furthermore, patients' capacity to give meaning to suffering and transcend it is intimately related to cultural beliefs and values (Chiu, 2000) (see Chapter 5 on cultural influences in cancer).

Culture is bound in language and ritual. The simple word *cancer* has widely varied meanings across cultures. Understanding culturally held beliefs, customs, language, and rituals will enable nurses to view the suffering experience closely from their patients' perspectives. In assessing cultural influences on suffering, nurses may find it helpful to explore patients' past illness experiences and ways of coping. Religion also is an important factor in cultural assessment because spirituality influences the personal interpretations of suffering, pain, and life after death (see Chapter 9 for more information on spiritual support).

## Suffering in the Family

Oncology nursing has been family-centered since the inception of this specialty, and nurses have recognized that suffering often is more intense for the family caregivers who observe the illness than for the patients with cancer. A diagnosis of cancer has been compared to a storm that blows through and burdens entire families with new responsibilities, limitations, and fears (Ferrell et al., 2003). Family caregivers often suffer from physical symptoms such as fatigue, which is an indication of the tremendous burden that caregivers carry in caring for their loved ones (Fujinami et al., 2015; Grant et al., 2013). Psychological sources of suffering may include caregivers' sense of helplessness, lack of control, and feelings of inadequacy as a caregiver. In a study by Ferrell (2002), fear of recurrence and the lingering effect of the initial diagnosis may exacerbate this stress. Family caregivers expressed distress concerning the intensive and prolonged side effects of the cancer therapy that their loved ones were receiving (Ferrell, 2002).

Family caregivers often express spiritual distress in feeling abandoned by a God who would allow their loved one to die of this disease. Thus, they may feel abandoned by a faith that might otherwise have provided them support in the caregiving tasks (Fujinami et al., 2015).

Just as peer support is important for patients, family caregivers may benefit from the support of other family caregivers. Support vehicles such as newsletters allow caregivers to share helpful experiences and information on treatment and symptom management techniques (Ferrell, 2002; Grant et al., 2013). Caregivers have acknowledged the "community of suffering" that occurs late at night in the children's hospital when parents congregate in the waiting room and share their experiences of having a child diagnosed with cancer (Ferrell, Rhiner, Shapiro, & Dierkes, 1994). The parents acknowledged this as one of the most helpful means of maintaining their strength in what was perceived to be an unendurable situation. Shifting from outpatient care to family care at home decreases the family caregivers' opportunity to seek support from other caregivers. Family caregivers' suffering likely is intensified by the fact that they suffer mostly in isolation (Fujinami et al., 2015). Family caregivers' suffering is closely related to their relationship with the patient. Those in various roles (e.g., daughter, parent, child, sibling) experience suffering differently. Parents often have described their feelings of having a child diagnosed with cancer as a terrible injustice to have an offspring face death before a parent (Battista & LaRagione, 2015).

## Nursing Interventions

A discussion of nursing interventions for suffering should begin by acknowledging the unique nature of suffering and the goals of nursing. For many symptoms of cancer, such as pain or nausea, the ultimate goal is elimination of the problem. However, nurses should realize that the goal with suffering is to support the sufferer through this process rather than to eliminate it. Nursing actions that attempt to stifle the voice of suffering only intensify it. Regarding suffering and care, the nursing process begins with an assessment of the sources of suffering. Through careful assessment, nurses recognize that a patient on escalating doses of morphine is, in fact, experiencing profound suffering not amenable to any opioid dose. Exploration of patients' beliefs and concerns often will reveal sources of suffering, such as an unresolved relationship or feelings of abandonment by God (Best et al., 2014; Kumasaka & Miles, 1996).

Careful diagnosis of the sources of suffering will help nurses distinguish between those that should be eliminated and those that should be supported. Patients have difficulty dealing with issues of transcendence and life meaning if their basic needs of pain and symptom management are ignored. Exploring and diagnosing sources of suffering will help nurses to determine the need for intervention by other professionals. Many sources of suffering are not attributable to the cancer diagnosis but rather result when the illness creates an urgency to resolve lifelong dilemmas.

Nursing intervention for suffering begins with simple presence, or "being with" the sufferer. Nurses frequently leave a home visit feeling frustrated that they have done little, only to be told by a patient of the value of their visit. Nurses play a unique role through their presence and through active listening to patients' concerns. Their presence creates an opportunity to intervene in the experience. Reich (1989) referred to this as *mute suffering*. In an interview, a Hispanic patient described a pivotal moment in her illness, when she was gradually confined to a recliner in the living room because of her uncontrolled pain and increasing weakness. Her daughter and grandchildren came to visit, and the young granddaughter ran through the room eager to visit her grandmother. As the child ran into the room, she slipped and fell. For the patient, this was the first time in her life that she was not able to rise to offer comfort to her grandchild. The suffering associated with this pivotal moment was far more intense than any physical pain she had experienced. This suffering was intertwined with cultural beliefs about her role as a grandmother, with her sense of purpose, and with a clear awareness of this loss as one of many that would eventually lead to her death. One of the most important nursing interventions for this patient was to allow her to describe this experience and to give voice to this intense personal crisis, which might have been viewed as a relatively insignificant event by others.

Spross (1996), an oncology nurse researcher, explored the concept of suffering using the metaphor of a coach supporting suffering patients. The role of the nurse as coach is to encourage, support, and provide direction and skills for the patient to meet the illness challenge. Spross equated the nurse's coaching role to other contexts, such as labor and delivery coaching and coaching roles in other professions.

Battenfield (1984), Coyle (2006), and other nurse authors have emphasized the nursing role in suffering as active listening and being present. One of the major contributions to this area of nursing practice is the work of Kahn and Steeves (1994). They described the nurse as a witness and moral agent. A witness is a special kind of moral agent with an obligation to speak out about what is witnessed. The role of a witness may be viewed in four common ways, each of which supports the importance of speaking out and the development of nursing's collective voice (Kahn & Steeves, 1994):

- **Firsthand observation:** Nurses are closest to the patient and have an opportunity to inform others of what was observed.
- **Ceremonial role:** Nurses reduce suffering by supporting or participating in rituals of transition or "rites of passage" that require witnesses to substantiate them.
- **Expert witness:** Expert witnesses testify or speak in public forums about the special knowledge their expertise brings to a public issue. Oncology nurses have spoken out in their own institutions and, increasingly, in public forums about issues such as unrelieved pain, cancer survivorship, and breast cancer.
- **Visionary:** Nursing's collective vision develops, as each nurse speaks out about the suffering he or she encounters, how best to respond to it, and the need for a future in which suffering is not ignored.

Nurses have emphasized that the process of finding meaning is a basic human endeavor (Borneman & Brown-Saltzman, 2015). Patients struggle with the questions "Why me?" and "Why now?" A patient with lung cancer may accept it as a result of smoking but then may struggle with guilt associated with the behavior that led to the disease. Research concerning suffering has led to nurses' understanding of the ways in which patients cope, such as the use of downward social comparison, in which patients compare themselves to others whose circumstances they believe are worse. Also, nurses now are speaking out about some of the burdens created by changes in the healthcare system. Figure 10-1 provides examples of nursing interventions for suffering and pain.

## Suffering Among Professionals

Oncology nursing has both rewards and demands that add to the unique nature of the specialty. In the current state of the ever-changing healthcare system, nurses transitioning into oncology from other areas of acute care may experience a sense of helplessness in rec-

---

- Provide aggressive pharmacologic pain management to achieve optimum pain relief.
- Include nonpharmacologic interventions that enhance a sense of control.
- Assist patients to verbalize and understand the cause of their pain; clarify physiologic causes of pain.
- Explore with patients and family members their images of pain, including metaphors and visions.
- Overcome barriers, such as fear of addiction, to optimum use of analgesics.
- Distinguish between the feelings or meaning attributed to pain and beliefs about death.
- Empower patients to assume an active role in pain assessment and management.
- Explore the losses associated with the illness and pain.
- Facilitate discussion between patients and family caregivers to acquire a shared meaning of pain.
- Encourage comparison of patients' pain to pain experienced by others.
- Identify limits to pain that patients perceive to be necessary or deserved.
- Facilitate spiritual interventions, including spiritual counseling, rituals, and prayer.
- Explore pain as a sign of hopelessness, and foster altered hope consistent with advancing disease.

**Figure 10-1. Nursing Interventions to Facilitate the Search for Meaning in Cancer Pain**

Note. From "The Meaning of Cancer Pain," by B.R. Ferrell and G. Dean, 1995, *Seminars in Oncology Nursing, 11,* p. 20. Copyright 1995 by W.B. Saunders. Reprinted with permission.

ognizing that suffering cannot be eliminated. Suffering also occurs across the trajectory of cancer, including with patients who are newly diagnosed, in active treatment, adjusting to survivorship, experiencing recurrence, or are at the end of life. Thus, nurses in all oncology settings encounter patients and families who are suffering and experience their own suffering and grief.

Vachon, Huggard, and Huggard (2015) have described the effects of witnessing suffering and the stress and compassion fatigue associated with it. The authors cited many factors influencing nurses' response to suffering in the workplace, such as lack of structures to offer emotional support. This can be counterbalanced by programs offering spiritual support and emphasis on self-care (Corless, 2015).

Nurses must receive support so that they can tend to their own suffering and not feel helpless in their attempts to care for their patients. Nurses can derive great meaning from their work if they are able to grow from their interactions with patients and families (Sabo & Vachon, 2011; Yoder, 2010).

## Case Study

Juan is a 42-year-old Latino man diagnosed with pancreatic cancer. He was separated from his wife Gloria for five years, but they reunited two years ago and now have twin sons who are aged 18 months. Juan was an auto mechanic but is now unemployed because of his cancer. His tumor has been unresponsive to chemotherapy, but he has insisted on participating in clinical trials. These regimens have greatly worsened his symptoms, but he insists on continuing treatment, as he wants his sons to know that he "never gave up and fought until the end."

Juan and his family have had to give up their home and move in with Gloria's father, Michael, who is 75 years old and has late-stage heart disease. Gloria's mother died one year ago from complications of diabetes. Michael and Gloria are both still grieving that loss.

The oncology nurses and clinical trial nurses are attempting to support Juan and his family as best they can. Juan accepts their offer to have the chaplain visit him during treatment. He shares that he knows he will "be punished in the next life" for the time he was separated from Gloria. He adds that, "Maybe my suffering now will help decrease my suffering later." Juan also shares that he still believes in miracles and seems to enjoy reaching out to other patients in the clinic to cheer them on and encourage them to also "keep fighting."

### Discussion
- What are the sources of Juan's suffering?
- How would you assess his needs based on the QOL domains of physical, psychological, social, and spiritual well-being?

## Conclusion

Suffering is an inherent aspect of life-threatening illness and clearly is within the domain of nursing. Attending to suffering requires skills that are distinct from other clinical competencies. The challenge to "be with" the sufferer sharply conflicts with the current emphasis on high-tech, aggressive care or "doing" in oncology. To truly help the suffering patient, the nurse must have the courage to open up, be vulnerable to, and be present for the needs of the patient. This is part of healthcare professionals' responsibilities if they are completely committed to every aspect of their patients' care. Kahn and Steeves (1994) stressed the importance of continuing to explore and value the role of nursing in suffering:

> One characteristic of nursing's development over the past decade is the discovery of its voice—the ability and willingness to express what nurses collectively know and understand about the nature of nursing practice. To continue the development of nursing's voice, it is crucial that we talk freely about what we know, including what we know about suffering. (p. 260)

# References

Battenfield, B.L. (1984). Suffering: A conceptual description and content analysis of an operational schema. *Image: The Journal of Nursing Scholarship, 16,* 36–41. doi:10.1111/j.1547-5069.1984.tb01382.x

Battista, V., & LaRagione, G. (2015). Pediatric hospice and palliative care. In B.R. Ferrell, N. Coyle, & J.A. Paice (Eds.), *Oxford textbook of palliative nursing* (4th ed., pp. 851–872). New York, NY: Oxford University Press.

Best, M., Aldridge, L., Butow, P., Olver, I., Price, M., & Webster, F. (2014). Assessment of spiritual suffering in the cancer context: A systematic literature review. *Palliative and Supportive Care, 13,* 1336–1361. doi:10.1017/S1478951514001217

Borneman, T., & Brown-Saltzman, K. (2015). Meaning in illness. In B.R. Ferrell, N. Coyle, & J.A. Paice (Eds.), *Oxford textbook of palliative nursing* (4th ed., pp. 554–563). New York, NY: Oxford University Press.

Borneman, T., Koczywas, M., Sun, V.C.-Y., Piper, B.F., Uman, G., & Ferrell, B.R. (2010). Reducing patient barriers to pain and fatigue. *Journal of Pain and Symptom Management, 39,* 486–501. doi:10.1016/j.jpainsymman.2009.08.007

Borneman, T., Koczywas, M., Sun, V., Piper, B.F., Smith-Idell, C., Laroya, B., ... Ferrell, B.R. (2011). Effectiveness of clinical barriers to pain and fatigue management in oncology. *Journal of Palliative Medicine, 14,* 197–205. doi:10.1089/JPM.2010.0268

Boston, P., Bruce, A., & Schreiber, R. (2011). Existential suffering in the palliative care setting: An integrated literature review. *Journal of Pain and Symptom Management, 41,* 604–618. doi:10.1016/j.jpainsymman.2010.05.010

Breitbart, W., & Applebaum, A. (2011). Meaning-centered group psychotherapy. In M. Watson & D. Kissane (Eds.), *Handbook of psychotherapy in cancer care* (pp. 137–148). West Sussex, United Kingdom: Wiley-Blackwell.

Cassell, E.J. (1982). The nature of suffering and the goals of medicine. *New England Journal of Medicine, 306,* 639–645. doi:10.1056/NEJM198203183061104

Cassell, E.J. (1999). Diagnosing suffering: A perspective. *Annals of Internal Medicine, 131,* 531–534. doi:10.7326/0003-4819-131-7-199910050-00009

Chiu, L. (2000). Transcending breast cancer, transcending death: A Taiwanese population. *Nursing Science Quarterly, 13*(1), 64–72. doi:10.1177/08943180022107302

Chochinov, H.M. (2012). *Dignity therapy.* New York, NY: Oxford University Press.

Cooke, L., Chung, C., & Grant, M. (2011). Psychosocial care for adolescent and young adult hematopoietic cell transplant patients. *Journal of Psychosocial Oncology, 29,* 394–414.

Copp, L.A. (1974). The spectrum of suffering. *Pain and Suffering, 74,* 491–495. doi:10.2307/3469642

Copp, L.A. (1990a). The nature and prevention of suffering. *Journal of Professional Nursing, 6,* 247–249. doi:10.1016/S8755-7223(05)80096-1

Copp, L.A. (1990b). Treatment, torture, suffering, and compassion. *Journal of Professional Nursing, 6,* 1–2. doi:10.1016/S8755-7223(05)80176-0

Corless, I. (2015). Bereavement. In B.R. Ferrell, N. Coyle, & J.A. Paice (Eds.), *Oxford textbook of palliative nursing* (4th ed., pp. 487–499). New York, NY: Oxford University Press.

Coyle, N. (2006). The hard work of living in the face of death. *Journal of Pain and Symptom Management, 32,* 266–274. doi:10.1016/j.jpainsymman.2006.04.003

Dow, K.H., Ferrell, B.R., Leigh, S., Ly, J., & Gulasekaram, P. (1996). An evaluation of the quality of life among long-term survivors of breast cancer. *Breast Cancer Research and Treatment, 39,* 261–273. doi:10.1007/BF01806154

Ferrell, B.R. (1993). To know suffering. *Oncology Nursing Forum, 20,* 1471–1477.
Ferrell, B.R. (1996). The quality of lives: 1,525 voices of cancer. *Oncology Nursing Forum, 23,* 907–916.
Ferrell, B.R., & Dean, G. (1995). The meaning of cancer pain. *Seminars in Oncology Nursing, 11,* 17–22. doi:10.1016/S0749-2081(95)80038-7
Ferrell, B.R., Rhiner, M., Shapiro, B., & Dierkes, M. (1994). The experience of pediatric cancer pain. Part I: Impact of pain on the family. *Journal of Pediatric Nursing, 9,* 368–379.
Ferrell, B.R., Smith, S., Cullinane, C., & Melancon, C. (2003). Psychological well-being and quality of life in ovarian cancer survivors. *Cancer, 98,* 1061–1071. doi:10.1002/cncr.11291
Ferrell, B.R., Sun, V., Hurria, A., Cristea, M., Raz, D., Kim, J., … Koczywas, M. (2015). Interdisciplinary palliative care for patients with lung cancer. *Journal of Pain and Symptom Management, 50,* 758–767. doi:10.1016/j.jpainsymman.2015.07.005
Ferrell, B.R., Wittenberg, E., Battista, V., & Walker, G. (2016a). Exploring the spiritual needs of families with seriously ill children. *International Journal of Palliative Nursing, 22,* 388–394. doi:10.12968/ijpn.2016.22.8.388
Ferrell, B.R., Wittenberg, E., Battista, V., & Walker, G. (2016b). Nurses' experiences of spiritual communication with seriously ill children. *Journal of Palliative Medicine, 19,* 1166–1170. doi:10.1089/jpm.2016.0138
Frankl, V. (1963). *Man's search for meaning: An introduction to logotherapy.* New York, NY: Pocket Books.
Fujinami, R., Sun, V., Zachariah, F., Uman, G., Grant, M., & Ferrell, B. (2015). Family caregivers' distress levels related to quality of life, burden, and preparedness. *Psycho-Oncology, 24,* 54–62. doi:10.1002/pon.3562
Grant, M., Sun, V., Fujinami, R., Sidhu, R., Otis-Green, S., Juarez, G., … Ferrell, B. (2013). Family caregiver burden, skills preparedness, and quality of life in non-small cell lung cancer. *Oncology Nursing Forum, 40,* 337–346. doi:10.1188/13.ONF.337-346
Kahn, D.L., & Steeves, R.H. (1994). Witnesses to suffering: Nursing knowledge, voice, and vision. *Nursing Outlook, 42,* 260–264. doi:10.1016/0029-6554(94)90046-9
Koch, L., Jansen, L., Brenner, H., & Arndt, V. (2013). Fear of recurrence and disease progression in long-term (≥ 5 years) cancer survivors—A systematic review of quantitative studies. *Psycho-Oncology, 22,* 1–11. doi:10.1002/pon.3022
Kumasaka, L., & Miles, A. (1996). My pain is God's will. *American Journal of Nursing, 96*(6), 45–47. doi:10.1097/00000446-199606000-00044
Montoya-Juárez, R., García-Caro, M.P., Schmidt-Rio-Valle, J., Campos-Calderón, C., Sorroche-Navarro, C., Sánchez-García, R., & Cruz-Quintana, F. (2013). Suffering indicators in terminally ill children from the parental perspective. *European Journal of Oncology Nursing, 17,* 720–725. doi:10.1016/j.ejon.2013.04.004
Morse, J.M., Bottorff, J.L., & Hutchinson, S. (1995). The paradox of comfort. *Nursing Research, 44,* 14–19. doi:10.1097/00006199-199501000-00004
Morse, J.M., & Carter, B. (1996). The essence of enduring and expressions of suffering: The reformulation of self. *Scholarly Inquiry for Nursing Practice, 10,* 43–60.
O'Sullivan, C.K., Bowles, K.H., Jeon, S., Ercolano, E., & McCorkle, R. (2011). Psychological distress during ovarian cancer treatment: Improving quality by examining patient problems and advanced practice nursing interventions. *Nursing Research and Practice, 2011,* Article ID 351642. doi:10.1155/2011/351642
Pinar, G., Ayhan, A., & Pinar, T. (2013). Emotions of gynecologic cancer patients dealing with permanent colostomy: A qualitative interview study. *Journal of Cancer Therapy, 4,* 1060–1067. doi:10.4236/jct.2013.46120
Reich, W.T. (1987). Models of pain and suffering: Foundations for an ethic of compassion. *Acta Neurochirurgica Supplementum, 38,* 117–122.
Reich, W.T. (1989). Speaking of suffering: A moral account of compassion. *Soundings, 72,* 83–108. doi:10.1007/978-3-7091-6975-9_20
Sabo, A.B., & Vachon, M.I.S. (2011). Care of professional caregivers. In M.P. Davis, P.C. Feyer, P. Ortner, & C. Zimmerman (Eds.), *Supportive oncology* (pp. 575–589). Philadelphia, PA: Elsevier.
Shapiro, B.S. (1996). The suffering of children and their families. In B.R. Ferrell (Ed.), *Suffering* (pp. 67–94). Burlington, MA: Jones & Bartlett Learning.
Spross, J.A. (1996). Coaching and suffering: The role of the nurse in helping people facing illness. In B.R. Ferrell (Ed.), *Suffering* (pp. 173–208). Burlington, MA: Jones & Bartlett Learning.
Sun, V., Grant, M., Koczywas, M., Freeman, B., Zachariah, F., Fujinami, R., … Ferrell, B. (2015). Effectiveness of an interdisciplinary palliative care intervention for family caregivers in lung cancer. *Cancer, 121,* 3737–3745. doi:10.1002/cncr.29567
Sun, V., Kim, J., Irish, T., Borneman, T., Sidhu, R., Klein, L., & Ferrell, B. (2015). Palliative care and spiritual well-being in lung cancer patients and family caregivers. *Psycho-Oncology, 25,* 1448–1455. doi:10.1002/pon.3987
Vachon, M., Huggard, P.R., & Huggard, J. (2015). Reflections on occupational stress in palliative nursing. In B.R. Ferrell, N. Coyle, & J.A. Paice (Eds.), *Oxford textbook of palliative nursing* (4th ed., pp. 969–986). New York, NY: Oxford University Press.

Wolfe, J., Grier, H.E., Klar, N., Levin, S.B., Ellenbogen, J.M., Salem-Schatz, S., ... Weeks, J.C. (2000). Symptoms and suffering at the end of life in children with cancer. *New England Journal of Medicine, 342,* 326–333. doi:10.1056/NEJM200002033420506

Wong, F.L., Francisco, L., Togawa, K., Bosworth, A., Gonzales, M., Hanby, C., ... Bhatia, S. (2010). Long-term recovery after hematopoietic cell transplantation: Predictors of quality-of-life concerns. *Blood, 115,* 2508–2519. doi:10.1182/blood-2009-06-225631

Yoder, A.E. (2010). Compassion fatigue in nurses. *Applied Nursing Research, 23,* 191–197. doi:10.1016/j.apnr.2008.09.003

# SECTION III

# Psychosocial Alterations

Chapter 11. Altered Mental Status
Chapter 12. Altered Sexuality
Chapter 13. Anger
Chapter 14. Anxiety
Chapter 15. Body Image Disturbance
Chapter 16. Denial
Chapter 17. Depression and Suicide
Chapter 18. Distress
Chapter 19. Grief
Chapter 20. Guilt
Chapter 21. Powerlessness

# CHAPTER 11

# Altered Mental Status

*Esther Muscari Desimini, RN, MSN, APRN, BC, MBA*

> *Cogito ergo sum. I think, therefore I am.*
> —René Descartes

Altered mental status, including delirium and dementia, is frequently seen in patients with cancer. Sometimes called *neurocognitive disorders* (American Psychiatric Association [APA] 2013), these changes may be caused by the cancer or its treatment or be completely unrelated. The effect of these disorders on patients, families, and healthcare professionals adds to the stress of coping with the cancer. Cognitive and behavioral changes can increase patients' and families' emotional distress, thereby affecting the time they spend together.

## Delirium

Delirium is a common condition or syndrome in which the patient is in a confused state that is acute in onset and can fluctuate. Delirium is unpredictable, usually temporary, almost always brief, treatable, and can sometimes go unrecognized (Centeno, Sanz, & Bruera, 2004; Harris, 2007; National Cancer Institute [NCI], 2016). Acute confusion is because of pathophysiologic insults of the central nervous system (CNS) and is observed as disordered cognition, attention, and behavior (Bond, Neelon, & Belyea, 2006). This syndrome is known by many names, including acute confusion; psychosis; acute organic brain syndrome; metabolic, toxic, or septic encephalopathy; and delirium. It is also sometimes incorrectly referred to as dementia. Delirium is sometimes referred to as terminal restlessness in the acute dying process. The diversity of names in the literature and among clinicians reflects imprecise and inconsistent identification and diagnosis of the problem. In the face of such confusing terminology, an awareness of the many labels used to describe a confused mental state is necessary in order to institute appropriate, timely intervention (NCI, 2016).

### Presentation

Delirium is often seen in the hospital setting and especially in the older patient. The literature reports a wide range of prevalence, which reflects the diverse and complex nature of it (Alici, Bates, & Breitbart, 2015). Delirium is reported in 14%–57% of hospitalized patients with cancer and up to 85% of terminally ill patients with cancer near the time of death (Bond et al., 2006; Breitbart & Alici, 2008; Harris, 2007). Because delirium develops over the course of a few hours to a few days, subtle early signs, such as a change in the ability to follow a conversation or the inability to remember the reason for hospitalization, can easily be missed.

Generally, the initial presentation of delirium involves some degree of confusion. Three types of delirium exist: hypoactive, hyperactive, and mixed (APA, 2013; Inouye, 2006; Maldonado, 2008; NCI, 2016). Hypoactive delirium is characterized by decreased psychomotor activity, decreased responsiveness, apathy, lethargy, withdrawal, and a flat affect, with patients appearing sleepy or tired. Because of its presentation, delirium is sometimes mistaken for depression or dementia. Hyperactive delirium is more easily recognized and is characterized by increased psychomotor activity, with an increased state of arousal, restlessness, agitation, and insomnia and the potential for combativeness (e.g., attempting to remove invasive equipment or monitoring devices). Hyperactive delirium is associated with disturbance in the sleep–wake cycle. Activity is disorganized and without purpose. Most people experience mixed delirium, which changes back and forth between hypoactive and hyperactive delirium because of the fluctuating nature of the syndrome. Untreated delirium can progress to a more permanent cognitive disorder (Bourgeois, Seaman, & Servis, 2008).

## Signs and Symptoms

Delirium is a medical diagnosis with the following signs and symptoms (APA, 2013; Siberski, 2014):
- Clouding of consciousness, awareness, and attention
- Global disturbance of cognition with perceptual distortions, illusions, and hallucinations not accounted for by a preexisting or evolving dementia
- Psychomotor disturbances that are reflected in either hypo- or hyperactive reaction times and flow of speech
- Disturbance of the sleep–wake cycle, with the disturbance developing over a short period of time and fluctuating during the course of the day
- Evidence from the history, physical examination, or laboratory findings that it is a consequence of another medical condition, medications, or intoxicating substances
- Neurologic symptoms can include dysphasia; dysarthria, tremor, or motor abnormalities; and asterixis associated with hepatic encephalopathy and uremia.

## Risk Factors and Etiologies

Children and older adults are at higher risk for delirium. Although age is a risk factor for the development of delirium, how much the association is independent from physical frailty is unclear. Various incidence and prevalence rates exist in different populations, with the incidence rate for a geriatric unit being 20%–29% and 47% for palliative care and cancer inpatient units (Bagri, Rico, & Ruiz, 2008; Gaudreau, Gagnon, Harel, Tremblay, & Roy, 2005; Gunther, Morandi, & Ely, 2008; Wilber, Carpenter, & Hustey, 2008).

Although the etiology of delirium usually is multifactorial in adults older than age 65, a single cause often is identifiable (Inouye, Westendorp, & Saczynski, 2014). Factors that predispose or contribute to experiencing delirium are outlined in Figure 11-1. Delirium is associated with six important risk factors: use of physical restraints, malnutrition, use of a bladder

| Predisposing and Contributing Factors | Precipitating Factors and Causes |
|---|---|
| • Alcoholism<br>• Brain radiation therapy<br>• Chemotherapy (e.g., vincristine, vinblastine, L-asparaginase, intrathecal methotrexate, interferon, interleukin, amphotericin)<br>• Dehydration<br>• Depression<br>• Emotional stress<br>• Hip fracture<br>• Immobility<br>• Intracerebral hemorrhage<br>• Metabolic abnormality<br>• Multitude of comorbidities<br>• Older age<br>• Pain<br>• Presence of dementia<br>• Prior cognitive impairment<br>• Severe/highly acute illness<br>• Surgery (postoperative)<br>• Unfamiliar environment<br>• Vision/hearing impairment | • Anemia<br>• Benzodiazepines<br>• Bladder catheter use<br>• Brain tumor—primary or metastasis<br>• Corticosteroids<br>• Disseminated intravascular coagulation<br>• $H_2$ blockers<br>• Hepatic failure<br>• High number of hospital procedures<br>• Hypercalcemia<br>• Hypercapnia<br>• Hyperglycemia<br>• Hypernatremia<br>• Hyperosmolality<br>• Hypoglycemia<br>• Hyponatremia<br>• Hypoxia<br>• Iatrogenic event<br>• Infection/sepsis<br>• Intensive care unit admission<br>• Metoclopramide<br>• Opioids<br>• Pain<br>• Physical restraint<br>• Renal failure<br>• Scopolamine<br>• Severe acute illness<br>• Tricyclic antidepressants |

**Figure 11-1. Causes Associated With Delirium**

*Note.* Based on information from American Psychiatric Association, 2013; Eubank & Covinsky, 2014; Gaudreau et al., 2005; Wilber et al., 2008.

catheter, any iatrogenic event, the use of three or more medications at one time, and dementia (Gunther et al., 2008). Catic (2011) noted a higher incidence of drug-induced delirium caused by the altered pharmacokinetics of aging, the high prevalence of polypharmacy, and the presence of comorbid disease. Although opioids, benzodiazepines, anticholinergics, and antidepressants are more often associated with the development of delirium, any medication can contribute to delirum in older adults (Bush & Bruera, 2009). Thus, a thorough medication history is valuable to determine if any new medications have been initiated or discontinued or if dosages have recently been adjusted. Underlying dementia has also been identified in 25%–50% of patients, increasing the risk of delirium two to three times (Maldonado, 2008).

## Pathophysiology

The pathophysiology of delirium lies in widespread disruption of the higher cortical functioning of the brain. Dysfunction is evident in diffuse areas, such as subcortical structures, the brain stem, the thalamus, the nondominant parietal lobe, the fusiform and prefrontal cortices, and the focal areas of the frontal and parietal cortex in the right hemisphere (Burns, Gallagley, & Byrne, 2004). Neurotransmitter abnormalities and altered cerebral metabolism, resulting in structural and physiologic insults that are often reversible, are believed to be the underlying pathophysiology of delirium (Clegg & Young, 2011; Pozuelo, 2015).

Delirium is the result of multiple complex and interactive biologic, psychological, and social factors (e.g., infectious processes, electrolyte imbalances, hematologic abnormalities, nutritional deficiencies, metabolic encephalopathy, sensory deprivation, sleep deprivation, anxiety, fear, inadequate social supports, body image changes, atypical environments found in the hospital) that interfere with normal neural transmissions in critical brain pathways. Delirium is attributable to temporary and often reversible neuronal tissue damage related to impaired cerebral oxygenation and neurochemical transmission.

The onset of acute confusion frequently signals a worsening of the primary illness or a complication of treatment. Patients who develop acute confusional states have higher morbidity and mortality during hospitalization and after discharge (Breitbart & Alici, 2012; NCI, 2016).

The clinical course of delirium in hospitalized adults is associated with adverse effects that often lead to safety issues and a loss of independence (Inyoue et al., 2014). It has been associated with impairments in motivation and compliance, urinary incontinence, and falls (Bond et al., 2006). Delirium contributing to prolonged hospitalizations first manifests itself before the seventh day of hospitalization. It includes mental signs of disorientation, memory loss, and impaired consciousness, followed by behavioral manifestations of falls, the need for restraints, incontinence, and pulled IV lines occurring within 24 hours of admission (Saravay et al., 2004). Delirium can persist into the post-acute setting, particularly if the patient is cognitively impaired or older than age 85 and experiences any of the following while hospitalized: severe delirium, disorientation, sleep disturbance, perceptual disturbance, attention disturbance, consciousness disturbance, incoherent speech, abnormal psychomotor activity, and fluctuating behavior (Kiely et al., 2004).

## Screening and Clinical Assessment

Considering delirium risk in hospitalized patients can contribute to a preventive care plan and possibly reduce the risk of injury or even occurrence of the syndrome. Early identification or suspicion needs in-depth assessment to prevent any potential adverse outcomes (Radtke, Gaudreau, & Spies, 2010).

Using tools for diagnosing delirium and dementia, such as the Mini-Mental State Examination (MMSE) (Folstein, Folstein, & McHugh, 1975), on hospitalized patients with cancer at risk for delirium or suspected of delirium is an effective strategy, especially when used in conjunction with assessment of other risk or precipitating factors, such as the presence of severe illness, frailty, and/or renal or hepatic dysfunction.

Careful review with healthcare providers, caregivers, and family members can provide important information as part of the assessment. Onset and timing of symptoms and consciousness assists in revealing the pattern of acuity and of fluctuation in the last few hours or days. Inquiring into the manifestations of disorientation, impaired attention/awareness, disordered thinking, altered memory, language or perception, hallucinations or delusions, inappropriate behavior, and/or emotional and psychomotor disturbances assists in reconstructing the original presentation of signs and symptoms. Note any disturbance in the sleep–wake cycle in the form of daytime drowsiness, insomnia, sleep fragmentation, or nocturnal worsening of symptoms. Soliciting family input regarding the patient's history of recent mental status condition and any changes in the patient's medical condition or drug prescriptions all contribute to an earlier and more accurate diagnosis and treatment initiation.

Hyperactivity combined with confusion can lead to self-injury. If patients are fearful or hallucinating, they may strike out at others. In patients who are critically ill, hypoactive behavior is difficult to differentiate from the illness or medication effects.

Delirium, if untreated, can severely complicate the course of patients who are critically ill. Because most cases of delirium are the result of physiologic, psychological, or environmental factors that are treatable with medical and nursing actions, the importance of early detection and accurate diagnosis cannot be overemphasized. Delirium is not a normal consequence of aging and can be reversible with treatment. Prompt assessment and management of symptoms, even when they are only mild, are crucial to the patient's optimal outcome.

## Delirium in Patients With Cancer

Delirium is the most common neuropsychiatric diagnosis among patients with cancer (Breitbart & Alici, 2012; Mehta & Roth, 2015). It is caused either by the direct effects of cancer on the CNS or by the indirect CNS complications of the disease and/or cancer treatment or other medical problems. The prevalence of delirium increases as cancer progresses. Patients with mild delirium can be misdiagnosed with anxiety or depression, with subsequent appropriate treatment being delayed. Patients should be evaluated for delirium if they exhibit acute onset of agitation, behavioral changes, impaired cognitive function, altered attention span, or fluctuating level of consciousness (Mehta & Roth, 2015). Consistent with other disease populations, the occurrence of delirium results in longer hospital stays (Breitbart & Alici, 2012). High-risk factors associated with the development of delirium in patients with cancer include multiple etiologies, such as advanced age (older than age 65), preexisting cognitive impairment, low albumin level, bone metastases, and the presence of a hematologic malignancy, with lymphoma being the most common (Breitbart & Alici, 2012; Bush & Bruera, 2009). These patients are more severely ill and functionally impaired than nondelirious patients with cancer (Bond et al., 2006). Agitation and difficulty in assessing pain and other symptoms have been found to be particularly challenging in palliative care patients with delirium and cancer (Şenel et al., 2015).

Delirium can occur as a direct result of cancer. Primary brain tumors or metastatic spread of disease to the brain by hematogenous or lymphatic routes may result in either delirium or dementia. However, by far the most frequent sources of delirium in patients with cancer are the indirect effects of organ dysfunction, electrolyte imbalances, sepsis, paraneoplastic syndromes, and nutritional deficiencies, as well as medication- and treatment-related side effects.

Hospitalized patients with cancer are most at risk of developing a narcotic- or steroid-induced confusional state, a metabolic encephalopathy related to the consequences of disease- or treatment-related side effects, infection, or recent surgery. Respiratory compromise causes cerebral hypoxia and confusion. Hepatic encephalopathy produces a neuropsychiatric disorder that may vary from mild alterations in mental status to coma. Uremia, as well as thyroid and adrenal dysfunction, also can produce mental status changes. Similar to the general medical population, patients with cancer may have multiple causes of delirium; the cancer population differs in that preexisting dementia as a contributory cause is considerably less likely. Resolution of delirium in patients with cancer can be expected in people with a new onset and an identifiable cause. Mortality associated with delirium in patients with cancer is related to the severity of the metabolic and structural abnormalities, hypoxia, critical organ failure (hepatic and renal), infection, and coagulopathies.

The variety of medications used to treat cancer and the side effects of treatment add to the risk for delirium in patients. Many medication dosages may need to be adjusted, especially in the older adult population (Burns et al., 2004). Some chemotherapy agents, as well as opioids, may increase the risk of delirium (Mehta & Roth, 2015). Corticosteroids sometimes given with chemotherapy administration are associated more with the risk of a "steroid psychosis" than are the chemotherapy agents themselves.

## Delirium in Patients With Terminal Cancer

Delirium is a frequent neuropsychiatric complication in the terminally ill oncology population (Breitbart & Alici, 2008). This adds to the distress experienced by patients and families. The presence of delirium may be a predictor of impending death for some patients (Pozuelo, 2015).

Factors that contribute to mental status changes and delirium during the terminal stage are the same as those in nonterminal patients with cancer. However, because of progressive disease, organ death, worsening hypoxemia, and increasing psychosocial stressors, terminally ill patients are at greater risk; therefore, the prevalence is greater than in the general oncology population. The main underlying pathologies of delirium in terminally ill patients with cancer include hepatic failure, medications, prerenal azotemia, hyperosmolality, hypoxia, disseminated intravascular coagulation, CNS damage, infection, and hypercalcemia (Breitbart & Alici, 2012).

The delirium seen in terminally ill patients can present as either hyperactive ("agitated"), hypoactive ("quiet, sedated"), or mixed behaviors, just as in other populations. Underlying pathologies most often associated with hyperactive psychomotor activity are hepatic failure, opioids, and steroids. Hypoactive delirium often is correlated with dehydration pathologies and electrolyte abnormalities such as hypercalcemia (Breitbart & Alici, 2012). Hyperactive delirium is identified more often in the clinical setting than other subtypes because the symptoms attract caregiver attention (Heidrich & English, 2015).

## Dementia

Dementia is a category of different syndromes characterized by gradual onset of memory deficits, changes in cognitive function, and behavior (National Institutes of Health [NIH], 2015). Changes in cognitive function can include executive functions (e.g., organizing) and language. Deterioration of intellectual functioning affects cognition, behavior, and social areas, resulting in grave disability. The *Diagnostic and Statistical Manual of Mental Disorders (DSM-V)* defines the neurocognitive disorder of dementia as having significant cognitive decline (for example, decline in memory, language, or learning) that interferes with independence in everyday activities (APA, 2013). Dementia, unlike delirium, does not involve any alteration in consciousness or alertness. Patients with dementia generally can be expected to have progressive deterioration of cognition and function.

Alzheimer disease (AD) is by far the most common form of dementia. Other less common types of dementia include the following (NIH, 2015):
- Vascular dementia
- Lewy body dementia
- Frontotemporal dementia
- Huntington disease–related dementia
- Toxic metabolic processes
- Alcohol abuse

- Creutzfeldt-Jakob disease
- HIV

Each of these types of dementia has a different etiology. In 2017, it was estimated that 5.5 million Americans had AD, with nearly all being older than age 65. This breaks down to 1 in 10 Americans older than age 65 who had AD in 2017. Because of the aging of the population, the annual number of new cases of AD and other dementias is projected to double by 2050 (Alzheimer's Association, 2017; Plassman et al., 2007).

## Signs and Symptoms

Neuropsychological impairment from dementia results in sufficient impairments in social functioning. Observed changes are seen in short- and long-term memory, language, speech, visuospatial ability, as well as mood and personality. The objective changes of dementia characteristically are an inability to learn and retain new information, short-term memory loss, and an inability to recall a list of items.

Declines in functioning or impaired abilities as previously observed in work or usual activities are suspect of dementia. Family members will notice the patient giving up behaviors and activities that were previously part of their routine. Activities of daily living are affected most often by memory loss. Changes are observed in the inability to complete usual, familiar tasks, such as bathing, dressing, using the bathroom, maintaining continence, eating, using the telephone, doing housework, taking prescribed medicines, managing one's personal finances, or preparing meals. In some cases, depression, and/or delirium can be misdiagnosed as dementia.

## Risk Factors and Etiologies

Dementia is a syndrome resulting from structural and metabolic changes rather than a specific disease. Dementias are caused by brain cell death, usually occurring over a course of time. It is important not to assume or label the dementia as AD but rather consider the possibility within the framework of other dementias and etiologies. The pathology of AD can, and often does, overlap with other pathologies that result in dementia. Figure 11-2 provides other distinguishing facts and clarifications about dementia.

Causes of dementia that are purely oncologic in nature usually result from brain and spinal column involvement. Musicco et al. (2013) studied a cohort of one million residents in Italy for development and correlation between AD dementia and cancer. The researchers reported that the risk of cancer in patients with AD dementia was halved, with the risk of AD dementia development in patients with cancer reduced by 35% (Musicco et al., 2013).

Important to note is that patients with dementia remain at risk for delirium. Duration of delirium in older adults with dementia tends to last longer than in those without dementia (McCusker, Cole, Dendukuri, Han, & Belzile, 2003).

## Nursing Care of Patients With Delirium and Dementia

### Assessment

Both delirium and dementia are associated with longer hospitalizations because of potentially deleterious events, such as falls, self-extubation, IV line removal, use of restraints, risk of cognitive and functional decline, increased use of healthcare services, nursing home admissions, risk of death, and increased healthcare costs. Because of this,

- Is not a global impairment of mental function: Some cognitive areas are spared with deterioration of other areas.
- Does not always impair memory: Memory may be spared early in the dementia course with other spheres of mental functioning affected.
- Does not always impair patients' insight into their condition: Despite insight being impaired early in the Alzheimer disease course, some patients with other types of dementia may be aware of their intellectual deterioration.
- Is not only a disorder of cognition but also a behavioral disorder: Some dementias manifest predominantly as changes in behavior and personality (such as frontotemporal lobar degenerations).
- Does not always occur in older adults: Dementia is not an inevitable occurrence for people older than age 65. The cognitive changes that occur because of aging are distinctly different than those associated with the pathology of the dementias.
- Is not synonymous with senility.
- Is not a predictable, constant progressive disorder: Dementia can plateau or be static at any point in the course of the syndrome and does not necessarily progress on any given schedule or course.
- Does not always have a delayed or gradual onset: Head trauma or hydrocephalus may result in acute dementia.
- Is treatable: Many dementias, including Alzheimer disease, are treatable or manageable. A few dementias are reversible, such as those caused by structural alterations from trauma or hydrocephalus.

**Figure 11-2. Characteristics of Dementia**

*Note.* Based on information from National Institutes of Health, 2015.

early diagnosis is key (Allen et al., 2011; Inouye, 2006; NCI, 2016; Waszynski, n.d.). A patient presenting with a confusional state needs to have a full assessment to identify the possible etiologies to help with determining treatment. At times, it can be difficult to distinguish between delirium and dementia, especially when evaluating new patients. Table 11-1 outlines these differences.

Knowledge of the baseline cognitive state is essential in making the correct diagnosis (Heidrich & English, 2015). Family members, possibly the patient, and primary care providers most likely will have noted behavioral and cognitive changes in the patient and will recall those early observations during worsening episodes. They can provide important information to obtain the correct diagnosis. Because delirium has precipitating factors, it is considered to be a medical emergency. Nurses and other healthcare professionals need to be educated regarding psychiatric assessment, differentiation of reversible and irreversible con-

**Table 11-1. Differentiating Features of Delirium and Dementia**

| Feature | Delirium | Dementia |
| --- | --- | --- |
| Onset | Acute | Insidious |
| Course | Fluctuating | Progressive, persistent |
| Duration | Days to weeks | Months to years |
| Consciousness | Altered, fluctuates | Clear until late stages |
| Attention | Impaired | Normal, except in severe dementia |
| Psychomotor changes | Increased or decreased | Often normal |
| Reversibility | Usually | Not usually; tends to be progressive |

*Note.* Based on information from Arnold, 2005; Heidrich & English, 2015.

ditions, and specific interventions. The most significant problem to overcome is delayed detection of mild, but important, signs and symptoms of impending delirium before a crisis occurs.

Frequent and systematic assessment of patients is important, including cognition, orientation, attention, wakefulness, mood, and psychomotor behavior. Because the patient's thinking will become acutely disorganized and fragmented as manifested in changed speech patterns and an inability to make decisions (e.g., what to eat, where to sit) or complete tasks, self-care deficits may be an early indication of delirium. Thinking processes in patients with dementia, however, are impoverished with decreases noted over time.

Nurses obtain a great deal of useful information about their patients during normal nursing interactions and may be the first to detect cognitive changes. These observations and impressions, along with the data collected by using a formal assessment tool, provide the information needed to make an accurate diagnosis and facilitate medical or psychiatric treatment.

Patients with memory problems cannot easily take in new information, and what new information they take in cannot be recalled. The initial signs of memory deficits may be repeated use of the call bell or forgetting the location of personal items (e.g., glasses, toothbrush). Short-term memory loss is seen early with both delirium and dementia. Long-term memory loss affects patients with severe delirium more often than those with dementia. For patients with dementia, memory loss is from the current point in time backward; therefore, these patients hold onto their long-term memory until the terminal stages. Patients can remain alert and conversant in the presence of serious memory impairment.

If patients cannot attend appropriately to what is occurring, decreased memory and disorganized thinking may result. Patients may have difficulty staying on topic during conversation, and they may not respond to others' attempts to refocus or redirect their attention. Patients with dementia tend not to exhibit extremes in behavior or speech, such as being hyper- or hypoalert, unless experiencing a compounding delirium. They also often have difficulty finding words. Deterioration in the speech of people with a dementing disease is more empty or sparse, with aphasia notable in many cases, especially in late stages.

Orientation is dependent on healthy cognitive functioning. Patients may be oriented to person, place, and day (global orientation) but may confuse the time of day, the length of hospitalization, or where familiar, simple things in their room are located. Although global orientation usually is not impaired until delirium is severe, immediate orientation to the surrounding environment may decrease significantly before it is noticed. Mild symptoms of disorientation may be overlooked as staff members attribute the behavior to the strange environment, anxiety, or sleepiness. Delirious patients usually experience impaired disorientation at times with the tendency to mistake unfamiliar for familiar places and people.

Sleep–wake cycles are disturbed in patients with delirium and dementia. In delirium, patients may have difficulty staying awake while being interviewed during the day but may be wide awake at night. Sundowning is seen in some neurocognitive disorders when symptoms worsen in the late afternoon or evening. Sundowning is typical in AD in the mid-stages (Alzheimer's Association, n.d.).

Because medication effects are the most common causes of delirium in both the general and terminally ill oncology population, patients' drug profiles require careful consideration. Numerous medications, including gastrointestinal drugs such as cimetidine, ranitidine, and metoclopramide, can contribute to delirium and may need to be tapered or stopped.

## Tools for Diagnosing Delirium and Dementia

Standardized cognitive assessments contribute to accurate diagnosis and monitoring of responses to interventions as well as disease progression over time. Without considering formalized testing results with other factors, dementia cannot be reliably differentiated from other diseases.

Mental status assessment with objective evaluations using bedside testing, clinical rating scales, or neuropsychological testing documents mental function compromise. Assessment of patients with altered mental status is best done at the bedside with careful attention being paid to deficits in attention and cognition. Patients with dementia have an alertness and attention that are relatively unaffected. People with delirium have reduced alertness and lack direction and selectivity, which can fluctuate throughout the course of the day. Standardized, objective measurement and reporting of delirium allow for quantification, evaluation of success of interventions, and communication to other clinicians. Objective tools assist in differentiating delirium and dementia from other causes of altered mental status. Once the correct diagnosis is made, potential treatable causes can be considered.

Standard mental status screening instruments have emerged for use at the bedside. Those most frequently described in the literature include the MMSE (Folstein et al., 1975), the Delirium Rating Scale (DRS) (Caeiro, Ferro, Albuquerque, & Figueira, 2004), the Confusion Assessment Method (CAM) (Inoyoue et al., 1990), and the Bedside Confusion Scale (BSCS) (Sarhill, Walsh, Nelson, LeGrand, & Davis, 2001).

The MMSE has the greatest advantage for early "flagging" of an abnormality because it is most familiar to clinicians and easy to conduct; it assists in distinguishing patients with and without dementia. The DRS uses a 10-point observational scale that rates temporal onset of symptoms (Caeiro et al., 2004). The CAM was designed to assist nonpsychiatric clinicians in their assessment of confusion (Morrison, 2003). The BSCS is a validated two-item instrument tested in patients with cancer that assesses level of alertness and attention, with totaled scores identifying borderline or confused mental states (Sarhill et al., 2001). Other tools are available in clinical practice. The Montreal Cognitive Assessment, a 10-minute screening test, assists in the diagnosis of mild cognitive impairment (Smith, Gildeh, & Holmes, 2007). The Mini-Cog™, a three-item recall followed by the clock drawing test, is sensitive in detecting dementia in the primary care setting (Borson, Scanlon, Brush, Vitaliano, & Dokmak, 2000). The Seven-Minute Screen is valuable in detecting AD and other dementias (Meulen et al., 2004). The Informant Questionnaire on Cognitive Decline in the Elderly and Memory Impairment Screen assist in detecting dementia and AD among adults in a community setting (Harrison et al., 2015). These assessment tools assist clinicians in distinguishing the intellectual changes of dementia from those associated with delirium, normal aging effects, and other conditions.

Wong, Holroyd-Leduc, Simel, and Straus (2010) reviewed delirium diagnostic tools to determine the accuracy of bedside instruments in diagnosing the presence of delirium in adults. The authors noted that instrument choice to evaluate delirium may be dictated by the amount of time available and the discipline of the examiner. The evidence is supported using CAM, which requires less than five minutes to complete. Another valuable resource is the review of delirium tools by Grover and Kate (2012).

Once staff members have observed changes in affect, behavior, and cognition, laboratory evaluation should be conducted to begin the process of ruling out specific conditions. Evaluation should include electrolytes, kidney function, liver function, blood glucose, and oxygen levels. Drug screening also may be needed. Other tests may include lumbar puncture, blood cultures, electroencephalogram, and computed tomography scans. An accurate assessment may include a psychiatric consultation, especially if no history of altered cognitive functioning exists.

## Differential Diagnosis

Despite its obvious nature, delirium often is unrecognized, underdiagnosed, and undertreated (Breitbart & Alici, 2012; Eubank & Covinsky, 2014). Differentiating between delirium and dementia can be difficult, especially early in the course of dementia. Delirium and dementia may be misdiagnosed as depression because of an emotional response to the cancer. Sometimes, these reactions can be misdiagnosed as mania, an acute schizophrenic reaction, depression, or even as part of normal aging (Eubank & Covinsky, 2014; Pozuelo, 2015). Therefore, the history of onset, presentation, and progression of signs and symptoms carry significant value in making an accurate diagnosis.

Dementia appears in a relatively alert individual and is associated with impaired short-term memory, judgment, and abstract thinking. Little or no clouding of consciousness occurs in people with dementia, and the onset is insidious (Bush & Bruera, 2009). Delirium, on the other hand, occurs in all ages and is characterized by fluctuating levels of consciousness (attention) and disordered orientation, with symptoms usually worsening at night with hyperactivity.

In older individuals who are physically ill, delirium and dementia both may be present and manifest clinically as delirium superimposed on dementia. Soliciting the patient's past medical history for depression, stroke or its risk factors, possible recent head trauma, or hospitalization in combination with a medication history can shed light on timing of events and contributors to the current condition. The challenge is to distinguish prior disease and reversible processes, such as an acute inflammatory process, that might be causing the dementia. Rapidly progressive dementia is suspected in patients whose physical functioning has declined within the past two years and is accompanied by prominent frontal release signs, such as the palmar grasp reflex, palmomental reflex, rooting, or suck reflexes (Rosenbloom & Atri, 2011).

Diagnostic dementia criteria require evidence of the following observations verified by a reliable informant and in combination with cognitive assessment: decline in memory evidenced by difficulty learning new information, impaired recall of previously learned tasks, and impaired reception of verbal and nonverbal information; decline in cognitive functions with general impairment of judgment and thinking along with a deterioration of general processing of information; lack of clouding of consciousness and delirium; decline in emotional control or social behavior as expressed by apathy, emotional liability, irritability, and/or inappropriate social behaviors; memory declines significant enough to interfere with ability to perform activities of daily living; and evidence of impairment of higher cortical functions that include aphasia, agnosia, and/or apraxia (Plassman et al., 2007).

## Management of Delirium and Dementia

Nursing recognition of delirium requires improvement; Rice et al. (2011) noted that nurses failed to identify delirium 75% of the time. Delay in diagnosis prolongs initiation of appropriate interventions necessary for supportive care and safety measures. Four major areas for interventions are environmental safety, interpersonal support, educational information, and biochemical manipulation. Because patients with delirium are especially sensitive to their surroundings, particular attention should be paid to lighting, noise, and activity. Rooms should be quiet and well lit. A night-light will decrease disorientation when visual stimuli are decreased. Minimize sensory input by limiting the number of staff members entering the patient's room, providing consistency with the same caregivers, and performing only required procedures (Hshieh et al., 2015).

Frequent, short contacts with a supportive family member who understands how to interact with the patient can be very helpful. Speaking in a calm, reassuring voice can set a quiet and orderly tone. The addition of a clock, a calendar, and a few small, familiar items from home can help to reorient the patient. Encouraging the patient to walk, read, or participate in personal care can promote orientation and awareness of reality. The most effective interpersonal intervention is the presence of a familiar companion or nurse who monitors the patient's behavior, provides a stable schedule, and explains noises, procedures, and equipment (Hshieh et al., 2015; Irwin, Pirrello, Hirst, Buckholz, & Ferris, 2013).

A careful review of the delirious patient's medication profile, noting the risks and benefits of drug treatment, should be considered before instituting new medications so that "deliriogenic" drugs can be avoided and medicine use reduced (NCI, 2016). Close monitoring of all the medications the patient is taking is required to determine whether they contribute to delirium. Neuroleptics/antipsychotics often result in patient improvement before the underlying causes are elucidated. Benzodiazepines usually are instituted in cases of drug withdrawal syndromes or are added to the regimen but have limited benefit alone. Because benzodiazepines are sedatives, use is not likely to improve sensorium or cognition. Antipsychotics such as haloperidol (0.5–10 mg/day) and risperidone (0.75 mg/day) are the mainstay of treatment and are effective with all types of delirium. The low incidence of cardiovascular and sedative side effects is another reason for choosing haloperidol. Haloperidol produces less orthostatic hypotension and fewer anticholinergic side effects while also providing the greatest degree of antipsychotic action. Risperidone and olanzapine are newer antipsychotic agents that have fewer neurologic side effects and can improve cognitive and behavioral symptoms in low doses (Mittal et al., 2004).

Other antipsychotics include chlorpromazine and thioridazine. A possible side effect of antipsychotics is extrapyramidal symptoms, including pseudoparkinsonism (shuffling gait, muscle twitching) and akathisia (the need to be in constant motion). Pretreating patients with diphenhydramine can assist in preventing these conditions but should be used carefully because this could contribute to lethargy. Sedation may be used for delirium at the end of life when the patient is near death or in pain depending on the goals of care.

Symptom management, safety precautions, and optimizing function are the goals in treating dementia. Cholinesterase inhibitors, such as donepezil, rivastigmine, and galantamine, increase levels of the chemical messenger involved in memory and judgment (Qaseem et al., 2008; Townsend, 2015). Another drug sometimes added to the cholinesterase inhibitor is memantine. It has been primarily used to treat AD but has also been used to treat Parkinson disease and Lewy body dementia.

Maintaining a consistent, stable environment is the cornerstone of managing dementia. The healthcare provider can help the patient by establishing a routine and providing cues around the environment (e.g., displaying a sign on bathroom door). If a patient with dementia is hospitalized, maintaining a consistent environment can be very difficult. Family members or outside caregivers may be able to give suggestions on the patient's routine that can be reinforced and communicated to the oncology team. See Figure 11-3 for more interventions.

Pain assessment and management are challenging with this population. Patients with delirium or dementia may be unable to provide self-report or give a response to a numerical pain scale. The American Society for Pain Management Nursing (2011) position statement on patient assessment when the patient is unable to self-report recommended seek-

Chapter 11. Altered Mental Status 195

**Assessment**
- Assess for physiologic and psychological factors that could contribute to cognitive impairment.
- Ensure that appropriate testing is completed.
- Monitor for signs of change in affect, behavior, and cognition. Consider performing a systematic mental status examination. Assess orientation on a regular basis.
- Determine patients' baseline personality and behavior.
- Identify current medication regimen, including dosages.
- Monitor sleep schedule.

**Nursing Diagnoses** (NANDA International, 2015)
- Disturbed sensory perception
- Disturbed thought processes
- Disturbed sleep pattern
- Risk for injury
- Risk for violence (self-directed or other-directed)
- Acute or chronic confusion

***DSM-V* Diagnoses** (American Psychiatric Association, 2013)
- Delirium due to another medical condition, medication-induced delirium
- Delirium due to multiple etiologies
- Major or mild neurocognitive disorder due to Alzheimer disease
- Sedative-, hypnotic-, or anxiolytic-induced neurocognitive disorder

**Expected Outcomes**
- Patients will demonstrate improved orientation and awareness of environment.
- Patients will experience an increase in frequency and length of sleep periods and increased periods of restful sleep.
- Patients will remain injury free.
- Patients will experience a decrease in frequency and severity of misperceptions, delusions, and hallucinations.

**Interventions: Patients**
- Use side rails appropriately, provide adequate lighting, and keep bed in lowest position.
- Orient patients to immediate environment at least every two hours; give cues such as name, time, and activities about to occur.
- Provide clock, calendar, and schedule of patients' daily routines.
- Provide simple, concise information related to patients' concerns.
- Reassure patients of the staff's attention to physical status and safety.
- Assess patients' feelings about hospitalization and treatment.
- Clarify and discuss worries and fears; provide reassurance when possible.
- Limit extraneous stimuli (e.g., intercom communications) as much as possible.
- Administer antipsychotic medication regimen as prescribed.
- Explain the purpose of psychotropic medication.
- Assess the effectiveness of psychotropic medication, and monitor for adverse side effects.
- Discuss with patients and families the rationale for physical restraints and the nursing care regimen.
- Assess patients' response to restraints to determine the continued need.

**Interventions: Family Members**
- Instruct family members about how to orient patients to time, place, and purpose of hospitalization as necessary; have them bring in photos or other personal items.
- Educate families regarding patterns of interactions with patients (e.g., simple, short explanations or directions, focus on one activity or problem at a time).
- Encourage families to reinforce information and communication from staff.
- Encourage family members to participate in patients' care according to their ability.
- Educate family members about the physical causes of an impaired mental state.
- Inform families about the purpose and expected outcomes of medications or restraints.
- Reassure families of the staff's concern for patients' safety.

**Figure 11-3. Plan of Care**

ing out proxy reporters (family members, private caregivers), closely monitoring behavior, and conducting an analgesic trial where pain medication is administered and the patient is observed for changes in behavior (Herr, Coyne, McCaffery, Manworren, & Merkel, 2011).

When all other methods of intervention fail, patient safety may require physical restraints if appropriate. Because many institutions are restraint-free environments, staff should be knowledgeable of alternative approaches to manage severe agitation. If restraints are used, frequent personal contact with the patient for support, reassurance, and orientation is essential. Special considerations are required if patients are dehydrated, have thrombocytopenia, have a fever, or are septic. Patients never should be threatened with restraints; however, when deemed necessary, they should be applied immediately and carefully according to institutional policies. Contrary to most nurses' concerns, restraints usually do not interfere with a good nurse–patient relationship when the reason for their use is explained appropriately to the patient and family members.

Additional management of delirium in the terminal phase may be different than in the general oncology population because families may choose sedation over alertness, thereby narrowing the treatment choices. Additionally, metabolic causes of the delirium may not be easily treatable or may be impossible to treat in the hospice setting; therefore, diagnostic and therapeutic decision making requires careful consideration and discussion with the family of what treatment could entail. Patients and families may not want to pursue further testing or treatment. Treatment of agitation symptoms includes antipsychotics, analgesics if pain is present, and a comfortable, safe environment for the patient and family.

## Psychosocial Response to Delirium and Dementia for the Patient and Family

Delirium and dementia take a heavy emotional toll on patients and their families. Patients experience anxiety when they are aware of being confused. Depression and anger, as well as fluctuating mixed moods are also common. For patients aware of losing their faculties, the fear of loss of control can be overwhelming. This loss may represent patients' greatest fears. Patients aware of mental changes are prone to anxiety, depression, and suicide attempts.

Family and friends usually are the first to notice changes in a patient's emotional state or behavior. Family members often see their loved one with a different personality, which is frightening and very distressing. Changes in behavior, including offensive behaviors such as foul language or sexual actions, are devastating. Sudden changes in mood, agitation level, and/or increasing care needs can be stressful. If the patient cannot participate in decision making, family members will have to assume new roles. If the patient is discharged with persistent delirium, thus requiring more assistance with self-care and close monitoring to prevent self-injury, the burden on the family is greatly increased.

The rapid onset of symptoms associated with delirium can add to the fear and anxiety of those caring for the patient. Family members may be at a loss to understand what is happening. Their initial response may be that the patient is reacting to the stress of the diagnosis or treatment. This can delay determining the etiology of the mental changes. Others may fear that the symptoms represent brain metastases and may become depressed or anxious at this prospect. Not realizing that the symptoms may be treated readily, family members may assume that the patient has advanced or terminal disease. Concerns about how to care for the patient, as well as the need for restraints or tranquilizers, add additional stress to an already difficult situation. Because communication with the patient is often impaired, family members are frequently left feeling helpless and frustrated as they try to determine the patient's needs. Patient explanation to family members, with an emphasis on understanding the differences between being uncomfortable and being confused, can assist them in coping and staying present for their loved one. Patients may recall more of the delirium experience than previously thought. Anecdotal reports have documented patients' awareness of profound disturbances in their consciousness and awareness (Burns et al., 2004).

Caring for a loved one with dementia can take a considerable physical and emotional toll on individuals because problems are ongoing and become more complex as the deterioration progresses. In addition, it is depressing for loved ones to anticipate the changes ahead because of the progressive and downward nature of dementia. Therefore, families require assistance and support with the acute needs of their loved one while also planning for future needs. Because they are instrumental in helping with appropriate nutrition and exercise, caregivers assume a vital role in the health and well-being of patients with dementia. Regular physical exercise such as walking or using an exercise bicycle can maximize patients' functioning and reduce their risk of falls.

An interprofessional approach comprising nursing, social work, spiritual direction, and ongoing medical intervention assists in meeting the complex needs of patients and families. Palliative care standards and hospice care both assist in meeting patients' needs during the terminal phase regardless of their cognition and are a necessary comfort and support for families. Respite care, either in the home or at a facility, should be encouraged for families who need a break. Families often need to be encouraged to trust respite care and be reminded that they are not abandoning their loved one but tending to the needs of their own bodies and minds.

## Healthcare Professionals' Responses to Delirium and Dementia

Because behavior, cognition, and mood can be unpredictable when patients are experiencing delirium, staff members may feel frustrated and angry about the situation. Most staff members have a more positive attitude and will take more active measures in caring for these patients if they believe the confusion and disorientation are reversible. Patients with more serious delirium or dementia may need constant repetition of instructions, tasks broken down into very small steps, or more time to accomplish activities of daily living. The staff may feel helpless to improve the patient's condition. Feeling as if their interventions do not make much difference in patients' outcomes may lead to low morale and decreased job satisfaction if staff members are responsible for a number of patients with these diagnoses. Staff members may detach emotionally and avoid those patients to decrease their own feelings of inadequacy. They may tend to give impersonal care and stop trying to communicate with confused or hostile patients. Staff members may be concerned about possible violence from confused patients. They mistakenly may believe that patients have control over their own behavior and become frustrated with negative, hostile, or impulsive patients who are slow to respond. Staff members need to be aware that these patients will take more time to provide care. The challenge of caring for these patients on top of the demands of providing the cancer treatment can be very difficult for healthcare professionals.

Healthcare staff should be encouraged to acknowledge the stress of caring for patients experiencing dementia or delirium and simultaneously be reminded that their response is normal and does not reflect negatively on them. Rotating care providers to these patients instead of a few primary care nurses repeatedly caring for the same patients injects forced breaks from constant care. Educating staff about causes, compounding factors, and management strategies can empower them so that they feel the support of working as a group for complex patients. Suggesting self-care activities such as exercise; time away; support groups; and sharing of feelings, frustrations, and concerns with a trusted colleague are ideas for relieving the constant stress.

## Case Study

Agnes is an 80-year-old woman admitted to the hospital with acute confusion and severe back pain. She has a history of breast cancer. Although Agnes had been living independently, her daughter recently hired a part-time caregiver at home because Agnes was weaker and having trouble caring for herself. Up to that point, Agnes had been maintaining her own household with little help, driving, and volunteering at the local hospital. Several days prior to admission, she became more withdrawn, irritable, and less interested in her usual activities. She reported not feeling like walking because of her arthritis. On the morning of admission, the caregiver called the daughter to report that the patient was screaming in pain and that she was talking about finding her late husband in the next room. The patient's daughter became frantic because her father had died of AD, and she feared her mother was presenting with that diagnosis. Agnes had told her daughter many times that she would not want to be kept alive if she was destined to live in a confused state.

On arrival to the emergency department, Agnes was screaming and disoriented. She knew her daughter but was unable to recognize her doctor of many years.

## Discussion

This patient presents with acute onset of confusion, which was diagnosed as delirium. Her history of breast cancer alerted the team to the possibility of metastatic disease among other etiologies. The daughter remained frantic and expressed that metastatic disease, along with dementia, was her mother's greatest fears. The nurse practitioner in the emergency department met with the daughter to explain that delirium was different from dementia and that the cause needed to be identified quickly so treatment could be initiated. The daughter was then more open to proceeding with the workup. After administration of haloperidol, the patient became more relaxed and the nurse practitioner was able to localize the patient's pain to her back. A trial of low-dose fentanyl was given, and the patient was able to acknowledge some relief of pain but remained confused. Once the pain was under control, the patient was admitted to the hospital. Initial laboratory work identified a high calcium level. The workup also identified bone metastasis in the vertebrae consistent with the location of the patient's pain. Other causes for delirium were ruled out. Upon treatment of the hypercalcemia and bone metastasis, the patient was able to return home in a week with a caregiver with her pain under control and the acute delirium resolved.

## Conclusion

Delirium and dementia are significant clinical problems because of their prevalence, the increasing age of society, and the subsequent likelihood that the problem will grow and continue to affect healthcare costs and care requirements. As a complication of cancer, delirium compromises treatment and causes significant distress for patients and families. Nurses are able to assess and intervene with the physiologic, psychological, and environmental causes of delirium and its cognitive, behavioral, and affective sequelae because of their frequent and close contact with patients and families. The staff of an oncology unit must be able to recognize and treat these complications. Early diagnosis and management of these serious clinical problems will enhance the quality of life for patients and family members, as fewer days will be lost to the disorientation, fear, disabilities, and confusion involved in the delirium and dementia experience.

## References

Alici, Y., Bates, A.T., & Breitbart, W.S. (2015). Delirium. In J.C. Holland, W.S. Breitbart, P.N. Butow, P.B. Jacobsen, M.J. Loscalzo, & R. McCorkle (Eds.), *Psycho-oncology* (3rd ed., pp. 304–316). New York, NY: Oxford University Press.

Allen, K.R., Fosnight, S.M., Wilford, R., Benedict, L.M., Sabo, A., Holder, C., … Hazelett, S. (2011). Implementation of a system-wide quality improvement project to prevent delirium in hospitalized patients. *Journal of Clinical Outcomes Management, 18,* 253–258. Retrieved from http://www.turner-white.com/pdf/jcom_jun11_delirium.pdf

Alzheimer's Association. (n.d.). Sleep issues and sundowning. Retrieved from http://www.alz.org/care/alzheimers-dementia-sleep-issues-sundowning.asp

Alzheimer's Association. (2017). *2017 Alzheimer's disease facts and figures.* Retrieved from https://www.alz.org/documents_custom/2017-facts-and-figures.pdf

American Psychiatric Association. (2013). *Diagnostic and statistical manual of mental disorders* (5th ed.). Washington, DC: Author.

American Society for Pain Management Nursing. (2011). Pain assessment in the patient unable to self-report: Position statement with clinical practice recommendations. *Pain Management Nursing, 12,* 230–250. doi:10.1016/j.pmn.2011.10.002

Arnold, E. (2005). Sorting out the 3 D's: Delirium, dementia, depression: Learn how to sift through overlapping signs and symptoms so you can help improve an older patient's quality of life. *Holistic Nursing Practice, 19,* 99–104. doi:10.1097/00004650-200505000-00004

Bagri, A.S., Rico, A., & Ruiz, J.G. (2008). Evaluation and management of the elderly patient at risk for postoperative delirium. *Clinical Geriatric Medicine, 24,* 667–686. doi:10.1016/j.cger.2008.06.002

Bond, S., Neelon, V.J., & Belyea, M.J. (2006). Delirium in hospitalized older patients with cancer. *Oncology Nursing Forum, 33,* 1075–1083. doi:10.1188/06.ONF.1075-1083

Borson, S., Scanlon, J., Brush, M., Vitaliano, P., & Dokmak, A. (2000). The Mini-Cog: A cognitive "vital signs" measure for dementia screening in multi-lingual elderly. *International Journal of Geriatric Psychiatry, 11,* 1021–1027. doi:10.1002/1099-1166(200011)15:11<1021::AID-GPS234>3.0.CO;2-6

Bourgeois, J.A., Seaman, J.S., & Servis, M.E. (2008). Delirium, dementia, and amnestic disorders. In R.E. Hales, S.C. Yudofsky, & G.O. Gabbard (Eds.), *Textbook of clinical psychiatry* (5th ed., pp. 303–363). Washington, DC: American Psychiatric Publishing.

Breitbart, W., & Alici, Y. (2008). Agitation and delirium at the end of life: "We couldn't manage him." *JAMA, 300,* 2898–2910. doi:10.1001/jama.2008.885

Breitbart, W., & Alici, Y. (2012). Evidence-based treatment of delirium in patients with cancer. *Journal of Clinical Oncology, 30,* 1206–1214. doi:10.1200/JCO.2011.39.8784

Burns, A., Gallagley, A., & Byrne, J. (2004). Delirium. *Journal of Neurology, Neurosurgery, and Psychiatry, 75,* 362–367. doi:10.1136/jnnp.2003.023366

Bush, S., & Bruera, E. (2009). The assessment and management of delirium in cancer patients. *Oncologist, 14,* 1039–1049. doi:10.1634/theoncologist.2009-0122

Caeiro, L., Ferro, J.M., Albuquerque, R., & Figueira, M.L. (2004). Delirium in the first days of acute stroke. *Journal of Neurology, 251*, 171–178. doi:10.1007/s00415-004-0294-6

Catic, A.G. (2011). Identification and management of in-hospital drug-induced delirium in older patients. *Drugs and Aging, 28*, 737–748. doi:10.2165/11592240-000000000-00000

Centeno, C., Sanz, Á., & Bruera, E. (2004). Delirium in advanced cancer patients. *Palliative Medicine, 18*, 184–194. doi:10.1191/0269216304pm879oa

Clegg, A., & Young, J.B. (2011). Which medications to avoid in people at risk of delirium: A systematic review. *Age and Ageing, 40*, 23–29. doi:10.1093/ageing/afq140

Eubank, K.J., & Covinsky, K.E. (2014). Delirium severity in the hospitalized patient: Time to pay attention. *Annals of Internal Medicine, 160*, 574–575. doi:10.7326/M14-0553

Folstein, M.F., Folstein, S.E., & McHugh, P.R. (1975). Mini-mental state: A practical method for grading the cognitive state of patients for the clinician. *Journal of Psychiatric Research, 12*, 189–198. doi:10.1016/0022-3956(75)90026-6

Gaudreau, J.-D., Gagnon, P., Harel, F., Tremblay, A., & Roy, M.-A. (2005). Fast, systematic and continuous delirium assessment in hospitalized patients: The nursing delirium screening scale. *Journal of Pain and Symptom Management, 29*, 368–375. doi:10.1016/j.jpainsymman.2004.07.009

Grover, S., & Kate, N. (2012). Assessment scales for delirium: A review. *World Journal Psychiatry, 2*, 58–70. doi:10.5498/wjp.v2.i4.58

Gunther, M.L., Morandi, A., & Ely, E.W. (2008). Pathophysiology of delirium in the ICU. *Critical Care Clinics, 24*, 45–65. doi:10.1016/j.ccc.2007.10.002

Harris, D. (2007). Delirium in advanced disease. *Postgraduate Medical Journal, 83*, 525–528. doi:10.1136/pgmj.2006.052431

Harrison, J.K., Fearon, P., Noel-Storr, A.H., McShane, R., Stott, D.J., & Quinn, T.J. (2015). Informant questionnaire on cognitive decline in the elderly (IQCODE) for the diagnosis of dementia within a secondary care setting. *Cochrane Database of Systematic Reviews, 2015*(3). doi:10.1002/14651858.CD010772.pub2

Heidrich, D.E., & English, N.K. (2015). Delirium, confusion, agitation and restlessness. In B.R. Ferrell, N. Coyle, & J.A. Paice (Eds.), *Oxford textbook of palliative nursing* (4th ed., pp. 385–403). New York, NY: Oxford University Press.

Herr, K., Coyne, P.J., McCaffery, M., Manworren, R., & Merkel, S. (2011). Pain assessment in the patient unable to self-report: Position statement with clinical practice recommendations. *Pain Management Nursing, 12*, 230–250. doi:10.1016/j.pmn.2011.10.002

Hshieh, T.T., Yue, J., Oh, E., Puelle, M., Dowal, S., Travison, T., & Inouye, S.K. (2015). Effectiveness of multicomponent nonpharmacological delirium interventions: A meta-analysis. *JAMA Internal Medicine, 175*, 512–520. doi:10.1001/jamainternmed.2014.7779

Inouye, S.K. (2006). Delirium in older persons. *New England Journal of Medicine, 354*, 1157–1165. doi:10.1056/NEJMra052321

Inouye, S.K., van Dyck, C., Alessi, C., Balkin, S., Siegal, A., & Horwitz, R. (1990). Clarifying confusion: The confusion assessment method. *Annals of Internal Medicine, 113*, 941–948. doi:10.7326/0003-4819-113-12-941

Inouye, S.K., Westendorp, R.G., & Saczynski, J.S. (2014). Delirium in elderly people. *Lancet, 383*, 911–922. doi:10.1016/S0140-6736(13)60688-1

Irwin, S.A., Pirrello, R.D., Hirst, J.M., Buckholz, G.T., & Ferris, F.D. (2013). Clarifying delirium management: Practical, evidenced-based, expert recommendations for clinical practice. *Journal of Palliative Medicine, 16*, 423–435. doi:10.1089/jpm.2012.0319

Kiely, D.K., Bergmann, M.A., Jones, R.N., Murphy, K.M., Orav, E.J., & Marcantonio, E.R. (2004). Characteristics associated with delirium persistence among newly admitted post-acute facility patients. *Journals of Gerontology Series A: Biological Sciences and Medical Sciences, 59*, M344–M349. doi:10.1093/gerona/59.4.M344

Maldonado, J.R. (2008). Delirium in the acute care setting: Characteristics, diagnosis and treatment. *Critical Care Clinic, 24*, 657–722. doi:10.1016/j.ccc.2008.05.008

McCusker, J., Cole, M., Dendukuri, N., Han, L., & Belzile, E. (2003). The course of delirium in medical inpatients: A prospective study. *Journal of General Internal Medicine, 18*, 696–704. doi:10.1046/j.1525-1497.2003.20602.x

Mehta, R.D., & Roth, A.J. (2015). Psychiatric considerations in the oncology setting. *CA: A Cancer Journal for Clinicians, 65*, 300–314. doi:10.3322/caac.21285

Meulen, E.F.J., Schmand, B., van Campen, J.P., de Koning, S.J., Ponds, R.W., Scheltens, P., & Verhey, F.R. (2004). The seven-minute screen: A neurocognitive screening test highly sensitive to various types of dementia. *Journal of Neurology, Neurosurgery, and Psychiatry, 75*, 700–705. doi:10.1136/mnnp.2003.021055

Mittal, D., Jimerson, N.A., Neely, E.P., Johnson, W.D., Kennedy, R.E., Torres, R.A., & Nasrallah, H.A. (2004). Risperidone in the treatment of delirium: Results from a prospective open-label trial. *Journal of Clinical Psychiatry, 65*, 662–667. doi:10.4088/JCP.v65n0510

Morrison, C. (2003). Identification and management of delirium in the critically ill patient with cancer. *AACN Clinical Issues, 14,* 92–111. doi:10.1097/00044067-200302000-00011

Musicco, M., Adorni, F., Di Santo, S., Prinelli, R., Pettenati, C., Caltagirone, C., … Russo, A. (2013). Inverse occurrence of cancer and Alzheimer disease: A population-based incidence study. *Neurology, 81,* 322–328. doi:10.1212/WNL.0b013e31829c5ec1

NANDA International. (2015). *Nursing diagnoses: Definitions and classification, 2015–2017.* Philadelphia, PA: Author.

National Cancer Institute. (2016). Delirium (PDQ®)—Health professional version. Retrieved from https://www.cancer.gov/about-cancer/treatment/side-effects/memory/delirium-hp-pdq

National Institutes of Health. (2015). *The dementias: Hope through research.* Retrieved from https://www.nia.nih.gov/alzheimers/publication/dementias/introduction

Plassman, B.L., Langa, K.M., Fisher, G.G., Heeringa, S.G., Weir, D.R., Ofstedal, M.B., …Wallace, R.B. (2007). Prevalence of dementia in the United States: The aging, demographics, and memory study. *Neuroepidemiology, 29,* 125–132. doi:10.1159/000109998

Pozuelo, L. (2015). Everyone owns delirium: A comprehensive approach to diagnosing and minimizing its impact. *Geriatric Times,* 12–13. Retrieved from http://my.clevelandclinic.org/ccf/media/Files/Geriatrics/Geriatric-Times/geriatric-times-2015.pdf?la=en

Qaseem, A., Snow, V., Cross, V., Forciea, M.A., Hopkins, R., Schekelle, P., … Owens, D. (2008). Current pharmacologic treatment of dementia: A clinical practice guideline from the American College of Physicians and the American Academy of Family Physicians. *Annals of Internal Medicine, 148,* 370–378. doi:10.7326/0003-4819-148-5-200803040-00008

Radtke, F.M., Gaudreau, J.D., & Spies, C. (2010). Diagnosing delirium. *JAMA, 304,* 2125. doi:10.1001/jama.2010.1616

Rice, K.L., Bennet, M., Gomez, M., Theall, K.P., Knight, M., & Foreman, M.D. (2011). Nurses' recognition of delirium in the hospitalized older adult. *Clinical Nurse Specialist, 25,* 299–311. doi:10.1097/NUR.0b013e318234897b

Rosenbloom, M.H., & Atri, A. (2011). The evaluation of rapidly progressive dementia. *Neurologist, 17,* 67–74. doi:10.1097/NRL.0b013e31820ba5e3

Saravay, S.M., Kaplowitz, M., Kurek, J., Zeman, D., Pollack, S., Novik, S., … Hoffman, L. (2004). How do delirium and dementia increase length of stay of elderly general medical inpatients? *Psychosomatics, 45,* 235–242. doi:10.1176/appi.psy.45.3.235

Sarhill, N., Walsh, D., Nelson, K.A., LeGrand, S., & Davis, M.P. (2001). Assessment of delirium in advanced cancer. The use of the bedside confusion scale. *American Journal of Hospice and Palliative Care, 18,* 335–341. doi:10.1177/104990910101800509

Şenel, G., Uysal, N., Ogus, G., Kaya, M., Kadiolullari, N., Koçak, N., & Karaca, S. (2015). Delirium frequency and risk factors among patients with cancer in palliative care unit. *American Journal of Hospice and Palliative Care, 34,* 282–286. doi:10.1177/1049909115624703

Siberski, J. (2014). Dementia and DSM-5: Changes, cost, and confusion. *Aging Well, 5,* 12. Retrieved from http://www.todaysgeriatricmedicine.com/archive/110612p12.shtml

Smith, T., Gildeh, N., & Holmes, C. (2007). The Montreal Cognitive Assessment: Validity and utility in a memory clinic setting. *Canadian Journal of Psychiatry, 52,* 329–332.

Townsend, M.C. (2015). *Psychiatric mental health nursing: Concepts of care in evidence-based practice* (8th ed.). Philadelphia, PA: F.A. Davis.

Waszynski, C.M. (n.d.). The Confusion Assessment Method (CAM). Retrieved from http://consultgeri.org/try-this/general-assessment/issue-13

Wilber, S.T., Carpenter, C.R., & Hustey, F.M. (2008). The six-item screener to detect cognitive impairment in older emergency department patients. *Academic Emergency Medicine, 15,* 613–616. doi:10.1111/j.1553-2712.2008.00158.x

Wong, C.L., Holroyd-Leduc, J., Simel, D.L., & Straus, S.E. (2010). Does this patient have delirium?: Value of bedside instruments. *JAMA, 304,* 779–786. doi:10.1001/jama.2010.118

CHAPTER 12

# Altered Sexuality

*Paula J. Anastasia, RN, MN, AOCN®*

> *Let someone love you just the way you are–as flawed as you might be, as unattractive as you sometimes feel, and as unaccomplished as you think you are. To believe that you must hide all the parts of you that are broken, out of fear that someone else is incapable of loving what is less than perfect, is to believe that sunlight is incapable of entering a broken window and illuminating a dark room.*
>
> —Marc Hack

Cancer affects an individual's total being, including the physical, emotional, spiritual, and sexual aspects of oneself. Sexuality in relation to cancer often is overlooked as a priority when treatment needs are assessed because of practitioners' and patients' reluctance to address the subject. Although all types of cancer can interfere with sexual health, the sexuality literature acknowledges gynecologic and breast cancers for women and genitourinary cancers for men as common cancers that potentially alter sexual function (Bober & Varela, 2012; Morreale, 2011). Human sexuality has no age restriction and, therefore, sexuality can be maintained until the end of life.

The most common sexual problem in men, especially geriatric men, is erectile dysfunction (ED), or the inability to maintain erection sufficient for sexual performance. Other types of dysfunction include loss of libido, and sexual bother, which is related to embarrassment or inability to enjoy life (Montorsi et al., 2010; Nelson, Deveci, Stasi, Scardino, & Mulhall, 2010; Saitz, Serefoglu, Trost, Thomas, & Hellstrom, 2013). Additional evidence-based longitudinal research studies for sexual dysfunction in the male and female populations are needed in order to obtain more accurate epidemiologic studies. The existing literature mainly focuses on ED in men and dysfunction in women. Among the general population, 40%–45% of women and 20%–30% of men report some type of sexual problem (Lewis et al., 2010). *Sexuality* refers not only to sexual intercourse but also to other facets of intimacy, such as body language, hugging, kissing, and touching. Self-esteem and body image are integral aspects of being sexual, and these are frequently affected by cancer and its treatment. Although cancer can alter a person's sexuality, it cannot take away one's sexual self.

## Important Principles About Sexuality

The American Psychiatric Association (APA, 2013) has defined sexual dysfunction as the inability to experience one of the four phases of the sexual response cycle: arousal, plateau, climax, and resolution. Recognizing that individuals are not one dimensional, the new updated definition includes gender-specific difficulties and subtypes that include lifelong versus acquired and generalized versus situational sexual problems. The *Diagnostic and Statistical Manual of Mental Disorders (DSM-V)* has simplified female sexual dysfunctions into three categories (sexual interest/arousal disorder, genito-pelvic pain/penetration, and female orgasmic disorder) and male sexual dysfunction into four categories (hypoactive sexual desire disorder, delayed ejaculation, erectile disorder, and premature ejaculation) (APA, 2013). Although individuals may experience alterations in sexual function, the *DSM-V* recognizes it as a disorder only if it is not associated with a medical condition such as cancer and if the duration is a minimum of six months, occurring at least 75% of the time and causing significant distress (APA, 2013). The World Health Organization (WHO) does not use the term *dysfunction* but refers to *sexual health* as a broad term to promote positive aspects of physical, emotional, and social well-being in relation to sexuality, which includes gender, sexuality, and sexual rights (WHO, 2015).

In both men and women, the frequency of sexual activity decreases with age and changes in sexual function and responses become more common (Coady & Kennedy, 2016; Lindau et al., 2007). Many external and internal variables can affect sexual functioning, including disease processes, health status, pain, emotions, stress, interpersonal relationships, and religious and cultural norms. An individual's background, culture, value system, past experiences, and current relationship will influence how he or she views sex (e.g., dirty, shameful). What is normal for one person may be viewed as abnormal to another (e.g., using a vibrator, oral stimulation, anal penetration). Therefore, the definition of altered sexual function (ASF) can have different meanings to individuals. It is documented that both physicians and nurses receive little training in addressing sexual problems with their patients (Association of Reproductive Health Professionals, 2008; Bober, Carter, & Falk, 2013). Lack of communication may convey to the patient that ASF is not important or that nothing can improve the issue (Bober et al., 2013; Bober & Varela, 2012; Coady & Kennedy, 2016).

## Altered Sexuality and Cancer

Communicating with patients and partners about possible changes in sexual function as a result of cancer treatment should be an ongoing assessment at each patient visit. Table 12-1 lists various cancers and types of sexual changes caused by surgical, chemotherapy, or radiation treatment. In addition to these factors, physiologic and psychological behaviors that alter sexuality can result from treatment side effects (e.g., nausea, pain) or the emotional response to cancer (e.g., anxiety, depression, fatigue). These reactions can negatively affect desire or libido and sexual functioning (National Comprehensive Cancer Network® [NCCN®], 2017b; Thygesen, Schjødt, & Jarden, 2012). It is reported that sexual issues are more common among female cancer survivors. It is estimated that 30%–100% of female patients with cancer experience sexual dysfunction. For men, the prevalence of ED following radical prostatectomy is estimated to be 27%–77%. For men who undergo external beam radiation, the prevalence is 30%–45% (Dizon & Katz, 2015). The incidence of ED in male survivors of colorectal cancer ranges from 45% to 75% (NCCN, 2017b). Other can-

## Table 12-1. Types of Treatment and Their Effect on Sexuality

| Malignancy | Intervention | Adverse Effects |
|---|---|---|
| Bladder | Surgical intervention<br>• Radical cystectomy<br>• Ileal conduit | Altered body image<br>Erectile dysfunction<br>Vaginal atrophy/shortening |
|  | Radiation | Fatigue<br>Pain |
|  | Chemotherapy/biotherapy | Urinary frequency<br>Diarrhea<br>Nausea<br>Alopecia |
| Breast | Surgical intervention<br>• Mastectomy<br>• Lumpectomy | Altered body image<br>Pain<br>Fatigue<br>Feelings of loss of femininity<br>Decreased nipple sensation |
|  | Radiation | Altered body image<br>Breast edema<br>Skin irritation<br>Fatigue |
|  | Chemotherapy/biotherapy | Nausea<br>Alopecia<br>Fatigue<br>Neuropathy<br>Decreased libido |
|  | Hormone therapy | Fluid retention<br>Hot flashes<br>Myalgia<br>Dyspareunia<br>Postmenopausal bleeding<br>Vaginal dryness |
| Colorectal | Surgical intervention<br>• Colectomy<br>• Colostomy | Altered body image<br>Pain |
|  | Radiation | Fatigue<br>Diarrhea |
|  | Chemotherapy/biotherapy | Nausea<br>Mucositis<br>Erectile dysfunction |
| Gynecologic | Surgical intervention<br>• Hysterectomy<br>• Oophorectomy<br>• Vaginectomy<br>• Vulvectomy<br>• Colostomy<br>• Ileal conduit | Fatigue<br>Pain<br>Decreased libido<br>Hot flashes<br>Altered body image<br>Vaginal atrophy<br>Vaginal stenosis |

*(Continued on next page)*

## Table 12-1. Types of Treatment and Their Effect on Sexuality *(Continued)*

| Malignancy | Intervention | Adverse Effects |
|---|---|---|
| Gynecologic *(cont.)* | Radiation | Fatigue |
| | Chemotherapy/biotherapy/hormone therapy | Chemotherapy-induced menopause<br>Alopecia<br>Nausea/vomiting<br>Neuropathy |
| Head and neck | Surgical resection<br>• Laryngectomy<br>• Tracheostomy | Altered body image<br>Fatigue<br>Facial disfigurement<br>Pain<br>Mucositis/xerostomia |
| Lung | Surgical intervention<br>• Pneumonectomy<br>• Lobectomy | Dyspnea<br>Pain |
| | Radiation | Fatigue |
| | Chemotherapy/biotherapy | Altered body image<br>Fatigue<br>Neuropathy<br>Nausea<br>Alopecia |
| Prostate | Surgical intervention: Prostatectomy | Altered self-esteem<br>Altered body image<br>Erectile dysfunction<br>Pain<br>Urinary incontinence |
| | Radiation | Fatigue |
| | Chemotherapy/hormone therapy | Hot flashes<br>Altered body image |
| Testicular | Surgical intervention: Orchiectomy | Altered self-esteem<br>Altered body image<br>Erectile dysfunction<br>Pain<br>Urinary incontinence |
| | Radiation | Fatigue |
| | Chemotherapy/hormone therapy | Hot flashes<br>Infertility |

*Note.* Based on information from Schover, 2001a, 2001b.

cers, including Hodgkin lymphoma and testicular cancer, have a reported 25% prevalence of long-term sexual problems (National Cancer Institute [NCI], 2017).

## The Impact of Surgery on Sexuality

Surgery can alter body image and self-esteem even if the surgical procedure does not interfere with sexual functioning and performance (Lehmann, Hagedoorn, & Tuinman, 2015).

Surgical intervention for head and neck cancer may cause scarring and facial disfigurement. Adjuvant radiation and chemotherapy can increase the risk for mucositis and xerostomia, causing difficulty with intimacy and kissing (Rhoten, Murphy, & Ridner, 2013). Other examples of altered body image caused by surgical intervention are stomas or ostomies as a result of colorectal or bladder cancer (Dunn, 2015). Lymphedema can occur in a variety of cancers, including breast and gynecologic, as well as melanoma and head and neck cancers (Fu, Deng, & Armer, 2014). Cancer-related lymphedema can occur years following cancer treatment, even with less invasive surgeries such as sentinel lymph node biopsy. The added assault to body image can interfere with an individual's self-esteem and desire to be intimate (see Chapter 15 for more information on body image disturbance).

### *Surgical Impact Related to Female Cancer*

A mastectomy may lead to inadequate body image and decreased feelings of attractiveness. Less invasive surgical approaches, such as lumpectomy, are alternatives to breast cancer surgical management that can achieve the same survival outcomes (American Cancer Society [ACS], 2017). Recent studies comparing radical mastectomy to lumpectomy and radiation therapy revealed that women who underwent lumpectomy had fewer issues related to altered body image and therefore reported fewer changes in frequency of intercourse and less sexual dysfunction (Morrelae, 2011). However, women who underwent a mastectomy compared to women who underwent breast-conserving surgery reported more sexual problems, including changes in libido and achieving an orgasm, up to a year after surgery (Aerts, Christiaens, Enzlin, Neven, & Amant, 2014). Reconstruction, which involves many months of procedures and discomfort, may assist in maintaining body image but can result in scarring and decreased nipple sensation. Some women do undergo nipple-sparing surgery, which maintains aesthetic appeal in select patients. However, nipple necrosis was reported in up to 7% in one study as well as locoregional and distant recurrences (Endara, Chen, Verma, Nahabedian, & Spear, 2013).

The three most common gynecologic cancers are endometrial, ovarian, and cervical (ACS, 2017). Sexual disruption from these types of cancers is caused by surgical treatments, including hysterectomy, bilateral salpingo-oophorectomy (BSO), and potential vaginal resection. Changes in sexual function can be acute or chronic and may manifest as dyspareunia and vaginal dryness caused by vaginal shortening, reduced lubrication, and fibrosis around the vaginal cuff (Coady & Kennedy, 2016; Lammerink, de Bock, Pras, Reyners, & Mouritis, 2012). The psychosexual adjustment for women with a gynecologic malignancy is complex. Psychologically, the removal of the reproductive organs can have devastating effects for all women, but more so if the woman is premenopausal (Levin et al., 2010). If both ovaries are removed in a premenopausal woman, menopause is immediate, and the potential vasomotor symptoms can interfere with sexual relationships due to hot flashes, mood changes, and insomnia resulting in fatigue. Long-term menopause without estrogen replacement can lead to vaginal thinning, dryness, and atrophy. Sexual desire or libido may decrease as a result of the stress from the initial diagnosis and manifest throughout the treatment phase. Menopause or absence of ovarian function may also accelerate changes in the libido (Dizon, Suzin, & McIlvenna, 2014). Some women may be hesitant to resume vaginal intercourse after postoperative healing, for fear of pain or the irrational belief that it will cause the cancer to spread. The function of the cervix with regard to sexual arousal has been controversial; most studies, however, do not support any difference in sexual satisfaction because of removal of the cervix (Komisaruk, Frangos, & Whipple, 2011). Women who had been treated for early-stage cervical cancer and received surgery and radiation therapy had more sexual dissatisfaction, such as vaginal dryness and decreased libido, lasting up to three years (Dizon et al., 2014). Lammerink et al. (2012) reviewed 20 studies over 12 years in women with cervical cancer. Most studies showed no difference in orgasmic function before and after treatment; however, change in sexual pain was noted and lasted longer after radiation therapy.

Pelvic exenteration, a radical surgery performed for curative treatment of recurrent cervical cancer, involves removal of the uterus, ovaries, vagina, bladder, and rectum. Although an uncommon procedure, the surgical outcome causes severe alterations in psychosexual functioning because of changes in body appearance (Mirhashemi et al., 2002; Rezk et al., 2013; Roos, de Graeff, van Eijkeren, Boon, & Heintz, 2004). A neovagina is constructed so that women can maintain vaginal intercourse. Many women continue to experience a lack of desire for sexual relation as well as the inability to have intercourse despite vaginal reconstruction in some situations (Hendren et al., 2007; Scott, Liu, & Mathes, 2010). Recent studies report more patients adapting to pelvic exenteration, especially if the healthcare provider has adequately counseled the patient on the procedure and subsequent long-term physical changes. Younger patients have the most difficulty adapting to daily life, with a poorer perception of body image (Rezk et al., 2013; Roos et al., 2004). Advanced or recurrent vulvar cancer requires a vulvectomy, which may involve minimal removal of the surrounding tissue or possibly an extensive disfiguring removal of the labia, clitoris, and lymph nodes. This can result in long-term or permanent edema, vulva hypersensitivity or discomfort, and potential inability to achieve an orgasm. Although less radical surgery is now the standard, disruption of sexual arousal still occurs. In a 10-year study of women with early-stage vulvar cancer followed by surgery, 43% were able to resume sexual intercourse. Of those, 50% reported their sexual outcome similar to presurgery baseline, and 42% reported it being worse (Hazewinkel et al., 2012).

### *Surgical Impact Related to Male Cancer*

Prostate cancer is the most prevalent cancer in men and the second leading cause of death after lung cancer (ACS, 2017). Regardless of treatment (e.g., radical prostatectomy, radiation, antiandrogen medication), numerous publications report changes in sexual function and performance for male cancer survivors (NCCN, 2017b). Men can have impotency problems that include desire, orgasm, or ejaculation (Bober & Varela, 2012). ASF will occur after prostatectomy, and despite improvement in outcomes with the nerve-sparing prostatectomy for localized prostate cancer, potency may take up to two years to return. The incidence of ED after prostatectomy in male cancer survivors is reported to be as high as 90% (NCCN, 2017c; Resnick et al., 2013). Men who have their prostate removed may still experience orgasmic pleasure but will experience a "dry ejaculation," which also results in infertility. Urinary incontinence, a side effect from prostatectomy, can alter self-esteem, cause feelings of shame or embarrassment, and decrease quality of life. A study comparing side effects of prostatectomy versus radiation showed that prostatectomy was more likely to cause urinary incontinence at the two- and five-year mark for patients. However, no difference was noted between the two groups at the 15-year mark (Resnick et al., 2013). In addition to ED, decreased libido and penile shortening are consequences of surgical intervention. Adverse effects of sexual dysfunction are factors in the treatment decision-making process for men and should be discussed with the patient and his partner at the time of diagnosis (Carlsson et al., 2012; Gontero et al., 2007). Men with a bladder cancer diagnosis are also at risk for ASF. Noninvasive bladder cancer may render the need for a transurethral resection of bladder tumor, causing temporary ASF. Advanced bladder cancer may require chemotherapy, radiation therapy, and prostatectomy (Dunn, 2015). Some men, regardless of age, relationship status, or gender preference, would choose a less aggressive treatment in exchange for more sexual function. Evaluating for emotional distress should be assessed at the time of diagnosis, during the treatment phase, and during surveillance follow-up care (NCCN, 2017c).

Testicular cancer occurs predominantly in younger men between the ages of 15 and 34 and is often curable with treatment (NCI, 2017). As with all cancers, sexual function and fertility issues need to be addressed upfront, especially in young men who may not have started dating or are thinking about conceiving a child in the future. Men undergoing retroperitoneal lymph node dissection (RPLND) and adjuvant therapy with platinum-based chemotherapy and/or radiation are at higher risk of sexual problems than those who only undergo RPLND (Steiner et al., 2008). However, nerve-sparing RPLND, which preserves ejaculation, has shown the same survival outcomes as standard RPLND and may be an option for early-stage disease (Beck, Bey, Bihrle, & Foster, 2010; NCCN, 2017b).

## The Impact of Radiation Therapy on Sexuality

Radiation therapy can have acute and delayed local effects, with fatigue as the most frequently reported. Sexual pain has been reported in as high as 45% of patients with gynecologic and rectal cancers treated with radiation therapy (Bregendahl, Emmertsen, Lindegaard, & Laurberg, 2015). Women undergoing radiation involving the rectum, bladder, uterus, or cervix may develop interruption of ovarian function, resulting in premature menopause. Although radiation treatment has become more specific and tissue targeted, the potential for scatter radiation always exists. Ovarian transposition may be performed to preserve fertility and prevent early menopause in women younger than age 40 (Hwang et al., 2012). Menopausal effects can lead to hot flashes and vaginal dryness that may indirectly interfere with sexual function and desire. Vaginal narrowing is possible after pelvic radiation, especially if the cervix is involved. Patients treated with pelvic radiation report more ASF than patients treated without radiation (Bjelic-Radisic et al., 2012; Mirabeau-Beale & Viswanathan, 2014). Lymphedema may occur after removal of or radiation to the lymph nodes. This commonly occurs following breast cancer treatment or groin dissection for gynecologic cancers. Lymphedema can affect appearance and self-esteem and decrease intimacy (Ferrandina et al., 2012; Fu et al., 2014). Enlargement of the thigh or arm can be deemed disfiguring to individuals. In addition to altered body image, lower leg edema can interfere with mobility, activities, and even style of dress in order to conceal the enlarged limb. Lymphedema of the lower limb can impair positioning of the legs comfortably for sex. Cervical cancer survivors have reported lymphedema to be the most disabling complication (Ferrandina et al., 2012).

Men treated with radiation therapy for prostate cancer have reported a cluster of side effects such as urinary urgency or leakage and decreased or absent orgasm, all contributing to ASF and decreased quality of life (Barnas et al., 2004).

## The Impact of Chemotherapy on Sexuality

High-dose chemotherapy, such as regimens used for bone marrow transplant (BMT), can cause short- and long-term ASF. Patients receiving high-dose chemotherapy report greater distress and dissatisfaction with sexual life after treatment than those receiving standard chemotherapy regimens (Thygesen et al., 2012). Lack of desire and alterations in body image are common to both genders receiving BMT. Specific chemotherapeutic agents may cause infertility or ovarian failure. Men are at risk for ejaculation difficulties and ED. These changes may be temporary or permanent and will depend on the cytotoxic agent, dosage, duration of chemotherapy, and patient's age. Alkylating agents is the drug class that most commonly causes ovarian failure (Thygesen et al., 2012).

Chemotherapy's common side effects (e.g., nausea, stomatitis, diarrhea, fatigue, depression) can inhibit sexual desire. Chemotherapy-induced peripheral neuropathy can impair the sense of touch, thereby negatively affecting intimacy. Alopecia alters patients' self-image and self-esteem, decreasing feelings of sexual attractiveness. Bone marrow suppression from chemotherapy also may cause side effects that affect sexual activity (Bober & Varela, 2012; NCI, 2017). For example, neutropenia increases the risk for vaginal infection and sexually transmitted infections. Fatigue may necessitate planning sexual activities to conserve energy, thereby reducing spontaneity. Lastly, bleeding risks secondary to thrombocytopenia must be addressed and sexual education should be provided if the patient has significant risk of bleeding or is engaging in aggressive sexual practices or anal intercourse (Thygesen et al., 2012).

Studies of long-term follow-up in women with breast cancer reported that women who received adjuvant chemotherapy had more sexual dysfunction as a result of vaginal dryness, dyspareunia, and decreased libido than those who did not receive chemotherapy (Ganz et al., 2002; NCCN, 2017c). Chemotherapy-induced menopause also can have a negative impact on the sexuality and quality of life of young women who have not yet entered natural menopause (Goetsch, Lim, & Caughey, 2014; Herbenick et al., 2011).

## The Impact of Hormonal Therapy

Endocrine therapies are prescribed in breast cancer, reproductive cancers, and prostate cancer. These medications may result in side effects that interfere with sexuality, desire, and function (Katz & Dizon, 2016). In breast cancer, steroidal or nonsteroidal aromatase inhibitors are used as maintenance in long-term follow-up, as well as for recurrent or stage IV disease. These medications can cause nausea, joint aches, hot flashes, vaginal dryness, urinary tract infections, and gastrointestinal upset contributing to loss of sexual desire and dyspareunia (Bober et al., 2013; Davison, 2012; Goetsch et al., 2014).

Men with advanced prostate cancer may receive androgen deprivation therapy in the form of luteinizing hormone–releasing hormone agonists, causing medical castration by preventing testosterone production in the testes. These treatments alter sexual function and self-esteem, with side effects that include hot flashes, gynecomastia, and decreased desire and erectile function. Nonsteroidal antiandrogen therapy blocks testosterone at the prostate and may cause fewer alterations in libido and arousal than luteinizing hormone–releasing hormones (NCCN, 2017b). Hot flashes occur in 80% of men receiving androgen deprivation therapy and can interfere with sleep, thus contributing to fatigue, low energy, and decreased sexual desire (Kaplan & Mahon, 2014). Ongoing nursing assessment of the patient's medication list is important because hormone therapies may be given as primary therapy or as adjuvant treatment for five years or more following standard treatment.

## Long-Term Treatment Impact on Sexuality

### *Menopause*

Menopause is the cessation of ovarian function, resulting in the permanent absence of menses. Although the average age of menopause is 52, premature menopause may result secondary to surgery (e.g., BSO), chemotherapy, or radiation therapy to the pelvis. It is estimated that women who undergo BSO experience an up to 50% reduction in testosterone from presurgical levels, and up to half of these women report a decrease in libido (Bober & Varela, 2012; Shifren, Monz, Russo, Segreti, & Johannes, 2008). Ovarian failure in a premenopausal female can cause distress in quality of life. Symptoms resulting from decreased estrogen production, such as hot flashes; mood changes (e.g., depression, irritability, fatigue, insomnia, memory loss); and loss of libido, resulting from decreased androgen production, may further affect the sexual self already threatened by the cancer diagnosis. The use of hormone replacement therapy has effectively managed vasomotor symptoms; however, long-term use is not without risk (Rossouw, Manson, Kaunitz, & Anderson, 2013).

### *Infertility*

For women with an intact uterus and at least one ovary, in vitro fertilization (IVF) may be a consideration. Alternatively, for women with an intact uterus and absence of both ovaries, IVF with donor oocytes is a possibility. The success of donor–recipient cycles is dependent on the quality of the oocyte. Embryo cryopreservation is an effective fertility-preservation intervention for young patients with cancer prior to starting chemotherapy. In order to participate in embryo cryopreservation, the patient needs a donor sperm. The patient also would require ovarian stimulation and a delay in starting chemotherapy (Misiewicz, 2012). Men with male factor infertility may inquire about intracytoplasmic sperm injection, in which a single sperm is injected into the cytoplasm of an egg. Sperm banking should be considered for young men who will be receiving surgery, radiation, or chemotherapy that may cause infertility (Williams, 2010). These techniques provide no guarantee of success and are expensive. However, they offer alternatives to infertility for patients with cancer. The pregnancy success rates of assisted reproductive technology are dependent on many factors, and each clinic will have its own statistics. Resources such as the Livestrong Foundation offer financial assistance for patients with cancer who are interested in IVF.

The nurse's role as an advocate for patients with potential infertility issues involves assessment and identification of patients interested in pursuing conception through IVF and/or childbirth. Because patients may not even realize infertility is a risk or that proactive options are available, the healthcare team needs to initiate the conversation about fertility. Young patients may not know if they want children in their future; however, a referral to a fertility specialist is essential so that the patient is informed of all the available options. Options potentially may be limited after initiating cancer therapy. Although ethical, cultural, and religious beliefs may challenge both nurses and patients, a discussion is still essential even if the patient chooses not to pursue any type of treatment. Adoption is a viable alternative that often is overlooked but should be discussed as a possible option for future parenting (Loren et al., 2013). Healthcare professionals should inform patients of the risks of infertility related to cancer treatments as part of the informed consent process. Nurses play a vital role in referring patients to social workers, therapists, and the appropriate technologic services for infertility support, sperm banking, and adoption. The American Society of Clinical Oncology guidelines recommend that healthcare providers advise patients regarding potential threats to fertility as early as possible to allow informed decision-making options (Loren et al., 2013).

### *Intimacy*

*Intimacy* refers to the physical or emotional closeness shared with another individual. Individuals dealing with a cancer diagnosis may experience a range of psychological responses, such as anxiety, depression, and anger, which may alter their feelings about intimacy and sexual activity. For instance, patients who have ostomies or alterations in elimination patterns may worry about the loss of control of bodily functions and refrain from intimate situations (Lehmann et al., 2015). Men may worry about the ability to have an erection, which may add to performance anxiety (Katz & Dizon, 2016). Cancer survivors who are single or involved in noncommitted relationships may face unique challenges when resuming their "new normal." Patients with cancer who are meeting potential dating partners are at greater risk for ASF than patients who are married (Katz, 2009). Uneasy feelings about when to tell a potential dating partner about their illness, and insecurities about attractiveness and acceptance are concerns that may prevent patients from starting a new relationship (Dizon et al., 2014). Support groups for single patients with cancer can be a therapeutic way to facilitate sharing of similar anxieties and issues. Online dating is an option that may allow the patient to be selective in choosing a partner, as the process can begin slowly with emails before face-to-face meetings. Topic-related dating sites also are available for people with specific illnesses, such as cancer or herpes.

Intimacy in older adults often is ignored because of society's perception that older people are not sexual or intimate. However, many older individuals remain sexually active in their later years. Physiologically, older patients may experience changes with sexuality caused by comorbid disease, such as menopause, or erectile and ejaculatory changes (Dunn, 2015). These changes may result in a couple needing to find ways to maintain intimacy without sexual intercourse. Older patients who are newly single, widowed, or divorced may have greater difficulty meeting new partners. In addition to their loss, grief, and sense of isolation, a cancer diagnosis may threaten their independence and self-esteem, especially if their spouse was a significant source of support (Hawkins et al., 2009). As the older adult population increases, these issues will become more apparent.

## Healthcare Professionals' Responses to Altered Sexuality

Sexuality is a difficult topic for most healthcare professionals to initiate with patients. Professionals must understand their own sexuality and preconceived notions about what constitutes acceptable or expected sexual behavior before attempting to assess and intervene with patients (Dunn, 2015). Research has revealed that nurses and physicians are comfortable discussing sexuality only if patients initiate the topic (NCCN, 2017c). Patients may be hesitant and embarrassed to broach the topic of sexuality with their healthcare team. By using principles of patient education, the nurse can identify patient readiness and recognize the patient's needs and willingness to discuss sexuality.

If the patient is in pain or experiencing other uncomfortable effects from the disease or treatment, discussing sexuality is not appropriate. Confidentiality and privacy are important to patients but not always available in a clinical setting (Bober & Varela, 2012). Barriers to discussion may include the patient's culture and values, age, gender, and sexual orientation. Information should be presented in a relaxed and nonjudgmental fashion so that the lines of communication remain open between the patient and nurse. However, this is a difficult and challenging aspect of care, and expertise comes only with personal insight, scientific understanding, and practice (Dunn, 2015). Nurses do not need to be sex therapists to assist patients who are experiencing sexual dysfunction. However, nurses need to be knowledgeable about the etiology and management of sexual dysfunction and how to make appropriate referrals.

# Nursing Care of Patients Experiencing Altered Sexuality

Identifying patients at risk for sexual dysfunction can assist the oncology team in facilitating counseling interventions in a timely manner. The literature has suggested that patients who have had sexual dysfunction or relationship discord prior to the cancer diagnosis will be at greater risk for sexual difficulties (Schover, 2001a, 2001b). However, identifying these patients may not be easy unless thorough assessment skills and questioning are employed. This begins with nurses understanding basic principles about sexuality and the psychological and physiologic factors that affect sexual functioning.

Nurses should be familiar with the four phases of the sexual response cycle: desire, excitement, orgasm, and resolution (see Figure 12-1). Patients most often will identify concerns with the phases of desire (decreased libido) and excitement (performance issues related to dyspareunia or ED). Patient education primarily will focus on these two areas. Andersen (1990) developed the ALARM model as a framework to assess sexual behaviors and the sexual response cycle (see Figure 12-2). Primary causes of sexual dysfunction can result from hypoactive sexual desire or secondary causes such as emotional disorders (anxiety, depression), psychosocial stressors (relationship stress, job conflict), or physical factors (diabetes, high blood pressure). Medications and substance abuse, including alcohol, also can interfere with sexual response (Davison, 2012; Shifren et al., 2008, Thygesen et al., 2012).

## Sexual History

A medical history should occur in the initial conversation and include mental health, sexual health, and medication use (e.g., prescription, nonprescription, recreation use). Providing privacy and confidentiality for patients and significant others is important in obtaining a successful sexual health history. Nurses must remember that some patients will react with embarrassment or resistance when they try to discuss sexual issues. Establishing a trusting and professional relationship will facilitate open communication. A health history that includes both the physical health and psychosocial and emotional health should be part of the sexual history. Personal questions related to sex will include asking about

---

1. Desire: Having an interest in sexual activity
2. Excitement: State of being aroused
3. Orgasm: Sexual climax
4. Resolution: Return to prearoused state

**Figure 12-1. Phases of Sexual Response**

*Note.* Based on information from Schover, 2001a, 2001b.

---

**A**ctivity: Frequency and type of sexual practice
**L**ibido/desire: Interest in sex
**A**rousal and orgasm: Ability to achieve orgasm
**R**esolution: Satisfaction with sexual activity
**M**edical history relevant to sexuality: Precipitating events

**Figure 12-2. ALARM Model for Sexual Functioning Assessment**

*Note.* Based on information from Andersen, 1990.

current sexual relationship, gender preference, sexually transmitted or acquired disease(s), problems performing or enjoying sex, safe sex practices and contraception, and sexual abuse. When taking the health history, it may be helpful to inform patients that although the questions appear to be personal, they are necessary to assess total well-being, which includes sexual health (NCCN, 2017c). Another recommendation is moving from less sensitive questions to more personal ones, such as first asking if they are in a sexual relationship and then inquiring about sexual difficulties. Another nonthreatening approach may be to ask, "How do you think your cancer and treatment will affect your sexual function and relationship?"

No standard screening procedures or questionnaires exist for sexual dysfunction in patients with cancer. The Female Sexual Function Index is the most widely used tool to assess sexual function and cancer-related ASF; however, its validation and reliability have been established only in healthy participants, not patients with cancer (Baser, Li, & Carter, 2012; Bober & Varela, 2012; Rosen et al., 2000). Numerous validated self-administered tools are available, including screening tools to identify patients with ASF, and outcomes measurement tools to evaluate treatment. The Derogatis Interview for Sexual Functioning measures five domains of sexual functioning: sexual fantasy, arousal, experience, drive, and orgasm (Derogatis, 1997). The Sexual Adjustment Questionnaire is a self-administered survey assessing desire, activity level, relationship, arousal, sexual techniques, and orgasm. This tool is used as an outcome measure for sexual functioning (Wilmoth, Hanlon, Ng, & Bruner, 2014). The International Index of Erectile Function was developed for use in clinical trials with sildenafil and has been validated in more than 32 languages (Rosen, Cappelleri, & Gendrano, 2002).

In the clinical setting, identifying patients at risk for sexual dysfunction can be simplified by asking straightforward questions such as, "Has your cancer or its treatment caused any changes in your sex life?" Another simple method is to use the NCCN Distress Thermometer when the patient presents for an appointment. The Distress Thermometer is a 0–10 scale asking patients to rank the areas of distress in their life. Categories include sexuality in addition to other physical, emotional, and social issues. The patient's baseline sexual health should be established at the initial visit prior to any cancer treatment (NCCN, 2017a).

## Differential Diagnosis

For some individuals, sexual expression is a release, a coping mechanism that validates closeness, reassurance, and love. For others, it is an extra stressor, an added responsibility, or pressure to "perform" in addition to the demands of the cancer treatment. Sexual dysfunction may manifest from physical behaviors or from an emotional response, such as depression, anxiety, or fear (see Table 12-2). Patients who are depressed may experience decreased desire or lack interest to engage in a relationship. Side effects from treatment (e.g., fatigue, pain, nausea) may compound an already depressed mood, further affecting desire, arousal, and orgasm. A thorough physical examination to rule out contributing causes such as diabetes or cardiovascular disease is essential (Gupta et al., 2011). Treatment of underlying symptoms is the first step to removing the barrier that is masking desires to respond sexually.

Reviewing patients' prescription and nonprescription medications is helpful in identifying other causes contributing to sexual dysfunction. Certain classifications of antidepressants (e.g., selective serotonin reuptake inhibitors [SSRIs]) suppress libido and the sexual response, including arousal and orgasm (Serretti & Chiesa, 2009). Some brands of antihypertensive

### Table 12-2. Psychological and Behavioral Responses That Affect Sexuality

| Response | Interventions |
| --- | --- |
| Anxiety | Assess anxiety and underlying fear.<br>Provide information and correct misconceptions about resuming or initiating sexual activity, including the following suggestions:<br>• Mood setting<br>• Warm bath with dim lights, candles, and music<br>• Relaxation tapes<br>• Massage<br>Suggest use of antianxiety medications or a glass of wine prior to activity if not contraindicated. (Note: May cause erectile dysfunction) |
| Depression | Assess cause (e.g., situational depression as a result of cancer, preexisting chronic depression).<br>Encourage verbalization of feelings with a focus on short-term positive outcomes.<br>Recommend involvement in a support group or referral to a therapist.<br>Recommend couples therapy as needed (e.g., partner is having difficulty coping with mastectomy, patient feels rejected).<br>Encourage discussion with patient and partner.<br>Consider antidepressants if necessary. (Note: May cause erectile dysfunction) |
| Fatigue | Recommend scheduling time for sexual activity. Suggest planning naps or conserving energy prior to sexual activity.<br>Provide illustrations of alternative, energy-conserving positions. |
| Pain | Schedule pain medication and monitor level of drowsiness prior to sexual activity.<br>Recommend use of vaginal lubricants and changing of position to reduce discomfort.<br>Recommend manual or oral stimulation. |
| Nausea | Time antiemetic dose according to expectation of nausea.<br>Monitor for drowsiness.<br>Provide a small snack and encourage relaxation activities (e.g., dim lights, music, massage).<br>Suggest passive sexual position if active movement causes nausea. |
| Decreased desire | Suggest initial use of intimacy without intercourse.<br>Recommend patient and partner use touch and stimulation to achieve arousal or increase desire (e.g., massage, hugging, kissing).<br>Remind patient to use strategies that have worked in the past to stimulate desire.<br>Recommend mood setting with lights and candles.<br>If not otherwise constrained, use a small amount of alcohol to increase desire.<br>Consider referral to a sex therapist for treatment of chronic problems or for testosterone injections. |

*Note.* Based on information from National Comprehensive Cancer Network, 2017a; Schover, 2001a, 2001b.

drugs cause ED. Other drugs that affect arousal and performance include antiadrenergic and anticholinergic agents, hormone therapies, and recreational drugs (NCI, 2017).

Patients may present with prior sexual dysfunction caused by a history of emotional or psychiatric illness, psychotropic medication use, or substance abuse. Low self-esteem, feelings of hopelessness, and body dysmorphic disorder can interfere with interpersonal relationships and sexual interest. Often, more than one variable is responsible for sexual dysfunction; therefore, psychosocial assessment and intervention are appropriate. An ongoing appraisal of individuals' physical and emotional health can assist in identifying secondary causes of sexual dysfunction.

## Interventions

One of the most common models for sexual counseling is the PLISSIT model, a four-step process used to guide nurses through information seeking and counseling for the patient (Annon, 1976) (see Figure 12-3). The first three phases of the model—permission, limited information, and specific suggestions—are interventions commonly used by nurses. The nurse should ask open-ended questions to assess if the patient is at risk for ASF. Validating and reassuring the patient that ASF is common, especially related to a cancer diagnosis, treatment, and survivorship, will often encourage patient dialogue. Questions and education should be patient centered. Asking the patient about goals of therapy and listening to the patient and repeating or rephrasing the issue for clarity will help reassure them. Resources that can assist patients include books, videos, teaching pamphlets, and support groups. ACS offers free booklets for men and women on sexuality and cancer (Schover, 2001a, 2001b). Support groups can be beneficial to patients, especially cancer-specific groups (e.g., breast cancer, prostate cancer) that allow patients to share similar areas of concern related to their disease and treatment.

Oncology nurses should regularly reassess patients' responses to suggestions and interventions based on their needs at each stage of the illness continuum. For example, at each follow-up appointment, nurses can intervene by again using the first three stages of the PLISSIT model and assisting patients to reevaluate their sexual needs and goals. The discussion should be done in a private space so that the patient feels comfortable talking. By asking patients if they have experienced any changes in sexual function since their prior visit or if they anticipate any changes, nurses are giving them permission to dialogue. The nurse should demonstrate active listening with eye contact if the patient chooses to engage in conversation. Prior to surgery, the patient's goal may be to reduce anxiety and enjoy alternative ways of expressing intimacy during recovery. The partner may benefit by accompanying the patient at healthcare visits and being involved with the conversation (Katz & Dizon, 2016). At later appointments, the nurse can follow up with the patient and discuss any alterations in sexual expression related to the surgery. Nurses can play a vital role in the ongoing assessment of patients' sexual health, making specific suggestions when appropriate and referring patients to a sex therapist if warranted by prolonged sexual dysfunction, the last phase of the PLISSIT model.

Men and women should be encouraged to maintain total body wellness with daily exercise. An adequate diet of increased fruit, vegetables, and water consumption, as well as relax-

---

**Permission:** The nurse provides an open and trusting environment for the patient that gives permission to discuss sexual feelings and behaviors. This is the initial assessment phase when the nurse identifies any potential for sexual dysfunction.

**Limited Information:** The nurse provides factual information regarding treatment and its effect on sexuality. The nurse should identify and clarify fears and misconceptions that the patient may be expressing (e.g., cancer is not contagious, intercourse will not cause the cancer to spread, fatigue from treatment may interfere with the desire for sexual activity).

**Specific Suggestions:** These are provided after a thorough sexual health history that includes baseline sexual functioning, attitudes, and beliefs. Comfort and knowledge in discussing strategies and options for improving sexual expression are important for this phase.

**Intensive Therapy:** This is recommended when the patient has prolonged or severe sexual dysfunction requiring referral to a sex therapist. Sexual dysfunction may be a preexisting condition or a result of the cancer treatment.

---

**Figure 12-3. The PLISSIT Model**

*Note.* Based on information from Annon, 1976.

ation, stress reduction activities, and proper sleep, may provide more energy. A plan of care is outlined in Figure 12-4, and available resources to support nursing interventions can be found in Figure 12-5.

## Female-Specific Considerations

Decreased libido, or hypoactive sexual desire disorder (HSDD), affects approximately 10% of women and can result from many variables (Davison, 2012). Validating how common the loss of libido is during diagnosis and treatment opens up communication with the patient. Menopausal women are more likely to experience HSDD because of changes in estrogen and androgens. Women should be reminded that desire and arousal can vary throughout different phases in life regardless of whether one is experiencing cancer. Encourage patients to talk about the positive aspects of what attracted them to their partner. For women without a current partner but who worry about long-term loss of libido, encourage self-discovery of arousal (e.g., erotic books, movies, self-stimulation).

In 2015, the U.S. Food and Drug Administration approved flibanserin (Addyi®) for premenopausal women with an acquired generalized HSDD as defined by the *DSM-V*, which excludes women with HSDD associated with a medical condition such as cancer. Flibanserin is a $5\text{-HT}_{1A}$ receptor agonist and $5\text{-HT}_{2A}$ receptor antagonist; however, the mechanism of action is unknown (Sprout Pharmaceuticals, 2016). Flibanserin has been shown to improve sexual desire as well as the number of satisfying events, thus reducing distress from loss of sexual desire. The most common side effects are dizziness, nausea, fatigue or insomnia, and dry mouth. Alcohol consumption is contraindicated, as it can increase hypotension and syncope (Sprout Pharmaceuticals, 2016).

The use of phosphodiesterase type 5 (PDE5) inhibitors, which are administered to men with ED, is currently being studied in women in the clinical trial setting for the treatment of sexual arousal. Chivers and Rosen (2010) reviewed 16 studies using PDE5 inhibitors in women with alterations in sexual arousal. The data remain mixed, reporting improved genital vasocongestion but few improvements in sexual arousal.

The side effects from menopause, whether naturally occurring or treatment related, can interfere with sexual pleasure on many levels. Vaginal atrophy or thinning of the vaginal lining can cause dryness, irritation, burning, and dyspareunia, which make vaginal penetration uncomfortable. Without intervention, women may resist sexual relations for fear of pain, causing their partner to feel rejected. Ask patients what they find most distressing. Ask what treatments have they tried that were or were not effective. Offer limited but specific suggestions for improvement.

Several options are available for treating vaginal dryness, including estrogen and non–estrogen-based preparations. Water-soluble, nonhormonal vaginal lubricants and nonhormonal vaginal moisturizers can effectively treat vaginal dryness but will not reverse vaginal atrophy. Vaginal moisturizers can be used as often as once a day or as little as once a week (Herbenick et al., 2011). Vaginal lubricants and moisturizers can be purchased without a prescription and can be used with sexual activity. A gynecologic examination should be performed to evaluate if the patient has atrophy or thinning of the vaginal wall or dryness. Atrophic changes are usually progressive over time and do not resolve spontaneously (Krychman, 2011).

Another therapy approved for vaginal atrophy and dyspareunia in postmenopausal women is ospemifene (Osphena®), a selective estrogen receptor modulator (SERM) (Shionogi, Inc., 2016). It is not indicated for women with known or suspected breast cancer or hormone-sensitive cancers. Similar to other SERMs (e.g., tamoxifen), ospemifene acts like estro-

**Assessment**
- Medical and sexual history
- Developmental age
- Learning needs regarding sexuality
- Nature of the sexual problem and its importance to the patient
- Partners' perceptions of the problem
- Extent of treatment- or cancer-related interference with normal sexual functioning
- Levels of anxiety and depression related to cancer or sexual alteration
- Patients' attitudes and beliefs regarding sexuality
- Additional life stressors that can impede sexual functioning

**Nursing Diagnoses** (NANDA International, 2015)
- Ineffective sexuality pattern
- Sexual dysfunction

***DSM-V* Diagnoses** (American Psychiatric Association, 2013)
- Other specified sexual dysfunction (followed by the specific reason [e.g., prostatectomy])
- Unspecified sexual dysfunction (symptoms cause significant distress but do not meet full criteria of a sexual dysfunctions diagnostic class)

**Expected Outcomes**
- Patients will verbalize perceptions of sexual concerns.
- Patients will identify ways to alter sexual functioning to adapt to physical changes.
- Patients will express satisfaction with sexual functioning.
- Patients will express satisfaction with ability to communicate sexual concerns with partners.

**Interventions**
- Be aware of own difficulties with discussion of sexual issues.
- Approach patients/partners with a nonjudgmental, accepting attitude.
- Encourage ongoing expression of sexual concerns, including personal meaning of changes to the patients.
- Provide information about the reasons for the sexual alteration; correct misconceptions regarding cancer or its treatment or any long-standing notions in general.
- Instruct patients/partners regarding contraindications to sexual activity (e.g., myelosuppression, thrombocytopenia).
- Address stress-related, depression-related, anxiety-related, or body image and self-esteem issues as necessary.
- Provide specific suggestions for overcoming treatment-related impediments to sexual functioning.
    - Fatigue: Take a nap prior to sexual activity; plan activity according to fatigue patterns.
    - Dyspareunia: Use water-soluble lubricants, increase time of foreplay, and change positions. Use vaginal dilators for vaginal stenosis.
    - Decreased libido: Fantasize. Discuss with the physician the use of estrogen or testosterone. Discover each other's erogenous areas with playful teasing techniques. Recommend mood setting with lights and candles, adult movies, sex toys, and magazines.
    - Erectile difficulty: Discuss probable etiology, including psychological and physical factors. Discuss available treatment options, such as prescription medications, vacuum devices, and penile prostheses. Discuss other forms of self- and/or partner pleasure.
- Discuss ways to experience intimacy or alternate forms of sexual gratification. Suggest initial use of intimacy without intercourse (e.g., kissing, cuddling, manual/oral gratification). Recommend patients and partners use touch stimulation to achieve arousal or increase desire. Make touch playful, and communicate what part of the body is aroused when touched or teased. Remind patients to use strategies that have worked in the past to stimulate desire.
- Encourage frank and open discussions with partners, provide support to initiate discussions, and ensure that partners have necessary knowledge regarding cancer- or treatment-related sexual effects.
- Consider referral to a sex counselor if correctable problems persist.

**Figure 12-4. Plan of Care**

**Organizations**
- American Association for Marriage and Family Therapy: www.aamft.org
- American Association of Sexuality Educators, Counselors and Therapists: www.aasect.org
- North American Menopause Society: www.menopause.org
- Sexuality Information and Education Council of the United States: www.siecus.org
- Society for Sex Therapy and Research: www.sstarnet.org

**Apps**
- Explore Women's Sex: Provides information on female anatomy and describes how women get turned on sexually
- My Sex Doctor: Addresses various topics and commonly asked questions about anatomy and sex
- Sexual Health Guide: Offers information and articles on how to be and stay sexually healthy

**Figure 12-5. Resources for Sexual Interventions**

gen on vaginal tissue and may cause proliferation of the endometrial lining; however, the incidence is low (Portman, Bachman, & Simon, 2013). The findings in a 52-week study of 426 postmenopausal women who were randomized to placebo or ospemifene confirmed efficacy and tolerability for those on the study drug in the treatment of vaginal atrophy (Goldstein et al., 2014).

Estrogen given systemically (transdermal or oral) or vaginally can effectively treat vaginal dryness and reduce vaginal atrophy, although vaginal estrogen may be more effective for dyspareunia. Urogenital symptoms are also responsible for dyspareunia and urinary tract infections (Krychman, 2011). Systemic estrogen is controversial in breast cancer survivors because of the risk of recurrence and is rarely, if ever, advised (Biglia, Maffei, Lello, & Nappi, 2010). Additionally, endometrial proliferation is a concern if the patient has an intact uterus, and estrogen alone should not be used; progesterone should be administered if systemic estrogen is prescribed. Systemic estrogen and progesterone replacement is indicated in individual cases because long-term use (greater than five years) can increase the risk of breast cancer and heart disease (Rossouw et al., 2013). The use of vaginal estrogen in breast cancer survivors is data challenged as to the degree of estrogen absorption. Women taking an aromatase inhibitor for breast cancer should not use vaginal estrogen products, even though systemic absorption is minimal. The mechanism of an aromatase inhibitor is to block the enzyme aromatase, which activates the peripheral conversion of androgens to estrogens in postmenopausal women. Because the risk of systemic absorption with vaginal estrogen is minimal, it is contraindicated for patients taking an aromatase inhibitor (Biglia et al., 2010).

Low-dose vaginal estrogen creams or tablets (inserted into the vagina) can be used daily for two to three weeks, then twice weekly after vaginal vascularization has occurred. Other estrogen preparations are extended-release ring formulations, which are inserted similar to a diaphragm every three months. Women who participate in regular sexual activity report fewer symptoms of vaginal atrophy. Offering the patient specific suggestions to alleviate initial symptoms of vaginal dryness and discomfort may result in more sexual relations.

Surgically induced menopause causes loss of all ovarian function and is believed to have a more significant symptomatology. Vasomotor symptoms, such as hot flashes, do not directly affect sexual function. However, intimacy and sexual stimulation may bring on a hot flash. Estrogen replacement was the treatment of choice for treating menopause-induced hot flashes for women without a uterus, but the addition of progesterone is required to prevent endometrial cancer. The long-term use of estrogen and progesterone is controversial and should be considered on an individual basis for women who have significant disruption in quality of life because of vasomotor symptoms (Rossouw et al., 2013).

Estrogen is not used in women with a history of breast cancer, so alternative remedies have been prescribed. SSRIs, a class of antidepressants, have been studied in women with breast cancer. In several randomized studies, the use of an antidepressant, especially venlafaxine, compared to placebo showed a significant decrease in hot flashes (Boekhout, Vincent, & Dalesio, 2011). Gabapentin compared to venlafaxine was equally effective in reducing hot flashes in a randomized crossover study in women with breast cancer (Kaplan & Mahon, 2014). Each patient must be evaluated individually because the use of antidepressants may cause nausea, dry mouth, constipation, and an inability to achieve orgasm.

In the scenario of dyspareunia in the vulvar vestibule area, the application of topical 4% aqueous lidocaine for three minutes to the tender site reduced painful symptoms in women with breast cancer, allowing speculum placement (Goetsch et al., 2014).

Vaginal stenosis, manifested by vaginal fibrosis, thickening, shortening, or obstruction, is associated with pelvic radiation or graft-versus-host disease from allogeneic hematopoietic stem cell transplantation (Thygesen et al., 2012). The effects of this complication can be delayed months to years after treatment. Women may be instructed to use vaginal dilators in the form of a cylinder or to practice vaginal intercourse to keep the vagina from further narrowing. Women should be counseled on having gynecologic examinations as part of their follow-up care (Park Kim, Lee, Chung, & Lee, 2013).

After their hysterectomy, some women may notice that the effects of vaginal shortening result in discomfort during sexual intercourse. Instruct patients to experiment with changes in sexual positioning, such as side-to-side or the woman on top, to control the amount of penetration from her partner (Schover, 2001b). The vagina will expand with use, so patients can be reassured that the discomfort is reversible. For women without a current partner, the use of a vaginal dilator can be used to decrease vaginal dryness, thinning, and stenosis (Carter, Goldfrank, & Schover, 2011).

## Male-Specific Considerations

Male patients will report ASF in the form of decreased libido, ED, and abnormal ejaculation. The nurse should provide privacy when asking the patient about any sexual changes since cancer diagnosis and treatment. Allow the patient to verbalize concerns and frustrations (Lehmann et al., 2015). Katz and Dizon (2016) noted that men may perceive themselves to be strong and self-sufficient and therefore resist communicating a problem. If the patient has a partner, education and discussion should be encouraged with both the patient and his partner. The nurse should rule out any underlying depression or anxiety in patients who report a decreased libido. Premature ejaculation may cause frustration and anger in the patient. Assessment is essential in knowing if ejaculatory problems are a result of the cancer treatment or a preexisting condition. Medications such as an SSRI, an anxiolytic, and topical analgesics may be helpful. Referral to a therapist also is an option.

ED may improve after one to two years, depending on the surgery and adjuvant use of medications (Barnas et al., 2004). However, this can also result in feelings of grief and altered body image (Nelson et al., 2010). Many therapeutic options are available for ED, including PDE5 inhibitors (Bober & Varela, 2012). The first of its kind, sildenafil, also known as Viagra®, revolutionized awareness of and opened communication about ED. Since then, several other products have been approved for ED. Patients should be counseled that it commonly takes 12–18 months postsurgery for recovery of nerve function, even with the use of a PDE5 inhibitor. If the patient is prescribed a PDE5 inhibitor, the nurse should be educated on adverse effects and drug interactions. For instance, sildenafil is metabolized by cytochrome P450 3A4; therefore, grapefruit juice should be avoided. The concomitant administration of a PDE5 inhibitor with nitrates can cause a significant drop in blood pressure. Patients should be assessed on an individual basis regarding their health history and medication history for possible drug interactions. Testosterone levels may need to be checked in men with low libido, especially in young men with testicular cancer who had normal libido prior to surgery (Steiner et al., 2008). Men undergoing hematopoietic cell transplantation experience gonad failure largely because of the chemotherapy and radiation administered prior to the transplant (Thygesen et al., 2012). Testosterone replacement may be an option. Nonpharmacologic treatments include vacuum erection devices, penile prostheses, and penile revascularization. This usually is reserved for men who do not respond to PDE5 inhibitor therapy and would entail referral to a urologist.

Androgen deprivation therapy is prescribed for advanced-stage prostate cancer to decrease the circulating plasma testosterone levels to that of castration levels. Side effects from hormone therapy include decreased libido, hot flashes, impotence, gynecomastia, and nausea. If gynecomastia is severe, low-dose radiation may be administered to reduce the size of the breast tissue. Liposuction also has been used. Similar to women with hot flashes, men who experience hot flashes can self-assess to understand what triggers the event. Beverages such as coffee or alcohol can stimulate a hot flash. Dressing in layers and using a fan or air conditioner can help patients control their environment. Medications such as venlafaxine and gabapentin may be helpful. Acupuncture and relaxation therapy have been tried with mixed results (Kaplan & Mahon, 2014).

## Case Study

Gilda is a 52-year-old, gravida 0, Caucasian woman who was diagnosed with stage IIIC ovarian cancer. She underwent an exploratory laparotomy, total abdominal hysterectomy, and BSO. Gilda will receive six cycles of IV chemotherapy of carboplatin and paclitaxel. Gilda was perimenopausal prior to her surgically induced menopause.

After surgery, Gilda reports hourly hot flashes and night sweats that interfere with sleep. However, if she takes a sleep aid, she can sleep most of the night. Gilda is vice president of a marketing firm and continues to work full time throughout her treatment. Her husband was recently laid off from his job and financial pressure was a concern for Gilda. Although her husband accompanies her to medical appointments and appears supportive, Gilda confides to her clinical nurse specialist (CNS) that he is having an affair. She is extremely distressed because, even though she is going through chemotherapy and is constantly tired, Gilda manages to take care of her husband's sexual needs.

Gilda verbalized that her marriage was vulnerable prior to her diagnosis, and once she realized she had a life-threatening illness, she coped by working and building her career. At the time, the CNS validated the life-altering changes caused by a cancer diagnosis, discussed how relationships are equally affected, and suggested couples counseling.

After her treatment, Gilda and her husband file for a mutual divorce. Even though she is devastated that her marriage is ending, Gilda verbalizes she is secretly relieved, as her husband had only been causing additional stress.

The CNS meets with Gilda after her sixth chemotherapy treatment and gives her the good news that her disease is currently in remission. Gilda states that she wants to date again, but she is concerned no one will want a relationship with a cancer survivor. In addition, at what point would she disclose she has cancer in remission, alopecia, low libido, and is divorced? She also questions her sexuality and femininity, stating, "Will I ever be viewed as desirable?" The CNS reassures Gilda that many women commonly share her feelings, even those without cancer.

The CNS listens to Gilda's concerns. They discuss the basics of any relationship. When trust and friendship are established with a companion, the CNS believes that Gilda can share her medical history. The CNS reminds Gilda that she is in the early stages of dating and that she should remove the pressure of viewing a "date" as a long-term relationship or marriage. Gilda verbalizes that it is helpful to be reminded not to overshare on a first date. The CNS identifies several issues with Gilda. First, Gilda is still grieving the loss of her marriage, and the CNS reinforces the need for Gilda to continue her private therapy sessions. Second, Gilda is also grieving her illness, which potentially alters her future goals. Finally, surgery and chemotherapy-induced side effects impacted her self-image. Her surgical debulking resulted in a vertical incisional scar. The CNS stresses that surgically induced menopause can decrease libido and cause hot flashes, insomnia, vaginal dryness, and sexual discomfort. Chemotherapy causes alopecia, fatigue, and body aches. Gilda is experiencing some of these negative effects.

Although apprehensive, Gilda starts slowly with online dating, which gives her more control over the who, where, and when. In a meeting with her CNS, Gilda confides that she has met someone she wants to become intimate with, but she is concerned that sex will be painful. The CNS feels confident in educating Gilda on supportive ways to promote comfort. A discussion ensues about interventions to assist a more pleasurable sexual intercourse and includes the use of lubricants for vaginal dryness and longer duration of foreplay and manual stimulation prior to penetration. Other suggestions include a side-lying position to aid in conserving energy and controlling the depth of penetration. Manual and oral stimulation are also discussed as means for sexual expression. The nurse recommends that Gilda and her partner use these if intercourse remains painful.

A discussion regarding estrogen replacement then ensues with Gilda, the CNS, and her gynecologist-oncologist. Gilda continues to be bothered by daily hot flashes and hourly night sweats that interrupt her sleep pattern and cause her to feel fatigued throughout the day. The pros and cons for estrogen replacement are discussed. Generally, short-term (e.g., two to five years), low-dose estrogen is considered if hot flashes are frequent and interfere with day-to-day activities and sleep, thus causing changes in quality of life. Gilda believes her busy job and sleep deprivation are reasons alone to try estrogen. The physician prescribes a low-dose estrogen patch with a return visit in one month to reevaluate.

## Discussion

Gilda's return visit included a positive attitude, as the estrogen patch effectively reduced most of her hot flashes. She felt more rested and energetic. Gilda reported a satisfied sexual relationship with an understanding partner after using the methods discussed at her last visit.

Gilda went through several phases of self-discovery after her cancer diagnosis and divorce. She had several life-altering stresses occurring all at once, but her determination and the follow-up support from her healthcare team helped her move forward with goals that ensured her quality of life.

This case illustrates complex themes that arise from helping patients to deal with some of the indirect effects of a cancer diagnosis and its treatment. A perimenopausal woman who was forced into menopause from a life-threatening diagnosis was faced with an unexpected end to her marriage. The CNS demonstrated expertise at assessing and identifying the underlying physical and emotional difficulties affecting Gilda's sexual concerns, including fatigue, body image changes, and fear of dating. Helping Gilda to understand the impact of her illness and encouraging her to reevaluate future goals enabled her to take care of herself physically and emotionally. The CNS also encouraged Gilda to continue her therapy sessions, which improved Gilda's ability to cope with rigorous but potentially effective cancer treatment.

## Conclusion

Research to support evidence-based interventions for sexual dysfunction is limited in the nursing and health-related literature. Thus, more randomized, controlled clinical trials are needed to test and support interventions to treat sexual dysfunction in patients with cancer. Patient-centered goals need to be identified to ensure that sexual wellness is part of patient education and survivorship care planning. Additional research on disease-specific cancers and disease-specific interventions is needed for individuals wanting to resume and achieve sexual functioning despite a cancer diagnosis. Prospective studies also are essential to identify the relationship between symptom management and sexual functioning and to identify effective education and counseling techniques for nurses and other healthcare professionals. Quality-of-life studies need to incorporate the benefits of sexuality and intimacy as possible factors in reducing emotional distress and improving psychosocial responses to illness.

Finally, nurses and physicians need to be aware of their own limitations in treating and counseling individuals with sexual dysfunction. Healthcare providers can gain more confidence through effective communication. Identifying practitioners and an interprofessional team to provide an interprofessional approach can improve patient care planning. Most patients need education pre- and post-treatment with routine evaluation and follow-up of interventions. There may be situations when a referral to another physician specialist, social worker, or sexual health therapist is appropriate after other interventions have been initiated and the patient is still in distress. The American Association of Sexuality Educators, Counselors and Therapists can provide referrals for patients needing more specialized education and assistance. Healthcare professionals are the advocates between patients and the resources that help guide patients back to sexual wellness. Through trust, skilled assessment techniques, and education, nurses can assist patients by providing information in the areas of sexuality and sexual rehabilitation, thus supporting their quality of life long after their cancer diagnosis.

## References

Aerts, L., Christiaens, M.R., Enzlin, P., Neven, P., & Amant, F. (2014). Sexual functioning in women after mastectomy versus breast conserving therapy for early-stage breast cancer: A prospective controlled study. *Breast, 23,* 629–636. doi:10.1016/j.breast.2014.06.012

American Cancer Society. (2017). *Cancer facts and figures 2017*. Atlanta, GA: Author.
American Psychiatric Association. (2013). *Diagnostic and statistical manual of mental disorders* (5th ed.). Washington, DC: Author.
Andersen, B. (1990). How cancer affects sexual functioning. *Oncology, 4,* 81–88.
Annon, J.S. (1976). The PLISSIT model: A proposed conceptual scheme for the behavioral treatment of sexual problems. *Journal of Sex Education and Therapy, 2,* 1–15.
Association of Reproductive Health Professionals. (2008). What you need to know talking to patients about sexuality and sexual health. Retrieved from https://www.arhp.org/uploadDocs/sexandsexfactsheet.pdf
Barnas, J.L., Pierpaoli, S., Ladd, P., Valenzuela, R., Aviv, N., Parker, M., ... Mulhall, J.P. (2004). The prevalence and nature of orgasmic dysfunction after radical prostatectomy. *BJU International, 94,* 603–605. doi:10.1111/j.1464-410X.2004.05009.x
Baser, R.E., Li, Y., & Carter, J. (2012). Psychometric validation of the female sexual function index (FSFI) in cancer survivors. *Cancer, 118,* 4606–4618. doi:10.1002/cncr.26739
Beck, S.D., Bey, A.L., Bihrle, R., & Foster, R.S. (2010). Ejaculatory status and fertility rates after primary retroperitoneal lymph node dissection. *Journal of Urology, 184,* 2078–2080. doi:10.1016/j.juro.2010.06.146
Biglia, N., Maffei, S., Lello, S., & Nappi, R.E. (2010). Tibolone in postmenopausal women: A review based on recent randomized controlled clinical trials. *Gynecological Endocrinology, 26,* 804–814. doi:10.3109/09513590.2010.495437
Bjelic-Radisic, V., Jensen, P.T., Vlasic, K.K., Waldenstrom, A.-C., Singer, S., Chie, W., ... Greimel, E. (2012). Quality of life characteristics in patients with cervical cancer. *European Journal of Cancer, 48,* 3009–3018. doi:10.1016/j.ejca.2012.05.011
Bober, S.L., Carter, J., & Falk, S. (2013). Addressing female sexual function after cancer by internists and primary care providers. *Journal of Sexual Medicine, 10*(Suppl. 1), 112–119. doi:10.1111/jsm.12027
Bober, S.L., & Varela, V.S. (2012). Sexuality in adult cancer survivors: Challenges and intervention. *Journal of Clinical Oncology, 30,* 3712–3719. doi:10.1200/JCO.2012.41.7915
Boekhout, A.H., Vincent, A.D., & Dalesio, O.B. (2011). Management of hot flashes in patients who have breast cancer with venlafaxine and clonidine: A randomized, double-blind, placebo-controlled trial. *Journal of Clinical Oncology, 29,* 3862–3868. doi:10.1200/JCO.2010.33.1298
Bregendahl, S., Emmertsen, K.J., Lindegaard, J.C., & Laurberg, S. (2015). Urinary and sexual dysfunction in women after resection with and without preoperative radiotherapy for rectal cancer: A population-based cross-sectional study. *Colorectal Disease, 17,* 26–37. doi:10.1111/codi.12758
Carlsson, S., Nilsson, A.E., Johansson, E., Nyberg, T., Akre, O., & Steineck, G. (2012). Self-perceived penile shortening after radical prostatectomy. *International Journal of Impotence Research, 24,* 179–184. doi:10.1038/ijir.2012.13
Carter, J., Goldfrank, D., & Schover, L.R. (2011). Simple strategies for vaginal health promotion in cancer survivors. *Journal of Sexual Medicine, 8,* 549–559. doi:10.1111/j.1743-6109.2010.01988.x
Chivers, M.L., & Rosen, R.C. (2010). Phosphodiesterase type 5 inhibitors and female sexual response: Faulty protocols or paradigms? *Journal of Sexual Medicine, 7,* 858–872. doi:10.1111/j.1743-6109.2009.01599.x
Coady, D., & Kennedy, V. (2016). Sexual health in women affected by cancer: Focus on sexual pain. *Obstetrics and Gynecology, 128,* 775–791. doi:10.1097/AOG.0000000000001621
Davison, S.L. (2012). Hypoactive sexual desire disorder. *Current Opinion in Obstetrics and Gynecology, 24,* 215–220. doi:10.1097/GCO.0b013e328355847e
Derogatis, L.R. (1997). The Derogatis Interview for Sexual Functioning (DISF/DISF-SR): An introductory report. *Journal of Sex and Marital Therapy, 23,* 291–304. doi:10.1080/00926239708403933
Dizon, D.S., & Katz, A. (2015, September 28). Overview of sexual dysfunction in male cancer survivors [Literature review current through June 2017]. Retrieved from https://www.uptodate.com/contents/overview-of-sexual-dysfunction-in-male-cancer-survivors
Dizon, D.S., Suzin, D., & McIlvenna, S. (2014). Sexual health as a survivorship issue for female cancer survivors. *Oncologist, 19,* 1–9. doi:10.1634/theoncologist.2013-0302
Dunn, M.W. (2015). Bladder cancer: A focus on sexuality. *Clinical Journal of Oncology Nursing, 19,* 68–73. doi:10.1188/15.CJON.68-73
Endara, M., Chen, D., Verma, K., Nahabedian, M.Y., & Spear, S.L. (2013). Breast reconstruction following nipple-sparing mastectomy: A systematic review of the literature with pooled analysis. *Plastic Reconstructive Surgery, 132,* 1043–1054. doi:10.1097/PRS.0b013e3182a48b8a
Ferrandina, G., Mantegna, G., Petrillo, M., Fuoco, G., Venditti, L., Terzano, S., ... Scambia, G. (2012). Quality of life and emotional distress in early stage and locally advanced cervical cancer patients: A prospective, longitudinal study. *Gynecologic Oncology, 124,* 389–394. doi:10.1016/j.ygyno.2011.09.041
Fu, M.R., Deng, J., & Armer, J.M. (2014). Putting evidence into practice: Cancer-related lymphedema. *Clinical Journal of Oncology Nursing, 18*(Suppl.), 68–79. doi:10.1188/14.CJON.S3.68-79

Ganz, P.A., Desmond, K., Leedham, A., Rowland, J.H., Meyerowitz, B.E., & Belin, T.R. (2002). Quality of life in long-term, disease-free survivors of breast cancer: A follow-up study. *Journal of the National Cancer Institute, 94,* 39–49. doi:10.1093/jnci/94.1.39

Goetsch, M.F., Lim, J.Y., & Caughey, A.B. (2014). Locating pain in breast cancer survivors experiencing dyspareunia: A randomized controlled trial. *Obstetrics and Gynecology, 123,* 1231–1236. doi:10.1097/AOG.0000000000000283

Goldstein, S.R., Bachman, G.A., Koninckx, P.R., Lin, V.H., Portman, D.J., & Ylikorkala, O. (2014). Ospemifene 12-month safety and efficacy in postmenopausal women with vulvar and vaginal atrophy. *Climacteric, 17,* 173–182. doi:10.3109/13697137.2013.834493

Gontero, P., Galzerano, M., Bartoletti, R., Magnani, C., Tizzani, A., Frea, B., & Mondaini, N. (2007). New insights into the pathogenesis of penile shortening after radical prostatectomy and the role of postoperative sexual function. *Journal of Urology, 178,* 602–607. doi:10.1016/j.juro.2007.03.119

Gupta, B.P., Murad, M.H., Clifton, M.M., Prokop, L., Nehra, A., & Kopecky, S.L. (2011). The effect of lifestyle modification and cardiovascular risk factor reduction on erectile dysfunction: A systematic review and meta-analysis. *Archives of Internal Medicine, 171,* 1797–1803. doi:10.1001/archinternmed.2011.440

Hawkins, Y., Ussher, J., Gilbert, E., Perz, J., Sandoval, M., & Sundquist, K. (2009). Changes in sexuality and intimacy after the diagnosis and treatment of cancer: The experience of partners in a sexual relationship with a person with cancer. *Cancer Nursing, 32,* 271–280. doi:10.1097/NCC.0b013e31819b5a93

Hazewinkel, M.H., Laan, E.T., Sprangers, M.A., Fons, G., Burger, M.P., & Roovers, J.-P. (2012). Long-term sexual function in survivors of vulvar cancer: A cross-sectional study. *Gynecologic Oncology, 126,* 87–92. doi:10.1016/j.ygyno.2012.04.015

Hendren, S.K., Swallow, C.J., Smith, A., Lipa, J.E., Cohen, Z., MacRae, H.M., ... McLeod, R.S. (2007). Complications and sexual function after vaginectomy for anorectal tumors. *Diseases of the Colon and Rectum, 50,* 810–816. doi:10.1007/s10350-006-0867-9

Herbenick, D., Reece, M., Hensel, D., Sanders, S., Jozkowski, K., & Fortenberry, J.D. (2011). Association of lubricant use with women's sexual pleasure, sexual satisfaction, and genital symptoms: A prospective daily diary study. *Journal of Sexual Medicine, 8,* 202–212. doi:10.1111/j.1743-6109.2010.02067.x

Hwang, J.H., Yoo, H.J., Park, S.H., Lim, M.C., Seo, S.S., Kang, S., ... Park, S.-Y. (2012). Association between the location of the transposed ovary and the ovarian function in patients with uterine cervical cancer treated with postoperative or primary pelvic radiotherapy. *Fertility and Sterility, 97,* 1387–1393. doi:10.1016/j.fertnstert.2012.02.052

Kaplan, M., & Mahon, S. (2014). Hot flash management: Update of the evidence for patients with cancer. *Clinical Journal of Oncology Nursing, 18*(Suppl.), 59–67. doi:10.1188/14.CJON.S3.59-67

Katz, A. (2009). My body my self: Body image and sexuality in women with cancer. *Canadian Oncology Nursing Journal, 19,* E1–E4. doi:10.5737/1181912x191E1E4

Katz, A., & Dizon, D.S. (2016). Sexuality after cancer: A model for male survivors. *Journal of Sexual Medicine, 13,* 70–78. doi:10.1016/j.jsxm.2015.11.006

Komisaruk, B.R., Frangos, E., & Whipple, B. (2011). Hysterectomy improves sexual response? Addressing a crucial omission in the literature. *Journal of Minimally Invasive Gynecology, 18,* 288–295. doi:10.1016/j.jmig.2011.01.012

Krychman, M.L. (2011). Vaginal estrogens for the treatment of dyspareunia. *Journal of Sexual Medicine, 8,* 666–674. doi:10.1111/j.1743-6109.2010.02114.x

Lammerink, E.A., de Bock, G.H., Pras, E., Reyners, A.K., & Mouritis, M.J. (2012). Sexual functioning of cervical cancer survivors: A review with a female perspective. *Maturitas, 72,* 296–304. doi:10.1016/j.maturitas.2012.05.006

Lehmann, V., Hagedoorn, M., & Tuinman, M.A. (2015). Body image in cancer survivors: A systematic review of case-control studies. *Journal of Cancer Survivorship, 9,* 339–348. doi:10.1007/s11764-014-0414-y

Levin, A.O., Carpenter, K.M., Fowler, J.M., Brothers, B.M., Andersen, B.L., & Maxwell, G.L. (2010). Sexual morbidity associated with poorer psychological adjustment among gynecological cancer survivors. *International Journal of Gynecological Cancer, 20,* 461–470. doi:10.1111/IGC.0b013e3181d24ce0

Lewis, R.L., Fugl-Meyer, K.S., Corona, G., Hayes, R.D., Laumann, E.O., Moreira, E.D., Jr., ... Segraves, T. (2010). Definitions/epidemiology/risk factors for sexual dysfunction. *Journal of Sexual Medicine, 7,* 1598–1607. doi:10.1111/j.1743-6109.2010.01778.x

Lindau, S.T., Schumm, L.P., Laumann, E.O., Levinson, W., O'Muircheartaigh, C.A., & Waite, L.J. (2007). A study of sexuality and health among older adults in the United States. *New England Journal of Medicine, 357,* 762–774. doi:10.1056/NEJMoa067423

Loren, A.W., Mangu, P.B., Beck, L.N., Brennan, L., Magdalinski, A.J., Partridge, A.H., ... Oktay, K. (2013). Fertility preservation for patients with cancer: American Society of Clinical Oncology clinical practice guideline update. *Journal of Clinical Oncology, 31,* 2500–2510. doi:10.1200/JCO.2013.49.2678

Mirabeau-Beale, K.L., & Viswanathan, A.N. (2014). Quality of life (QOL) in women treated for gynecologic malignancies with radiation therapy: A literature review of patient-reported outcomes. *Gynecologic Oncology, 134,* 403–409. doi:10.1016/j.ygyno.2014.05.008

Mirhashemi, R., Averette, H.E., Lambrou, N., Penalver, M.A., Mendez, L., Ghurani, G., & Salom, E. (2002). Vaginal reconstruction at the time of pelvic exenteration: A surgical and psychosexual analysis of techniques. *Gynecologic Oncology, 87,* 39–45. doi:10.1006/gyno.2002.6780

Misiewicz, H.M. (2012). Fertility issues of breast cancer survivors. *Journal of the Advanced Practitioner in Oncology, 3,* 289–298.

Montorsi, F., Adaikan, G., Becher, G., Khoury, S., Sharlip, I., Althof, S.E., …Wasserman, M. (2010). Summary of the recommendations on sexual dysfunction in men. *Journal of Sexual Medicine, 7,* 3572–3588. doi:10.1111/j.1743-6109.2010.02062.x

Morreale, M.K. (2011). The impact of cancer on sexual function. *Advances in Psychosomatic Medicine, 31,* 72–82. doi:10.1159/000328809

NANDA International. (2015). *NANDA nursing diagnoses: Definitions and classification, 2015–2017.* Philadelphia, PA: Author.

National Cancer Institute. (2017). Testicular cancer–Patient version. Retrieved from https://www.cancer.gov/types/testicular

National Comprehensive Cancer Network. (2017a). *NCCN Clinical Practice Guidelines in Oncology (NCCN Guidelines®): Distress management* [v.2.2017]. Retrieved from https://www.nccn.org/professionals/physician_gls/pdf/distress.pdf

National Comprehensive Cancer Network. (2017b). *NCCN Clinical Practice Guidelines in Oncology (NCCN Guidelines®): Prostate cancer* [v.1.2017]. Retrieved from https://www.nccn.org/professionals/physician_gls/pdf/prostate.pdf

National Comprehensive Cancer Network. (2017c). *NCCN Clinical Practice Guidelines in Oncology (NCCN Guidelines®): Survivorship* [v.2.2017]. Retrieved from https://www.nccn.org/professionals/physician_gls/pdf/survivorship.pdf

Nelson, C.J., Deveci, S., Stasi, J., Scardino, P.T., & Mulhall, J.P. (2010). Sexual bother following radical prostatectomy. *Journal of Sexual Medicine, 7,* 129–135. doi:10.1111/j.1743-6109.2009.01546.x

Park, J., Kim, T.-H., Lee, H.-H., Chung, S.-H., & Lee, D. (2013). Gynecological complication of chronic graft-versus-host disease: Vaginal obstruction. *Obstetrics and Gynecology Science, 56,* 277–280. doi:10.5468/ogs.2013.56.4.277

Portman, D.J., Bachman, G.A., & Simon, J.A. (2013). Ospemifene, a novel selective estrogen receptor modulator for treating dyspareunia associated with postmenopausal vulvar and vaginal atrophy. *Menopause, 6,* 623–630. doi:10.1097/gme.0b013e318279ba64

Resnick, M.J., Koyama, T., Fan, K.-H., Albertsen, P.C., Goodman, M., Hamilton, A.S., … Penson, D.F. (2013). Long-term functional outcomes after treatment for localized prostate cancer. *New England Journal of Medicine, 368,* 436–445. doi:10.1056/NEJMoa1209978

Rezk, Y.A., Hurley, K.E., Carter, J., Dao, F., Bochner, B.H., Aubey, J.J., … Chi, D.S. (2013). A prospective study of quality of life in patients undergoing pelvic exenteration: Interim results. *Gynecologic Oncology, 128,* 191–197. doi:10.1016/j.ygyno.2012.09.030

Rhoten, B.A., Murphy, B., & Ridner, S.H. (2013). Body image in patients with head and neck cancer: A review of the literature. *Oral Oncology, 49,* 753–760. doi:10.1016/j.oraloncology.2013.04.005

Roos, E.J., de Graeff, A., van Eijkeren, M.A., Boon, T.A., & Heintz, A.P. (2004). Quality of life after pelvic exenteration. *Gynecologic Oncology, 93,* 610–614. doi:10.1016/j.ygyno.2004.03.008

Rosen, R.C., Brown, C., Heiman, J., Leiblum, S., Meston, C., Shabsigh, R., … D'Agostino, R. (2000). The Female Sexual Function Index (FSFI): A multidimensional self-report instrument for the assessment of female sexual function. *Journal of Sex and Marital Therapy, 26,* 191–208. doi:10.1080/009262300278597

Rosen, R.C., Cappelleri, J.C., & Gendrano, N., III. (2002). The International Index of Erectile Function (IIEF): A state-of-the-science review. *International Journal of Impotence Research, 14,* 226–244. doi:10.1038/sj.ijir.3900857

Rossouw, J.E., Manso, J.E., Kaunitz, A.M., & Anderson, G.L. (2013). Lessons learned from the Women's Health Initiative trials of menopausal hormone therapy. *Obstetrics and Gynecology, 121,* 172–176. doi:10.1097/AOG.0b013e31827a08c8

Saitz, T.R., Serefoglu, E.C., Trost, L.W., Thomas, R., & Hellstrom, W.J.G. (2013). The pretreatment prevalence and types of sexual dysfunction among patients diagnosed with prostate cancer. *Andrology, 1,* 859–863. doi:10.1111/j.2047-2927.2013.00137.x

Schover, L.R. (2001a). *Sexuality and cancer: For the man who has cancer and his partner.* Atlanta, GA: American Cancer Society.

Schover, L.R. (2001b). *Sexuality and cancer: For the woman who has cancer and her partner.* Atlanta, GA: American Cancer Society.

Scott, J.R., Liu, D., & Mathes, D.W. (2010). Patient-reported outcomes and sexual function in vaginal reconstruction: A 17-year review, survey, and review of the literature. *Annals of Plastic Surgery, 64,* 311–314. doi:10.1097/SAP.0b013e3181af8fca

Serretti, A., & Chiesa, A. (2009). Treatment-emergent sexual dysfunction related to antidepressants: A meta-analysis. *Journal of Clinical Psychopharmacology, 29,* 259–266. doi:10.1097/JCP.0b013e3181a5233f

Shifren, J.L., Monz, B.U., Russo, P.A., Segreti, A., & Johannes, C.B. (2008). Sexual problems and distress in United States women: Prevalence and correlates. *Obstetrics and Gynecology, 112,* 970–978. doi:10.1097/AOG.0b013e3181898cdb

Shionogi, Inc. (2016). *Osphena® (ospemifene).* Retrieved from http://osphena.com

Sprout Pharmaceuticals. (2016). *Addyi® (flibanserin).* Retrieved from http://www.addyi.com

Steiner, H., Zangerl, F., Stohr, B., Granig, T., Ho, H., Bartsch, G., & Peschel, R. (2008). Results of bilateral nerve sparing laparoscopic retroperitoneal lymph node dissection for testicular cancer. *Journal of Urology, 180,* 1348–1352. doi:10.1016/j.juro.2008.06.040

Thygesen, K.H., Schjødt, I., & Jarden, M. (2012). The impact of hematopoietic stem cell transplantation on sexuality: A systematic review of the literature. *Bone Marrow Transplantation, 47,* 716–724. doi:10.1038/bmt.2011.169

Williams, D.H. (2010). Sperm banking and the cancer patient. *Therapeutic Advances in Urology, 2,* 19–49. doi:10.1177/1756287210368279

Wilmoth, M.C., Hanlon, H.L., Ng, L.S., & Bruner, D.W. (2014). Factor analysis of the modified sexual adjustment questionnaire–male. *Journal of Nursing Measurement, 22,* 241–254. doi:10.1891/1061-3749.22.2.241

World Health Organization. (2015). Sexual and reproductive health. Retrieved from http://www.who.int/reproductivehealth/en

CHAPTER 13

# Anger

*Liz Cooke, RN, MN, AOCN®, PMHNP-BC, AGPCNP-BC*

> *It is easy to fly into a passion–anybody can do that–but to be angry with the right person to the right extent and at the right time and with the right object and in the right way–that is not easy, and it is not everyone who can do it.*
>
> —Aristotle

Every human being has the capacity to feel and express anger. *Anger* is defined as a fundamental normal complex emotion with a complicated range of expression. It typically is generated as a response to a perceived threat or frustration when goals are blocked (Shahsavarani & Nouhi, 2014; Speilberger & Reheiser, 2009; Turner, 2007). The emotion of anger often is confused with other behavioral manifestations, such as hostility, violence, impulsiveness, and aggression; however, anger remains distinct as a construct. Unlike hostility and aggression, anger does not inherently imply a negative harmful act. Unlike impulsiveness, it does not necessarily imply limited forethought. Unlike violence, it does not necessarily coexist with power or physical force (Menninger, 2007; Shahsavarani & Nouhi, 2014).

## Theories on Anger

Theories about the construct of anger continue to be debated in the literature. In the early years of psychoanalytic theory, Sigmund Freud labeled anger as a defense mechanism, and most recent neurobiologic evidence focuses on the activated structures in the brain, such as the amygdala and cerebral cortex. Theories of anger include psychoanalytic, behavioral, anthropologic, and sociocultural, as well as neurobiologic, which encompasses genetic components (Deater-Deckard & Wang, 2012; Ratner, 2002; Thomas, 1990).

### Psychoanalytic Theory

According to psychoanalytic theory, anger is a powerful instinct, emotion, and drive. Under the tenets of this theory, suppressing drives is considered to be unhealthy to the goal of pleasure-seeking, ego-focused actions. Therefore, to maintain psychological health, mastery, and control over the environment, anger is a common means to attain desired base objectives (Menninger, 2007). Nevertheless, anger displayed as a passive-aggressive behavior is thought of as an immature defense (Sadock & Sadock, 2015). It is thought that if anger is held in and turned inward toward the ego, feelings of guilt, hopelessness, depression, and perhaps suicide may develop.

## Behavioral Theory

Behavioral theory and learning theory include identifying whether anger is learned either as a stimulus-response mechanism (classic behavioral/operant) or as a modeling (social learning) component. Classic behavioral learning theory holds that anger is a learned response to environmental stimuli. In contrast, social learning theorists argue that anger is an emotion that is learned through observation and has reinforcement value and individual behavior potential. The psychological situation is based on the individual's analysis (Fortinash & Holoday-Worret, 2011). In other words, the same stimuli in different situations and under different conditions in different individuals could cause emotional reactions other than anger.

Cognitive behavioral therapists have suggested that anger, like all emotions, is created by the individual's cognitive perception of an event. Therefore, an emotional response and subsequent behavior can be modified by teaching the individual to recognize and change maladaptive cognitions. The efficacy of cognitive behavioral interventions has been shown to be effective in modifying anger (Hofmann, Asnaani, Vonk, Sawyer, & Fang, 2012).

## Anthropologic and Sociocultural-Related Theories

Interest has increased in the view of behavior and emotions from a social and medical anthropology perspective. This is the study of universal human behavior and cross-cultural distinctions. Sociocultural theory believes that mental functioning is mediated by cultural values, concepts, and beliefs (Ratner, 2002). Within this perspective, the context of anger includes the following variables: interpersonal relationships between the parties, level of perceived justice or injustice of the situation, social status and gender of the parties, nature of the environment, and specific values and beliefs of the sociocultural group. The nature of angry behavior must be studied within the context of the social event and cannot be separated from the cultural experience. For example, Deater-Deckard and Wang (2012) discussed how individuals learn to express anger based on socialization within the family system.

## Neurobiologic Theory

Research on behavior and the connection to brain neurobiology is increasing. Studies continue to indicate that neurochemical and neurostructural areas in the brain modulate anger and impulsive aggression. Emotions and drives, including anger, are centered in two main areas of the brain: the amygdala and the cerebral cortex. The amygdala of the limbic system of the brain is the location of integration of internal and external stimuli and internal drives and more primitive emotions (anxiety, fear, aggression, and panic) (Sadock & Sadock, 2015). An interplay exists between the amygdala and the frontal lobe, or cerebral cortex, in which anger is modulated. Actual physical changes have been found in the brains of those who are impulsively aggressive (Denson, 2013). Neurochemical mediation of aggression is carried out by neurotransmitters: serotonin, dopamine, norepinephrine, gamma-aminobutyric acid, and acetylcholine. Other substances, such as steroids, glucose, and neuropeptides, are thought to influence aggressive behavior. Increasingly, genetic factors are thought to play a role in aggression. Research has recently focused on the genetic contribution to anger, which has been studied in twins (Saudino & Wang, 2012). Rapid advances in knowledge about the brain and its function likely will revolutionize future treatment approaches toward anger management.

Other theories, such as humanistic and developmental, have little empirical evidence tied to the explanation of anger as an emotion but provide some conceptual explanations.

## General Expressions of Anger

Anger can be displayed on a continuum, from mild annoyance to extreme rage, and has been conceptualized as both a state and personality trait. Although anger is a natural and universal emotion, higher levels of anger may stimulate physiologic arousal of the sympathetic division of the autonomic nervous system and can lead to a number of bodily responses in those who are angry. Physiologic symptoms may include increased blood pressure, elevated pulse rate and body temperature, clenched jaw, tense muscles, cognitive disturbances, gastrointestinal disturbances, and sweating.

## Constructive and Destructive Anger in Patients With Cancer

The cancer experience can bring on a variety of expressions of anger, and patients with cancer may display anger openly or in more guarded ways (see Figure 13-1). Although various individuals display anger differently in regard to intensity and onset, managing anger appropriately is an interpersonal skill that can be developed. The expression of anger as a constructive mechanism can be helpful to patients with cancer as they demonstrate speaking openly and setting boundaries. Those who act assertively may receive better medical care as a direct result of advocating for themselves. Taking control can promote a feeling of empowerment, thus increasing a sense of personal control while reducing feelings of helplessness and hopelessness. Nevertheless, anger can be expressed destructively through various indirect expressions of anger (e.g., suppression, displacement, passive-aggression, denial, repression) and through expressions of anger disproportionate to the event. Anger also can lead from an internal state to a physical act of aggression in which others are hurt (Wilkowski & Robinson, 2010). Unfortunately, if the patient is in the clinical environment and displays

| Overt Behavior | Covert Behavior |
|---|---|
| • Verbally abuses others<br>• Criticizes; displays hostility<br>• Explodes with little or no provocation<br>• Intimidates; threatens<br>• Curses; calls others names<br>• Strikes or throws objects<br>• Is sarcastic, demanding<br>• Is frequently irritated or annoyed<br>• Has defensive or aggressive body language (e.g., tense, clenched fists) | • Is silent, moody, withdrawn<br>• Acts bitter, apathetic<br>• Asks loaded questions<br>• Attempts to control everything<br>• Refuses to see visitors, eat, or drink<br>• Repeatedly breaks institutional rules<br>• Is overly nice<br>• Displays indecisiveness or ambivalence; procrastinates<br>• Detaches emotionally from others<br>• Forgets to do important things |

**Figure 13-1. Expression of Anger**

aggressive behavior, it may affect treatment decision making when clinicians decide an optimum treatment course in the face of reservations about compliance and coping with treatment stress (Shahsavarani & Nouhi, 2014).

## The Influence of Anger on Cancer Development

Researchers are interested in the possibility that anger as a personality trait or emotional state may be a contributing variable to either the initiation of cancer or cancer progression (Thomas et al., 2000). The effect of personality and stress on the development of cancer is unclear. However, early studies have indicated that preexisting personality traits and the lack of emotional expression, particularly that of anger, may interact with biologic and environmental factors to promote the development of cancer, influence its progression, and affect survival outcomes (Grossarth-Maticek, Bastiaans, & Kanazir, 1985; Thomas, 1988). In fact, early researchers described a "type C" personality as characterized by passive coping, pleasant and self-sacrificing demeanor, and a marked inability to express emotion, especially fear and anger (Temoshok, 1985; Temoshok & Dreher, 1994). This behavior was labeled as a lifelong repressive coping style. Other early studies have linked anger to coping styles, benign and malignant disease, childhood factors, survival, and expression ability (Butow, Coates, & Dunn, 1999; Derogatis, Abeloff, & Melisaratos, 1979; Greer & Morris, 1975; Kune, Kune, Watson, & Bahnson, 1991; Levy, 1984; Morris, Greer, Pettingale, & Watson, 1981).

The link from anger to cancer continues to indicate mixed results. Dalton, Boesen, Ross, Schapiro, and Johansen (2002) found inconsistent evidence of psychological factors as risk factors for the development of cancer. This was because of the many methodological issues of confounding variables and the difficulty with defining and measuring concepts such as personality and emotion. Butow et al. (2000) reviewed empirical evidence for a relationship between psychosocial factors and breast cancer development. Although they found few well-designed studies that explored the association between life events and breast cancer, the authors discovered that anger suppression was a predictor of cancer risk, with the strongest evidence suggesting that younger women are at increased risk. Rationality/antiemotionality predicted cancer risk, but social support, chronic anxiety, and presence of depression did not affect breast cancer development. The authors concluded that emotional repression and severe life events were the strongest predictors in the development of breast cancer; in this study, the sample of patients with breast cancer who appeared to repress emotions and had experienced severe life events seemed to have a higher incidence of breast cancer development.

Garssen (2004) reviewed 30 years of research on whether psychological factors affect cancer and concluded that no psychological factor, including anger, convincingly demonstrated an influence on cancer development. Nevertheless, some factors, such as loss, chronic depression, and low level of social support, hinted to negative emotional states. The author recommended more research in examining demographic, biologic, and psychological risk factors.

Rather than searching for a causal relationship between cancer and anger, current research is more focused on the role that anger plays in patient outcomes. Gerhart et al. (2016) found that anger proneness in patients with prostate cancer was linked to pessimism. Schlatter and Cameron (2010) investigated the role of anger in symptom management in patients undergoing chemotherapy and were able to indicate that anger suppression had independent relationships to symptom and mood processes. Anger has been shown to be negatively associated with coping. Barinková and Mesároová (2013) noted that a lower level of anger was linked to better coping and improved quality of life.

# Anger as a Response to Cancer

Anger is not an uncommon emotion, as patients and families navigate through the trajectory of cancer diagnosis, treatment, disease recurrence, survivorship, and end-of-life issues. Nurses who are aware of these potential emotional points may have the opportunity to implement therapeutic interventions to assist patients.

## Integrating the Diagnosis

After the initial shock and disbelief, anger is the emotion that most patients exhibit at the time of diagnosis (Thomas et al., 2000). The diagnosis of cancer frequently disrupts one's belief in a fair and safe world, and people often express the subsequent disorientation and confusion as anger. Some people believe that if they lead a good life, behave morally, and follow "the rules," they should be protected from the harm of life-threatening illness. Patients may strongly feel that it is unfair that they are sick. "Why me?" and "How did I get it?" are difficult questions to answer. Healthcare providers may try to offer answers, but the existential issues of responsibility, guilt, punishment, and atonement need to be addressed at a deeper and more spiritual level. The values and beliefs of individuals and families can affect subsequent acceptance of the diagnosis and agreement to participate in a prescribed treatment program. Finding and integrating a new self-image that includes catastrophic illness is a task that patients with cancer must address. In fact, high levels of suppressed anger in both the patient and family members significantly predicted negative perceived partner support at the time of diagnosis (Julkunen, Gustavsson-Lilius, & Hietanen, 2009). During this time of crisis, involving the patient and family in interventions may influence all involved with subsequent coping along the cancer trajectory.

Receiving a diagnosis of cancer is a trigger that may rekindle old feelings of sadness, loss, unfairness, and sometimes anger. Patients' perceptions of how they are being "mistreated" by healthcare professionals may parallel and reflect how they were mistreated as children (Kübler-Ross, 1969). In fact, a recent book by Hall and Hall (2016) on medical trauma lists cancer as the top diagnosis that can trigger medical trauma. Unresolved feelings of loss and unfairness may escalate into overt expressions of anger displaced onto people who are perceived as being healthy, including family members, friends, and coworkers. Feelings of unworthiness, guilt, or shame can lead to anger toward the self that manifests as depression. Holding onto feelings of unfairness may impede the process of mourning the losses associated with cancer. If these feelings are not resolved, they may manifest as ongoing dissatisfaction and anger with everything surrounding the illness, including the nursing care being received. Data suggest that anger that is not expressed will increase emotional distress at diagnosis (Ando et al., 2009). Subsequently, if people involved with a patient do not understand the origin of the anger and distress, they may react to it personally and begin to reject the patient even more, thus reinforcing the patient's experience of rejection and unfairness. It is often best to ask, "What is behind the anger?" Some possibilities for the reaction of anger could be fear, loss of control, shattered dreams/goals, or a sense of unfairness. This question often is helpful to stabilize the response of the nurse so that the anger is not seen as a threat but as a symptom of angst that is much deeper.

## Preparing for and Facing Treatment

Patients newly diagnosed with cancer not only must come to terms with the loss of desired goals but also must focus on life-saving treatments rather than life-enhancing achievements.

Patients and their families may find that old ways of coping are inadequate in helping to deal with the physical and psychological pain associated with the illness (e.g., loss of health, mobility, independence). Major lifestyle changes that revolve around treatment schedules and doctors' visits can create major disruptions in the lives of family members. The presence of cancer in an individual's life immediately curtails or modifies the achievement of both short- and long-term goals. Carver and Harmon-Jones (2009) described anger as an approach-related emotion, meaning that as goals are blocked by the cancer and treatment, anger is manifested from the person trying to "approach" the barrier and being unable to restore to the desired state. One method to channel this type of anger is to manifest it as a "fighting spirit" and visualize the cancer cells as the enemy. Data suggest that this method of coping during treatment actually may improve survival (Thomas et al., 2000).

The combination of having a severe life-threatening illness, being identified as a "patient," and having to acquiesce to the demands of an impersonal hospital environment contributes significantly to patients' and family members' feelings of loss of control and competence (Simms, 1995; Williams, Dawson, & Kristjanson, 2008). Prolonged waiting times for unfamiliar procedures, separation from family and friends, and disconnection from their world all contribute to patients feeling frustrated and powerless. Hospital and clinic settings often are structured to be efficient rather than warm and inviting. Routines are designed to serve the masses, not necessarily to address the needs of individuals. Patients can feel unimportant, frightened, and neglected—feelings that may precede an outburst of anger. In these situations, patients may express anger in a variety of ways. Patients and family members may direct abusive language or aggressive behavior at each other or toward others, express negative feelings about the hospital staff, or refuse to participate in the plan of care.

Anger as part of the mourning process often is felt most profoundly in those who experience disfiguring surgery, loss of body parts, and loss of control of the body (Simms, 1995; Slatman, Halsema, & Meershoek, 2015). However, it is important to remember that the perception of the injury to patients' physical and emotional integrity should guide the therapeutic response. Those who face months or even years of intensive, life-threatening therapies (e.g., those undergoing treatment for leukemia) may be at greater risk for experiencing fear, isolation, alienation, and anger. Factors that can affect expression of these emotions during treatment include patients' and family members' need to "protect" one another from bad news, the pressure to think positive and not "jinx" the treatment response, and not wanting to burden others by admitting that one has negative thoughts or fears. In addition to treatment concerns, socioeconomic concerns may include worrying about keeping one's job and housing, gaining or maintaining health insurance, paying large out-of-pocket medical expenses, and taking care of other family members while participating in treatment. Some patients may respond to the experience by outwardly raging toward others, using verbal threats and name calling, and showing other negative responses to deal with their emotions. Others may turn their anger inward, seething quietly while cooperating with the designated protocol. Either way, patients' anger often is a mask for other feelings and is used as a coping mechanism for dealing with deeper, more frightening emotions.

Nurses can address the underlying feelings with reflective statements. A statement such as, "It sounds like you are worried about the side effects of the chemotherapy; tell me what you know about it" will help patients to gain control and focus on the real issue. Nurses should provide factual information as needed but continue to focus on the patient's underlying feelings of anxiety, fear, and frustration.

When patients refuse to comply with a treatment protocol, nurses should try to ascertain the underlying reason. It is important to understand patients' and families' perceptions of the problem as well as the other factors contributing to the refusal (e.g., physical limitations, family problems, environmental stressors). Explore alternatives and, in a nonintimidating manner, explain the possible consequences of not following medical advice. Educating patients about their condition empowers them to identify personal goals of care. Collaborating with patients and giving them the opportunity to participate in decisions about their care affirm their value and competence.

## Becoming a Survivor and Returning to Normalcy

Survivors of cancer have several tasks to accomplish when treatment is complete. They must negotiate a return to normalcy that includes regaining previous familial, occupational, and social roles. They must cope with and manage the anxiety associated with the possibility that the cancer may return. Through a constantly evolving process, they must integrate and find meaning in a new identity as a cancer survivor.

Survivors may experience difficulty in returning to old roles. Family members may have become comfortable in carrying out those roles and may not want to give them up. Survivors may not be willing to perform tasks that caregivers expect the now "healthy" individual to do. These are potential sources of conflict within the family. Some families will transition easily; others will have a more difficult time.

With their lifeline to the treatment team newly cut, survivors must learn to handle their fears of recurrence. For some, it is the first time during the experience that they have allowed themselves to deal with the full impact of cancer on their lives. They may feel many emotions—fear, relief, sadness, anxiety, and anger. Most will be able to manage these feelings without professional assistance. Others, especially those who find that their ability to function has been affected, may require further support and skills training to manage these difficult emotions.

Anger can be a demand for change or a passionate wish for things to be different. It can be an expression of the loss of dreams and hopes that the cancer diagnosis irrevocably changed. Survivors can channel their anger in positive ways, reestablishing important boundaries, challenging their grief into meaningful benefits for others, and asserting personal integrity in the face of the body- and life-altering disease. Therefore, many survivors become active in cancer advocacy groups (e.g., National Coalition for Cancer Survivorship, American Cancer Society) that promote legislative, societal, and healthcare system changes to benefit those facing cancer.

## Experiencing Progression or Recurrence and Making Difficult Decisions

Facing the real possibility that the cancer cannot be cured, only forestalled, may elicit strong negative emotions from patients and families. They often express disappointment and anger at this time. Patients and families may express dismay that the cancer has returned, insisting, "But they said they got it all." Perhaps physicians were not overtly direct in telling the family about the small likelihood of cure. Despite all efforts by professionals to communicate the gravity of the situation, patients and families may not yet accept that death is inevitable.

A major task that must be accomplished at this juncture is weighing the risks and benefits of further treatment while appraising the value of quality of life and what it means to the individual and family. At this time, patients and family members may wish to participate in clinical trials, some maintaining unrealistic hope for cure, others seeing this as the last chance to stay alive, and still others wishing to perform an altruistic act to benefit others. When the trial is unsuccessful or patients are found to be ineligible to participate, team members must be prepared to deal with the resulting anger, even rage, that patients and families may display.

## Preparing for End of Life

It is important at this time to put one's affairs in order, designate a proxy to make healthcare decisions, and begin the difficult process of letting go. Awareness of dying can precipitate expression of anger, as individuals and family members mourn the loss of health, career, income, lifestyle, relationships, independence, and unattained goals. Individuals struggle to find meaning and purpose in life yet must face being deprived of a future. Everyone and everything must be given up, and the short time remaining may be filled with emotional and physical pain. The bereaved and the dying patient may have difficulty acknowledging and accepting the presence of anger. Writing a last will and testament or accepting hospice may be too painful because these are concrete indicators that life is coming to a close. Terminally ill patients may vent anger at God, doctors, nurses, close family members, and others who are healthy; they also may direct anger at themselves. Kübler-Ross (1969) summed up the anger phase of the grieving process as the patient's last loud cry: "I am alive, do not forget that. You can hear my voice; I am not dead yet!" (p. 52).

When anger is present in the terminal stages of illness, patients have little energy to expend in angry outbursts. Silent bitterness, indifference, or apathy may replace open anger and aggressive behavior (Kübler-Ross, 1969). Family members often become openly angry toward one another, particularly when they disagree about the loved one's treatment or end-of-life decisions. Family members may voice anger toward medical and nursing personnel as a reaction to overwhelming stress and feelings of helplessness, frustration, and the anticipatory loss of their loved one.

## Death

At the time of death, many families who have prepared for this moment are able to quietly accept the outcome and begin preparation for family rituals of grief and bereavement. They easily accept the nursing staff's offer of support and assistance. However, when facing the death of a loved one, some families may exhibit loud verbal or physical outbursts. These "outbursts" may have nothing to do with anger, and the nurse may confuse the behaviors with anger and feel uncomfortable around them. Anger at the time of death can also be an emotional reaction of grief, which can be manifested as blame to the patient or staff. These irrational expressions of anger can induce guilt (Tyrie & Mosenthal, 2012). Nursing staff need to be aware that in certain ethnic groups and cultures, overt displays of grief are accepted, even expected. These demonstrative behaviors include shouting, screaming, loud crying, rocking and wailing, "fainting" or "seizing," and self-flagellation (striking oneself). They may vent distress in a number of ways, including striking themselves, other objects (windows and furniture), or other people. Nursing staff should carefully assess the context of these situations. Nonintrusive nursing interventions should focus on promoting comfort; providing safety; and preventing self-harm, harm to others, or destruction of furniture or equipment during this difficult time. Further intervention may not be required. In very rare cases, nurses may need to set kind but firm limits on these behaviors. If ineffective, parties can be asked to leave the area to collect themselves. In rare instances, security personnel may need to be called.

# Nurses' Responses to Anger

When nurses become targets of patients' anger, they may respond to this anger in a variety of ways. Although violence is difficult to predict, nurses can be better prepared if the potential for aggressive behavior has been fully assessed.

## Step 1: Assess the Situation

Look for factors that may elicit patients' and family members' anger (see Table 13-1). Anger is one of many normal human reactions to the diagnosis of cancer. Nurses may feel intimidated by the anger and worry about aggression. Although anger is internal, aggression, the actual act of hurting others, is uncommon (Wilkowski & Robinson, 2010). Nevertheless, any emotion that affects the physical or psychological functioning of the patient needs intervention. On a busy oncology unit, bedside nurses can perform a basic clinical interview with the patient and family: Is the patient easily angered or slow to anger? What situations trigger anger? Does the patient tend to hold in anger and then explode? How does the patient control anger or cool down? Has the patient hurt others or him- or herself when angry? How do family members respond to the anger? What events have created anxiety and frustration during this and other hospitalizations? Is the patient experiencing pain or other symptoms (Hulbert-Williams, Neal, Morrison, Hood, & Wilkinson, 2012; Sela, Bruera, Conner-Spady, Cumming, & Walker, 2002)? Is the family experiencing social and financial stressors (Cano & Vivian, 2003)? Has there been a history of alcohol abuse (Aviles, Earleywine, Pollock, Stratton, & Miller, 2005; Parrott & Zeichner, 2002) or psychiatric disorder? The bedside nurse also may call on other resources to assess and intervene with angry patients and families, including advanced practice psychiatric nurses, social workers, chaplains, psychologists, and psychiatrists.

### Table 13-1. Factors That Elicit Patients' Anger

| Experience | Reaction |
| --- | --- |
| Physiologic/metabolic<br>• Chemical imbalances<br>• Metastatic disease<br>• Treatment effects | Cognitive impairment<br>Physical effects on body |
| Environmental/institutional<br>• Powerlessness, vulnerability<br>• External stimuli (noise, lights, loss of privacy, interruptions)<br>• Frustrating people and situations<br>• Loss of control | Unfamiliar treatments, tests, and routines<br>Long waiting periods<br>Lack of control, competence, and decision making |
| Sociocultural/economic<br>• Isolation, aloneness, abandonment<br>• Humiliation, shame<br>• Past anger, grief, unfairness | Feeling out of control, unable to manage emotions<br>Asking "Why me?" |
| Psychological<br>• Overwhelmed, confused<br>• Unmet expectations<br>• Fear, anxiety | Expression of vulnerability or little or no control<br>Hypersensitive/overreactive |

## Step 2: Ask Questions

Ask this question: "How do I feel about being with the patient?" Feelings of fear, anger, inadequacy, being manipulated, or the desire to avoid the patient are signs that the therapeutic relationship needs to be examined more closely, as anger may be the problem.

## Step 3: Self-Assessment

Continuing with further self-assessment, ask, "How do I express and manage my own anger?"; "Is it constructive in this case?"; "Am I denying my angry feelings toward this patient?"; "Is it helping the patient?"; "Does it help me to achieve my desired goals, or does it defeat me?"; "What type of patients are problems for me?"; and "What situations push my buttons?" Self-awareness is an important component of assessment. Keeping an anger log can help nurses to identify themes, patterns, and the types of patients that provoke angry feelings.

## Step 4: Identify Triggers

Identify early signs that indicate an escalation in anger. Increased frustration, a raised voice, rapid speech, agitated or rigid and tense body movements, demanding and aggressive statements, increased motor activity, and sudden silence are warning signs that anger is escalating. Understanding the progression of anger in both patients and family members helps nurses to assess and intervene early in the process to possibly defuse anger and prevent aggression.

# Interventions During an Angry Episode

Each patient is an individual. One patient may respond better to an anger intervention method than another. Flexibility and careful deep listening may reveal foundational emotions (fear, loss, out of control) that may need to be named and addressed. Some simple interventions and combination interventions include the following:

- Care must always be taken to realize that the anger is an internal emotional expression to the experience of cancer. It may be a way to cope with helplessness, express control, combat fear, and "fight" the disease (Thomas et al., 2000). Be aware that the anger itself may be a "sacred" space that patients have chosen, and interventions should be as supportive and therapeutic as possible.
- Patients vent their anger verbally. Therefore, waiting until they have calmed down on their own may be all that is needed. Stay calm and maintain eye contact with patients. Do not set limits, argue, or try to intervene during the outburst because patients are not likely to hear them, nor are they likely to benefit from what is said. It may be helpful to take deep breaths, perform positive self-talk (e.g., "I can handle this."), count to 10 before responding, or remember words of wisdom from others (see Figure 13-2). Becoming defensive or argumentative may only worsen the situation. Face the person and the anger and define the situation, not the person, as the problem. Express concern and compassion.
- When patients have calmed down, acknowledge their feelings, express regret about the situation, and confirm, "Yes, having to wait 30 minutes for your pain medication is a problem." Understand that family members are acting as advocates for their loved ones. Use this knowledge to collaborate with patients and families on ways to address the problem. Do not justify the situation (e.g., "We are short-staffed today."). This only makes the situ-

**Assessment**
- Identify the presence of risk factors that could lead to violent behavior.
- Identify patients who feels powerless.
- Recognize increasing signs of frustration, anger, and anxiety.
- Assist patients to identify anger triggers.
- Include families in the assessment and risk factors for anger.
- Understand where patients stand in the trajectory of cancer.
- Assess typical coping mechanisms and helpful supportive interventions.
- Assess for physical symptoms which may make patients more vulnerable to psychological symptoms.

**Nursing Diagnoses** (NANDA International, 2015)
- Risk for other-directed violence
- Other relevant associated diagnoses: Powerlessness, anxiety, fear, dysfunctional grieving, pain, chronic low self-esteem, social isolation, ineffective coping

***DSM-V* Diagnoses** (American Psychiatric Association, 2013)
- Depressive disorders
- Anxiety disorders
- Trauma and stressor-related disorders
- Disruptive, impulse control, and conduct disorders
- Personality disorders

**Expected Outcomes**
- Patients will acknowledge and express angry feelings appropriately.
- Patients will identify sources of frustration that trigger angry feelings.
- Patients will identify underlying feelings that contribute to angry outbursts.

**Interventions: Patients**
- Stay calm and quiet when patients are expressing anger and express posture of openness.
- Speak calmly with a low voice and do not argue with or threaten patients.
- Make eye contact, call patients by name, and do not cross arms or have hands on hips; do not touch patients. Keep the exit open.
- Acknowledge patients' feelings, express regret about the problem, and show empathy.
- Identify patients' perception of the problem.
- Discern the triggering event and any underlying feelings.
- Provide factual information if patients feel uninformed.
- Focus on the underlying feelings using reflective statements.
- If patients are refusing a treatment or procedure, ascertain the reason for their refusal to comply with the medical regimen.
- Find ways to empower patients that give them control over the situation.
- Advocate for patients; discuss with the team possible options that allow for maximum patient control and accomplishment of treatment goals.
- Call for assistance if it appears that patients may lose behavioral control. (A show of force may prevent further escalation.)
- Use chemical or physical restraints as a last resort.
- Consider the underlying feeling that is fueling the anger (loss, fear, control).

**Interventions: Family Members**
- Share information with family members so that they are informed of treatment schedules and expected outcomes.
- Allow family members to vent feelings of anger over the potential or impending loss of their loved one.
- Recognize that some families will be strong advocates for their loved ones; avoid defensive responses.
- Address underlying feelings of anxiety, fear, grief, and guilt.
- Educate family members about the grieving process and the phases that they and patients can expect to experience.
- If appropriate, refer family members for support group/individual grief counseling.

**Figure 13-2. Plan of Care**

ation worse. When possible, allow patients and families to consider the options and select the action they would like to take. In some cases, nurses may find it helpful to leave the situation to calm down first and then return to address patient or family concerns.
- Support groups can offer a shared experience for many patients. Although anger can be expressed at these support groups, it is a complex emotion, and steering those patients to support groups managed by a clinician may be a better fit than those managed by peer counselors (Thomas et al., 2000).
- Because nurses might expect anger to be common, they may not refer patients to mental health professionals. This lack of referral may not be best for this patient population. Saini (2009) recommended a combination approach of both individual psychologically based approaches (cognitive behavioral, psychodynamic, and relaxation) with medication. In addition, Sanini demonstrated that at least eight sessions of evidence-based psychological treatment had significant results and are highly effective in anger treatment. Creative psychological interventions, such as therapeutic treatments through the expression of music, art, and drama, have also been shown to help anger (Archer, Buxton, & Sheffield, 2015).
- Nurses and physicians may commonly react to anger by distancing behavior rather than through empathetic connection (Alexander et al., 2011; Finset, 2012; Mjaaland, Finset, Jensen, & Gulbrandsen, 2011). This reaction may be because of one's own attitude toward anger as a negative emotion (Berkowitz & Harmon-Jones, 2004). However, these patients need a connection and understanding. Data indicate that expressed strong emotions of empathy and understanding can have a powerful effect on the situation and may lead to positive psychophysiological activation (Finset, 2012). Efforts to change the situation may help patients to regulate their emotions (Rivers, Brackett, Katulak, & Salovey, 2007). Nurses should guard their own desire to flee and face the emotion for the patient's benefit. Patients need the continuing relationship of providers for support of their own well-being and physical distress (Gerhart, Sanchez Varela, Burns, Hobfoll, & Fung, 2015). While studying anger in transplant patients and its effect on providers, Gerhart et al. (2015) found that higher levels of patient anger were associated with higher levels of perceived negative interactions and clinical outcomes, as the anger eroded the support between the provider and patient.
- Another focus that may be helpful is that of the desire to problem solve. The patient's own ability to cope with emotions may be inadequate to deal with the overwhelming stressor of a cancer diagnosis. Nurses may promote collaborative problem solving rather than focusing blame on others. Empathize and show understanding without being patronizing (e.g., "I know you feel discouraged about your cancer relapse. I really cannot imagine how that feels, but I am here to try and help and understand. What can we do together to help your feelings?"). Simple education often can give patients more perspective on their treatment, symptoms, and expectations of future events.
- Psychological and physical domains are linked; if patients have many symptoms, their ability to cope decreases. Make sure to address all the physical symptoms possible to strengthen patients' ability to cope.
- Research indicates that partner/family support seems to mediate anger for the patient and affect long-term quality of life (Julkunen et al., 2009). Remember to include family, caregivers, and partners in any referrals and discussions. A family-centered approach will strengthen the coping of the entire system.
- Nurses can manage their own responses, particularly anger (see Table 13-2), by taking advantage of "anger busters," including talking to other nurse confidants; attending stress management, anger management, and conflict resolution classes; participating in assertiveness training; learning cognitive restructuring skills (e.g., reframing perceptions of an

### Table 13-2. Patients' Anger and Nurses' Responses

| Patients' Behavior as Interpreted by Nurse | Nurses' Feelings |
| --- | --- |
| Insolent, entitled | Feels unappreciated, like a servant |
| Abusive, threatening | Feels fearful, anxious |
| Intimidating, hypercritical | Feels inadequate, defensive |
| Controlling | Feels manipulated, becomes controlling |
| Angry | Takes personally, becomes angry in return |

*Note.* Based on information from Thomas, 1998.

event to decrease anger, using cognitive self-control techniques); and augmenting relaxation and focused breathing skills.

## When Violence Occurs

Expressing anger is not the same as acting aggressively. In very rare cases, patients or family members may lose control and become physically violent. Nurses must ensure the safety of themselves, others, and the violent patient or family member. If they have any concern about violence occurring, nurses should keep the door open and position themselves so that they can quickly leave. Stay at least a few arm lengths away, with arms loosely folded or hands clasped, and maintain direct eye contact to anticipate aggressive movement and to exert some control. Maintain a quiet and confident voice, and tell the patient or family member that this behavior is unacceptable. Healthcare professionals should let the patient know that they will not allow anyone, including the patient, to get hurt. Nurses should maintain their composure to give the violent patient or family member less control over them and others. However, if violence or the threat of violence continues, retreat to safety and call for adequate help. As a last resort, physical restraints or medication and intervention by appropriate personnel (e.g., security) may be necessary to control the situation.

### Case Study

Henry is a 25-year-old patient with acute leukemia with poor prognostic features. He has gone through two induction chemotherapy regimens but continues to have persistent disease and did not achieve a remission. Henry was recently admitted to the hematology unit for fever, cough, and shortness of breath and was started on fluids and broad-spectrum antibiotics. Because his bone marrow is in relapse, he receives platelets daily for a platelet count less than 10,000/mm$^3$, and frequently needs blood transfusions when his hemoglobin drops below 8 g/dl. Henry complains of bone pain and requires narcotics for management of pain. After a few days, his pulmonary symptoms worsen, with a severe drop in blood pressure, and he is transferred to the intensive care unit (ICU). He is in the ICU for four days and returns to the general hematology unit.

When Henry returns to the unit, his nurses note a big difference in his mood. He is withdrawn, irritable, and snappy. Although his respiratory symptoms have improved, he still has considerable pain and is asking for pain medication on a regular basis. Henry also has developed renal insufficiency and is getting dialysis every other day. The hope is to discharge him in one week's time. Although he is still eating, his appetite has decreased. Henry also seems to have difficulty sleeping and sits up in bed and stares out the window in darkness. When the nurses try to engage him, he throws silverware in the corner and yells, "Stop bugging me! Just leave me alone and get me my pain medication." Henry has a supportive family, friends, and girlfriend, but the nurses notice that they are visiting less and less during his hospitalization. Some nurses begin asking not to be assigned to him, and there is frustration among the nursing staff about his swearing and generally abusive behavior.

The nurses call in the psychologist, social worker, nurse practitioner, and physician for a team meeting to discuss Henry and how to help him. It is clear that his family has distanced themselves somewhat, probably in response to his anger. The team meeting is very helpful for the nurses to discuss what services Henry and his family might need. The physician says he has broached the subject of comfort care with the patient and his family and was met with silence. The psychologist wonders if the patient was experiencing some sense of regression and disconnection from his peers similar to other young adult patients with cancer. The social worker asks if family and friends need to connect with support systems within the organization in the form of support groups, and a session is suggested for staff for assessment of caregiver burnout, grief, and suffering. The nurses want advice on how to deal with Henry's anger and depression as well as their own distancing behavior. The nurse practitioner on the case asks if Henry's distress over his physical symptoms is compounding him psychologically and if he uses the pain medication, in part, as a coping mechanism.

## Discussion

A team plan was enacted to provide psychological and community services for Henry and his family members who were facing resistant disease and end-of-life issues. The physician and nurse practitioner made a concerted effort to manage his symptoms and involved the palliative care team. The nurses specifically felt a great deal of support by hearing the different viewpoints from the team. They also realized that the distancing behavior that they manifested was actually counterproductive to the patient's needs. With some coaching, the nurses were able to set some limits on his cussing and troublesome behavior of throwing objects in the corner. A care plan was created that assigned consistent nurses who were able to establish a sense of trust and compassion despite Henry's anger. The nurses eventually realized that he was facing an existential crisis, and his way of coping was manifested in symptoms of possible depression and anger. He continued to be a difficult patient, but the nurses felt a great deal of support from the entire team of professionals and were better equipped to understand Henry's suffering despite his anger.

# Conclusion

Nurses often are targets of patients' and families' anger. Oncology nurses who understand that this anger can be a mask for more frightening underlying feelings of powerlessness, confusion, grief, anxiety, and fear will be more effective in providing important therapeutic support to others, helping them to defuse anger successfully, and assisting those experiencing cancer to constructively deal with their anger.

*The author would like to acknowledge Ashby C. Watson, APRN, BC, OCN®, for her contribution to this chapter from the previous edition of this book.*

# References

Alexander, S.C., Pollak, K.I., Morgan, P.A., Strand, J., Abernethy, A.P., Jeffreys, A.S., … Tulsky, J.A. (2011). How do non-physician clinicians respond to advanced cancer patients' negative expressions of emotions? *Supportive Care in Cancer, 19,* 155–159. doi:10.1007/s00520-010-0996-5

American Psychiatric Association. (2013). *Diagnostic and statistical manual of mental disorders* (5th ed.). Washington, DC: Author.

Ando, N., Iwamitsu, Y., Kuranami, M., Okazaki, S., Wada, M., Yamamoto, K., … Miyaoka, H. (2009). Psychological characteristics and subjective symptoms as determinants of psychological distress in patients prior to breast cancer diagnosis. *Supportive Care in Cancer, 17,* 1361–1370. doi:10.1007/s00520-009-0593-7

Archer, S., Buxton, S., & Sheffield, D. (2015). The effect of creative psychological interventions on psychological outcomes for adult cancer patients: A systematic review of randomised controlled trials. *Psycho-Oncology, 24,* 1–10. doi:10.1002/pon.3607

Aviles, F., Earleywine, M., Pollock, V., Stratton, J., & Miller, N. (2005). Alcohol's effect on triggered displaced aggression. *Psychology of Addictive Behaviors, 19,* 108–111. doi:10.1037/0893-164X.19.1.108

Barinková, K., & Mesároová, M. (2013). Anger, coping, and quality of life in female cancer patients. *Social Behavior and Personality, 41,* 135–142. doi:10.2224/sbp.2013.41.1.135

Berkowitz, L., & Harmon-Jones, E. (2004). Toward an understanding of the determinants of anger. *Emotion, 4,* 107. doi:10.1037/1528-3542.4.2.107

Butow, P.N., Coates, A.S., & Dunn, S.M. (1999). Psychosocial predictors of survival in metastatic melanoma. *Journal of Clinical Oncology, 17,* 2256–2263.

Butow, P.N., Hiller, J.E., Price, M.A., Thackway, S.V., Kricker, A., & Tennant, C.A. (2000). Epidemiological evidence for a relationship between life events, coping style, and personality factors in the development of breast cancer. *Journal of Psychosomatic Research, 49,* 169–181. doi:10.1016/S0022-3999(00)00156-2

Cano, A., & Vivian, D. (2003). Are life stressors associated with marital violence? *Journal of Family Psychology, 17,* 302–314. doi:10.1037/0893-3200.17.3.302

Carver, C.S., & Harmon-Jones, E. (2009). Anger is an approach-related affect: Evidence and implications. *Psychological Bulletin, 135,* 183. doi:10.1037/a0013965

Dalton, S.O., Boesen, E.H., Ross, L., Schapiro, I.R., & Johansen, C. (2002). Mind and cancer: Do psychological factors cause cancer? *European Journal of Cancer, 38,* 1313–1323. doi:10.1016/S0959-8049(02)00099-0

Deater-Decard, K., & Wang, Z. (2012). Anger and irritability. In M. Zentner & R.L. Shiner (Eds.), *Handbook of temperament* (pp. 124–144). New York, NY: Guilford Press.

Denson, T.F. (2013). The multiple systems model of angry rumination. *Personality and Social Psychology Review, 17,* 103–123. doi:10.1177/1088868312467086

Derogatis, L., Abeloff, M., & Melisaratos, N. (1979). Psychological coping mechanisms and survival time in metastatic breast cancer. *JAMA, 242,* 1504–1508. doi:10.1001/jama.1979.03300140020016

Finset, A. (2012). "I am worried, Doctor!" Emotions in the doctor–patient relationship. *Patient Education and Counseling, 88,* 359–363. doi:10.1016/j.pec.2012.06.022

Fortinash, K.M., & Holoday-Worret, P.A. (2011). *Psychiatric mental health nursing.* St. Louis, MO: Mosby.

Garssen, B. (2004). Psychological factors and cancer development: Evidence after 30 years of research. *Clinical Psychology Review, 24,* 315–338. doi:10.1016/j.cpr.2004.01.002

Gerhart, J.I., Sanchez Varela, V., Burns, J.W., Hobfoll, S.E., & Fung, H.C. (2015). Anger, provider responses, and pain: Prospective analysis of stem cell transplant patients. *Health Psychology, 34,* 197–206. doi:10.1037/hea0000095

Gerhart, J.U., Schmidt, E., Lillis, T., O'Mahony, S., Duberstein, P., & Hoerger, M. (2016). Anger proneness and prognostic pessimism in men with prostate cancer. *American Journal of Hospice and Palliative Medicine, 34,* 497–504. doi:10.117/104990911663658

Greer, S., & Morris, T. (1975). Psychological attributes of women who develop breast cancer: A controlled study. *Journal of Psychosomatic Research, 19,* 147–153. doi:10.1016/0022-3999(75)90062-8

Grossarth-Maticek, R., Bastiaans, J., & Kanazir, D. (1985). Psychosocial factors as strong predictors of mortality from cancer, ischaemic heart disease and stroke: The Yugoslav prospective study. *Journal of Psychosomatic Research, 29,* 167–176. doi:10.1016/0022-3999(85)90038-8

Hall, M.F., & Hall, S.E. (2016). *Managing the psychological impact of medical trauma: A guide for mental health and health care professionals.* New York, NY: Springer.

Hofmann, S.G., Asnaani, A., Vonk, I.J., Sawyer, A.T., & Fang, A. (2012). The efficacy of cognitive behavioral therapy: A review of meta-analyses. *Cognitive Therapy and Research, 36,* 427–440. doi:10.1007/s10608-012-9476-1

Hulbert-Williams, N., Neal, R., Morrison, V., Hood, K., & Wilkinson, C. (2012). Anxiety, depression and quality of life after cancer diagnosis: What psychosocial variables best predict how patients adjust? *Psycho-Oncology, 21,* 857–867. doi:10.1002/pon.1980

Julkunen, J., Gustavsson-Lilius, M., & Hietanen, P. (2009). Anger expression, partner support, and quality of life in cancer patients. *Journal of Psychosomatic Research, 66,* 235–244. doi:10.1016/j.jpsychores.2008.09.011

Kübler-Ross, E. (1969). *On death and dying.* New York, NY: Macmillan.

Kune, G., Kune, S., Watson, L., & Bahnson, C. (1991). Personality as a risk factor in large bowel cancer: Data from the Melbourne Colorectal Cancer Study. *Psychological Medicine, 21,* 28–41. doi:10.1017/S0033291700014628

Levy, S.M. (1984). Emotions and progression of cancer: A review. *Advances, 1,* 10–15.

Menninger, W.W. (2007). A psychoanalytic perspective on violence. *Bulletin of the Menninger Clinic, 71,* 115–131. doi:10.1521/bumc.2007.71.2.115

Mjaaland, T.A., Finset, A., Jensen, B.F., & Gulbrandsen, P. (2011). Physicians' responses to patients' expressions of negative emotions in hospital consultations: A video-based observational study. *Patient Education and Counseling, 84,* 332–337. doi:10.1016/j.pec.2011.02.001

Morris, T., Greer, S., Pettingale, K., & Watson, M. (1981). Patterns of expression of anger and their psychological correlates in women with breast cancer. *Journal of Psychosomatic Research, 25,* 111–112. doi:10.1016/0022-3999(81)90098-2

NANDA International. (2015). *NANDA nursing diagnoses: Definitions and classification, 2015–2017.* Philadelphia, PA: Author.

Parrott, D.J., & Zeichner, A. (2002). Effects of alcohol and trait anger on physical aggression in men. *Journal of Studies in Alcohol, 63,* 196–204. doi:10.15288/jsa.2002.63.196

Ratner, C. (2002). *Cultural psychology: Theory and methods.* New York, NY: Springer.

Rivers, S.E., Brackett, M.A., Katulak, N.A., & Salovey, P. (2007). Regulating anger and sadness: An exploration of discrete emotions in emotion regulation. *Journal of Happiness Studies, 8,* 393–427. doi:10.1007/s10902-006-9017-2

Sadock, B.J., & Sadock, V.A. (Eds.). (2015). *Kaplan and Sadock's synopsis of psychiatry: Behavioral sciences/clinical psychiatry.* Philadelphia, PA: Wolters Kluwer Health/Lippincott Williams & Wilkins.

Saini, M. (2009). A meta-analysis of the psychological treatment of anger: Developing guidelines for evidence-based practice. *Journal of the American Academy of Psychiatry and the Law Online, 37,* 473–488.

Saudino, K.J., & Wang, M. (2012). Quantitative and molecular genetic studies of temperament. In M. Zentner & R.L. Shiner (Eds.), *Handbook of temperament* (pp. 347–367). New York, NY: Guilford Press.

Schlatter, M.C., & Cameron, L.D. (2010). Emotional suppression tendencies as predictors of symptoms, mood, and coping appraisals during AC chemotherapy for breast cancer treatment. *Annals of Behavioral Medicine, 40,* 15–29. doi:10.1007/s12160-010-9204-6

Sela, R.A., Bruera, E., Conner-Spady, B., Cumming, C., & Walker, C. (2002). Sensory and affective dimensions of advanced cancer pain. *Psycho-Oncology, 11,* 23–34. doi:10.1002/pon.551

Shahsavarani, A.M., & Nouhi, S. (2014). Explaining the bases and fundamentals of anger: A literature review. *International Journal of Medical Reviews, 1,* 143–149. Retrieved from http://journals.bmsu.ac.ir/ijmr/index.php/ijmr/article/view/56/102

Simms, C. (1995). How to unmask the angry patient. *American Journal of Nursing, 95*(4), 36–40.

Slatman, J., Halsema, A., & Meershoek, A. (2015). Responding to scars after breast surgery. *Qualitative Health Research, 26,* 1–13. doi:10.1177/1049732315591146

Spielberger, C.D., & Reheiser, E.C. (2009). Assessment of emotions: Anxiety, anger, depression, and curiosity. *Applied Psychology: Health and Well-Being, 1,* 271–302. doi:10.1111/j.1758-0854.2009.01017.x

Temoshok, L.R. (1985). Biopsychosocial studies on cutaneous malignant melanoma: Psychosocial factors associated with prognostic indicators, progression, psychophysiology, and tumor-host response. *Social Science and Medicine, 20,* 833–840. doi:10.1016/0277-9536(85)90338-7

Temoshok, L.R., & Dreher, H. (1994). Disconnects in understanding "the type C" connection. *Advances, 10,* 64–72.

Thomas, C.B. (1988). Cancer and the youthful mind: A forty-year perspective. *Advances, 5,* 42–58.

Thomas, S.P. (1990). Theoretical and empirical perspectives on anger. *Issues in Mental Health Nursing, 11,* 203–216. doi:10.3109/01612849009014555

Thomas, S.P. (1998). *Transforming nurses' anger and pain: Steps toward healing.* New York, NY: Springer.

Thomas, S.P., Greer, M., Davis, M., Droppleman, P., Mozingo, J., & Pierce, M. (2000). Anger and cancer: An analysis of the linkages. *Cancer Nursing, 23,* 344–349. doi:10.1097/00002820-200010000-00003

Turner, M.M. (2007). Using emotion in risk communication: The anger activism model. *Public Relations Review, 33,* 114–119. doi:10.1016/j.pubrev.2006.11.013

Tyrie, L.S., & Mosenthal, A.C. (2012). Care of the family in the surgical intensive care unit. *Anesthesiology Clinics, 30,* 37–46. doi:10.1016/j.anclin.2011.11.003

Wilkowski, B.M., & Robinson, M.D. (2010). The anatomy of anger: An integrative cognitive model of trait anger and reactive aggression. *Journal of Personality, 78,* 9–38. doi:10.1111/j.1467-6494.2009.00607.x

Williams, A.M., Dawson, S., & Kristjanson, L.J. (2008). Exploring the relationship between personal control and the hospital environment. *Journal of Clinical Nursing, 17,* 1601–1609. doi:10.1111/j.1365-2702.2007.02188.x

CHAPTER 14

# Anxiety

*Nancy Jo Bush, DNP, RN, MN, MA, AOCN®, FAAN*

> *To venture causes anxiety, but not to venture is to lose one's self.
> And to venture in the highest sense is precisely to be conscious of
> one's self.*
>
> —Søren Kierkegaard

One of the most common psychological responses to the cancer experience is anxiety. Cancer is perceived as a threat to well-being (Greer, MacDonald, & Traeger, 2015). Feelings of fear and apprehension are normal when patients with cancer are confronted with possible losses and their own mortality. Acute stress is a common response to a life-threatening illness, and normal anxiety reactions present at different points along the cancer continuum (Pasacreta, Minarik, Nield-Anderson, & Paice, 2015). Anxiety is not of itself pathologic but is a response to perceived threats (Levin & Alici, 2010). The associated anxiety in response to cancer may also be helpful to motivate the individual's efforts to seek evaluation, treatment, and support (Greer et al., 2015). However, a minority of individuals may experience elevated levels of anxiety, causing marked distress and interference with normal functioning (Greer et al., 2015). If uncontrolled anxiety develops, it can be disabling for the patient, interfering with both treatment response and psychosocial functioning. Of importance when working with patients with cancer are recognizing signs and symptoms of anxiety, differentiating between normal or expected anxiety responses, and intervening appropriately to prevent dysfunctional or abnormal reactions. A clear distinction does not always exist between the normal fears that cancer initiates and other anxiety reactions that are intense enough to meet the criteria for pathologic anxiety. Disease and treatment-related side effects can also make the differential diagnosis for anxiety challenging in patients with cancer (Cohen & Bankston, 2011; Greer et al., 2015).

## Important Principles Related to Anxiety

*Anxiety* has been termed by Levin and Alici (2010) as a psychobiologic emotion that is part of one's defensive structure. Anxiety motivates a person to mobilize resources to reduce the threat of perceived danger. It activates the primal fight, flight, freeze, and faint reactions

(Levin & Alici, 2010). Therefore, threats to an individual's physical and psychological safety will cause fear and anxiety. Fear is an affective response to a *real* threat or danger, whereas anxiety is an affective response to a *perceived* threat or danger. Fear is the cognitive appraisal that an actual danger exists in a given situation, and anxiety involves the emotional response to that appraisal (Beck & Emery, 1985; Levin & Alici, 2010). Fear leads to the stress response of "fight or flight" in contrast to anxiety, which reduces one's ability to act. Anxiety also can cause psychosomatic symptoms. It is a state of arousal that can present as specific symptoms ranging from palpitations and shortness of breath (as in acute stress situations) to more diffuse symptoms, such as fatigue, insomnia, and restlessness (as with generalized anxiety disorders [GADs]). Therefore, fear and anxiety affect every system of the body: physiologic, cognitive, emotional, and behavioral (Beck & Emery, 1985; Levin & Alici, 2010). The somatic symptoms of anxiety overlap with many of the symptoms of cancer and side effects of treatment; healthcare professionals must recognize the psychological symptoms of anxiety to make an accurate diagnosis.

Anxiety is experienced universally with both positive and negative ramifications (Levin & Alici, 2010). Normal anxiety often occurs when individuals face a new obstacle or challenge. For example, going off to college is an exciting yet anxiety-provoking experience. Normal or mild to moderate anxiety can motivate people by enhancing learning, problem solving, and attention. Normal anxiety may, therefore, serve an adaptive or "positive" function, preparing individuals physically and psychologically to meet challenges and avoid harm (Beck & Emery, 1985; Levin & Alici, 2010). As a transient arousal state, normal anxiety may signal coping responses to deal with any outside threat (e.g., the diagnosis of cancer). Severe, sustained anxiety interferes with coping efforts by immobilizing individuals with associated symptoms (Levin & Alici, 2010). In fact, avoidance coping is considered to be a chief behavioral component of clinical anxiety—avoidance being the "negative" dimension of anxiety. Individuals overwhelmed by anxiety also have a reduced sense of self-efficacy to problem solve (Levin & Alici, 2010).

Although fear and anxiety are differentiated, they often are similar. Individuals experiencing anxiety usually describe a subjective feeling of fear that includes dread, apprehension, and impending doom. Patients may be especially anxious and fearful at the time of initial diagnosis and treatment, with concerns mostly focused on existential issues of life and death (Pasacreta et al., 2015). Patients with cancer experience fear when they are confronted with real threats (e.g., poor prognosis). Anxiety closely follows as patients face the perceived threats most often associated with cancer: pain, disfigurement, and multiple physical and psychosocial losses. Despite many shared fears, each patient with cancer will experience different levels of anxiety. A diagnosis of stage I cancer with a good prospect for cure will create a different level of distress than the initial diagnosis of metastatic disease with a limited prognosis (Strada & Sourkes, 2015).

Anxiety may be a psychological response to the cancer or a chronic problem that is intensified by the disease or treatment. Genetic influences and environmental factors are increasingly being recognized as contributing to the risk of anxiety disorders (Levin & Alici, 2010). In childhood, early experiences lead to the development of coping behaviors, personality traits, and defense mechanisms. Some of these behaviors, traits, or mechanisms serve to relieve anxiety; however, if they fail, intense emotional or physical discomfort ensues (Gorman & Sultan, 2008). If a person has trait anxiety (a personality characteristic), he or she is predisposed to more frequent intense reactions to stressful events. In other words, normal anxieties experienced with cancer treatments may be exacerbated if the individual has pre-existing trait anxiety (e.g., anticipatory nausea and vomiting) (Levin & Alici, 2010). Many patients who present with anxiety, such as GAD, will have a history of clinically significant anxiety that is reactivated by the cancer experience (Greer et al., 2015). These normal or expected anxious responses to cancer and treatment include feelings of apprehension, tension, nervousness, and worry. Heightened levels of arousal and anxiety proneness have been associated with the diagnosis of cancer. If individuals have a past coping history of generalized anxiety or a history of an anxiety disorder, such as panic attacks, they may experience more intense anxiety with a cancer diagnosis than the general population. Other factors, such as prior coping history, emotional stability, social support, symptom distress, and sense of control, also will influence how much anxiety individuals experience (Pasacreta et al., 2015). A predictor of psychological adjustment to a chronic illness such as cancer is the individual's emotional stability and coping strategies used prior to diagnosis. Those with a major psychiatric history or psychiatric hospitalization are particularly vulnerable to decompensate (Pasacreta et al., 2015). In addition, anxiety often is associated with other psychiatric symptoms, such as depression, and may occur as a component of cancer pain, fatigue, treatment, or metabolic side effects. Severe anxiety reduces the threshold for patients' physical distress, especially pain, and can exacerbate the side effects of treatment agents (Pasacreta et al., 2015).

Anxiety is an affective response to stress. According to Selye's (1956) stress theory, the symptoms of anxiety can put wear and tear on the body because of the physical and psychological energy required to support these symptoms. Most importantly, anxiety negatively affects coping (Levin & Alici, 2010) and may indirectly have a negative effect on immune function (Fawzy, Fawzy, Hyun, & Wheeler, 1997). "Be it stress, anxiety, or worry, all are related to important neuroendocrine changes, which may account in part for the poorer survival among patients with cancer who experience heightened stress" (Anderson et al., 2014, p. 1617).

## Cultural Influences on the Experience and Expression of Anxiety

The health- and illness-related responses and behaviors of patients with cancer develop through lifelong socialization. Nursing responses to a patient's expression of anxiety may seem judgmental or accusatory if they are not offered in the context of the individual's sociocultural background (Grassi, Nanni, Donovan, & Jacobsen, 2015). "How crisis experiences are manifested varies vastly, and a patient's own culture can account for some of this variation" (Chase, 2013, p. 337). In some cultures, anxiety may be expressed through somatic symptoms rather than affective/behavioral symptoms (Pasacreta et al., 2015). Nurses must recognize that symptomatic complaints such as weakness, dizziness, palpitations, and tension may be masking an underlying anxiety disorder. In Latino and Mediterranean cultures, patients may complain of "nerves" or headache, whereas in Asian cultures, the complaint may be of weakness, tiredness, or feeling "imbalanced" (Pasacreta et al., 2015).

Expressions of feelings such as anxiety also may go undetected because of communication barriers. Cancer is a very frightening experience, and anxiety may be intensified when patients find themselves unable to express their emotional distress to their caregivers. In addition, language barriers have been found to interfere with patients' abilities to integrate the distressing experiences that cancer imposes. In some cultures, communicating openly about a cancer diagnosis or prognosis is seen as unethical because it is perceived as taking away hope (Grassi et al., 2015). Emotional expressions of uncertainty, anxiety, and grief vary across cultures. For example, in some cultures, the display of intense emotions may be expected at times (e.g., bereavement), whereas stoic reactions and the development of somatic symptoms may be more appropriate in other groups. Stoic behavior serves to minimize discomfort and may reflect a cultural value learned and validated throughout one's lifetime. Patients may feel anxious and worried but hesitate to share these feelings because of embarrassment or shame. In contrast, some patients may appear overly angry and raged, intimidating and alienating those around them. Individuals' exaggerated emotional responses may not necessarily be indicative of abnormal behavior but instead a cultural norm (Grassi et al., 2015; Pasacreta et al., 2015). Therefore, emotional and coping responses (i.e., anxiety) must be assessed within the framework of patients' cultural values, attitudes, and normative behaviors. Assessment also should include prior coping history, social support, religious beliefs, and other life stressors. Providing a safe environment for patients to express anxiety within their own perspective of the cancer experience will ensure that they receive the appropriate help.

## Classifications of Anxiety Disorders in Patients With Cancer

### Adjustment Disorder

The *Diagnostic and Statistical Manual of Mental Disorders (DSM-V)* contains a number of classifications of anxiety disorders (American Psychiatric Association [APA], 2013). The most common disorder requiring psychiatric referral in the cancer population is adjustment disorder (Li, Hales, & Rodin, 2015). In reference to anxiety, adjustment disorder is classified in the *DSM-V* as *adjustment disorder with anxiety* (APA, 2013). However, symptoms of anxiety in patients with cancer most often coexist with depression and other mixed states more commonly than anxiety existing alone (Greer et al., 2015). An adjustment disorder is defined as emotional or behavioral symptoms that occur in response to an identifiable stressor(s) (e.g., cancer, treatment) that develops within three months of the onset of the stressor(s) (APA, 2013). The predominant manifestations of anxiety are symptoms such as nervousness, worry, or jitteriness. Again, this diagnosis often coexists with depressed mood. Therefore, *adjustment disorder with mixed anxiety and depressed mood* also encompasses depressive symptoms such as tearfulness and feelings of hopelessness (APA, 2013).

The normal fears associated with cancer occur and change along the illness trajectory. Patients commonly feel overwhelmed at the time of diagnosis and at other transition points: onset of treatment, the end of treatment, recurrence, and terminal phases. Even during phases of remission, fears of cancer recurrence may overshadow individuals' psyche. The difference between these normal and expected fears and a diagnosis of adjustment disorder is based on the duration and intensity of symptoms, as well as the functional impairment caused by the anxiety symptoms. An adjustment disorder has been defined as an intermediary psychological state that falls between normal coping under the stress of cancer and a major mental disorder (Li et al., 2015). Clinical indicators for an adjustment disorder are under the realm of maladaptive responses, which affect quality-of-life issues (e.g., interference with relationships, work, activities). An enduring pattern of anxiety can lead to significant clinical distress, thus preventing adaptation, impairing problem solving and coping, and interfering with compliance to the cancer treatment. Levin and Alici (2010) noted that a diagnosis of adjustment disorder with anxiety carries the risk of minimizing the severity of anxiety and may preclude the use of psychotherapy or pharmacotherapy.

## Preexisting Anxiety Disorder

Different than reactive or situational anxiety, preexisting anxiety disorders can recur and be exacerbated by the cancer diagnosis and treatment. Individuals with a history of anxiety (e.g., GAD, panic disorder) may be at a greater risk for appraising the stressor of cancer as more threatening and overwhelming than individuals without such history (Levin & Alici, 2010; Pasacreta et al., 2015).

### *Generalized Anxiety Disorder*

GAD is defined as excessive anxiety and worry regarding events or activities of daily living. Symptoms of GAD include restlessness, fatigue, difficulty concentrating, irritability, tension, and sleep disturbances (APA, 2013). Common to GAD and other preexisting anxiety disorders (e.g., panic disorder, phobias) is the extreme fear of losing control and being overwhelmed and vulnerable to threatening experiences. "The intensity, duration, or frequency of the anxiety or worry is out of proportion to the actual likelihood or impact of the anticipated event" (APA, 2013, p. 222). Genetics, temperament, and environment all may play a role in the development of GAD and other anxiety disorders (APA, 2013). When asked, adult patients often can confirm that anxious behaviors and emotions have been identifiable from an early age or earlier experience (APA, 2013). Patients with cancer have multiple worries that range from prognosis, treatment, fear of recurrence, and quality-of-life issues (e.g., role changes, dependency, occupational stressors). Thus, the cancer journey may uniquely color the anxiety experienced in GAD (Levin & Alici, 2010).

### *Panic Disorder*

Reactivation of preexisting anxiety disorders may interfere with cancer treatment and overwhelm the coping abilities of the individual. Panic in patients experiencing cancer may occur for the first time or may reflect an exacerbation of preexisting panic disorder (Levin & Alici, 2010). Panic disorder is the sudden and unpredictable attack of intense fear or discomfort, causing individuals to have an overwhelming urge to escape (APA, 2013). Panic attacks are associated with symptoms that range from trembling, palpitations, shortness of breath, and chest pain to fears of losing control, "going crazy," or dying (APA, 2013). These terrifying feelings are an abrupt surge of fear or intense discomfort that peaks in minutes and are followed by constant fears of recurring attacks (APA, 2013). Often, patients may change their behavior, such as avoiding actions related to the attacks (e.g., exposure to a painful or frightening procedure such as bone marrow biopsy may cause the person to abruptly terminate treatments) (APA, 2013).

### *Panic Disorder With Phobia*

Panic attacks may occur with agoraphobia (the fear of being in places or situations from which escape may be difficult) or claustrophobia (the fear of being in closed places) (APA, 2013). Agoraphobic patients may have difficulty being in strange hospital environments and treatment rooms; claustrophobic patients may have difficulty with magnetic resonance imaging (MRI) scans or radiation therapy. A past history of phobias may complicate the care of patients with cancer because of the numerous medical procedures that patients must confront, such as receiving injections with a needle, seeing blood, or undergoing other invasive medical procedures. These specific phobias are described in the *DSM-V* and are termed *blood-injection-injury* phobias (APA, 2013). This subtype is highly familial and characterized by a strong vasovagal response (e.g., bradycardia, hypotension, fainting) to the feared object or treatment (APA, 2013). Although the individual recognizes that the fear is unreasonable, avoidant behaviors, anxious anticipation, or distress become inevitable (APA, 2013).

## Anxiety Disorders Caused by Medical Conditions

The *DSM-V* separately classifies anxiety disorders caused by medical factors associated with cancer or treatment (APA, 2013). This classification is a direct physiologic consequence of a medical disorder and not accounted for by a mental disorder (APA, 2013). The most common medical problems that place patients with cancer at risk for anxiety include uncontrolled pain, cognitive deficits, central nervous system disorders, medication side effects, and metabolic abnormalities. A common but preventable cause of anxiety related to cancer is uncontrolled pain (Levin & Alici, 2010). Patients experiencing acute pain may exhibit symptoms associated with generalized anxiety (e.g., restlessness, irritability, diaphoresis, muscle tension). Chronic pain may contribute to both chronic anxiety and depression. If the pain is unrelenting and severe, anxiety and agitation can lead to dissociative episodes or suicidal ideation (see Chapter 8 for information related to pain).

Medications commonly used in the cancer setting also can contribute to symptoms of anxiety. Steroids (e.g., dexamethasone, prednisone) can place patients at risk for psychiatric symptoms that range from anxiousness, irritability, and agitation to psychosis. Steroid-induced anxiety often is difficult to differentiate from other anxiety-producing medications (e.g., bronchodilators); therefore, nurses must pay close attention to the onset of symptoms related to steroid treatment. Antiemetics (e.g., metoclopramide, prochlorperazine) can contribute to motor restlessness (akathisia) several hours to days after chemotherapy treatment (Levin & Alici, 2010). Withdrawal symptoms will precipitate anxiety with the discontinuation of certain drugs, such as alcohol, street drugs (e.g., heroin, methamphetamine), narcotics, and anxiolytics. If alcohol is stopped abruptly for illness or hospitalization, some patients may exhibit severe anxiety within the first day. Prominent anxiety, panic attacks, obsessions, or compulsive behaviors can predominate this clinical picture of substance-induced anxiety disorder (APA, 2013). Other substances that often go unrecognized include benzodiazepines, barbiturates, opioids, and nicotine. Withdrawal may present with sudden, intense anxiety and agitation (Levin & Alici, 2010).

Changes in metabolic, hormonal, or cognitive status can cause anxiety in patients with cancer. Abnormal metabolic states that cause anxiety include hypoxia, sepsis, hypoglycemia, hypocalcemia, and undetected bleeding (Levin & Alici, 2010). Anxiety also may exacerbate preexisting respiratory distress (Levin & Alici, 2010). A most common metabolic change causing anxiety in patients with cancer is hypoxia. Hypoxia is a very fearful experience for patients because of its frightening symptoms of restlessness, agitation, and the feeling of being smothered. Pulmonary embolism and coronary occlusion are examples of underlying medical problems that must be ruled out when anxiety appears with hypoxia and chest pain. Anxiety and restlessness often accompany the chills and fever associated with sepsis and may signal early delirium. Changes in electrolyte status resulting from endocrine abnormalities (e.g., hypoglycemia) or disease (e.g., metastatic hypercalcemia) cause anxiety, as well as hormone-secreting tumors (e.g., thyroid and parathyroid tumors) (Levin & Alici, 2010). Paraneoplastic syndromes associated with certain malignancies (e.g., adrenocorticotropic-producing lung cancer) can cause anxiety, and pheochromocytoma (a rare tumor of the adrenal medulla) has been associated with panic symptoms (Paice, 2011). Patients with pancreatic cancer have been known to manifest symptoms of distress, anxiety, and depression that may be related to a false neurotransmitter released from the tumor (Paice, 2011). Existential and spiritual distress, as well as the fear of the unknown, may manifest as anxiety at the end of life (Paice, 2011).

## Post-Traumatic Stress Disorder

The *DSM-IV* classified post-traumatic stress disorder (PTSD) as an anxiety disorder and included life-threatening illnesses such as cancer as risks for precipitating the event (APA, 2000). A PTSD response of intense fear or horror could result from individuals witnessing (e.g., death of a loved one from cancer) or experiencing (e.g., personal injury from a previous cancer treatment) events that involved actual or threatened death or serious injury (APA, 2000). Based on the *DSM-IV* criteria, the National Cancer Institute (NCI, 2015) estimated that the incidence of PTSD in early-stage patients ranged from 3%–4% and was 35% in recently diagnosed patients evaluated after treatment. For patients presenting with PTSD-like symptoms, incidence rates were estimated to be 20% in patients with early-stage disease to 80% in those with recurrent disease (NCI, 2015). Because of differences in assessment methods between studies (e.g., questionnaire vs. interview), assessment time points (e.g., postdiagnosis vs. posttreatment), and sample characteristics (e.g., severity of disease), efforts to determine prevalence rates have been difficult (Abbey, Thompson, Hickish, & Heathcote, 2015).

The *DSM-V* changed the classification of PTSD to trauma and stressor-related disorders, removing the criteria of life-threatening illness. According to the *DSM-V*, medical incidents that qualify as traumatic events involve sudden, catastrophic events such as waking during surgery or anaphylactic shock (APA, 2013). Therefore, it is less likely that a diagnosis of PTSD will be given to patients with cancer (and survivors) in favor of the *DSM-V's* adjustment disorder (Abbey et al., 2015). Because the literature does not signify the presence or absence of catastrophic events during the cancer experience that would make the diagnosis one of trauma, it has been recommended that clinicians consider the full range of "discrete events" that would warrant a diagnosis of PTSD and, if absent, consider the diagnosis of adjustment disorder (Abbey et al., 2015). If the patient experiences a traumatic event along the continuum of disease and treatment, the nurse may observe symptoms of intrusion (e.g., distressing memories, recurrent dreams), avoidance of stimuli associated with the trauma, negative alterations in cognitions or mood, and marked alterations in arousal or reactivity (e.g., hypervigilance) (APA, 2013). In a meta-analysis of prevalence rates and moderating factors for cancer-related PTSD, Abbey et al. (2015) found that the experience of cancer may be traumatic enough to bring about a PTSD diagnosis. Especially at risk may be younger patients, those with advanced disease, and those who have recently completed treatment (Abbey et al., 2015). As children with cancer survive into adulthood, as adults survive cancer, and as chronic illness becomes more common, the risks of PTSD in these populations will need to be further studied.

## The Response of Healthcare Professionals to Anxious Patients

Anxiety is a highly transferable emotion from patient to professional (Pasacreta et al., 2015). Nurses may experience apprehension when caring for patients who are visibly anxious or experiencing panic attacks. If the nurse has not had adequate training or experience in dealing with these intense reactions, feelings of inadequacy or fear may surface. Nurses also may experience frustration if constant reassurances and interventions do not appear to calm the patient. In these situations, nurses may have difficulty being consistent and supportive. If patients' anxiety is not controlled, the feelings most likely will surface and be exhibited by family members. Anxious patients and family members may appear to healthcare providers to be too demanding and unreasonable, adding further stress to an already difficult situation. Resentment and hostility may develop if nurses or physicians believe that patients and family members require more attention than the situation warrants. Anxiety may not be recognized as a priority for nursing care, especially if nurses consider the anxiety to be a weakness or failure of patients to adequately cope. All of the aforementioned situations warrant further support for patients as well as the professionals involved in their care. A consultation with the psychiatric clinical nurse specialist could result in more in-depth assessment of patients' situations. In addition, a consultation could support nurses by helping them to understand and address their own concerns and frustrations. Therapeutic effectiveness can be compromised if nurses fail to recognize and manage their own anxiety (Pasacreta et al., 2015).

# Nursing Care of Patients Experiencing Anxiety

## Assessment

Oncology nurses play a vital role in identifying patients' symptoms of anxiety and implementing appropriate interventions (see Figure 14-1). Within effective psycho-oncology treatment, assessment of anxiety has been defined as a standard of practice (Anderson et al., 2014; Levin & Alici, 2010). Assessing the "function" or role of anxiety for patients is important. Nurses must distinguish whether the vague, uneasy feelings described as anxiety are normal and expected or negative and disabling. The plan of care outlines criteria for assessment and intervention. Initially, patients should be evaluated for normal or expected anxiety symptoms at diagnosis and at stressful transition points along the disease continuum. Initial, early emotional reactions to the cancer experience have proved to be predictive of later adaptation and helpful in identifying patients at high-risk for future psychiatric disorders (Anderson et al., 2014; Pasacreta et al., 2015). Patients particularly vulnerable to psychological distress are those who are diagnosed with late-stage disease or with no hope for cure (Pasacreta et al., 2015). Anxiety has also been shown to be the most common psychological health issue among long-term cancer survivors (Anderson et al., 2014).

A cancer diagnosis or treatment may trigger a new onset of anxiety, or patients may report an exacerbation of an existing problem with anxiety (Greer et al., 2015). Anxiety also appears to persist over time, remaining a valid concern for long-term cancer survivors (Greer et al., 2015). A thorough assessment will begin with patients' health history to determine any preexisting anxiety or related psychiatric disorders. A thorough physical examination must follow to determine whether any medical conditions (e.g., uncontrolled pain) are underlying the symptoms of anxiety. It is not possible to accurately evaluate anxiety unless medical symptoms such as pain have been addressed and controlled. Nurses should assess all physical symptoms, emotions, cognitive changes, behavioral responses, and the stage of illness to determine the level of patients' anxiety and differentiate the contributing causes on which to base interventions.

### *Physical Symptoms*

Anxiety affects every system of the body; disease and treatment-related effects may make the differential diagnosis of anxiety challenging (Greer et al., 2015; Traeger, Greer, Fernan-

### Assessment
- Recognize the signs and symptoms of anxiety.
- Validate patients' perceptions of the anxiety experience.
- Assess for anxiety at major transition points along the cancer continuum.
- Differentiate between normal or expected anxiety responses and abnormal responses.
- Assess for previous anxiety disorders (e.g., generalized anxiety disorder [GAD], panic, phobias, post-traumatic stress disorder [PTSD]).
- Assess for underlying medical conditions (e.g., pain, sepsis, medications, cognitive disruptions, metabolic imbalances, hormonal imbalances) that may be contributing to anxiety symptoms.
- Assess for concurrent symptoms of depression.

### Nursing Diagnoses (NANDA International, 2015)
- Anxiety
- Ineffective coping
- Fear
- Impaired verbal communication
- Low self-esteem (e.g., chronic, situational)

### *DSM-V* Diagnoses (American Psychiatric Association [APA], 2013)
- Acute stress disorder
- GAD
- Adjustment disorder with anxiety
- Adjustment disorder with mixed anxiety and depressed mood
- Panic disorder
- Specific phobia (e.g., blood-injection-injury type)
- PTSD (APA, 2000)
- Anxiety disorder due to another medical condition
- Substance- or medication-induced anxiety disorder

### Expected Outcomes
- Patients will identify feelings associated with anxiety.
- Patients will identify causative factors for anxiety.
- Patients will problem solve and develop ways to recognize and control anxiety.
- Patients will participate in strategies to relieve anxiety (e.g., relaxation techniques), if appropriate.

### Interventions
- Provide a safe, supportive environment.
- Reduce environmental stimuli.
- Educate patients regarding the disease and treatment.
- Inform patients of impending tests and procedures.
- Answer questions, and provide time for patients to reflect.
- Encourage verbalization of fears and anxieties.
- Normalize feelings for patients at each crisis point of the disease continuum.
- Assess present and past coping mechanisms.
- Assist patients to identify anxiety-provoking stimuli and the positive and negative ways to deal with it.
- Teach cognitive behavioral techniques to decrease anxiety (e.g., relaxation exercises, cognitive reframing).
- Provide positive reinforcement for adaptive coping strategies.
- Administer anxiolytic medications, and educate patients about their purpose and effects.
- Refer patients for psychiatric evaluation, if necessary.
- Provide supportive resources for patients' coping (e.g., refer to support groups).
- Evaluate patients' outcomes, and revise the plan of care, when appropriate.

**Figure 14-1. Plan of Care**

dez-Robles, Temel, & Pirl, 2012). Cardiovascular effects include palpitations and chest pain combined with respiratory symptoms of hyperventilation and dyspnea (Cohen & Bankston, 2011). Patients experiencing anxiety may describe feelings of suffocation. Medical conditions such as pulmonary embolism, congestive heart failure, and pleural effusion may bring about similar symptoms (Greer et al., 2015). Common gastrointestinal symptoms include anorexia, nausea, and diarrhea. Other symptoms include difficulty swallowing and heartburn. Patients may describe feelings of choking or may complain of vague stomach ailments. Dizziness, weakness, headaches, confusion, and fine tremors are common neurologic symptoms. Breathlessness may be caused by a panic disorder (Greer et al., 2015). Medications such as steroids or antiemetics (e.g., prochlorperazine) may also cause anxiety symptoms (Greer et al., 2015). The sympathetic "fight or flight" energy that anxiety demands leaves individuals physically and emotionally exhausted.

### *Emotional Responses*

Anxiety may intensify the physical symptoms associated with cancer, thereby negatively affecting quality of life (Anderson et al., 2014). Patients experiencing anxiety appear to be tense and worried, and they may complain of feeling nervous. With anxiety disorders, patients' moods may be dominated by unrealistic worries, fears, and helplessness, or they may "worry about being worried" (Levin & Alici, 2010). Patients may worry about prognosis, uncertainty, or recurrence, which has been described metaphorically as "the sword of Damocles suspended above the patient's head" (Levin & Alici, 2010, p. 325). Irritability and fatigue commonly occur and are related to the physiologic energy that anxiety consumes. Impaired communication (e.g., rapid, pressured speech; repetitive questioning; silence and withdrawal) may also be a symptom of anxiety.

Noncompliance with medical treatment may be another emotional response of anxiety and may cause patients to refuse tests, treatments, or procedures out of fear and apprehension. This warrants psychiatric evaluation, as excessive worry may worsen cancer outcomes (Levin & Alici, 2010). Assessment for depressive symptoms is important because depression and anxiety commonly occur together in patients with cancer. A clinical indicator that distinguishes between depression and anxiety is that depressed patients predominantly feel hopeless, whereas anxious patients predominantly feel helpless. The association between depression and suicide is well known; however, anxiety is also a risk factor for suicide (Levin & Alici, 2010).

### *Cognitive Changes*

An anxious patient will have difficulty concentrating and maintaining attention (Pasacreta et al., 2015). Memory may be affected, and the patient may be unable to focus on the conversation or task at hand. Problem-solving abilities may be impaired, which, in turn, may negatively affect coping. An adaptive response to stressful situations requires problem-solving activities to manage and solve the threat. Cognitive deficits from the disease or treatment also may contribute to anxiety and feelings of helplessness.

### *Behavioral Responses*

Patients experiencing anxiety will demonstrate changes in behavior such as restlessness, pacing, wringing of hands, and nail biting. Other symptoms that may occur without a physiologic cause include irritability or outbursts of anger; trembling or shaking; recurrent and persistent ideas, thoughts, or impulses; and repetitive behaviors to prevent discomfort (Pasacreta et al., 2015). Anxiety can be immobilizing and interfere with patients' ability to perform activities of daily living, solve problems, and interact with others. Treatments may be affected if the patient has blood, injection, and injury phobias or claustrophobia (Traeger et al., 2012). Other behavioral responses to the cancer experience may be linked to anxiety. Preexisting anxiety may be a causative factor in patients with anticipatory nausea and vomiting. Evaluating other behaviors that may be linked to anxiety are important but often overlooked; risky behaviors and substance abuse are common when individuals try to mitigate the stressor and self-medicate (e.g., smoking, alcohol/drug abuse). Anxious patients must be assessed for signs of withdrawal from these substances or other medications when treatment or hospitalization interferes with self-medication regimens.

### *Phases of Illness*

Different stages along the disease continuum require assessment of anxiety responses that are unique to the demands confronted at particular phases of disease and treatment. The stage of diagnosis is one of shock and disbelief, and acute stress reactions are more common at this time. Reactivation of these same feelings has been reported at the time of recurrence but with more intensity (Pasacreta et al., 2015). In a longitudinal study of survivors, Boyes et al. (2013) found that early psychological morbidity was predictive of survivors who would benefit most from routine screening across the disease trajectory.

Anxiety appears to increase with disease progression. As functional ability is lost, dependency on others increases, pain is experienced, quality of life diminishes, and psychological symptoms are potentiated (Pasacreta et al., 2015). During the terminal stages of cancer, fear and anxiety are related to existential concerns, loss of control, unrelieved pain, burden on family, and separation from loved ones (Pasacreta et al., 2015). Anxiety has been described as interpersonally contagious (Pasacreta et al., 2015); therefore, healthcare professionals should not overlook the anxiety experienced by family members at the patient's end of life.

## Differential Diagnosis

In patients experiencing excessive anxiety, factors other than their psychological state must be ruled out first. A differential diagnosis must address the possibility of underlying metabolic imbalances, pain, hypoxia, medications, or other medical states contributing to patients' anxious symptoms. The major challenge in diagnosing anxiety or coexisting depression is the overlap of somatic symptoms related to the cancer, its treatment, and those that are syndromes of these psychological disorders (e.g., anorexia, weight loss, restlessness) (Pasacreta et al., 2015). Once nurses have ruled out medical conditions contributing to anxiety (e.g., pain is adequately controlled), they must then address direct psychosocial causes. If anxious behaviors are severe (e.g., patients are immobilized by fear) or interfere with treatment (e.g., noncompliance, avoidant coping), patients should be evaluated for underlying or preexisting anxiety disorders. Differentiating normal or expected anxiety responses from abnormal responses depends on the intensity, extent, and duration of symptoms (Pasacreta et al., 2015). If abnormal anxiety is suspected, patients must again be asked about a history of chronic fear, phobias, or panic attacks. Specific questions should address patients' subjective feelings and fears. Examples include "What are the sensations you feel when you begin your chemotherapy treatment?" and "What particular situations in the past made you feel that the world was closing in on you?"

## Interventions

The first step in the management of anxiety is to determine its exact cause. A thorough assessment can provide the necessary information for identifying causative factors, the duration and intensity of symptoms, and the resources needed to assist the patient. Interventions often are grouped into psychotherapeutic or pharmacologic but may be most effective when used simultaneously. If individuals are immobilized by anxiety, pharmacologic intervention may be used to manage the physiologic symptoms, enabling patients to have the physical and emotional energy to focus on the beneficial psychotherapeutic interventions. Anxiolytic medications help patients gain control over agonizing anxiety (Pasacreta et al., 2015). For example, the use of anxiolytic medications may help to control ruminating thoughts and worries enough to assist patients in working through fears and anxieties in psychotherapy, thus providing more permanent control over long-standing anxiety. Different types of interventions may be beneficial at different transition points across the disease continuum. Psychoeducational approaches have proved to be beneficial at the time of diagnosis (Fawzy, Fawzy, Arndt, & Pasnau, 1995), and palliative, psychotherapeutic interventions are most beneficial at the end of life (Pasacreta et al., 2015). Anxiety that occurs at the terminal stages of cancer often is related to hypoxia and/or untreated pain. Therefore, oxygen and IV opiates are effective treatments (Pasacreta et al., 2015). Feelings of vulnerability are also common at the stage when treatment ends, therefore warranting psychosocial assessment (Boyes et al., 2013). Nurses are in a key position to assess patients for anxiety, provide evidence-based interventions, and refer patients, if necessary, to the appropriate resource. The primary physician should be notified if an underlying medical cause needs to be ruled out. If symptoms are severe enough to require psychotherapy or medication management, a psychiatric referral is warranted. This may be the case if patients are at risk of harm to themselves or others, are experiencing severe anxiety or agitation, or are exhibiting psychosis or confusion (delirium) (Anderson et al., 2014).

### *Psychotherapeutic Interventions*

Nondrug treatment of anxiety provides cognitive and behavioral interventions intended to help patients to develop the skills needed to cope effectively with anxiety. The types of psychotherapeutic interventions studied have ranged from behavioral training, education, individual psychotherapy, and group therapy support, with small to moderate effects shown in research that has addressed the influence of specific interventions and changes in anxiety levels (Levin & Alici, 2010). Cognitive interventions begin with cognitive restructuring, or the process of helping patients to understand how thought processes (e.g., constant worrying) can negatively influence mood (Baker & Emery, 1985). Interventions can teach patients how to take control over their worries, including initiating behaviors such as keeping a diary of daily concerns, setting aside a time each day to worry, and sharing concerns with supportive people for validation. These interventions will help patients to gain insight into the relationship between thinking and feeling. Working on changing negative thought patterns helps patients to regain a feeling of control over what is causing them anxiety and helps them to differentiate between realistic and unrealistic fears (Cope et al., 2016).

Another major component of psychotherapeutic interventions are relaxation techniques, including progressive relaxation, which comprises breathing exercises, guided imagery, music, yoga, biofeedback, and meditation (see Chapter 25). The effectiveness of these distraction techniques in directly decreasing anxiety responses demands further study, but they have shown promise for managing procedural pain, chemotherapy-related nausea and vomiting, and specific phobias. A regular exercise regimen can provide relaxation, stress reduction, and a time for cognitive restructuring. In severe cases of anxiety that involve phobias and panic, patients may find desensitization techniques useful. The goal is for patients to remain relaxed when confronted with the feared stimuli or thoughts of the feared stimuli. Psychotherapy can be accomplished using a variety of methods, including short-term psychoeducational formats (e.g., American Cancer Society's "I Can Cope" classes), support groups (e.g., Cancer Support

Community), and individual therapies of longer duration if patients have a past history of psychiatric problems or earlier trauma. Concurrent use of an antianxiety agent to support patients until cognitive and behavioral changes are learned may enhance any of these interventions.

Review of evidence-based practice strongly supports psychoeducational, psychosocial (e.g., cognitive behavioral therapy), and support group approaches as effective in managing anxiety (Cope et al., 2016; Sheldon, Swanson, Dolce, Marsh, & Summers, 2008). In a systematic review of the effects of psychosocial strategies on anxiety and depression in prostate cancer, researchers found that psychosocial strategies were more effective than routine care in decreasing psychological morbidity, although the effect was not sustainable (Chien, Liu, Chien, & Liu, 2014). This suggests the importance of introducing these interventions prior to therapy and continuing thereafter to maintain effectiveness.

## *Pharmacologic Interventions*

Pharmacologic treatment for anxiety in patients with cancer includes benzodiazepines for acute short-term management of symptoms, as well as selective serotonin reuptake inhibitors (SSRIs) and serotonin–norepinephrine reuptake inhibitors for long-term management (Greer et al., 2015). The most commonly used drugs for acute anxiety are those of the benzodiazepine group, which includes alprazolam, lorazepam, and clonazepam. All are useful for treating short-term anxiety related to cancer treatment, GAD, and panic disorders. Because of their short half-life, alprazolam and lorazepam are the preferred drugs for older adult patients. They also are useful for their sedative and muscle-relaxing effects and are effective in treating insomnia. Because of its potentially beneficial side effect of transient amnesia, lorazepam has been used to treat anxiety in pre-chemotherapy regimens or prior to anxiety-producing treatments (e.g., claustrophobia related to MRI). Lorazepam can help patients to forget other unpleasant experiences, such as nausea and vomiting, which is an important intervention for any patients with a prior history of trait anxiety. Lorazepam is available parenterally, allowing patients with cancer to premedicate to mitigate apprehension prior to treatments. A cautionary side effect of these short-acting benzodiazepines is rebound anxiety between doses (Pasacreta et al., 2015). Patients who exhibit rebound anxiety may benefit from a switch to a longer-acting benzodiazepine (e.g., diazepam). If longer-acting diazepam is used in older adults or those with liver disease, dosages should be decreased and intervals increased (Pasacreta et al., 2015). Another caution with benzodiazepines is the possibility of respiratory depression. Patients with pulmonary disease or lung metastasis may instead benefit from an antihistamine. Benzodiazepines have dependence and abuse potential and the possibility of withdrawal symptoms when discontinued and therefore must be used with careful consideration (Pasacreta et al., 2015). The choice and dosage of anxiolytic medication must be made in accordance with patients' medical history (e.g., liver and cardiopulmonary function), age, symptoms, and goal of treatment.

Other drug classifications have been found to be clinically useful in treating anxiety. Buspirone is beneficial in treating chronic anxiety (e.g., GAD) and phobia because of its nonaddictive quality, but it may take two to three weeks to become effective (Pasacreta et al., 2015). Other advantages of buspirone include its lack of sedative effects, its limited effect on liver disease, and its lack of effect on cognition (Pasacreta et al., 2015). Tricyclic antidepressants have more sedative effects and have been used to treat anxiety-related insomnia and depression. A common example is amitriptyline. The antipsychotic drug chlorpromazine has more sedative effects. Antihistamines such as diphenhydramine have been used for their calming effects and to relieve the akathisia associated with phenothiazines used as antiemetics. Combining a medication with sedative effects with the analgesic may relieve anxiety associated with painful procedures (e.g., hydroxyzine, fentanyl). For patients who present with mixed symptoms of anxiety and depression, an antidepressant with sedative effects may be the treatment of choice. Many of the tricyclic antidepressants (e.g., imipramine) and SSRIs (e.g., paroxetine) have sedative effects for treating the anxiety component of depression and appear to be well-tolerated by patients. If an SSRI is chosen, the potential for drug–drug interactions must be taken into consideration (e.g., fluoxetine may decrease serum levels of tamoxifen) (Greer et al., 2015).

A major concern in pharmacologic management is using appropriate medication(s) to treat the correct symptom, and all agents must be monitored for effectiveness and side effects. At times, patients with cancer may appear agitated or restless because of underlying medical problems, including pain, nausea, or dyspnea. Careful assessment is needed to ensure that the correct medication is being used to treat the appropriate symptom and that the underlying medical problem is being addressed. For example, if pain is controlled adequately with around-the-clock administration, anxiety symptoms should diminish if pain is the causative factor. In addition, pharmacologic management of anxiety often is underutilized, or prescribed doses are too low because of fears of addiction. These fears generally are unwarranted in those with cancer, and patients most often discontinue the use of these medications when symptoms abate. Other concerns of pharmacologic treatment include unwanted side effects such as sedation and cognitive impairment, requiring cautionary use in older adults. When discontinued, these drugs must be tapered on a schedule to avoid withdrawal symptoms or rebound anxiety. Pharmacotherapy is likely to be effective in the treatment of anxiety but should always be combined with psychosocial interventions (Sheldon et al., 2008).

## Case Study

Sally is a 41-year-old Caucasian woman being treated for stage III ovarian carcinoma. Diagnosed unexpectedly because of subtle symptoms on presentation, Sally was initially treated with a total abdominal hysterectomy. Six weeks after surgery, she presents to the clinic to begin six cycles of paclitaxel/carboplatin. Upon greeting Sally in the infusion room, the chemotherapy nurse notices that she is tearful and shaky as she sits down. The nurse begins to review the plan of care for the regimen with Sally in an attempt to calm her. When asked if she has any questions, Sally bursts into tears and exclaims, "I do not know if I can go through with this!" The nurse gently put her hand on Sally's and inquires, "What worries you the most?" Sally expresses that she could not sleep at all the night before because of "nerves." She felt "physically and emotionally drained" since her diagnosis and surgery, and her fear of chemotherapy is "intense." Acutely aware of Sally's anxiety, the nurse escorts her into a treatment room for privacy and asks if someone accompanied her to the clinic. Sally tearfully states that she is a recent divorcée with two young children who are in school. "My best friend offered to take time off work to be with me today, but I thought I could do this on my own. I wanted to be brave and I did not want to burden anyone," Sally explains.

The nurse spends several minutes reassuring Sally that she will be fine while gently encouraging her to reach out to others for support. The nurse realizes that she needs to carry out a thorough psychosocial assessment of Sally's medical and psychological history. Upon review, Sally informs the nurse that she has not emotionally recovered from her divorce when she was diagnosed. Sally explains that she has battled anxiety and depression since youth and has been on and off antidepressants at different stressful times of her life. She has gone on the antidepressant venlafaxine after surgery. Her physician felt that in addition to supporting her history of situational depression, it would also help the mood changes and hot flashes that Sally was experiencing related to surgically induced menopause. Sally started the medication only two weeks ago, and she has yet to feel any change in mood. Sally also expresses that her "nerves feel out of control." Everything is making Sally "nervous," especially the thought of chemotherapy. She dreads the idea of hair loss and fears feeling nauseated and sick. She is also on a leave of absence from her job as an elementary school teacher and misses her "life before cancer."

### Discussion

The nurse's interventions with Sally were both appropriate and supportive. When confronted with a tearful and nervous patient, the nurse pulled Sally aside to do a thorough psychosocial assessment. Finding out that Sally had a history of depression and anxiety and had come to the clinic unaccompanied, the nurse began to change the plan of care. She spoke unhurriedly and gently to Sally in order to ease her anxiety and fear and reassured her that the healthcare team was available to support her through the treatments. She also encouraged Sally to change her appointment to the following day in order to have someone accompany her to the clinic. The nurse spoke with Sally about obtaining a wig when treatment commenced so that her hair loss would not be as devastating. She also reviewed the protocol with Sally and assured her that antiemetics would be given before, during, and following the chemotherapy to prevent nausea and vomiting. A benzodiazepine was also prescribed for Sally's acute anxiety and insomnia. The nurse instructed Sally that this medication would be administered along with the chemotherapy to help her relax during treatment. The physician instructed Sally to continue the antidepressant, which was expected to take another few weeks to take effect. This would hopefully treat both Sally's mood changes and her anxiety long term. The nurse also encouraged Sally to join a local Cancer Support Community support group, which could provide her with a safe place to share her feelings and concerns.

The nurse's role proved to be pivotal in the ongoing assessment and treatment plan of this patient. An interprofessional treatment plan was set in motion that would include the physician, advanced practice nurse, infusion nurses, and office staff. Continued evaluation of Sally's anxiety would be necessary in addition to ongoing assessment for signs of depression. Short-acting anxiolytics were to be used initially to control Sally's acute anxiety related to chemotherapy but then discontinued once the antidepressant took effect. The nursing staff responded to Sally's emotional needs by creating a structured, safe environment and by providing reassurance as part of their interventions.

## Conclusion

Anxiety is a normal response that appears at different transition points along the cancer trajectory. Although the experience of anxiety is a normal reaction to the threat of cancer, it is an uncomfortable and distressing emotion for most patients. For patients at high risk, anxiety can become overwhelming, disabling, and even pathologic. Anxiety has been shown to have a strong independent relationship with worse health-related quality of life (Greer et al., 2015). Oncology nurses are in key positions to assess patients' anxiety, implement and test for evidence-based interventions, and evaluate effective outcomes (Sheldon et al., 2008). Validating anxiety in patients with cancer and testing interventions require future research to support evidence-based practice. Clinical practice recommendations include using follow-up visits as a source of reassurance, particularly for fears of recurrence and suffering (Traeger et al., 2012). To decrease anxiety, it is most helpful for a nurse to elicit specific concerns, explore perceived threats that patients attach to symptoms or test results, and correct misinformation (Traeger et al., 2012).

Intervention programs aimed at reducing levels of distress and anxiety and programs developed to support coping require further investigation in controlled clinical trials. Inherent in these programs are strategies for psychological support and education, which are major components of psychosocial oncology nursing. Standards of practice and outcome criteria exist to guide oncology nurses in the treatment of patient anxiety and call upon nursing to identify its role in providing effective anxiety interventions needed to enhance the coping and adaptation of patients with cancer.

# References

Abbey, G., Thompson, S.B.N., Hickish, T., & Heathcote, D. (2015). A meta-analysis of prevalence rates and moderating factors for cancer-related post-traumatic stress disorder. *Psycho-Oncology, 24,* 371–381. doi:10.1002/pon.3654

American Psychiatric Association. (2000). *Diagnostic and statistical manual of mental disorders* (4th ed.). Washington, DC: Author.

American Psychiatric Association. (2013). *Diagnostic and statistical manual of mental disorders* (5th ed.). Washington, DC: Author.

Anderson, B.L., DeRubeis, R.J., Berman, B.S., Gruman, J., Champion, V.L., Massie, M.J., ... Rowland, J.H. (2014). Screening, assessment, and care of anxiety and depressive symptoms in adults with cancer: An American Cancer Society of Clinical Oncology guideline adaptation. *Journal of Clinical Oncology, 32,* 1605–1619. doi:10.1200/JCO.2013.52.4611

Beck, A.T., & Emery, G. (1985). *Anxiety disorders and phobias: A cognitive perspective.* New York, NY: Basic Books.

Boyes, A.W., Girgis, A., D'Este, C.A., Zucca, A.C., Lecathelinais, C., & Carey, M.L. (2013). Prevalence and predictors of the short-term trajectory of anxiety and depression in the first year after a cancer diagnosis: A population-based longitudinal study. *Journal of Clinical Oncology, 31,* 2724–2729. doi:10.1200/JCO.2012.44.7540

Chase, E. (2013). Crisis intervention for nurses. *Clinical Journal of Oncology Nursing, 17,* 337–339. doi:10.1188/13.CJON.337-339

Chien, C.-H., Liu, K.-L., Chien, H.-T., & Liu, H.-E. (2014). The effects of psychosocial strategies on anxiety and depression of patients diagnosed with prostate cancer: A systematic review. *International Journal of Nursing Studies, 51,* 28–38. doi:10.1016/j.ijnurstu.2012.12.019

Cohen, M.Z., & Bankston, S. (2011). Cancer-related distress. In C.H. Yarbro, D. Wujcik, & B.H. Gobel (Eds.), *Cancer nursing: Principles and practice* (7th ed., pp. 667–684). Burlington, MA: Jones & Bartlett Learning.

Cope, D.G., Fulcher, C.D., Berkowitz, A., Coignet, H., Conley, S., Drapek, L., ... Walker, D.K. (2016). Putting evidence into practice: Anxiety. PEP recommendations. Retrieved from https://www.ons.org/practice-resources/pep/anxiety

Fawzy, F.I., Fawzy, N.W., Arndt, L.A., & Pasnau, R.O. (1995). Critical review of psychosocial interventions in cancer care. *Archives of General Psychiatry, 52,* 100–112. doi:10.1001/archpsyc.1995.03950140018003

Fawzy, F.I., Fawzy, N.W., Hyun, C.S., & Wheeler, J.G. (1997). Brief, coping-oriented therapy for patients with malignant melanoma. In J.L. Spira (Ed.), *Group therapy for medically ill patients* (pp. 133–163). New York, NY: Guilford Press.

Gorman, L.M., & Sultan, D.F. (Eds.). (2008). *Psychosocial nursing for general patient care* (3rd ed.). Philadelphia, PA: F.A. Davis Company.

Grassi, L., Nanni, M.G., Donovan, K.A., & Jacobsen, P.B. (2015). Cross-cultural considerations in screening and assessment. In J.C. Holland, W.S. Breitbart, P.N. Butow, P.B. Jacobsen, M.J. Loscalzo, & R. McCorkle (Eds.), *Psycho-oncology* (3rd ed., pp. 411–416). New York, NY: Oxford University Press.

Greer, J.A., MacDonald, J., & Traeger, L. (2015). Anxiety disorders. In J.C. Holland, W.S. Breitbart, P.N. Butow, P.B. Jacobsen, M.J. Loscalzo, & R. McCorkle (Eds.), *Psycho-oncology* (3rd ed., pp. 296–303). New York, NY: Oxford University Press.

Levin, T.T., & Alici, Y. (2010). Anxiety disorders. In J.C. Holland, W.S. Breitbart, P.B. Jacobsen, M.S. Lederberg, M.J. Loscalzo, & R. McCorkle (Eds.), *Psycho-oncology* (2nd ed., pp. 324–339). New York, NY: Oxford University Press.

Li, M., Hales, S., & Rodin, G. (2015). Adjustment disorders. In J.C. Holland, W.S. Breitbart, P.N. Butow, P.B. Jacobsen, M.J. Loscalzo, & R. McCorkle (Eds.), *Psycho-oncology* (3rd ed., pp. 274–280). New York, NY: Oxford University Press.

NANDA International. (2015). *Nursing diagnoses: Definitions and classification, 2015–2017*. Philadelphia, PA: Author.

National Cancer Institute. (2015). Cancer-related post-traumatic stress (PDQ®) [Health professional version]. Retrieved from http://www.cancer.gov/about-cancer/coping/survivorship/new-normal/ptsd-hp-pdq

Paice, J.A. (2011). Care during the final days of life. In C.H. Yarbro, D. Wujcik, & B.H. Gobel (Eds.), *Cancer nursing: Principles and practice* (7th ed., pp. 1829–1841). Burlington, MA: Jones & Bartlett Learning.

Pasacreta, J.V., Minarik, P.A., Nield-Anderson, L., & Paice, J.A. (2015). Anxiety and depression. In B.R. Ferrell, N. Coyle, & J.A. Paice (Eds.), *Oxford textbook of palliative nursing* (4th ed., pp. 366–384). New York, NY: Oxford University Press.

Selye, H. (1956). *The stress of life*. New York, NY: McGraw-Hill.

Sheldon, L.K., Swanson, S., Dolce, A., Marsh, K., & Summers, J. (2008). Putting evidence into practice. Evidence-based interventions for anxiety. *Clinical Journal of Oncology Nursing, 12,* 789–797. doi:10.1188/08.CJON.789-797

Strada, A.E., & Sourkes, B.M. (2015). Principles of psychotherapy. In J.C. Holland, W.S. Breitbart, P.B. Jacobsen, M.S. Lederberg, M.J. Loscalzo, & R. McCorkle (Eds.), *Psycho-oncology* (3rd ed., pp. 397–401). New York, NY: Oxford University Press.

Traeger, L., Greer, J.A., Fernandez-Robles, C., Temel, J.S., & Pirl, W.F. (2012). Evidence-based treatment of anxiety in patients with cancer. *Journal of Clinical Oncology, 30,* 1197–1205. doi:10.1200/JCO.2011.39.5632

# CHAPTER 15

# Body Image Disturbance

*Joan R. Schleper, MS, RN, GNP-BC, CNS*

> *Each one has a scar of distortion,*
> *Yet each has this sermon to sing,*
> *"The presence of what would deface me,*
> *Has made me a beautiful thing."*
>
> —Frank H. Keith

Body image is the individual perception of one's own body. It was first defined by neurologist Paul Ferdinand Schilder in the 1920s as "the picture of our own body which we form in our mind, that is to say, the way in which the body appears to ourselves" (Schilder, 1950, p. 11). Schilder was the first to identify body image as multidimensional. From 1969–1990, Shontz's research and publications shifted body image into cognitive and perceptual dimensions (Shontz, 1990). Body image is now viewed as encompassing neurologic, psychological, and sociocultural elements. It is recognized as being a factor in eating disorders, obesity, disfigurement, functional loss, disability, rehabilitation, and reconstructive and cosmetic surgery (Cash & Smolak, 2011; Grogan, 2008; Thompson, 2004).

Although the view of body image has now expanded well beyond Schilder's initial description, no universally accepted definition currently exists. Dropkin (1999) defined body image as "the dynamic perception of one's own bodily appearance, function, and sensations as well as feelings associated with this perception. It occurs largely at a subconscious level and is normally regulated by the condition of the body" (p. 310). Berlucchi and Agliotì (2010) expanded the definition of body image to include two concepts: body schema and body image. *Body schema* is defined as the unconscious system of physiologically formed sensory perceptions of an individual's body limits and extension that is used for control and orientation. *Body image* is the system of conscious perceptions involving a group of thoughts, feelings, perceptions, beliefs, and attitudes, as related to an individual's body (Berlucchi & Agliotì, 2010). Both of these systems are involved in body image disturbances. Perhaps the most consistent consensus of the definition of body image is that it is a complex, multidimensional construct that encompasses an individual's assessment of their body, thoughts, perceptions, and feelings and behaviors about not only appearance, but of function and physical competence as well (Cash & Pruzinsky, 2004; Dropkin, 1997; Fingeret, 2010; Pruzinsky, 1996). The American Psychiatric Association

(APA, 2013) identifies problems related to body image dysfunction to include diagnoses such as eating and feeding disorders, body dysmorphic disorder, sexual disorders, and adjustment disorder.

The concepts of body control and body boundary are also important in understanding body image. People generally value the ability to be in control, whether it is to control normal bodily functions or daily schedules. Correctly assessing one's ability to be in control enhances self-perception, self-concept, and self-esteem and supports a more positive body image (Ervik & Asplund, 2012; NANDA International, 2015; Snöbohm, Friedrichsen, & Heiwe, 2010).

Loss of body control is often reported by patients and noted as "body betrayal." Body boundary includes the entire physical appearance, which varies in importance to each individual. Men or women who choose to wear certain clothing, jewelry, hairstyles, or makeup portray their own perceived body image to all observers. A person's outward appearance dictates how well defined their body boundaries are; an immaculate outward image depicts body control and well-defined body boundaries. The multidimensional construct of body image encompasses an individual's assessment of their body—not just of appearance but also function and physical competence—in the following dimensions: thoughts, perceptions, feelings, and behaviors (Cash & Pruzinsky, 2004).

Cash's (2011) cognitive behavioral model has been widely accepted as a framework for treatment interventions of body image difficulties. In this model, two body image attitudes are theorized to influence feelings, thoughts, and behaviors: body image evaluation and body image investment. Body image evaluation addresses to what degree one is satisfied with their appearance as well as the discrepancy between one's desired body characteristic and one's self-perceived body appearance and characteristics. Body image investment addresses the importance of one's appearance and body characteristics (Cash, 2011; Fingeret, Teo, & Epner, 2014).

As people mature, they begin to assimilate individual, unique qualities into their personality. An individual's talents, traits, and abilities make him or her distinct from others. Interpersonal, sociocultural, and physical characteristics can affect thoughts, feelings, and actions contributing to body image. This idea supports Cash's (2011) cognitive behavioral model. Individuals who value their self-image see themselves as worthy and tend to have a more positive body image. Body image is also associated with self-consciousness during sexual activity, which is linked to sexual functioning. Therefore, measures of body image are correlated with sexual function, satisfaction, and self-esteem (Wiederman, 2011).

# Body Image Development

Development of body image is caused by multiple factors derived from a combination of one's social, cognitive, emotional, and physical development. These influences interact to create an individual's body image (see Table 15-1).

Body image is also influenced by society. In Western societies, body image and physical appearance are strongly promoted by all forms of mass media. Tiggemann (2011) described a conceptual sociocultural model for investigating body image dissatisfaction and eating disorders. It includes societal or sociocultural ideals of beauty promoted by a variety of mass media outlets and social media platforms. Cohen and Blaszczynski (2015) demonstrated that Facebook use was linked to a higher baseline body image dis-

## Table 15-1. The Development of Body Image

| Developmental Stage | Influences |
|---|---|
| Infancy (0–12 months old) | Newborns detect visual-tactile intersensory synchrony in relation to their own bodies, providing evidence that body perception is present at birth (Filippetti et al., 2013). Separation of self from mother and father is a first step in formation of body boundaries. |
| Young childhood (2–4 years old) | By age 2, children develop a sense of "I" or "me" in photos or mirrors, and a demonstration of pride and shame is evident (Smolak, 2011). Mastery of physical/motor tasks becomes the foundation for feelings of control of self and environments and toward positive feelings of self. |
| Early childhood (5–10 years old) | Children compare themselves first to one child, then many other children. Appearance is one of their social comparisons, with self-evaluation of physical/athletic skills and physical appearance becoming their initial foundation of body image—the latter more pronounced in girls. By age 6, clear evidence exists of children becoming concerned about weight and shape that is similar to those of adolescents and adults (Smolak, 2011). By age 8, boys are more prone to producing and maintaining an unrealistically positive belief that their attributes and abilities are better than average—a self-serving bias (Ricciardelli & McCabe, 2011). Children begin to recognize maleness and femaleness without any real recognition of the physical sexual characteristics present in each gender. Sex differentiation must develop prior to further boundary expansion. |
| Adolescence: Onset of puberty | Body image is constantly changing, especially skin (acne), body hair distribution, voice change, height, weight, shape, strength, fitness, and muscularity, all of which can produce lack of control over body and self (Wertheim & Paxton, 2011). Interactions with and opinions of peers often are more important than those with parents. Adolescents are aware of changes in their own bodies and in friends/peers; timing of puberty can affect body image. Adolescents may feel threatened with feelings of insecurity or fear as they compare their bodies to others; there is a strong desire to fit in (Wertheim & Paxton, 2011). Body changes and egocentrism result in concerns about the way they view and compare themselves with others (Larouche & Chin-Peuckert, 2006). Peer acceptance heavily influences self-acceptance; teasing and sarcastic comments about weight, shape, or other features negatively influence body image. Sexual harassment can cause adolescents, especially girls, to objectify their body as it is observed and evaluated; this is correlated with shame of one's body (Wertheim & Paxton, 2011). |
| Adulthood | Body image becomes more stable but is never fully constant or formed (e.g., weight gain, wrinkling, less muscle tone and strength with age). Societal double standard of aging affects body image evaluation of physical appearance/attractiveness/sexuality, with a generally more positive view in adult men and a more critical view in adult women (Grogan, 2011). As maturity increases, adults face recognition of physiologic adaptation in the body caused by aging, with some findings that older women attach less importance to appearance and looks and more to their roles in family/society (Tiggemann, 2004). Decreased association with body image satisfaction and self-esteem exists in older versus younger men and women; appearance does not predict self-esteem. Men are more likely to be satisfied with body image than women, and appearance concerns decrease more so in men than in women. A focus on health, fitness, and body function is more prevalent in men (Baker & Gringart, 2009). |

*Note.* Based on information from Baker & Gringart, 2009; Filippetti et al., 2013; Grogan, 2011; Larouche & Chin-Peuckert, 2006; Ricciardelli & McCabe, 2011; Smolak, 2011; Stern, 1990; Tiggemann, 2004; Wertheim & Paxton, 2011.

satisfaction and increased risk of eating disorder. Exposure to all types of media results in ideals being internalized by individuals, thereby affecting their satisfaction or dissatisfaction in meeting this desired societal view of beauty, size, weight, and proportion. The promotion of a thin body has been associated with beauty, success, and happiness. According to Tiggemann (2011), 90% of girls aged 3–10 own at least one Barbie doll, which depicts a very unrealistic body proportion. In one study, girls aged 5–8 were shown images of a Barbie doll. The girls reported an increased desire for thinness and lower self-esteem; however, these effects were less prevalent in older girls (Dittmar, Halliwell, & Ive, 2006). Action figures with a "V-shaped" muscular physique (e.g., Superman, G.I. Joe) are marketed to young boys and their parents as toys that promote the thin, muscular ideal body to male children. However, this is not to the same degree that the "thin" ideal is promoted to young girls (Levine & Chapman, 2011). To challenge the impact of society on body image in young people, parents, peers, friends, coaches, and mentors can influence children's body image verbally, through actions and behaviors, and by example (Field et al., 2001).

Adolescents gain 50% of their adult body weight during puberty, with girls experiencing widening of the hips and increased body fat, further removing them from society's view of the ideal body weight. Conversely, pubertal changes in boys usually bring more height, musculature, and wider shoulders, which tend to conform more to projected media images (McCabe, Ricciardelli, & Finemore, 2002). In terms of body image, children and adolescents are influenced by television, magazines, movies, video games, the Internet, and social media (e.g., Facebook). These influences continue into young adulthood, with adolescent and young adult women having more body dissatisfaction after exposure to the ideal unattainable body image in television commercials and magazines. These media images can result in more body dissatisfaction, with a resultant decrease in self-esteem and self-concept, along with increased anxiety, anger, depression, ridicule, shame, rejection, exclusion, and isolation (Cho, Kwak, & Lee, 2013; Fallon & Hausenblas, 2005; Hargreaves & Tiggemann, 2004; Levine & Chapman, 2011; Silva, Taquette, & Coutinho, 2014). Despite already having an underweight body mass index, even professional models and ballet dancers have shown a greater desire for thinness (Swami & Szmigielska, 2013; Zoletić & Duraković-Belko, 2009).

One of the most important aspects of body image is physical attractiveness. In American society and Western culture, the standard of physical attractiveness often is based on youth, vitality, and sexual attraction. Societies create meaning; in Western societies, a dichotomy has been created where women are associated with the body and men with the mind. Consequently, men frequently place great importance on the physical attractiveness of a possible mate, which relates to the "objectification" of women more so than men. Originating in objectification theory, the message to women, from multiple sources, is that the female body is to be observed, evaluated, possessed by men, and viewed as an object, thus devaluing women (Levine & Smolak, 2002; McKinley, 2002). Although objectification of women is not as pervasive as in the past, it is still ongoing. This is evidenced by Heflick and Goldenberg's (2014) findings that an emphasis is placed on women's physical characteristics by others, causing them to act like and be perceived as objects without a mind.

Although illness and deformity hold fewer stigmas today, a natural human tendency still exists to label or avoid people who are different or perceived as vulnerable and weak. Therefore, people with chronic conditions or illnesses, especially those that cause visible symptoms, must be prepared to develop ways to deal with stigmas such as avoidance, discrimination, hostility, fear, disgust, condescension, isolation, and simple curiosity.

## Body Image and Illness

Trauma, major illness or injury, or other physical conditions can cause an alteration in body image. Stages of adaptation to body image changes depend on the age and performance status of the individual, nature of the illness or condition, the individual's thoughts and perception of the alteration, duration of the alteration, the person's previous coping abilities, and support systems (see Table 15-2).

Responses to body image disturbance caused by illness may be subtle. Morse, Bottorff, and Hutchinson (1995) characterized four different types of reactions:

1. **The deceiving body:** Some patients have reported a sadness because their body has deceived them. It acted normal with no symptoms, but then disease was discovered during a routine examination. Trust in their body is lost.

### Table 15-2. Stages of Adaptation

| Stage | Descriptors |
| --- | --- |
| Impact—The patient experiences initial encounter with illness or injury. | An awareness develops of changes in body part, structure, function, appearance, or sexuality.<br>The patient enters a state of shock, as irreversibility becomes evident (sudden alterations create longer impact).<br>Anxiety and fear become dominant expressions and threaten health and function and cause discomfort.<br>A sense of depersonalization may be assumed.<br>The patient becomes self-centered, owing to situational loss of control of his or her body.<br>A developmental regression may occur.<br>The patient may feel a sense of failure in own body and have a preoccupation with change or loss. |
| Retreat—The patient attempts to return to the stable feelings of self that existed before the critical event. | The patient may indulge in wishful thinking and avoid reality through fantasy.<br>The process begins of reorganization and strengthening.<br>The patient starts to sort and reorganize his or her shattered self-image. |
| Acknowledgment—The patient actively mourns the loss and experiences a sense of hopelessness. | The patient experiences a "self-not-self" sensation.<br>A new body is forcibly recognized.<br>The patient clings to a strong image of the old body and avoids looking at or touching one's self.<br>The patient begins to resolve conflicts resulting from the newly formed or altered self.<br>The patient continues to be self-centered, focusing on the needs of the self.<br>The patient may feel that relationships are threatened and may feel abandonment. The patient may avoid or change social interactions because of fear of reactions from others.<br>The family may feel grief for the patient's lost body image. |
| Reconstruction—The patient replaces the need to mourn with the decision to try new approaches to living. | The patient reintegrates positive life experiences.<br>The patient reintegrates altered body image, reorganizes social values, and redefines support systems.<br>The patient adjusts to technical devices or procedures and finds satisfaction with body image and thoughts about self. The patient's strengths are emphasized. |

*Note.* Based on information from Ervik & Asplund, 2012; NANDA International, 2015; Snöbolm et al., 2010; Stern, 1990.

2. **The vulnerable body:** Because of the violation of disease and treatment, some patients report feeling vulnerable and fear future experiences. Patients wage a constant vigil to watch for signs of impending pain or discomfort. They feel fragile and move cautiously and hesitantly to protect the self that is left.
3. **The violated body:** Boundaries often are violated, not only through the indignity of exposing intimate and private parts to strangers but also when caregivers enter a room without knocking or ask patients whether their bowels have moved. Although patients experience anger, embarrassment, and a loss of personhood, they passively participate in diagnostic or treatment procedures as if they have no choice, believing this simply is part of their care.
4. **The betraying body:** Patients often feel that their body has betrayed them. They have taken good care of themselves, eaten all the right foods, exercised, and had regular medical checkups, but they still have become ill. A once strong, beautiful, and healthy self-image can vanish as treatment or disease progresses.

Some additional reactions particularly related to cancer include the following:
- Loss of control of one's body and subsequent uncertainty; for example, the individual cannot control their body. Rather, disease and treatment side effects seem to control the individual's body, contributing to a greater sense of uncertainty (Foster & Stern, 2014).
- Feeling different from others, which can result in the sense of being "damaged" or stigmatized (Carpentier, Fortenberry, Ott, Brames, & Einhorn, 2011)
- Loss of body part or loss of normal body function, with resultant simulated grieving process of denial or disbelief, anger, and depression

Chronic illness can bring on new challenges to one's body image. Some patients may have to make major lifestyle changes, including changes in how they perceive their own bodies. Examples of these patients include those with diabetes who must endure daily glucose monitoring, constant dietary restrictions, or insulin injections; those with impaired memory, movement, or speech following cerebral vascular accident; patients with partial or complete spinal cord injury with immobility; and those with epilepsy receiving daily medication that can affect driving or cause uncertainty of future seizure occurrence and sequelae, such as falls, fractures, or other trauma. Moreover, many medications (e.g., antipsychotics, beta blockers) affect libido and sexual functioning, which are inextricably associated with body image because of resultant appearance and/or functional changes.

A self-image that integrates the illness is necessary for the individual's adjustment. This transition is easier if self-image and ego are strong before the illness (Dropkin, 1999). Patients who have a poor self-image and a weaker ego prior to a major change in life or body integrity may not be as open and flexible during the adaptation process because of fewer personal resources. Furthermore, failure to address self-image with patient education and during treatment can result in less effective treatment outcomes (Brotto, Yule, & Breckon, 2010).

Some important considerations regarding body image and illness include the following:
- Sudden physical changes are more difficult than change over time, and increased physical changes have been associated with a worsened body image (Foster & Stern, 2014).
- The illness or untoward side effects can influence appearance appraisal, thereby affecting the cognitive processing of one's thoughts, emotions, interpretations, and comparisons. This influences one's coping and self-regulating strategies and behaviors (Cash, 2011).
- Personality characteristics such as risk-taking behavior, tendency to experience negative emotions, or resilience may influence an individual's body image attitudes (Cash, 2011).

Concerns about body image are not always related to changes in physical appearance. Even if a change is not visible, patients still may feel damaged and stigmatized and must learn to cope with the fact that they will never be quite the same physically or psychologically (Foster & Stern, 2014). For example, feeling less feminine after a hysterectomy can affect how a woman perceives her body. Difficulty arises if a loss of uniqueness of the self accompanies the change. Even though a body normally undergoes continual change, a crisis can occur if a person experiences a change in some characteristic that he or she attributes to their uniqueness and individuality (Laken & Laken, 2002). For example, a woman who views her long, red hair as a key component to her individuality and beauty may experience more distress with alopecia from chemotherapy. Illness breeds uncertainty; whether dealing with an unexpected improvement in or a worsening of a condition, the patient must adapt and learn to cope. When a patient's health changes frequently or extensively, the sense of integration among past, present, and future images of oneself may be lost (Schover, 2005).

Changes in the patient's health will affect the family and partner's perceptions of the individual, and their reactions will have an impact on the patient's body image. Family members may suffer feelings of loss, disorientation, aversion, and fear that, in turn, may evoke sensations of rejection and undesirability on the part of the person who has changed. Does the spouse continue to reach out with an affectionate touch or hold hands in public? Are family members willing to participate in rehabilitation efforts?

Feelings of acceptance and attractiveness will be negatively influenced if friends, coworkers, or strangers avert their gaze, look with pity, or use too much kindness when interacting with the affected person.

It may seem like a Herculean task for a patient to relinquish an image of health, invulnerability, and competence and replace it with something equally acceptable; however, this is what happens when disease changes create a need to generate a new body image from one that has taken a lifetime to create.

## Body Image and Cancer

A cancer diagnosis is highly feared because it can be life-threatening and often results in multimodality treatments that present many challenges. In a study by Bellizzi et al. (2012), roughly 60% of participants aged 15–39 reported that cancer negatively affected the appearance of their body. The disease and/or treatment can contribute to many body changes, including alopecia, skin changes, surgical scars, wounds, disfigurement, cachexia, and weight gain. Alterations in sensations such as taste or smell may occur, and difficulty chewing may persist. The patient may require devices such as an artificial eye or tracheostomy. Colostomy, artificial limbs, prostheses, and/or implanted catheters may be required. These and many other results of cancer or its treatment may be visible (e.g., amputation) or invisible (e.g., orchiectomy, vulvectomy). All of these factors and resulting treatment effects can influence the extent of body image changes and disturbances. Loss of control of body functions, such as bowel or bladder, can result in a sense of feeling loss of control of one's life and can have a major impact on self-esteem and feelings about one's body. Despite these potential concerns, body image may not be addressed adequately by oncology professionals. It is not uncommon for a patient with cancer to worry about being seen as "vain" and experience shame and embarrassment about having body image concerns while facing such a serious illness (Fingeret, Vidrine, Reese, Gillenwater, & Gritz, 2010).

Hair loss is one of the most common indicators to others that a person likely has cancer. Alopecia, which can include the loss of all body hair, including pubic hair, can be embarrassing and cause feelings of unattractiveness. It is often dismissed by healthcare professionals by statements such as, "Do not worry. The hair will grow back." Rasmussen, Hansen, and Elverdam (2010) studied 23 cancer survivors of various solid tumors, leukemia, and lymphoma. Of these survivors, nearly 75% described perceptions of being stared at in a very specific manner. Because of the stigma of having a cancer diagnosis, these perceptions were felt regardless of whether visible changes were evident or not (e.g., wearing a wig, artificial eyelashes, penciled eyebrows). A changed physical appearance, such as having very short hair, caused participants to feel avoided by others or as though they were greeted with a specific compliment. The survivors perceived these social effects as a way to maintain silence or secrecy about their diagnosis, thus making it impossible for them to discuss their cancer experience (Rasmussen et al., 2010).

## Specific Cancers and Body Image

### Head and Neck Cancer

Head and neck cancers (HNCs), including oral cavity and larynx, account for approximately 4% of all cancers (Siegel, Miller, & Jemal, 2017). HNCs are most commonly treated with surgery and/or radiation. To a lesser degree, chemotherapy and targeted therapies may be used. Resultant side effects of these treatments can produce visible and disfiguring body image changes. Difficulties with speech and sensory or nerve deficits are but the beginning of adverse treatment effects. Some permanent or temporary side effects can include loss of teeth, chewing problems, trismus, xerostomia, weight loss, swallowing or aspiration difficulties, and/or altered feeding needs via gastrostomy and facial disfigurement. Altered breathing with either tracheostomy or laryngeal stoma may also result from treatment and contribute to embarrassment and intimacy problems. In a study by Fingeret et al. (2012), it was estimated that up to 75% of surgically treated patients for HNC of the skin had body image and embarrassment concerns that persisted over one year. Speech and eating dysfunctions increased body image dissatisfaction compared to either dysfunction alone. Patients with both speech and eating dysfunctions tended to avoid social activities (Fingeret et al., 2012). In a study of patients with HNC (N = 522), Wong et al. (2013) noted that those with increased treatment and symptom side effects had the most significant negative stereotype of patients with cancer. This created a stigma that affected body image, thus resulting in behavioral avoidance and social isolation. In another study of patients with HNC (Chen et al., 2014), speaking less after surgery was noted in 71% of patients compared to before surgery, and more body image distress was evident in those with laryngeal, hypopharyngeal, and facial area tumors. Interestingly, distress in those who had reconstructive surgery also contributed to social isolation and depression (Chen et al., 2014). However, Dooks, McQuestion, Goldstein, and Molassiotis (2012) found that support from family, friends, and professionals, along with email and video messaging and support groups, improved communication and social integration of patients who underwent total laryngectomy surgery.

### Skin Cancer

Skin cancers comprise both melanoma and nonmelanoma tumors. Basal cell cancer is the most common nonmelanoma skin cancer, with 70% occurring on the face (American

Cancer Society [ACS], 2015; Erba et al., 2007). Because both nonmelanoma skin cancers, basal and squamous cell carcinomas, tend to occur in sun-exposed areas of the body, treatment can ultimately lead to scars or loss of an eye, nose, or ear. This can result in disfigurement, functional deficits, and body image problems that contribute to the patient's preoccupation with appearance. In patients with nonmelanoma cancer, appearance regarding visibility of the scar and scar size were the most prevalent reported body image concerns (Radiotis, Roberts, Czajkowska, Khanna, & Körner, 2014). When people were shown photos with large central or peripheral facial skin cancer lesions versus small central facial skin cancers, it was reported that the larger lesions were more disturbing, thus providing evidence that other's perceptions of those affected with facial scarring or disfigurement are apparent (Godoy et al., 2011). One study noted that after melanoma treatment, 64% of women reported worsened appearance, and 23% were dissatisfied with the appearance of their surgical site (Atkinson, Noce, Hay, Rafferty, & Brady, 2013).

## Breast Cancer

Breast cancer has been the most thoroughly researched of all cancer sites and is the most common cancer affecting women (Siegel et al., 2017). Many patients are treated with radiation therapy, which can produce changes in breast appearance and sensitivity, skin color alterations, breast shrinkage, or firmness from fibrosis. Radiation may also affect the arm, shoulder, and hand, producing swelling, pain, and stiffness. In addition, some patients may experience difficulty with raising the treated arm. Small permanent ink tattoos are applied to mark the radiation field. However, new advances in applying fluorescent dye tattoos allow the markings to be visible only under special fluorescent lights. For patients, invisible markings seem to further improve body image because there are no visible signs of having received radiation treatments (Azvolinsky, 2015). After a five-year follow-up randomized trial of 2,236 female patients, up to 40% noted significant breast changes after radiation therapy, and roughly one-third reported arm and shoulder pain. However, body image concerns and other breast symptoms lessened over time (Hopwood et al., 2010).

Breast cancer surgery treatment effects may include scarring, loss of the breast, change in breast appearance (e.g., contour, shape, loss of nipple), lymphedema, and sensory changes in the affected breast, arm, or hand. Reconstruction after surgery has implications for body image. Immediate reconstruction is a way to minimize the impact of losing the breast. A discrepancy may exist between the perceptions of what a surgeon's impression of a "good outcome" is from that of a patient who wishes to "look like I used to" (Harcourt & Rumsey, 2011; Mulders, Vingerhoets, & Breed, 2008). Teo et al. (2015) found that those who delayed reconstruction surgery were at particular risk for body image distress. In a rare prospective study of 98 women with breast cancer who delayed reconstruction, body image and sexual relationship satisfaction improved after the reconstruction. Poorer general mental health, higher cancer distress, and less partner relationship satisfaction contributed to a negative effect on body image with delayed reconstruction (Gopie, ter Kuile, Tinman, Murear, & Tibben, 2014).

An important sequela of breast cancer surgery is lymphedema. Although lymphedema can affect the upper or lower extremity (e.g., melanoma, gynecologic or urologic, surgical oncologic procedures), upper extremity lymphedema in surgically treated patients with breast cancer affects body image and appearance. In two recent studies, those with an increased volume of lymphedema reported greater appearance disturbance and body image dissatisfaction. Pain intensity and body integrity beliefs were positively associated with depressive symptoms. Higher levels of pain from lymphedema led to a higher state of body image dissatisfaction, which, in turn, led to greater depressive symptoms (Teo, Fingeret, Liu, & Chang, 2015; Teo, Novy, Chang, Cox, & Fingeret, 2015). Lymphedema's permanence has been reported as a constant reminder of cancer and loss of health, function, and normalcy, affecting patients' sense of self and social activities (Fu et al., 2012; Thomas & Hamilton, 2014). Healthcare professionals often lack awareness of this disorder, which produces frustration for patients. Physicians tend to dismiss lymphedema because "nothing can be done about it." In addition to the weight and discomfort of lymphedema, it places patients at an increased risk of infection. Lymphedema can be visible if affecting an upper extremity. It is more invisible in a lower limb; however, both sites can contribute to patients' feelings of embarrassment about their appearance (Thomas & Hamilton, 2014).

## Gynecologic Cancer

Gynecologic cancer's most common site is the uterine corpus, affecting 7% of all female cancers (Siegel et al., 2017). It also includes the uterine cervix, ovary, vulva, and vagina, affecting about 68,000 women per year (ACS, 2015). These cancers often are perceived as "invisible" and sometimes referred to as "silent cancers." The treatment side effects from surgery, radiation, and chemotherapy are objective side effects. The thoughts, perceptions, emotions, and behaviors of patients are the subjective treatment effects and are often neglected. Moreover, treatment effects threaten femininity and the perception of physical appearance in addition to all realms of sexual and reproductive function and sexual desirability (Giacomoni, Venturini, Hoarau, Guyon, & Conri, 2014).

Body image was also found to be associated with sexual functioning in patients with ovarian and vulvar cancer (Barlow, Hacker, Hussain, & Parmenter, 2014; Liavaag et al., 2008). With radical and multiple vulvar excisions or the development of lower extremity lymphedema, more body dissatisfaction was noted. The reverse effects were reported in those treated for early-stage disease. Furthermore, the invisibility of the treatment effects to the vulva appeared to protect patients' body image (Barlow et al., 2014). Abnormal Pap smear results or a positive human papillomavirus (HPV) test may produce guilt, self-blame, distress, and anxiety in those affected. These results also affect body image and relationships with partners and raise sexual and reproductive issues (Herzog & Wright, 2007). In those treated for cervical cancer, 2- to 5-year survivors reported worse body image and more sexual concerns than the 6- to 10-year survivors. This suggests that body image concerns last well into survivorship but do gradually decrease over time. These results may be reflective of more treatment-related side effects in those treated with radiation therapy compared to surgery alone (Korfage et al., 2009). In a rare prospective study of 16 patients undergoing a pelvic exenteration (anterior, posterior, or en bloc pelvic resection, resulting in urinary and bowel diversions) for advanced cervical cancer, physical and psychological measurements were taken preoperatively, and at 3, 6, and 12 months following surgery. Body image and sexual function declined at 3 months, but declines returned near baseline at 12 months (Rezk et al., 2013). These results contrasted with those of another longitudinal prospective research study conducted by Hawighorst-Knapstein et al. (2004) where 31 patients undergoing pelvic exenteration had worse body image scores over time; however, more of these patients received adjuvant treatments than in the previous study.

## Genitourinary Cancer

Genitourinary malignancies include prostate, bladder, kidney, testicular, and penile cancers and comprise almost 370,000 new cases every year (ACS, 2017). Prostate cancer is the most common malignancy among men (Siegel et al., 2017). Treatments may include surgery that can result in incontinence or erectile dysfunction, with the latter continuing to be problematic even with nerve-sparing surgical procedures. Because of urethral resection during prostatectomy, a patient's penis length is shortened. Surprisingly, this often is not communicated to patients preoperatively, creating postprocedure body image distress (Oliffe, 2005). Radiation may produce feelings of exposure, decreased erectile function, and a poor self-perception (Hedestig, Sandman, Tomic, & Widmark, 2005). Depending on the stage or extent of disease, androgen deprivation therapy (ADT) also can be used. Inducing castration levels of testosterone to interrupt this hormone's effects on the prostate is the goal, but side effects of ADT are numerous and include decreased libido, impotence, fatigue, hot flashes, mood swings, change in fat deposition or body shape, gynecomastia, bone loss, and loss of masculinity (Chapple & Ziebland, 2002). Given the profound effects of ADT, significant body image dissatisfaction was reported in men undergoing ADT (Ervik & Asplund, 2012; Harrington, Jones, & Badger, 2009). Furthermore, Taylor-Ford et al. (2013) reported that dissatisfaction persisted over a two-year period.

Penile and testicular cancers account for about 3% of all genitourinary cancers (Siegel et al., 2017). Side effects of radiation and surgery can produce erectile and ejaculatory dysfunction, and sexual discomfort may negatively affect sexual enjoyment and orgasm. In those who underwent partial penectomy, significantly more problems were reported with orgasm, appearance, and urinary function than in those who were treated with penile-sparing surgery (Kieffer et al., 2014). In 401 patients treated for germ cell testicular cancers three years earlier, body image changes were independently associated with all measures of sexual dysfunction, and increased levels of erectile dysfunction were linked with negative changes in body image (Rossen, Pedersen, Zachariae, & von der Masse, 2012). Similar results were found in stage I and II testicular patients treated with orchiectomy and radiation therapy: 61% noted changes in their body, and 48% expressed fertility concerns. Furthermore, sexual dysfunction was associated with changes in body image (Wortel, Alemayehu, & Incrocci, 2015). Of the 161 patients noted in a study by Wortel et al. (2015), 48% received information about testicular prosthesis, while 44% were not informed. Consequently, only 9% had received prosthesis; these patients were significantly younger. In the prosthesis patients, no problems were reported with body image, sexual contacts, or undressing in locker rooms (Wortel et al., 2015). Incrocci, Hop, Wijnmaalen, and Slob (2002) demonstrated that implantation of testicular prostheses is virtually without complications and has provided many patients with improved body image.

Patients with bladder cancer noted distress in their appearance interfering with daily activities (Gilbert et al., 2010). Being embarrassed about the visibility of a stoma appliance and surgical scars, in addition to alopecia and weight loss from chemotherapy, resulted in impaired body image in those with more advanced disease (Palapattu et al., 2004). In a comparison of radical cystectomy and urinary diversion procedures for bladder cancer in 37 female cancer survivors over an average of five years, physical and emotional perception of body image was found to be worse in survivors who underwent cutaneous ureterostomy than in those treated with Bricker or Paduan ileal neobladder (Gacci et al., 2013). Only the latter surgical technique does not result in an external stoma placement. In another study examining surgical techniques and body image, Aboumohamed et al. (2014) investigated 182 patients with bladder cancer who underwent urinary diversion with stoma placement. This procedure was done via open radical cystectomy or robot-assisted radical cystectomy, using either intracorporeal or extracorporeal surgical technique. No differences were reported in body image or urinary or bowel function among these groups in a retrospective case analysis. Interestingly, sexual function was better in the open radical cystectomy group; measurements were done preoperatively and twice postoperatively (Aboumohamed et al., 2014).

## Colorectal Cancer

Colorectal cancers are the third most common cancer. They affect both genders and can result in either a temporary or permanent stoma following surgery, therefore affecting both body image and sexual functioning (ACS, 2015). In their study, Sharpe, Patel, and Clarke (2011) found that patients with stomas for treatment of colorectal cancer had poorer body image, which worsened over time. They also found that body image was a strong predictor of initial levels of anxiety, depression, distress, and subsequent anxiety and distress. Cotrim and Pereira (2008) studied a sample of 153 patients and 96 informal caregivers. Patients who had a stoma reported lower overall quality of life, lower body image, poorer health-related quality of life, and poorer social activity when compared with patients who had colorectal cancer and no stoma. McKenzie et al. (2006) reported that 33% of participants with ostomies withdrew from social and leisure activities; this may have further contributed to depression. A large randomized European Union study of 617 participants undergoing either open or laparoscopic surgery for rectal cancer used one of several measures, including the European Organisation for Research and Treatment of Cancer Quality of Life questionnaire. This instrument measures body image, sexual function and problems, sexual enjoyment in males and females, stoma-related and/or elimination problems, and future perspectives. The study found that the type of procedure (i.e., open or laparoscopic surgery) had similar results (Andersson et al., 2013).

# Nursing Care of Patients With Body Image Disturbance

## Assessment

Because body image disturbances may adversely affect a patient's recovery from a life-threatening illness, nurses have a responsibility to assess and identify adverse changes in body image and begin appropriate interventions. Nurses, rather than physicians, spend more time with patients and their families; therefore, they are at the forefront of identifying patients with body image difficulties.

Assessment tools are identified in the literature to measure body image. However, tools developed for the purpose of screening patients for body image are lacking (Fingeret et al., 2014). The most frequently used instrument in body image research is the Body Image Scale (BIS), which was originally developed to discern changes in satisfaction with body image appearance in patients with breast cancer (Hopwood, Fletcher, Lee, & Al Ghazal, 2001). This instrument is a 10-item self-rated Likert scale that addresses general body image issues and body image related to the cancer experience. Worse body image problems are associated with higher scores on the BIS (Hopwood et al., 2001; Kim et al., 2015).

Other body image scales have been developed. Many of these are geared to specific populations, such as a particular age group (e.g., for young people with cancer), a specific ethnic group or disease site (e.g., breast cancer, hematologic malignancies), or specific culture (Patt, Lane, Finney, Yanek, & Becker, 2002).

Nurses, even advanced practice nurses, often fail to address body image dissatisfaction. Questions about the patient's perception of their body image need to be incorporated in routine assessment, and specialized questions need to be added to identify issues for patients at high risk for body image distress. Reluctance to address feelings and concerns about physical appearance can inhibit patient disclosure (Konradsen, Krikevold, & Zoffman, 2009). Maguire, Faulkner, Booth, Elliot, and Hillier (1996) noted that nurses' reluctance in inquiring about their patients' feelings and concerns was caused by their own fear of damaging patients psychologically and their feelings of inadequacy in addressing patients' issues. Fingeret et al. (2014)

offered observations to nurses in recognizing potential body image difficulties in patients (see Figure 15-1). Nurses often feel a decided discomfort in discussing emotions and personal or intimate details with their patients. However, with further education emphasizing therapeutic communication, continued practice, and recognition of the importance of these issues in the clinical setting, these fears of inadequacy and uncomfortable feelings will subside.

- Unrealistic expectations about treatment outcomes for appearance and functioning
- Preoccupied with concerns about upcoming appearance changes
- Difficulties making treatment decisions due to concerns about appearance/body changes
- Difficulties with or avoidance of viewing oneself after treatment
- Highly dissatisfied with appearance outcome following treatment
- Preoccupied with perceived or actual physical flaws resulting from cancer and/or its treatment
- Avoidance of social situations due to appearance/body changes
- Romantic relationship distress due to body image changes
- Considerable time and effort spent in appearance-fixing behaviors
- Persistent distress, anxiety, or depression due to body image changes

**Figure 15-1. Observations Indicating Possible Body Image Difficulties in Patients With Cancer**

Note. From "Managing Body Image Difficulties of Adult Cancer Patients: Lessons From Available Research," by M.C. Fingeret, I. Teo, and D.E. Epner, 2014, *Cancer, 120*, p. 637. Copyright 2014 by American Cancer Society. Reprinted with permission.

## Differential Diagnosis

Body image disturbance may be only a symptom of a much broader group of issues. These may include the ability to learn to use the maximum amount of self-reliance to problem solve, the ability to accept a certain level of physical dependence, and the ability to develop certain social skills to deal with society's stigmas and attitudes toward individuals with an altered physical appearance.

Body image disturbance may involve more serious psychiatric diagnoses, including mood disorders (e.g., depression); body dysmorphic disorder (when the individual is preoccupied with perceived defects or flaws in physical appearance), now classified as a type of obsessive-compulsive disorder; and other anxiety disorders and sexual dysfunctions (e.g., sexual aversion, erectile dysfunction, male hypoactive sexual desire disorder, female sexual interest/arousal disorders, genito-pelvic pain or penetration disorder) (APA, 2013).

An individual's response to a body alteration will be determined, in part, by the meaning of the change for the person. This may include loss of control, change in appearance, altered sexual functioning, or a change in self-esteem and self-identity. Body image problems can masquerade as denial, depression, shame, or casual indifference (Carpenito-Moyet, 2006).

## Interventions

Because the effect of disease on body image is closely bound to psychological symptoms and the physical effects of the illness and its treatment, nurses must be able to address body image dysfunction with timely interventions.

Fingeret et al. (2014) categorized five types of body image interventions: cognitive behavioral therapy, psychological interventions that focus on psychosexual therapy and expressive-supportive therapy, education interventions, cosmesis-focused interventions to correct or hide perceived defects like scars, and physical fitness interventions.

Fingeret et al. (2014) also provided a conceptual framework called "The Three C's":
1. Remind patients that body image difficulties are very "common." Normalizing concerns in this way reduces shame, embarrassment, and stigma.
2. Inquire about specific body image "concerns" through open-ended questions that elicit patient narrative.
3. Ask about the "consequences" of body image difficulties in daily functions, such as social, emotional, occupational, and recreational.

An important first step is to establish open communication with the patient so that he or she is able to share concerns about body image changes. If the patient is open to this, the nurse needs to be ready to actively engage the patient in this conversation. Other times, the nurse will need to be more active in addressing the topic. Nurses may ask particular questions or make statements when providing supportive interventions. For example, nurses may begin a conversation with a comment such as, "It's a rough surgery or treatment that you have been through," and then respond to the patient's concerns to encourage him or her to keep talking. Use of reflective techniques, open-ended statements, and validation of responses encourages patients to express feelings and promotes open communication. Nurses also may begin statements about emotions and body image concerns with, "Tell me how you're doing" and "How are things at home or work?" Responses beginning with "This must be very difficult for you. Tell me more about your concerns" can be helpful as well (see Table 15-3).

Fingeret et al. (2014) provided four additional examples of specific strategies for addressing body image concerns: educate patients about what to expect in terms of appearance and functional outcomes, connect patients with relevant community resources, refer patients to a mental health specialist for brief or intensive therapy if needed, and follow up with patients with known body image issues about their concerns at each clinic visit. Numerous community resources are available to assist patients in dealing with body image (Fingeret et al., 2014). A variety of support groups and education programs are available to address body image distress. Many of these are accessible on the Internet as well as in person. Brief counseling and support groups are sometimes not enough to address body image disturbance, and more formal psychotherapy may be suggested.

Rancour and Brauer (2003) gave patients a homework assignment and encouraged them to write a letter to the affected body part and describe their reactions to its impending loss. This exercise enabled patients to focus on their strengths, which included the qualities that would be recovered and helped them to grieve for those abilities that would be lost forever. Nurses can help to normalize feelings of sadness and anger by restating patients' frustrations, which can help patients through this difficult process.

Fingeret et al. (2012) reported that body image dissatisfaction was greater in younger patients, with 25%–44% dissatisfied with the information they received related to body image. Furthermore, 34% wanted assistance either in written format (e.g., pamphlets, print resources) or in counseling services, if available, within the facility. These patients preferred not to be referred to an outside mental health specialist (Fingeret et al., 2012). This suggests that patients need more than a brochure or a website to address their body image concerns. These findings support nursing's role in the education and referral processes for patients with body image concerns. See Figure 15-2 for more interventions.

## Evidence-Based Practice

Research is limited in identifying interventions to promote healthy body image in patients with cancer. The use of cognitive behavioral therapy (CBT) as an intervention

### Table 15-3. Examples of Communication Strategies for Addressing Body Image Concerns

| | Body Image Challenge | Typical Approaches | Preferred Approaches — Exploratory Phrases | Preferred Approaches — Empathic Phrases |
|---|---|---|---|---|
| Example #1 | "I can't stand to look in the mirror or show my body to my husband since my mastectomy." | Premature reassurance: You look great! Don't worry, your swelling will continue to go down, and things will look even better in a few weeks. | What do you see when you look in the mirror? Have you discussed your concerns with your husband? | This must be a huge adjustment for you, since you used to be more comfortable with your body. |
| Example #2 | "I rarely leave the house since my surgery. I don't like when people stare at me or talk about my appearance or garbled speech. I worry about what others think of me, especially my grandkids." | Cheerleader: You need to get out more, and you will feel better. Your family needs you and loves you just the way you are. | What do you think your grandkids think of you now? Do you think your friends and family miss seeing you? | You obviously love your grandkids tremendously. It must be very difficult for you to not spend time with them like you used to. |
| Example #3 | "I had beautiful hair down to my waist before I started chemotherapy. I can't stop crying about my hair falling out." | Cheerleader: Don't give up! You're nearly done with chemo. | Tell me more about what this is like for you. Do you have any close friends or family you feel comfortable talking to about your concerns? | I know how much pride you take in your appearance, so this must be very difficult for you. |
| Example #4 | "There is no way I'm getting a (colostomy) bag. Everyone will be able to see it through my clothes, and my wife will never sleep with me again." | Premature reassurance: Ostomy bags these days are easily concealable beneath your clothes. Education, scare tactic: If you don't get proper treatment, you will die of your cancer. | Tell me more about your concerns. Have you discussed this issue with your wife? | I can imagine the thought of having a colostomy bag must be shocking and can be difficult to accept at first. I understand that you have a lot of concerns. |

*Note.* From "Managing Body Image Difficulties of Adult Cancer Patients: Lessons From Available Research," by M.C. Fingeret, I. Teo, and D.E. Epner, 2014, *Cancer, 120*, p. 639. Copyright 2014 by American Cancer Society. Reprinted with permission.

**Assessment**
- Recognize that body image includes more than the physical body alone.
- Consider the variables that may have an impact on body image (e.g., loss of a body part, change or loss of function, immediate versus prolonged change).
- Use the Body Image Scale or other tools available to assess the extent of possible concern or dysfunction.
- Be aware if patients are making treatment decisions based on anticipating body image changes.
- Identify the following:
  - Feelings of anger, sadness, frustration, and guilt
  - The nature of the threat
  - Patient's support system
- Continue to reassess patients' responses at all stages (e.g., diagnosis, treatment, recovery).
- Evaluate the need for more in-depth assessment and counseling.

**Nursing Diagnoses** (NANDA International, 2015)
- Disturbed body image
- Disturbed personal identity
- Sexual dysfunction
- Readiness for enhanced self-concept

***DSM-V* Diagnoses** (American Psychiatric Association, 2013)
- Adjustment disorder
- Anxiety disorders
- Depressive disorders
- Body dysmorphic disorder
- Sexual dysfunction

**Expected Outcomes**
- Patients/partners will accept help or care.
- Patients/partners will acknowledge and discuss body loss/changes.
- Patients/partners will look at the affected area.
- Patients/partners will reject feelings of being dirty or defiled and contaminated.
- Patients will not feel stigmatized.
- Patients/partners will resume sexual activity as appropriate.
- Patients/spouses/families will resume social and recreational activities.

**Interventions**
- Acknowledge loss.
- Provide opportunity for discussion of body changes.
- Maintain modesty and privacy to show patients that they are valued.
- Demonstrate acceptance of an altered body and change in functions.
- Focus on abilities rather than disabilities or loss.
- Provide/assist with meticulous personal care.
- Offer realistic compliments.
- Assist partners to accept change.
- Assist patients to strengthen a newly reorganized sense of self.
- Help patients to view and touch the changed area as appropriate.
- Provide necessary strategies (e.g., wig, prosthesis) for dealing with anticipated changes.
- Provide access to specific group therapy resources, support groups, and other services (e.g., Reach to Recovery; Look Good Feel Better; Y-ME) (see Appendix).

**Figure 15-2. Plan of Care**

approach has been studied most (Fingeret et al., 2014). These studies involved group sessions where the focus was on addressing dysfunctional thoughts, emotions, and behaviors through goal setting, cognitive restructuring, systematic desensitization, and skills training conducted by a mental health professional (Cash, 2011). Several studies have demonstrated improvements for participants using the CBT approach (Fadaei et al., 2011; Fingeret et al., 2014).

Evidence-based clinical practice guidelines do not exist per se for body image disturbance. However, both the Agency for Healthcare Research and Quality (www.guideline.gov) and the National Comprehensive Cancer Network® (www.nccn.org) provide guidelines that indirectly may affect body image.

## Case Study

Steve is a 58-year-old man who is married and has one adult daughter. He was working as an engineer when he was diagnosed with HPV-positive oropharyngeal cancer on the base of his tongue that extended into the floor of his mouth. He underwent a surgical resection with a split thickness skin graft taken from his left thigh. He also had a right neck dissection and a tracheostomy with copious secretions and a gastrostomy tube. He was discharged with both the tracheostomy and gastrostomy and required radiation and chemotherapy because of the high incidence of recurrence.

Upon his first clinic visit in preparation for chemotherapy, Steve's nurse observes he is not making eye contact and appears depressed. His wife reports that he is very irritable. Steve is started on an antidepressant at his wife's request. In subsequent clinic visits for chemotherapy, Steve remains depressed. He has lost 15 pounds since surgery and tells the nurse that he does not want to leave his house except to go to the doctor or walk his dog. His nurse attempts to engage him in more conversation, but verbalization is very difficult due to Steve's tracheostomy. He generally only speaks one-word answers when asked a direct question. The nurse feels at a loss as to how to help.

Some months later, after completion of his chemotherapy and radiation, Steve's tracheostomy is removed. At a follow-up visit, he rarely speaks during the consultation. His wife tells the nurse that he remains very depressed and does not want to go out in public. He has had several episodes of choking when around other people and continues to have a lot of secretions. He underwent swallowing therapy, but his wife reports he has continued to be very fearful of oral intake. Steve's wife tells the nurse, "I never realized how social eating and drinking was before this."

### Discussion

Steve clearly was depressed and socially isolated. He most likely felt overwhelmed by his body image deficits and embarrassed by not being able to control his secretions when swallowing, which resulted in prolonged coughing. This led to avoidance of social situations, which increased his isolation and depression. As a male engineer, Steve may have had a strong need to be able to "fix" his own situation, which led to further feelings of helplessness and isolation.

Steve was presented at the clinic's psychosocial rounds, and the advanced practice nurse (APN) scheduled an individual appointment with the patient. The APN opened the consultation by acknowledging all the life changes Steve had experienced since the initial surgery. He acknowledged feeling "untouchable, dirty, and inadequate." He said, "I am always spitting and hacking, and I cannot eat or drink anything without choking." Steve has felt that people are uncomfortable around him because of his difficulty in swallowing his saliva. Steve explained he has been feeling this way since his surgery but had been unable to acknowledge these feelings until now. After further discussion, Steve agreed to share his feelings with his wife to reduce his sense of isolation. The APN also referred Steve to a local support group for patients with HNC so that he could learn how others are coping with the body image changes in eating and swallowing from treatment. Steve remained on the antidepressant and agreed to an appointment with the clinic psychologist for his social avoidance and his persistent depression. At the appointment, he benefitted from acknowledging what he was feeling rather than hiding and avoiding contact with others. With this new awareness, Steve's family could reinforce their love and caring for him by demonstrating affection and physical contact. Steve benefitted from this support and could make more efforts to be around others. He started slowly by increasing his socialization, first with family, then with a few close friends.

## Conclusion

Body image is how people think, feel, and see. It also comprises attitudes, beliefs, and self-evaluations about themselves and their own bodies, including bodily and sexual function. Body image is a mental and attitudinal impression formed by past or historical experiences and current situations. This self-evaluation is determined by mental and attitudinal impressions that can be influenced by family, friends, occupation, society, and culture, thus affecting behaviors. Body image perception and self-evaluation are dynamic processes that are ever changing (Cash, 2011). A chronic physical illness such as cancer can create a complex array of thoughts, perceptions, self-evaluations, and behaviors that translate into changes and distortions in body image. These changes will vary depending on the cancer site and treatment and will be affected by the patient's age, sex, life experience, support systems, and usual or pre-illness coping mechanisms.

Continued research will be necessary to define and describe the effect of cancer and its treatment on body image and function, as this relates to all specific cancer sites. Investigators must perform more prospective studies examining body image before cancer treatments and must follow up for longer periods to further describe, assess, and test specific interventions related to body image. Interventions to improve body self-esteem as it relates to body image must also be investigated. Through continued efforts encompassing assessment and interventions guided by evidence-based practice, nurses will be able to be more sensitive to the ways in which patients maintain or restore an orientation to their bodies and body function. With therapeutic communication, empathy, and compassionate interventions, patients may be able to look forward with realistic hope to the whole range of individual relationships with themselves, as well as to richer human interrelationships, including with spouses and partners, parents, children, siblings, and friends. In addition, patients enhance social, occupational, and recreational relationships with an accepting, revised, and renewed body image.

*The author would like to acknowledge Carol Campbell-Norris, BA, MS, and Judith A. Shell, PhD, LMFT, RN, AOCN®, for their contributions to this chapter from the previous edition of this book.*

## References

Aboumohamed, A.A., Raza, S.J., Al-Daghmin, A., Tallman, C., Creighton, T., Crossley, H., ... Guru, K.A. (2014). Health-related quality of life outcomes after robot-assisted and open radical cystectomy using a validated bladder-specific instrument: A multi-institutional study. *Urology, 83,* 1300–1308. doi:10.1016/j.urology.2014.02.024

American Cancer Society. (2017). *Cancer facts and figures, 2017.* Retrieved from https://www.cancer.org/content/dam/cancer-org/research/cancer-facts-and-statistics/annual-cancer-facts-and-figures/2017/cancer-facts-and-figures-2017.pdf

American Psychiatric Association. (2013). *Diagnostic and statistical manual of mental disorders* (5th ed.). Washington, DC: Author.

Andersson, J., Angenete, E., Gellerstedt, M., Angeras, U., Jess, P., Rosenberg, J., ... Haglind, E. (2013). Health-related quality of life after laparoscopic and open surgery for rectal cancer. *British Journal of Surgery, 100,* 941–949. doi:10.1002/bjs.9144

Atkinson, T.M., Noce, N.S., Hay, J., Rafferty, B.T., & Brady, M.S. (2013). Illness-related distress in women with clinically localized cutaneous melanoma. *Annals of Surgical Oncology, 20,* 675–679. doi:10.1245/s10434-012-2635-5

Azvolinsky, A. (2015). Breast irradiation therapy innovations forgo permanent marks, minimize treatment. *Journal of the National Cancer Institute, 107.* doi:10.1093/jnci/djv067

Baker, L., & Gringart, E. (2009). Body image and self-esteem in older adulthood. *Aging and Society, 29,* 977–995.

Barlow, E.L., Hacker, N.F., Hussain, R., & Parmenter, G. (2014). Sexuality and body image following treatment for early-stage vulvar cancer: A qualitative study. *Journal of Advanced Nursing, 70,* 1856–1866. doi:10.1111/jan.12346

Bellizzi, K.M., Smith, A., Schmidt, S., Keegan, T.H.M., Zebrack, B., Lynch, C.F., ... Simon, M. (2012). Positive and negative psychosocial impact of being diagnosed with cancer as an adolescent or young adult. *Cancer, 118,* 5155–5162. doi:10.1002/cncr.27512

Berlucchi, G., & Aglioti, S.M. (2010). The body in the brain revisited. *Experimental Brain Research, 200,* 25–35. doi:10.1007/s00221-009-1970-7

Brotto, L.A., Yule, M., & Breckon, E. (2010). Psychological interventions for the sexual sequelae of cancer: A review of the literature. *Journal of Cancer Survivorship, 4,* 346–360. doi:10.1007/s11764-010-0132-z

Carpenito-Moyet, L.J. (Ed.). (2006). *Nursing diagnosis: Application to clinical practice* (11th ed.). Philadelphia, PA: Lippincott Williams & Wilkins.

Carpentier, M.Y., Fortenberry, J.D., Ott, M.A., Brames, M.J., & Einhorn, L.H. (2011). Perceptions of masculinity and self-image in adolescent and young testicular cancer survivors: Implications for romantic and sexual relationships. *Psycho-Oncology, 20,* 738–745. doi:10.1002/pon.1772

Cash, T.F. (2011). Cognitive-behavioral perspectives on body image. In T.F. Cash & L. Smolak (Eds.), *Body image: A handbook of science, practice, and prevention* (2nd ed., pp. 39–47). New York, NY: Guilford Press.

Cash, T.F., & Pruzinsky, T. (Eds.). (2004). Future challenges for body image theory, research, and clinical practice. In T.F. Cash & T. Pruzinsky (Eds.), *Body image: A handbook of theory, research, and clinical practice* (pp. 509–516). New York, NY: Guilford Press.

Cash, T.F., & Smolak, L. (Eds.). (2011). Understanding body images: Historical and contemporary perspectives. In T.F. Cash & L. Smolak (Eds.), *Body image: A handbook of science, practice, and prevention* (2nd ed., pp. 3–11). New York, NY: Guilford Press.

Chapple, A., & Ziebland, S. (2002). Prostate cancer: Embodied experience and perceptions of masculinity. *Sociology of Health and Illness, 24,* 820–841. doi:10.1111/1467-9566.00320

Chen, S.-C., Yu, P.-J., Hong, M.-Y., Chen, M.-H., Chu, P.-Y., Chen, Y.-J., ... Lai, Y.-H. (2014). Communication dysfunction, body image, and symptom severity in postoperative head and neck cancer patients: Factors associated with the amount of speaking after treatment. *Supportive Care in Cancer, 23,* 2375–2382. doi:10.1007/s00520-014-2587-3

Cho, A., Kwak, S.-M., & Lee, J.-H. (2013). Identifying attentional bias and emotional response after appearance-related stimuli exposure. *Cyberpsychology, Behavior, and Social Networking, 16,* 50–55. doi:10.1089/cyber.2012.0223

Cohen, R., & Blaszczynski, A. (2015). Comparative effects of Facebook and conventional media on body image dissatisfaction. *Journal of Eating Disorders, 3,* 1–11. doi:10.1186/s40337-015-0061-3

Cotrim, H., & Pereira, G. (2008). Impact of colorectal cancer on patient and family: Implications for care. *European Journal of Oncology Nursing, 12,* 217–226. doi:10.1016/j.ejon.2007.11.005

Dittmar, H., Halliwell, E., & Ive, S. (2006). Does Barbie make girls want to be thin? The effect of experimental exposure to images of dolls on the body image of 5- to 8-year-old girls. *Developmental Psychology, 42,* 283–292. doi:10.1037/0012-1649.42.2.283

Dooks, P., McQuestion, M., Goldstein, D., & Molassiotis, A. (2012). Experiences of patients with laryngectomies as they integrate into their community. *Supportive Care in Cancer, 20,* 489–498. doi:10.1007/s00520-011-1101-4

Dropkin, M.J. (1997). Postoperative body image in head and neck cancer patients. *Quality of Life–A Nursing Challenge, 4,* 110–113.

Dropkin, M.J. (1999). Postoperative body image in head and neck cancer patients. *Cancer Practice, 7,* 309–313.

Erba, P., Farhadi, J., Wettstein, R., Arnold, A., Harr, T., & Pierer, G. (2007). Morphoeic basal cell carcinoma of the face. *Scandanavian Journal of Plastic Reconstructive and Hand Surgery, 41,* 184–188. doi:10.1080/02844310701282138

Ervik, B., & Asplund, K. (2012). Dealing with a troublesome body: A qualitative interview study of men's experiences living with prostate cancer treated with endocrine therapy. *European Journal Oncology Nursing, 16,* 103–108. doi:10.1016/j/ejon.2011.04.005

Fadaei, S., Janighorban, M., Mehrabi, T., Ahmadi, S.A., Mokaryan, F., & Gukizade, A. (2011). Effects of cognitive behavioral counseling on body image following mastectomy. *Journal of Research in Medical Sciences, 16,* 1047–1054.

Fallon, E.A., & Hausenblas, H.A. (2005). Media images of the "ideal" female body: Can acute exercise moderate their psychological impact? *Body Image, 2,* 62–73. doi:10.1016/j.bodyim.2004.12.001

Field, E.A., Camargo, C.A., Jr., Taylor, C.B., Berkey, C.S., Roberts, S.B., & Colditz, G.A. (2001). Peer, parent, and media influences on the development of weight concerns and frequent dieting among preadolescent and adolescent girls and boys. *Pediatrics, 107,* 54–60. doi:10.1542/peds.107.1.54

Filippetti, M.L., Johnson, M.H., Lloyd-Fox, S., Dragovic, D., & Farroni, T. (2013). Body perception in newborns. *Current Biology, 23,* 2413–2416. doi:10.1016/j.cub.2013.10.017

Fingeret, M.C. (2010). Body image and disfigurement. In J. Duffy & A. Valentine (Eds.), *MD Anderson manual of psychosocial oncology* (pp. 271–288). New York, NY: McGraw-Hill.

Fingeret, M.C., Teo, I., & Epner, D.E. (2014). Managing body image difficulties in adult cancer patients: Lessons from available research. *Cancer, 120,* 633–641. doi:10.1002/cncr.28469

Fingeret, M.C., Vidrine, D.J., Reece, G.P., Gillenwater, A.M., & Gritz, E.R. (2010). Multidimensional analysis of body image concerns among newly diagnosed patients with oral cavity cancer. *Head and Neck, 32,* 301–309. doi:10.1002/hed.21181

Fingeret, M.C., Yuan, Y., Urbauer, D., Weston, J., Nipomnick, S., & Weber, R. (2012). The nature and extent of body image concerns among surgically treated patients with head and neck cancer. *Psycho-Oncology, 21,* 836–844. doi:10.1002/pon.1990

Foster, R.H., & Stern, M. (2014). Peer and romantic relationships among adolescent and young adult survivors of childhood hematological cancer: A review of challenges and positive outcomes. *Acta Haematologica, 132,* 375–382. doi:10.1159/000360239

Fu, M.R., Ridner, S.H., Hu, S.H., Stewart, B.R., Cormier, J.N., & Armer, J.M. (2012). Psychosocial impact of lymphedema: A systematic review of literature from 2004 to 2011. *Psycho-Oncology, 22,* 1466–1484. doi:10.1002/pon.3201

Gacci, M., Saleh, O., Tommaso, C., Gore, J.L., D'Elia, C., Minervini, A., ... Carini, M. (2013). Quality of life in women undergoing urinary diversion for bladder cancer: Results of a multicenter study among long-term disease-free survivors. *Health and Quality of Life Outcomes, 11,* 43. doi:10.1186/1477-7525-11-43

Giacomoni, C., Venturini, E., Hoarau, H., Guyon, F., & Conri, V. (2014). How women with gynaecological cancer deal with treatment: Issues of visibility and invisibility. *Gynécologie Obstétrique et Fertilité, 42,* 795–799. doi:10.1016/j.gyobfe.2014.09.013

Gilbert, S.M., Dunn, R.L., Hollernbeck, B.K., Montie, J.E., Lee, C.T., Wood, D.P., & Wei, J.T. (2010). Development and validation of the Bladder Cancer Index: A comprehensive, disease specific measure of health related quality of life in patients with localized bladder cancer. *Journal of Urology, 183,* 1764–1769. doi:10.1061/j.juro.2010.01.013

Godoy, A., Ishii, M., Byrne, P.J., Boahene, K.D.O., Encarnacion, C.O., & Ishii, L.E. (2011). How facial lesions impact attractiveness and perception: Differential effects of size and location. *Laryngoscope, 121,* 2542–2547. doi:10.1002/lary.22334

Gopie, J.P., ter Kuile, M.M., Timman, R., Murear, M.A.M., & Tibben, A. (2014). Impact of delayed implant and DIEP flap breast reconstruction on body image and sexual satisfaction: A prospective follow-up study. *Psycho-Oncology, 23,* 100–107. doi:10.1002/pon/3377

Grogan, S. (2008). *Body image: Understanding body dissatisfaction in men, women, and children* (2nd ed.). East Sussex, United Kingdom: Routledge.

Grogan, S. (2011). Body image development in adulthood. In T.F. Cash & L. Smolak (Eds.), *Body image: A handbook of science, practice, and prevention* (2nd ed., pp. 93–100). New York, NY: Guilford Press.

Harcourt, D., & Rumsey, N. (2011). Body image and biomedical interventions for disfiguring conditions. In T.F. Cash & L. Smolak (Eds.), *Body image: A handbook of science, practice, and prevention* (2nd ed., pp. 404–412). New York, NY: Guilford Press.

Hargreaves, D.A., & Tiggeman, M. (2004). Idealized media images and adolescent body image: "Comparing" boys and girls. *Body Image, 1,* 351–361. doi:10.1016/j.bodyim.2004.10.002

Harrington, J.M., Jones, E.G., & Badger, T. (2009). Body image perceptions in men with prostate cancer. *Oncology Nursing Forum, 36,* 167–172. doi:10.1188/09.ONF.167-172

Hawighorst-Knapstein, S., Fusshoeller, C., Franz, C., Trautmann, K., Schmidt, M., Pilch, H., ... Vaupel, P. (2004). The impact of treatment for genital cancer on quality of life and body image: Results of a prospective longitudinal 10-year study. *Gynecologic Oncology, 94,* 398–403. doi:10.1016/j.ygyno.2004.04.025

Hedestig, O., Sandman, P.O., Tomic, R., & Widmark, A. (2005). Living after external beam radiotherapy of localized prostate cancer: A qualitative analysis of patient narratives. *Cancer Nursing, 28,* 310–317. doi:10.1097/00002820-200507000-00013

Heflick, N.A., & Goldenberg, J.L. (2014). Seeing eye to body: The literal objectification of women. *Current Directions in Psychological Science, 23,* 225–229. doi:10.1177/0963721414531599

Herzog, T.J., & Wright, J.D. (2007). The impact of cervical cancer on quality of life—The components and means for management. *Gynecologic Oncology, 107,* 572–577. doi:10.1016/j.ygyno.2007.09.019

Hopwood, P., Fletcher, I., Lee, A., & Al Ghazal, S. (2001). A body image scale for use with cancer patients. *European Journal of Cancer, 37,* 189–197. doi:10.1016/S0959-8049(00)00353-1

Hopwood, P., Haviland, J.S., Sumo, G., Mills, J., Bliss, J.M., & Yarnold, J.R. (2010). Comparison of patient-reported breast, arm, and shoulder symptoms and body image after radiotherapy for early breast cancer: 5-year follow-up in the randomized Standardization of Breast Radiotherapy (START) trials. *Lancet Oncology, 11,* 231–240. doi:10.1016/S1470-2045(09)70382-1

Incrocci, L., Hop, W.C., Wijnmaalen, A., & Slob, A.K. (2002). Treatment outcome, body image, and sexual functioning after orchiectomy and radiotherapy for stage I–II testicular seminoma. *International Journal of Radiation Oncology, Biology, Physics, 53,* 1165–1173. doi:10.1016/S0360-3016(02)02849-3

Kieffer, J.M., Djajadiningrat, R.S., van Muilekom, E.A.M., Graafland, N.M., Horenblas, S., & Aaronson, N.K. (2014). Quality of life for patients treated for penile cancer. *Journal of Urology, 192,* 1105–1110. doi:10.1016/j.juro.2014.04.014

Kim, M.K., Kim, T., Moon, H.G., Jin, U.S., Kim, K.J., Kim, J.W., ... Han, W. (2015). Effect of cosmetic outcome on quality of life after breast cancer surgery. *European Journal of Surgical Oncology, 41,* 426–432. doi:10.1016/j.ejso.2014.12.002

Konradsen, H., Kirkevold, M., & Zoffman, V. (2009). Surgical facial cancer treatment: The silencing of disfigurement in nurse–patient interactions. *Journal of Advanced Nursing, 65,* 2409–2418. doi:10.1111/j.1365-2648.2009.05102.x

Korfage, I.J., Essink-Bot, M.-L., Mols, F., van de Poll-Franse, L., Kruitwagen, R., & van Ballegooijen, M. (2009). Health-related quality of life in cervical cancer survivors: A population-based survey. *International Journal of Radiation Oncology, Biology, Physics, 73,* 1501–1509. doi:10.1016/j.ijrobp.2008.06.1905

Laken, V., & Laken, K. (2002). *Making love again: Hope for couples facing loss of sexual intimacy.* East Sandwich, MA: North Star Publications.

Larouche, S.S., & Chin-Peuckert, L. (2006). Changes in body image experienced by adolescents with cancer. *Journal of Pediatric Oncology, 23,* 200–209. doi:10.1177/1043454206289756

Levine, M.P., & Chapman, K. (2011). Media influences on body image. In T.F. Cash & L. Smolak (Eds.), *Body image: A handbook of science, practice, and prevention* (2nd ed., pp. 101–109). New York, NY: Guilford Press.

Levine, M.P., & Smolak, L. (2004). Body image development in adolescence. In T.F. Cash & L. Pruzinsky (Eds.), *Body image: A handbook of theory, research, and clinical practice* (pp. 74–82). New York, NY: Guilford Press.

Liavaag, A.H., Dørum, A., Bjøro, T., Oksefjell, H., Fosså, S.D., Tropé, C., & Dahl, A.A. (2008). A controlled study of sexual activity and functioning in epithelial ovarian cancer survivors. A therapeutic approach. *Gynecologic Oncology, 108,* 348–354. doi:10.1016/j.ygyno.2007.10.009

Maguire, P., Faulkner, A., Booth, K., Elliot, C., & Hillier, V. (1996). Helping cancer patients disclose their concerns. *European Journal of Cancer, 32,* 78–81. doi:10.1016/0959-8049(95)00527-7

McCabe, M.P., Ricciardelli, L.A., & Finemore, J. (2002). The role of puberty, media and popularity with peers on strategies to increase weight, decrease weight and increase muscle tone among adolescent boys and girls. *Journal of Psychosomatic Research, 52,* 145–153. doi:10.1016/S0022-3999(01)00272-0

McKenzie, F., White, C.A., Kendall, S., Finlayson, A., Urquhart, M., & Williams, I. (2006). Psychological impact of colostomy pouch change and disposal. *British Journal of Nursing, 15,* 308–316. doi:10.12968/bjon.2006.15.6.20678

McKinley, N.M. (2004). Feminist perspectives of objectified body consciousness. In T.F. Cash & L. Pruzinsky (Eds.), *Body image: A handbook of theory, research, and clinical practice* (pp. 55–62). New York, NY: Guilford Press.

Morse, J.M., Bottorff, J.L., & Hutchinson, S. (1995). The paradox of comfort. *Nursing Research, 44,* 14–19. doi:10.1097/00006199-199501000-00004

Mulders, M., Vingerhoets, A., & Breed, W. (2008). The impact of cancer and chemotherapy: Perceptual similarities and differences between cancer patients, nurses, and physicians. *European Journal of Oncology Nursing, 12,* 97–102. doi:10.1016/j.ejon.2007.10.002

NANDA International. (2015). *Nursing diagnoses: Definitions and classification, 2015–2017.* Philadelphia, PA: Author.

Oliffe, J. (2005). Constructions of masculinity following prostatectomy-induced impotence. *Social Science and Medicine, 60,* 2249–2259. doi:10.1016/j.socscimed.2004.10.016

Palapattu, G.S., Haisfield-Wolfe, M.E., Walker, J.M., Brintzenhoffeszoc, K., Trock, B., Zabora, J., & Schoenberg, M. (2004). Assessment of perioperative psychological distress in patients undergoing radical cystectomy for bladder cancer. *Journal of Urology, 172,* 1814–1817. doi:10.1097/01.ju.0000141245.08456.1a

Patt, M.R., Lane, A.E., Finney, C.P., Yanek, L.R., & Becker, D.M. (2002). Body image assessment: Comparison of figure rating scales among urban black women. *Ethnic Disease, 12,* 54–62.

Pruzinsky, T. (1996). Social and psychological effects of facial disfigurement: Quality of life, body image and surgical reconstruction. In R.W. Weber, H. Goepfert, & M.J. Miller (Eds.), *Basal and squamous cell skin cancers of the head and neck* (pp. 357–362). Philadelphia, PA: Lippincott Williams & Wilkins.

Radiotis, G., Roberts, N., Czajkowska, Z., Khanna, M., & Körner, A. (2014). Nonmelanoma skin cancer: Disease-specific quality-of-life concerns and distress. *Oncology Nursing Forum, 41,* 57–65. doi:10.1188/14.ONF.57-65

Rancour, P., & Brauer, K. (2003). Use of letter writing as a means of integrating an altered body image: A case study. *Oncology Nursing Forum, 30,* 841–846. doi:10.1188/03.ONF.841-846

Rasmussen, D.M., Hansen, H.P., & Elverdam, B. (2010). How cancer survivors experience their changed body encountering others. *European Journal of Oncology Nursing, 14,* 154–159. doi:10.1016/j.ejon.2009.10.001

Rezk, Y.A., Hurley, K.E., Carter, J., Dao, F., Bochner, B.H., Aubey, J.J., ... Maker, V. (2013). A prospective study of quality of life in patients undergoing pelvic exenteration: Interim results. *Gynecologic Oncology, 128,* 191–197. doi:10.1016/j.ygyno.2012.09.030

Ricciardelli, L.A., & McCabe, M.P. (2011). Body image development in adolescent boys. In T.F. Cash & L. Smolak (Eds.), *Body image: A handbook of science, practice, and prevention* (2nd ed., pp. 85–92). New York, NY: Guilford Press.

Rossen, P., Pedersen, A.F., Zachariae, R., & von der Maase, H. (2012). Sexuality and body image in long-term survivors of testicular cancer. *European Journal of Cancer, 48,* 571–578. doi:10.1016/j.ejca.2011.11.029

Schilder, P. (1950). *The image and appearance of the human body.* New York, NY: International Universities Press.

Schover, L.R. (2005). Sexuality and fertility after cancer. *American Society of Hematology Education Program Book, 2005, 523*–527. doi:10.1182/asheducation-2005.1.523

Sharpe, L., Patel, D., & Clarke, S. (2011). Relationship between body image disturbance and distress in colorectal cancer patients with and without stomas. *Journal of Psychosomatic Research, 70,* 395–403. doi:10.1016/j.jpsychores.2010.11.003

Shontz, R.C. (1990). Body image and physical disability. In T.F. Cash & T. Pruzinsky (Eds.), *Body image: Development, deviance, and change* (pp. 149–169). New York, NY: Guilford Press.

Siegel, R.L., Miller, K.D., & Jemal, A. (2017). Cancer statistics, 2017. *CA: A Cancer Journal for Clinicians, 67,* 7–31. doi:10.3322/caac.21387

Silva, M.L.A., Taquette, S.R., & Coutinho, E.S.F. (2014). Senses of body image in adolescents in elementary school. *Revista de Saúde Pública, 48,* 438–444. doi:10.1590/S0034-8910.2014048005083

Smolak, L. (2011). Body image development in childhood. In T.F. Cash & L. Smolak (Eds.), *Body image: A handbook of science, practice, and prevention* (2nd ed., pp. 67–75). New York, NY: Guilford Press.

Snöbohm, C., Friedrichsen, M., & Heiwe, S. (2010). Experiencing one's body after a diagnosis of cancer—A phenomenological study of young adults. *Psycho-Oncology, 10,* 863–869. doi:10.1002/pon.1632

Stern, C. (1990). Body image concerns, surgical conditions, and sexuality. In C. Fogel & D. Lauver (Eds.), *Sexual health promotion* (pp. 498–516). Philadelphia, PA: Elsevier Saunders.

Swami, V., & Szmigielska, E. (2013). Body image concerns in professional fashion models: Are they really an at-risk group? *Psychiatry Research, 20,* 113–117. doi:10.1016/j.psychres.2012.09.009

Taylor-Ford, M., Meyerowitz, B.E., D'Orazio, L.M., Christie, K.M., Gross, M.E., & Agus, D.B. (2013). Body image predicts quality of life in men with prostate cancer. *Psycho-Oncology, 22,* 756–761. doi:10.1002/pon.3063

Teo, I., Fingeret, M.C., Liu, J., & Chang, D.W. (2015). Coping and quality of life of patients following microsurgical treatments for breast cancer–related lymphedema. *Journal of Health Psychology, 21,* 2983–2993. doi:10.1177/1359105315589801

Teo, I., Novy, D.M., Chang, D.W., Cox, M.G., & Fingeret, M.C. (2015). Examining pain, body image, and depressive symptoms in patients with lymphedema secondary to breast cancer. *Psycho-Oncology, 24,* 1377–1383. doi:10.1002/pon.3745

Teo, I., Reece, G.P., Christie, I.C., Guindani, M., Markey, M.K., Heinberg, L.J., ... Fingeret, M.C. (2015). Body image and quality of life of breast cancer patients: Influence of timing and stage of breast reconstruction. *Psycho-Oncology, 25,* 1106–1112. doi:10.1002/pon.3952

Thomas, R., & Hamilton, R. (2014). Illustrating the (in)visible: Understanding the impact of loss in adults living with secondary lymphedema after cancer. *International Journal of Qualitative Studies on Health and Well-Being, 9.* doi:10.3402/qhw.v9.24354

Thompson, J.K. (Ed.). (2004). *Handbook of eating disorders and obesity.* New York, NY: John Wiley & Sons.

Tiggemann, M. (2011). Sociocultural perspectives on human appearance and body image. In T.F. Cash & L. Smolak (Eds.), *Body image: A handbook of science, practice, and prevention* (2nd ed., pp. 12–19). New York, NY: Guilford Press.

Wertheim, E.H., & Paxton, S.J. (2011). Body image development in adolescent girls. In T.F. Cash & L. Smolak (Eds.), *Body image: A handbook of science, practice, and prevention* (2nd ed., pp. 76–84). New York, NY: Guilford Press.

Wiederman, M.W. (2011). Body image and sexual functioning. In T.F. Cash & L. Smolak (Eds.), *Body image: A handbook of science, practice, and prevention* (2nd ed., pp. 271–278). New York, NY: Guilford Press.

Wong, F.L., Francisco, L., Togawa, K., Kim, H., Bosworth, A., Atencio, L., ... Bhatia, S. (2013). Longitudinal trajectory of sexual functioning after hematopoietic cell transplantation: Impact of chronic graft-versus-host disease and total body irradiation. *Blood, 122,* 3973–3981. doi:10.1182/blood-2013-05-499806

Wortel, R.C., Alemayehu, W.G., & Incrocci, L. (2015). Orchiectomy and radiotherapy for stage I–II testicular seminoma: A prospective evaluation of short-term effects on body image and sexual function. *Journal of Sexual Medicine, 12,* 210–218. doi:10.1111/jsm.12739

Zoletić, E., & Duraković-Belko, E. (2009). Body image distortion, perfectionism and eating disorder symptoms in risk group of female ballet dancers and models and in control group of female students. *Psychiatria Danubina, 21,* 302–309.

# CHAPTER 16

# Denial

*Linda M. Gorman, RN, MN, PMHCNS-BC, CHPN, FPCN*

> *A great deal of intelligence can be invested in ignorance when the need for illusion is deep.*
>
> —Saul Bellow

Faced with a diagnosis of cancer, a man maintains the staunch belief that his doctor has made a mistake. At the time of diagnosis of metastasis, a family member tries to persuade the patient to refuse therapy because he does not believe the patient really has cancer. A patient who is dying refuses home hospice care because she plans to "beat this thing." All of these scenarios can exemplify varying degrees of denial. Although literature related to this subject exists, the concept of denial remains confusing and elusive. Denial can be confused with hope, wisdom, positive attitude, avoidance, contradiction, escape, misinformation, and delusion (Borneman, Irish, Sidhu, Koczywas, & Cristea, 2014; Kreitler, 1999; Weisman, 1989). Clinicians frequently use the term *denial* in clinical practice, even though its meaning sometimes can be unclear.

Strictly speaking, denial is a form of self-deception. It is a defense against anxiety because of a threat. It is a means to achieve psychological equilibrium, even if the defense creates more dysfunction (Block, 2006). Originally, denial was identified in psychoanalytic theory as a pathological reaction to unacceptable thoughts and feelings. Over time, it has been broadened to be viewed as a coping mechanism that can be adaptive or maladaptive (Vos, Putter, van Houwelingen, & de Haes, 2008). It is complex, multilayered, and difficult to measure.

In a sense, all defense mechanisms use denial to the extent that reality is distorted to cope with a stressor. Individuals deal with emotional conflict from internal or external stressors by refusing to acknowledge some painful aspect of the reality or subjective experience that would be apparent to others (McIntyre, Norton, & McIntyre, 2009). In a psychiatric sense, complete denial is a primitive unconscious defense that is viewed as pathologic. It can be seen in some personality disorders, psychoses, and periods of regression (Kernberg, 2009). Complete denial may be viewed as a delusion when reality is completely distorted. For example, a patient with cancer may think, *I was well before I came to the doctor; he made me sick.*

Denial is commonly viewed as a way to temporarily minimize a threat and protect oneself from intolerable thoughts, such as a threat to one's existence. This is especially common in life-threatening illnesses (Block, 2006). Denial generally fluctuates and can be viewed on a continuum. Given the situation and level of threat at a particular moment, denial can be present or absent (Vos et al., 2008). This may explain why a person can appear to be using denial one minute but is able to acknowledge the stressor the next. Rousseau (2000) defined denial as an unconscious mechanism aimed at negating a disease-oriented threat to the integrity of personhood and daily life. Denial can be pathologic when the individual remains out of touch with reality and makes poor decisions based on this altered reality.

As an initial response to bad news, denial is considered to be a normal and an adaptive response to any loss (Kreitler, 1999; Stephenson, 2004). Hearing that a breast lump is malignant or that a loved one suddenly has died may represent such overwhelming stress to individuals that blocking it out becomes a protective mechanism. It is recognized as a common reaction in acute grief. For example, upon hearing news of the death of a loved one, a denial response may be "That's not true. He's getting better, not worse." Denial is the first stage of grief identified by Elisabeth Kübler-Ross (1969). This first stage of grief is sometimes referred to as shock and disbelief (Engle, 1962). In some cases, its presence has been shown to increase the length of the bereavement period (Buckley et al., 2015).

## Denial and Coping

Denial is an adaptive coping mechanism to temporarily reduce stress. It is woven into many coping mechanisms. Weisman's (1972) early research on denial suggested that excessive use of denial is a sign of poor coping. Good copers have confidence in their abilities to deal with problems, not avoid them.

Denial protects the integrity of one's self-concept by distorting reality in a self-enhancing way. It promotes a sense of mastery and control that, in turn, leads to lowered anxiety, which may enhance decision making under stress (Russell, 1993). Denial functions as a positive reaction because initially, the person's coping resources are insufficient to adequately deal with the stress. Minutes, hours, or days later, when the individual has had an opportunity to develop some coping resources, he or she usually will begin to face the meaning of the information. During this time, individuals can gain a sense of control that can inhibit the very distressing feelings of powerlessness and use the time to cope with their serious realities (Block, 2006). Denial can be intermittent; individuals may have brief periods of awareness of a painful reality and then a short time later deny its existence.

Continuation of denial over a long period of time usually is considered to be maladaptive coping because the psychic energy required to maintain the defense becomes a physical and emotional drain that can have a negative impact on the person (Kreitler, 1999). A negative outcome of extensive use of denial can interfere with getting support to face the stressor. This can lead to increased isolation and reinforcement of the use of denial as a defense. Individuals who maintain a strong denial defense over months or even years are more likely to be exhibiting a pathologic process because they are never able to attain a sense of mastery over the loss. Nevertheless, for some, ongoing denial may be the only way to maintain functioning. Major denial can also be a marker for depression (Block, 2006).

The circumstances under which people use denial will determine its positive or negative value. For example, avoiding treatment for a skin lesion or breast lump for months could be life-threatening. In these situations, denial not only shields the patient from facing the possible meaning of the lesion but also becomes destructive because treatment is delayed. In contrast, refusing to believe a terminal prognosis may allow the patient to maintain hope and feel less anxious. Appearing cheerful or emotionally detached but still pursuing cancer treatment would not have life-threatening implications and may help patients and their families to cope. Denial can present a barrier to decision making and planning. For example, it can impair or delay the development of a realistic treatment plan, lead to delays in treatment, or impair communication with professionals. This is maladaptive denial characterized by rigidity of belief (Block, 2006).

Short-term or less encompassing denial may offer some short-term benefits and be adaptive to the situation without promoting other problems. In adaptive denial, for example, a patient may recognize having a terminal illness but consciously set that awareness aside to focus on living. This allows the patient an opportunity to maintain a better quality of life and at the same time save energy to deal with future issues (see Figure 16-1).

Weisman (1989) described the process of identifying denial to include some information (reality) being given, the rejection of all or part of this information, a more acceptable replacement concept, reorientation to the new reality, and finally, some recognition by another that the person has misinterpreted the obvious reality. This final part is necessary, as denial is generally recognized by others but not by the individual experiencing it.

---

**Adaptive Denial**
- Temporary, short-lived
- Intermittent
- Allows time to develop coping mechanisms
- Does not influence major decisions
- Others rally around the person until he or she can cope

**Maladaptive Denial**
- Lasts much longer than expected
- Persistent use of denial, even in the face of obvious truth
- No indication of use or new development of more adaptive coping skills
- Influences major decisions
- Isolates person from others
- Rigid beliefs
- May be an indicator of depression
- Impairs adjustment

**Figure 16-1. Characteristics of Adaptive and Maladaptive Denial**

*Note.* Based on information from Block, 2006; Rousseau, 2000; Stephenson, 2004.

---

# Denial and Illness

Much of the early clinical research related to denial has been conducted on patients with cardiac disease (Hackett, Cassem, & Wishnie, 1968; Levine et al., 1987; Lowery, 1991). These researchers found that denial was critical in the adjustment period after a myocardial infarction (MI). Denial was identified as a factor in lowering a patient's heart rate and blood pressure. Patients fearing the implications of their condition have a higher heart rate and blood pressure. "Deniers" were identified as individuals who were able to admit to having had a heart attack but described little awareness of fear. At the other extreme, however, were patients who did not seek treatment for chest pain (calling it "indigestion") or who were found doing push-ups in the coronary care unit in an effort to maintain they were healthy. In addition, deniers resumed work and sexual activity sooner than non-deniers. The initial research by Hackett et al. (1968) revealed that denial reduced distress and was associated with lower mortality following a heart attack. More recent studies also identified that denial may play a protective role during and shortly after hospitalization for acute MI (McKinley, Moser, & Dracup, 2000; Mosher, Dracup, & Wu, 2012; Perkins-Porras, Whitehead, Strike, & Steptoe, 2008; Zerwic & Ryan, 2004). However, if these patients are less adherent, they may have worse long-term outcomes. Perkins-Porras et al. (2008) found that previous experience with heart disease was not a predictor of seeking help earlier.

Denial has been identified as a common symptom in addictive disorders (Williams, Olfson, & Galanter, 2015). It is a prime symptom, as the individual is unable to acknowledge the impact of the addiction on oneself and others.

## Denial and Cancer

Denial is a useful and healthy initial response to a crisis such as a cancer diagnosis (Rabinowitz & Peirson, 2006). Self-deception in the face of a cancer diagnosis is a natural protective mechanism. It is expected initially in the presence of a serious cancer diagnosis (Vos et al., 2008). A certain level of denial in patients with lung cancer can have a protective effect on social and emotional outcomes (Vos, Putter, van Houwelingen, & de Haes, 2011).

Because cancer represents many people's worst fear, overwhelming anxiety caused by a symptom that could indicate cancer or the idea of facing cancer treatment certainly is understandable. Weisman (1989) identified cancer as the most dreaded of diseases.

Specific fears that have been identified over the years include cancer representing terrible pain and suffering and then death; disfigurement; loss of role, financial security, or job; separation from or rejection by loved ones; and tremendous threat to self-concept, especially in individuals who associate cancer with guilt and punishment for past "sins" (e.g., promiscuity, drug use) (Holland, 2003; Holland & Wiesel, 2015).

A cancer diagnosis represents uncertainty. To counteract the discomfort and anxiety of uncertainty, it is natural for people to focus on a positive outcome (Borneman et al., 2014). Because potential negative outcomes are not being addressed, focusing on a positive outcome can be viewed as denial. This is where clinicians may assume that a patient who does not acknowledge negative news is in denial; however, it may also be an expression of positive thinking or hope. Borneman et al. (2014) suggested that the longer one lives beyond the prognosis, the more the awareness of death becomes tangential. Life becomes ambiguous and uncertain. The authors speculated that uncertainty of a serious cancer diagnosis such as lung cancer can promote the use of hope as a way to deal with the uncertainty. Although a form of denial, hope can be a healthy coping strategy for patients to enjoy the moment. Jacobsen et al. (2014) reported that some patients with healthy coping are not always realistic and may give the impression of not understanding the prognosis.

Studies have examined denial and its impact on the diagnosis of cancer. Denial has been identified as a factor in delaying diagnosis and treatment (Khalili, Farajzadegan, Mokarian, & Bahrami, 2013; Panzarella et al., 2014; Reich, Gaudron, & Penel, 2009). Extreme denial at the first sign of symptoms can lead to late diagnosis and contributes to the need for more aggressive treatment when the disease becomes advanced. It also can contribute to delays in beginning treatment (Singer, 2014). Whether this denial protects people from awareness of suffering and pain caused by the disease and its symptoms is open for debate. Little research exists on these patients because they often are at the end stage of disease when they finally seek care.

Denial in regard to cancer treatment also can manifest itself as noncompliance with treatment when patients fail to complete a course of chemotherapy or radiation. Acknowledging the reality of treatment and side effects may force patients to face the threat of cancer for the first time. Patients may be so overwhelmed that the only way to deal with the threat is to refuse more treatment. Patients in denial may be less likely to attend support groups or educational programs because they have convinced themselves that the information would not apply to them. No one knows how much suffering is created by advanced symptoms of pain, bowel obstructions, or pathologic fractures because patients with cancer who are in denial are unable to acknowledge symptoms and do not seek treatment. These areas are all understudied.

With advanced disease, some patients are able to maintain an upbeat, hopeful outlook that may be associated with denial. This response can give patients energy to continue trying new therapies or can lessen anxiety and depression, which positively affects patients and those around them.

## Denial and Death

Although death is an inevitability that all people must face, imagining one's own nonexistence is nearly impossible (Weisman, 1972). Combined with the taboo of discussing and facing death in Western culture, this adds to the prevalent use of denial at the end of life. Death is a reminder of a person's ultimate powerlessness, and denial often is used when facing death because the idea of nonexistence is so threatening.

Some terminally ill individuals may maintain denial until the very end, even in the face of advanced disease. Denial can hinder acceptance of and preparation for death (e.g., estate planning, end-of-life care decisions) as well as cause isolation from family and friends who are fearful of saying the "wrong thing" around the patient (Cotter & Foxwell, 2015). They are being prevented from saying goodbye. On the other hand, some individuals retain a strong sense of what gives their lives meaning. Not all patients with an upbeat, hopeful attitude with advanced disease are in denial. This may be patients' normal personality or the result of true acceptance.

For terminally ill individuals, denial represents the last effort to control an uncontrollable situation. Nurses may be concerned that patients will suffer more because they are not participating in end-of-life decisions. This is a concern that has not been proven in the literature but should be considered (Cotter & Foxwell, 2015).

## Impact of Denial on the Patient's Family

A study by Kogan, Dumas, and Cohen (2013) found that a patient's denial can add additional burdens for the family (e.g., feeling discouraged from seeking information to better manage the patient's care, feeling powerlessness and guilt). Caregivers described feeling frustrated and burdened by the denial. In many cases, they recognized it as a long-standing coping pattern for the patient. The denial prevented families from acknowledging their own needs and seeking more support. These family members were more likely to develop solitary coping strategies and employ denial themselves.

Denial also may allow families to maintain a normal routine while not being overwhelmed with the realities of their loved one's illness. Not thinking about what could happen in the future may give family members a respite.

Family members also can exhibit denial when the patient is not. In this case, family members may avoid facing the reality of the disease and may make efforts to convince the patient of this as well. This can contribute to conflict and avoidance of each other unless each person can understand and accept the other's perspective.

## Healthcare Professionals' Responses to Denial

When faced with patients in denial, healthcare professionals often react with concern. Nurses may feel that patients are not coping effectively and need intervention. Denial can inhibit the therapeutic relationship when patients are unable to talk about their emotional response to an illness or tolerate necessary teaching about chemotherapy because of the inability to believe that treatment is needed.

Clinicians may interpret seemingly unreasonable hopes (e.g., "I will beat the cancer."; "I believe in miracles!") as denial, which is often labeled as unhealthy coping. However, these statements often are an effective coping strategy to defend against a painful reality. Rather than trying to bypass the denial, the clinician may be more helpful by supporting the patient. By understanding that these statements do not reflect a dense denial, but rather an effective coping strategy that defends against a painful reality, clinicians can better support the patient (Jacobsen et al., 2014).

Healthcare professionals can even inadvertently promote denial by such questions as "You're doing OK today, right?" This can be a way to maintain hope that the patient is improving. Clinicians also can perpetuate denial in a mistaken belief that it is supporting the patient. Singer (2014) reported that reinforcing patient denial communicates to them that their prognosis must be even worse than expected if the healthcare provider cannot face it either.

At times, cultural beliefs or language barriers can mimic denial. For example, some cultures may have taboos against mentioning a certain disease, so patients may appear to be in denial when, in reality, they simply do not believe in verbally acknowledging the condition. Taboos about acknowledging cancer can also exist. Also, if a patient has not been given a diagnosis in a way that easily can be understood, their reaction may be misinterpreted as denial.

Families may go to great lengths to avoid letting the patient hear the word *cancer*, and this easily could be misidentified as denial. If a language barrier exists, patients could act as if they understood the information when they actually did not comprehend the implications. Patients who might not react as expected could also be mistakenly labeled as being in denial. Healthcare professionals need to take such instances into account to better understand their patients' responses.

## Evidence-Based Practice

Weisman (1972) remains the seminal research on the use of denial in patients with cancer. This study is based on multiple interviews with people in different stages of illness. His work became the basis for much future research. Recent research on this topic is very limited. Small studies with cancer populations, particularly lung cancer, have demonstrated the regular presence of denial.

Vos et al. (2008) studied patients with lung cancer and found that the greatest use of denial was in the four to eight months after diagnosis. At this point, the initial diagnosis is faced and treatment started. Once some period of adjustment to the disease has occurred, the increase in denial may reflect a way to maintain balance and sense of normalcy in life in the presence of a potentially life-limiting illness. Moreover, the permanent realization that one's prospects for the future include pain and dyspnea and the potential imminence of death is difficult for some patients to bear. The level of denial expressed reflects a decision to "make the best of things" and disregard the illness and its impact as much as possible. In a study of 195 patients with lung cancer, those who rated higher in denial reported a better quality of life, including less anxiety and higher social functioning, than those with lower levels of denial (Vos et al., 2011).

## Nursing Care of Patients in Denial

### Assessment

Nurses need to be alert to the many different forms denial can take. Often, the first sign of denial is when a patient refutes awareness of information the nurse knows they have received. For example, after the doctor has told the patient about a new metastasis, the patient tells the nurse they just heard everything is going well. Other signs might include not asking questions when questions normally are expected, absence of signs of an expected normal emotional response to bad news, or inappropriate responses such as laughing and joking.

More subtle signs might include changing the subject when the illness is discussed, avoiding use of the word *cancer*, or minimizing or hiding symptoms in an effort to maintain the denial (e.g., referring to respiratory distress from a pleural effusion as a cold, refusing to acknowledge pain). The patient may exhibit dismissive gestures or comments when distressing events are discussed or imply that the distressing events are not applicable.

Once nurses determine that the patient is using denial, they should try to identify factors that may contribute to the patient's need to use this defense and recognize that denial can be a response to anxiety, stress, and feelings of loss of control (Doenges, Moorhouse, & Murr, 2013). Collecting information on the patient's current stresses and past coping styles may provide that information.

More extreme maladaptive behaviors may include refusing to see the physician or follow through with treatment. Patients may be unable to acknowledge or minimize even obvious complications (e.g., a pathologic fracture, bleeding).

Denial also could be a factor when patients pursue unconventional therapy. A particular concern is when very ill patients refuse conventional therapy and seek unproven methods, including special diets or unusual drugs that may be promoted by unscrupulous providers.

A family in denial may exhibit the same types of behaviors as patients, such as going to great lengths to dismiss new symptoms, encouraging the patient not to listen to healthcare professionals, becoming angry if the nurse talks about cancer or chemotherapy, or exhibiting a lack of expected emotions regarding the patient's illness.

## Differential Diagnosis

Differentiating adaptive denial from denial with deleterious effects is an important part of the assessment. Although both forms protect individuals emotionally, maladaptive denial can be dangerous because the disease can progress when treatment is avoided. In addition, emotional sequelae of maladaptive denial include isolation of family members from the patient because they fear saying the wrong thing around the patient, inhibition of emotional growth when the individual never deals with a major loss, and the risk of future emotional problems. Anxiety and depression also can resemble denial in some situations. In addition, poor communication about the disease and prognosis can cause unexpected or unanticipated patient reactions.

Psychotic thought processes, dementia or other conditions with memory impairment, delirium, or other psychiatric disorders could be incorrectly labeled as denial. If patients refuse to believe a diagnosis because of confusion or delusional thoughts, denial is not the mechanism. Further psychiatric evaluation must be provided. In addition, neurologic impairments (e.g., stroke, brain tumor) can mimic denial if they cause a neglect syndrome in which patients disavow a symptom or even a part of the body.

## Interventions

Denial is sometimes viewed as an obstacle to care rather than a symptom that requires further exploration (Williams et al., 2015). Because denial is often not static, care needs to be taken to consider the circumstances when it is evident. A nonintrusive, supportive approach should be the initial intervention. Incorporate statements and questions such as, "Tell me what the doctor told you about your condition," "What adjustments have you had to make with your illness?" and "What are you concerned about?" into the nursing assessment. Answers to these questions will provide information about the patient's perspective. Reassessment using these same questions will help to establish the firmness of the denial. Once the nurse has this information, consideration needs to be given on how this coping mechanism is achieving its goal of protecting the patient. The nurse's role is not to take away denial but rather to ensure that destructive outcomes do not occur because of it.

When approaching a patient who has a history of or is suspected of using denial, nurses must ensure that they know what the patient has been told and in what words. Be aware of discrepancies between what the patient says and what the professionals have told the patient. Initially, use the same words the patient uses to describe the condition in an effort to establish rapport. For example, if the patient uses the word "growth" or "lump" to describe the disease, initially use this word, too.

Nurses should not confront an individual with information they believe he or she should have; rather, they should recognize the need that denial serves and consider the patient's fears, the issues that need to be addressed, and the role that teaching and support play in addressing the denial. Spend time listening to the person and provide support to build a trusting relationship. Confronting the patient with the truth may lead to extreme reactions of anger, anxiety, and distress. Patients may react with more denial and be able to ignore the information. The nurse risks isolating the patient further because the patient could feel that the staff is cruel, harsh, or negative and untrustworthy.

Providing information to patients in small amounts is important. Provide some information about side effects or the treatment plan, and observe the response. Reinforce the information, and ask patients to repeat what they understand. Presenting information in small amounts produces much less anxiety than presenting the whole picture at one time.

If patients focus on unrealistic goals or hopes, listen to them but avoid agreeing with or reinforcing them. Focus instead on specific, potentially achievable goals. For example, if the patient is bedbound, do not focus on the ability to play tennis soon but rather direct the discussion to identify ways to increase muscle strength. Sometimes, developing a backup plan for patients can help. For example, if a patient refuses home care because he or she believes help is unnecessary, arrange a one-time evaluation visit "just in case." Another suggestion is to ask the patient how he or she would handle a specific situation (e.g., "What would you do if you were too weak to answer the door?").

For patients who demonstrate denial and will not accept any teaching or assistance, give family members information on what to expect. Work with them to establish a plan of action if the patient's condition deteriorates. Ensure that they know how to set up home care, have keys to the patient's home, and have the doctor's telephone number. Educate them regarding signs of pain or other indications of deterioration. Provide support to family members about the difficulty of the current situation and review the reasons the patient needs this defense.

If family members are using extensive denial, try to encourage them to participate in the patient's care to increase their understanding of the extent of the patient's illness or disability. Engage family members in a discussion about observations regarding the patient's condition and needs. Assist them in identifying their fears about the patient's illness. Families may need help to support a patient using denial. Encourage family members to avoid pushing the reality onto the patient. Too aggressive an approach at this critical time could lead to further patient withdrawal (Mayo Clinic, 2014).

If patients are using denial that has life-threatening implications, the healthcare team may consider a psychiatric consultation. The consultant may be able to determine if a psychiatric disorder is inhibiting patients' recognition of the illness. If patients do not have a psychiatric disorder and have the capacity to make medical decisions, they have the right to refuse medical treatment. As difficult as this can be for the families and healthcare professionals, patients have the right to use denial to protect themselves from the information and cannot be forced into treatment (see Figure 16-2).

---

**Assessment**
- Recognize the various forms denial can take.
- Reassess patients' responses at different points of the disease or hospital stay.
- Consider variables that may be causing patients to use denial.
- Determine adaptive and maladaptive effects of the use of denial.
- Identify possible differential diagnoses.

**Nursing Diagnoses** (NANDA International, 2015)
- Ineffective coping
- Ineffective denial

**DSM-V Diagnoses** (American Psychiatric Association, 2013)
- Adjustment disorder with anxiety
- Adjustment disorder with depressed mood: Major depression

**Differential Diagnoses**
- Neurologic impairment
- Psychosis
- Depression

---

**Figure 16-2. Plan of Care**

*(Continued on next page)*

**Expected Outcomes**
- Patients will seek and follow through with medical interventions.
- Patients will accurately describe implications of the illness.
- Patients will acknowledge emotional responses to the diagnosis.
- Patients will verbalize realistic expectations of the illness.

**Interventions: Patients**
- Determine the degree of denial and effectiveness of denial as a coping strategy.
- Observe patients' responses to information given by the healthcare team.
- Give patients information about their condition in small amounts without being threatening.
- Avoid confronting patients' denial directly.
- Take time to encourage a trusting, supportive relationship.
- Recognize patients' need for extra support.
- Reinforce possible positive outcomes of treatment.
- Consider psychiatric consultation if the denial has life-threatening implications.

**Interventions: Family Members**
- Include family members in patients' care so they can see the extent of the disease.
- Identify which family members can tolerate even a little information about the patients.
- Help families to establish an action plan if patients' condition deteriorates.

**Figure 16-2. Plan of Care** *(Continued)*

## Case Study

Jean is a 68-year-old Caucasian woman who is admitted to an oncology unit with a huge fungating mass on her chest that has been undiagnosed and untreated for years. She was brought to the emergency department by her daughter because she was too weak to get out of bed and had a high fever. When her daughter helped her up, she smelled a strong unpleasant odor and realized that Jean had placed multiple thick dressings under her dress to absorb drainage. On examination in the emergency department, the nurse realizes that Jean has a large untreated breast cancer. Her daughter is shocked. Jean shows no reaction at hearing the diagnosis and instead claims that she has an infection.

The daughter begins thinking back to the recent past. Jean had been noted by family and friends to be more isolated over the previous year. She had refused social events and asked her family not to visit. She had not seen a doctor in some years. Her daughter recently realized that when she saw her mother, she was wearing loose-fitting clothes and heavy perfume. Putting this all together, the daughter realizes that her mother had been hiding this diagnosis for some time. Jean's mother had died of breast cancer 40 years earlier, and she had always described an intense fear of the diagnosis.

On the oncology unit, Jean remains passive and does not participate in any of her care. She appears depressed and does not acknowledge her diagnosis. Her daughter has assumed medical decision-making authority to begin treatment for the infection and eventual surgery. When the oncology clinical nurse specialist comes to the room to educate on surgery and further treatment, Jean says she is too tired to listen and to talk to her daughter.

## Discussion

Jean exhibited maladaptive denial of her symptoms for an extended period of time, indicating a profound disturbance in her coping ability. She was aware at some level that the mass was growing and creating drainage and odor. However, this awareness did not lead her to seek action. She was unable to acknowledge it to others and did not seek medical care. Intense fear of cancer based on past experience with her mother, along with impaired coping strategies for this stress, contributed to the denial. Considering her ongoing coping strategies, Jean's lack of reaction to finally hearing her diagnosis probably was expected. This patient would be high risk for serious depression once the reality of the situation was acknowledged. The oncology team recommended that the advanced practice nurse (APN) from the psychosocial oncology team meet with Jean to further assess her. The patient was started on antidepressants. The APN made several brief visits to give the patient an opportunity to develop a relationship but not overwhelm her or raise expectations. Jean eventually was able to acknowledge her fear of cancer. With support from her family as well as her oncology team, the patient was able to participate in the treatment plan.

## Conclusion

Denial tends to occur frequently at times of stress during the cancer experience. It is particularly evident at the onset of cancer symptoms, diagnosis, metastasis/recurrence, and end-stage disease. The initial appearance of denial symptoms should be considered to be normal, adaptive behavior. Denial indicates that the person is overwhelmed with the emotional impact of this stress and, at least initially, does not have adequate coping mechanisms to deal with the anxiety. Denial provides protection from an overwhelming threat. If denial behavior persists, healthcare professionals must evaluate whether it is adaptive or maladaptive. Maladaptive denial may require more intensive assessment and intervention but should never be approached in a harsh manner as something that must be "fixed." The impact of maladaptive denial may include late diagnosis, incomplete treatment, and isolation from family and healthcare professionals. Whatever the extent of the denial, healthcare professionals must continue to support patients without reinforcing its maladaptive aspects. Denial remains an elusive and sometimes confusing behavior that is difficult to measure and study.

## References

American Psychiatric Association. (2013). *Diagnostic and statistical manual of mental disorders* (5th ed.). Washington, DC: Author.

Block, S. (2006). Psychological issues in end of life care. *Journal of Palliative Medicine, 9*, 751–772. doi:10.1089/jpm.2006.9.751

Borneman, T., Irish, T., Sidhu, R., Koczywas, M., & Cristea, M. (2014). Death awareness, feelings of uncertainty, and hope in advanced lung cancer patients: Can they coexist? *International Journal of Palliative Nursing, 20*, 272–277. doi:10.12968/ijpn.2014.20.6.271

Buckley, T., Spinaze, M., Bartrop, R., McKinley, S., Whitfield, V., Havyatt, J., ... Tofler, G. (2015). The nature of death, coping response and intensity of bereavement following death in the critical care environment. *Australian Critical Care, 28*, 64–70. doi:10.1016/j.aucc.2015.02.003

Cotter, V.T., & Foxwell, A.M. (2015). The meaning of hope in the dying. In B.R. Ferrell, N. Coyle, & J.A. Paice (Eds.), *Oxford textbook of palliative nursing* (4th ed., pp. 475–486). New York, NY: Oxford University Press.

Doenges, M.E., Moorhouse, M.F., & Murr, A.C. (2013). *Nursing diagnosis manual: Planning, individualizing, and documenting client care* (4th ed.). Philadelphia, PA: F.A. Davis.

Engle, G. (1962). *Psychological development in health and disease*. Philadelphia, PA: Elsevier Saunders.

Hackett, T.P., Cassem, N.H., & Wishnie, H.A. (1968). The coronary-care unit: An appraisal of its psychologic hazards. *New England Journal of Medicine, 279,* 1365–1370. doi:10.1056/NEJM196812192792504

Holland, J.C. (2003). American Cancer Society Award lecture. Psychological care of patients: Psycho-oncology's contribution. *Journal of Clinical Oncology, 21*(Suppl. 23), 253S–265S. doi:10.1200/JCO.2003.09.133

Holland, J.C., & Weisel, T.W. (2015). Introduction: History of psychosocial oncology. In J.C. Holland, W.S. Breitbart, P.N. Butow, P.B. Jacobsen, M.J. Loscalzo, & R. McCorkle (Eds.), *Psycho-oncology* (3rd ed., pp. xxv–xxxv). New York, NY: Oxford University Press.

Jacobsen, J., Kvale, E., Rabow, M., Rinaldi, S., Cohen, S., Weissman, D., & Jackson, V. (2014). Helping patients with serious illness live well through the promotion of adaptive coping: A report from the Improving Outpatient Palliative Care (IPAL-OP) Initiative. *Journal of Palliative Medicine, 17,* 463–468. doi:10.1089/jpm.2013.0254

Kernberg, O.F. (2009). Psychoanalysis: Freud's theories and their contemporary development. In M.G. Gelder, N.C. Andreasen, J.J. López-Ibor, & J.R. Geddes (Eds.), *New Oxford textbook of psychiatry* (2nd ed., pp. 294–312). New York, NY: Oxford University Press.

Khalili, N., Farajzadegan, Z., Mokarian, F., & Bahrami, F. (2013). Coping strategies, quality of life and pain in women with breast cancer. *Iranian Journal of Nursing and Midwifery Research, 18,* 105–111.

Kogan, N.R., Dumas, M., & Cohen, S.R. (2013). The extra burdens patients in denial impose on their family caregivers. *Palliative and Supportive Care, 11,* 91–99. doi:10.1017/S1478951512000491

Kreitler, S. (1999). Denial in cancer patients. *Cancer Investigation, 17,* 514–534. doi:10.3109/07357909909032861

Kübler-Ross, E. (1969). *On death and dying.* New York, NY: Macmillan.

Levine, J., Warrenburg, S., Kerns, R., Schwartz, E.G., Delaney, R., Fontana, A., ... Casione, R. (1987). The relationship of denial to the course of recovery in coronary heart disease. *Psychosomatic Medicine, 49,* 109–117. doi:10.1097/00006842-198703000-00001

Lowery, B.J. (1991). Psychological stress, denial and myocardial infarction outcomes. *Image, 23,* 51–55. doi:10.1111/j.1547-5069.1991.tb00635.x

Mayo Clinic. (2014). Denial: When it helps, when it hurts. Retrieved from http://www.mayoclinic.org/healthy-lifestyle/adult-health/in-depth/denial/art-20047926

McIntyre, K.M., Norton, J.R., & McIntyre, J.S. (2009). Psychiatric interview, history and mental status examination. In B.J. Sadock, V.A. Sadock, & P. Ruiz (Eds.), *Kaplan and Sadock's comprehensive textbook of psychiatry* (9th ed., pp. 886–906). Philadelphia, PA: Wolters Kluwer Health/Lippincott Williams & Wilkins.

McKinley, S., Moser, D.K., & Dracup, K. (2000). Treatment-seeking behavior for acute myocardial infarction symptoms in North America and Australia. *Heart and Lung, 29,* 237–247. doi:10.1067/mhl.2000.106940

Mosher, D.K., Dracup, K., & Wu, J.-R. (2012). Cardiac denial and delay in treatment for myocardial infarction. In R. Allan & J. Fisher (Eds.), *Heart and mind: The practice of cardiac psychology* (2nd ed., pp. 305–326). Washington, DC: American Psychological Association.

NANDA International. (2015). *Nursing diagnoses: Definitions and classification, 2015–2017.* Philadelphia, PA: Author.

Panzarella, V., Pizzo, G., Calvino, F., Compilato, D., Colella, G., & Campisi, G. (2014). Diagnostic delay in oral squamous cell carcinoma: The role of cognitive and psychological variables. *International Journal of Oral Science, 6,* 39–45. doi:10.1038/ijos.2013.88

Perkins-Poros, L., Whitehead, D.L., Strike, P.C., & Steptoe, A. (2008). Causal beliefs, cardiac denial and prehospital delays following the onset of acute coronary syndromes. *Journal of Behavioral Medicine, 31,* 498–505. doi:10.1007/s10865-008-9174-3

Rabinowitz, T., & Peirson, R. (2006). "Nothing is wrong, doctor": Understanding and managing denial in patients with cancer. *Cancer Investigations, 24,* 68–72. doi:10.1080/07357900500449678

Reich, M., Gaudron, C., & Penel, N. (2009). When cancerphobia and denial lead to death. *Palliative and Supportive Care, 7,* 253–255. doi:10.1017/S1478951509000327

Rousseau, P. (2000). Death denial. *Journal of Clinical Oncology, 18,* 3998–3999.

Russell, G.C. (1993). The role of denial in clinical practice. *Journal of Advanced Nursing, 18,* 938–940. doi:10.1046/j.1365-2648.1993.18060938.x

Singer, S. (2014). Psychosocial impact of cancer. In U. Goerling (Ed.), *Psycho-oncology* (pp. 1–10). doi:10.1007/978-3-642-40187-9_1

Stephenson, P.S. (2004). Understanding denial. *Oncology Nursing Forum, 31,* 985–988. doi:10.1188/04.ONF.985-988

Vos, M.S., Putter, H., van Houwelingen, H.C., & de Haes, H.C. (2008). Denial in lung cancer patients: A longitudinal study. *Psycho-Oncology, 17,* 1163–1171. doi:10.1002/pon.1325

Vos, M.S., Putter, H., van Houwelingen, H.C., & de Haes, H.C. (2011). Denial and social and emotional outcomes in lung cancer patients: The protective effect of denial. *Lung Cancer, 72,* 119–124. doi:10.1016/j.lungcan.2010.07.007

Weisman, A.D. (1972). *On dying and denying.* New York, NY: Behavioral Publications.

Weisman, A.D. (1989). Denial, coping, and cancer. In E.L. Edelstein, D.L. Nathanson, & A.M. Stone (Eds.), *Denial: A clarification of concepts and research* (pp. 251–260). New York, NY: Plenum Press.

Williams, A.R., Olfson, M., & Galanter, M. (2015). Assessing and improving clinical insights in patients "in denial." *JAMA Psychiatry, 72,* 303–304. doi:10.1001/jamapsychiatry.2014.2684

Zerwic, J.J., & Ryan, C.J. (2004). Delays in seeking MI treatment: Chances of survival increase if symptoms are treated within two hours of onset. *American Journal of Nursing, 104*(1), 81–83. doi:10.1097/00000446-200401000-00027

CHAPTER 17

# Depression and Suicide

*Angela V. Albright, RN, APRN, PhD, and*
*Sharon M. Valente, RN, APRN, BC, PhD, FAAN*

> *Melancholy*
> *Sits on me as a cloud along the sky,*
> *Which will not let the sunbeams through, nor yet*
> *Descend in rain and end; but spreads itself*
> *'Twixt heavens and earth, like envy between man*
> *And man–an everlasting mist.*
>
> —Lord Byron

The sadness and dysphoric mood that patients with cancer experience upon receiving their diagnosis and while coping with treatment are not surprising. In addition to "normal" affective reactions, many cancer drugs, the disease process itself, or physical discomfort can induce depressive symptoms. Depression occurs two to three times more often in patients with cancer than in the general population (Krebber et al., 2014). Depression diagnosis and higher levels of depressive symptoms are associated with higher mortality. This was true in studies that assessed depression before cancer diagnosis, and in those that assessed depression following cancer diagnosis (Pinquart & Duberstein, 2010). These depressions, however, often are overlooked and not treated when healthcare workers assume that depression is "normal." Patients with cancer are at higher risk for suicide as well (Valente, 2010, 2011). Wishing to die might be confused with the desire for a "rational suicide" (i.e., when the patient has understandable motives with unimpaired mental processes) and may not be properly evaluated (Schramme, 2013). Identifying and treating depression, therefore, is an essential part of oncology nurses' roles. They are in a prime position to identify patients who are at risk and to carry out preventive and restorative measures surrounding this issue. Rigorously conducted intervention studies show that depression treatment programs, even for those with a poor prognosis, are effective (Rodin, 2014).

## Assessment of Depression

According to the *Diagnostic and Statistical Manual of Mental Disorders (DSM-V)* (American Psychiatric Association [APA], 2013), in order to be accurately diagnosed with a major depressive episode, the patient must have suffered from a depressed mood or loss of interest or pleasure in nearly all activities for at least two weeks. In addition, four of the following conditions must exist: (a) changes in appetite, weight, sleep, and psychomotor activity, (b) decreased energy, (c) feelings of worthlessness or guilt, (d) difficulty thinking, concentrating, or making decisions, and (e) recurrent thoughts of death or suicidal ideation, plans, or attempts. Physical symptoms such as loss of appetite, decreased energy, and insomnia could be related to the cancer disease process or to treatment modalities such as medications. Hence, the definitive diagnosis of depression is challenging in people with cancer. Practitioners need to be more aware of depressive symptoms and depressive disorders of patients with cancer (Pinquart & Duberstein, 2010). Some researchers have suggested that criteria for the diagnosis of depression in patients with cancer should exclude physical symptoms and focus only on psychological ones because physical symptoms can reflect both depression and oncology disorders (Akechi et al., 2009). Others have argued that including the physical symptoms does not necessarily result in a false positive diagnosis. More risk may be involved in not looking at all the signs and symptoms (Muehlbauer, 2013). One option is to exclude the physical criteria for research purposes. For clinical purposes, however, the more inclusionary approach will prevent underdiagnosing depression.

Another category of diagnosis in the *DSM-V* (APA, 2013), depressive disorder due to another medical condition, addresses depression with a clear etiology in a medical illness. A greater understanding of the biology of cancer includes recognition of the role of cytokines in inducing sickness behaviors that parallel symptoms of depression (Musselman, 2011). Whether from a biologic condition, from treatment for a medical condition, or from a psychological process, the depressed patient needs intervention to improve coping or alleviate the depressive condition.

Nonpsychiatric clinicians often lack skill in detecting major depression (Blair, 2012). Valente (2010) found that nurses underestimated the level of moderate or severe depressive symptoms in patients. Nurses were most influenced by crying, depressed mood, and physical symptoms (e.g., anorexia, insomnia, constipation, fatigue), which are often not reliable indicators of depression in a medically ill population. Most physicians and nurses underdiagnose depression on a medical service, and a limited number of these patients receive appropriate treatment for depression (Rodin, 2014). Nurses were more likely to focus on physical symptoms, were concerned with their lack of training in identifying psychiatric symptoms, and were frustrated in their inability to convince medical staff to seek further assessment or antidepressant medication (Valente, 2010). However, short training sessions for nurses and physicians have increased confidence and skill in assessing depression in both nurses and oncologists.

For screening purposes, the Patient Health Questionnaire-9, the Hopkins Symptom Checklist, the Hamilton Rating Scale, the Beck Depression Inventory, the Hospital Anxiety and Depression Scale (HADS), and the Zung Self-Rating Depression Scale have been used to identify patients with cancer with depressive symptoms who may need further evaluation and treatment (Sharpe et al., 2014). Another useful tool is the National Comprehensive Cancer Network® (NCCN®) Distress Thermometer, which allows patients to rank symptoms of distress over the previous week on a visual scale of 1–10 (NCCN, 2017) (see Chapter 18). The U.S. Preventive Services Task Force (USPSTF) recommendation statement on screening for depression in adults supports the use of screening adults who receive care in clinical practice (Siu & USPSTF, 2016). Careful consideration should be given to routine screens for depression as part of the interprofessional assessment of patients with cancer (Lloyd-Williams, Shiels, & Dowrick, 2007). Although these self- and observer-rated scales may render false positives, they can be useful tools for the nurse because they can be administered quickly and efficiently. Used as an adjunct to a thorough psychosocial history, these scales will help identify people who are in need of additional intervention from the time of diagnosis and throughout their treatment course. It is often found that staff members tend to estimate anxiety and depression at higher rates than patients do and that identification of clinically significant depression with HADS was inaccurate. This emphasizes the need for nurses to use objective criteria in assessment and to be very aware of the emotional issues of self so as not to confuse their own emotions with those of the patients. Providers need to acquire and maintain skill in accurate detection of depression (Valente, 2011).

## Depression in Special Populations

The clinical features of major depressive episodes are more similar than different when compared among pediatric, adolescent, adult, and older adult patients; men and women; and ethnic groups. Because children may be unable to express or verbalize their feelings, other signs may need to be analyzed (e.g., acting-out behaviors, not meeting developmental tasks, withdrawal, self-destructive behaviors). In older adult patients, the clinical presentation is similar to that used for adults but may be more likely to include memory loss and poor concentration, which can be confused with dementia (Pignone et al., 2002). Depression can be undiagnosed or misdiagnosed in some cultural and ethnic groups because of healthcare professionals' stereotypes about the expected behaviors, language barriers, and lack of access to mental health services among the groups (Zager & Yancy, 2011). The *DSM-V* suggests that some cultures may differ in their judgments about the seriousness of depressive symptoms or may express depressive symptoms as "nerves" (Latino) or "imbalances" (Asian). It is always important to base any assessment on an individual's own "normal."

## Risk Factors for Depression

To assess for depression, the nurse must be able to identify factors that might contribute to depression. Several psychological and physical variables have been identified that may affect the level of distress that accompanies a cancer diagnosis.

### Severity of Illness

Patients with advanced cancer are especially prone to depression. It might be more difficult to detect yet very important to treat (Massie, Lloyd-Williams, Irving, & Miller, 2011). For reasons that are currently unclear, depression rates have been found to be higher in certain types of cancer, such as pancreatic, gastric, breast, brain, lung, and head and neck (Massie et al., 2011). Williams and Payne (2003) also found a greater incidence of depression than anxiety in patients who were terminally ill compared to those who survived chemotherapy. The overall psychological distress was highest for those undergoing treatment.

Nurses need to determine what patients understand about their disease and the associated beliefs about what will happen next. At times, patients are not told about their prognosis, or it is discussed with them in an oblique way (Given & Given, 2012). Uncertainty cannot be avoided in the treatment of cancer; however, the anxiety it can cause can be minimized by giving as much information as patients seem to need rather than ignoring or skirting the issues. Patients' perceptions of their illness are important for nurses to elicit and understand so that they can identify areas that need clarification. Interventions aimed at providing choices and a sense of control are important to combat the demoralization that can come with setbacks and disappointing progress (Yennurajalingam et al., 2011).

## Stressful Life Events

Coping with the diagnosis of cancer is expected to be stressful. Nurses should not forget to find out what else might be happening in patients' lives. Because cancer often brings thoughts about one's mortality, nurses can also increase patients' control by initiating a therapeutic discussion of patients' wishes for end-of-life care and considering wishes for a surrogate decision maker or advance directives.

Experiencing recent losses is associated with depression. When a diagnosis of cancer occurs, it might be accompanied by loss of body image and self-concept following disfiguring surgery or the physical effects of chemotherapy. Individuals also might be considering the possibility of loss of job, status, income, or relationships.

A cancer diagnosis might raise existential issues. Because it is associated with loss of life, the diagnosis might trigger a crisis of meaning. To the extent that a person has difficulty reconciling their condition within a belief system, the result could be a sense of futility. The belief system that sustained a person in the past might be challenged and found to be lacking.

## History of Depression in Self or the Family

People who have experienced a major depressive episode are at risk for recurrent episodes (APA, 2013). People with cancer who have had a depressive episode in the past should be carefully evaluated throughout the course of their disease. A previous suicide attempt greatly increases the risk for a subsequent attempt (Leung et al., 2013).

A genetic predisposition to depression has been established. Therefore, even if a person has not had a previous depressive episode, a family history of depression, especially recurrent depression, might indicate a risk.

## Medications

Many chemotherapeutic agents that fight cancer as well as other commonly used drugs have side effects that include depression (see Figure 17-1). If depression is severe, the drug's benefits should be weighed against the risks and suffering of the depression, and modifications in dose or drug selection should be made accordingly.

## Socioeconomic Pressures

Fear of or actual inability to hold a job or position that provides income because of the illness can be overwhelming, depending on the individual and their financial situation. Losing a job also might result in loss of social status.

## A Tendency to Pessimism

People who have developed a pessimistic outlook on life are more prone to depression (Manicavasagar, Perich, & Parker, 2012). With the added stress of a cancer diagnosis, the pessimism might seem additionally validated and reinforce a negative worldview. Accord-

- Acyclovir
- Benzodiazepines/sedatives/hypnotics
- Beta-blockers/calcium channel blockers
- Clonidine
- Corticosteroids
- Digoxin
- Diuretics
- Estrogens/oral contraceptives
- Hydralazine
- Levodopa
- Methyldopa
- Opioids
- Reserpine

**Figure 17-1. Examples of Drugs That May Cause Depressive Side Effects**

*Note.* Based on information from Sadock & Sadock, 2007; Townsend, 2015.

ing to cognitive therapy, depression arises primarily from negative distortions in cognitive processes of thinking, knowing, and perceiving. The person believes that he or she is worthless, the world is barren, and the future is bleak. They see cancer as a catastrophe. In a cross-sectional and a follow-up study, Degner, Hack, O'Neil, and Kristjanson (2003) found that most women with breast cancer described the meaning of cancer as "challenge" or "value." However, those who described it as "enemy," "loss," or "punishment" were more likely to have depression and anxiety, as well as a poorer quality of life. In addition, patients who catastrophized their illness had greater emotional distress. These distortions and irrational pessimistic beliefs automatically guide thoughts and shape emotional responses, but these thinking patterns can be changed (Hack et al., 2011).

## Alcohol or Substance Abuse

Depression may be an outcome of chronic alcohol intake and/or alcohol and substance abuse. Another possibility might be that people who use alcohol or other substances as regular coping mechanisms have not developed more positive, affirming methods of coping (Cosci, Fava, & Sonino, 2015).

## Poorly Controlled Pain

Investigations into the relationship between cancer pain and depression have suggested that depression enhances pain and that pain and its treatment can contribute to depression (Smith, 2011). Despite advances in the assessment and treatment of pain, undertreatment occurs from lack of knowledge, fear of addiction, and failure of the healthcare system to facilitate delivery of proper pain management care. The presence of pain and suffering has a profound effect on quality of life (Lovell, Phillips, Luckett, & Agar, 2015).

## Differential Diagnosis

Before planning interventions for a diagnosis of depression, nurses need to evaluate the possibility that other disorders may present similar symptoms. These would include central nervous system (CNS) diseases (e.g., Parkinson disease, dementia, multiple sclerosis, neoplastic lesions); endocrine disorders (e.g., hyperthyroidism, hypothyroidism); drug-related conditions (e.g., cocaine abuse, side effects of some CNS depressants); infectious disease (e.g., mononucleosis); sleep-related disorders (e.g., sleep apnea, insomnia); other psychiatric disorders such as dysthymia (with low mood for two years); and anxiety, which can include panic disorder, generalized anxiety, phobias, bipolar disorders (depression alternates with manic states), and trauma (e.g., post-traumatic stress disorder). Screening tools often will help to establish data for the diagnosis.

Symptoms of depression may coexist with other major psychological diagnoses (e.g., anxiety) (see Chapter 14). Uncontrolled symptoms related to disease and treatment also may contribute to or exacerbate depression (e.g., fatigue). Metabolic statuses (e.g., electrolyte imbalances) that increase the risk of confusional states (e.g., psychosis, delirium) need to be differentiated from depressive symptoms. When depression seems likely, nurses need to consider the possibility of chronic alcohol intake and alcohol and substance abuse, which may also lead to a deficit in coping mechanisms.

Depression and cancer pain are a two-way street; each can contribute to or enhance the other. Despite advances in the assessment and treatment of pain, clinical experience shows that undertreatment occurs because of a lack of knowledge, fear of addiction, and lack of proper pain management care.

## Interventions for Depression

Oncology nurses need to be aware of the importance of their relationship with patients in case finding, intervening directly, and making proper referrals. Nurses must know what resources and treatment modalities are available to assist the depressed patient with cancer. Oncology nurses who are in frequent contact with their patients are in a prime position to identify emotional issues, support positive behaviors, assist in mobilizing support systems, and restore hope. A treatment plan should include not only the establishment of a trusting and caring relationship but also the facilitation of additional help when needed (see Figure 17-2). This plan should be made in the context of a collaborative treatment team. A depression care team (e.g., a nurse care manager, a primary care physician, a psychiatrist, an oncologist) has been effective in treating people with cancer. This team provides a unified and consistent approach to patient care because all professionals have agreed on the treatment plan (Rodin, 2014). The Oncology Nursing Society Putting Evidence Into Practice guidelines (Cope et al., 2017) recommend the following interventions for depression in patients with cancer: antidepressants, cognitive behavioral interventions, integrated or collaborative behavioral healthcare model, mindfulness-based stress reduction, and psychoeducational interventions (see Chapter 25 for information on or therapeutic modalities).

Psychiatric consultation is necessary for patients with severe depression and suicidal thoughts (Walker, Sawhney, et al., 2014). Cognitive, behavioral, and psychotherapy have been shown to be beneficial in meta-analyses (Raingruber, 2011). Other treatments for depression include education and in recalcitrant cases, electroconvulsive therapy.

Psychotherapy for depression provides an opportunity for patients to explore issues that arise (e.g., existential questions of the meaning of life, death, and loss of control; impact on relationships; vulnerable feelings). Management of affect and behavior is possible with cognitive behavioral approaches that teach patients to recognize the triggers for nonproductive and self-defeating thinking. Once the pattern is recognized, the patient is assisted in devel-

## Assessment
- Identify presence of risk factors for depression and suicide.
- Determine previous coping methods.
- Identify the meaning of the illness to patients.
- Consider confounding factors (e.g., illness, medications).
- Identify physical and emotional symptoms of depression.
- Explore degree and length of symptoms.
- See Table 17-3 for significant indicators of suicide risk in clinical practice.

## Nursing Diagnoses (NANDA International, 2015)
- Powerlessness
- Ineffective coping
- Complicated grieving
- Spiritual distress
- Risk for suicide

## *DSM-V* Diagnoses (American Psychiatric Association, 2013)
- Major depressive disorder
- Mood disorder because of a general medical condition
- Cognitive mental disorder because of a general medical condition

## Expected Outcomes
- Patients will experience an increased sense of control and self-efficacy.
- Patients will verbalize hope about quality of life and current relationships.
- Patients will name at least three sources of support for emotional and physical needs.
- Patients will replace automatic negative thoughts and distortions with two or three alternative explanations.

## Interventions
- Correct cognitive distortions by discussing irrational thoughts and automatic and negative thinking patterns.
- Offer support.
- Assist in setting attainable goals. Avoid becoming discouraged with patients' responses, as this reinforces their negativity.
- Encourage maximum possible participation in self-care activities.
- Mobilize support systems, including family, friends, professionals, and spiritual leaders.
- Alleviate physical suffering and physical symptoms that impede the quality of life.
- Use a therapeutic relationship to facilitate dialogue, ventilation, and exploration of feelings and thoughts.
- In moderate to severe cases of depression or cases of attempted suicide, refer for psychiatric consultation for psychotherapy or pharmacologic interventions.
- Refer for pain management, social support, pastoral counseling, palliative care, or hospice care as appropriate.
- Create and monitor no-suicide contracts as needed.
- Refer for music or other adjunctive therapies (e.g., self-hypnosis, positive thinking, problem solving).

**Figure 17-2. Plan of Care**

oping new thought patterns that lead to more positive behaviors and outcomes. Oncology nurses can take an active role in helping patients to identify self-defeating behaviors. Nurses who have formed a therapeutic relationship with their patients can coach positive thoughts and behaviors.

Relaxation skills can help to prevent aggravating anxiety and tension. Patients can learn simple, progressive muscle relaxation as a form of self-regulation. Visualization exercises also are effective and can be easily conducted. Relaxation to counter anxiety and tension is effective in reducing pain. Pain always should be addressed, and every avenue of relief should be pursued.

Sleep hygiene education can help to address sleep disturbances that often accompany chemotherapy. Lack of sleep increases fatigue and pain and decreases quality of life (Davis & Goforth, 2014). Outcome studies for alternative and complementary therapies, such as mindfulness, therapeutic touch, massage, aromatherapy, yoga, and acupuncture, and exercise programs are yet to be conclusive because of methodological issues; however, these interventions may contribute to overall well-being (Mishra et al., 2012; Sharma & Haider, 2013).

Family therapy can provide a forum where family members can identify and address unresolved conflicts. The therapist can help family members to voice their sense of the strain brought on by the disease. This can be crucial in that the depression that exists might be mutual among all parties (Given & Given, 2012). Family members who are caregivers may feel resentful and guilty about those feelings. The patient senses the resentment and feels guilty. A chance to discuss the circular effects that family members and patients have on one another could bring increased understanding and relief. Exactly who to include in the therapy should be explored carefully; the significant others who comprise the support system should be identified and included in the therapy. Oncology nurses also might make the effort to include family members in care planning meetings to solicit their support and give them a chance to identify needs that arise while caring for a loved one.

Group counseling is an excellent modality that provides patients with a chance to improve their outlook via sharing their experiences with others and gaining feedback in an accepting atmosphere. Educational programs (e.g., American Cancer Society's "I Can Cope") can clarify misconceptions about the disease and its treatment and contribute to an awareness of the ability of patients to engage in self-care and improve their sense of control and mastery over their situation. Other psychoeducational programs have shown to increase survival times and compliance with medical treatment and to reduce mood disturbance (Yennurajalingam et al., 2011).

A variety of psychosocial interventions have been found to be effective. The key is to determine which interventions are most appropriate, depending on patient preference and availability of services. The goal is to match the intervention with the patient. Nurses can suggest individual or group counseling, mindfulness, or hypnosis and recognize patients' preferences for some modalities over others. Patients who want one-on-one attention or are nervous in group settings may not find group counseling helpful.

## Antidepressants

Antidepressant medications can be a very useful adjunct to psychotherapy by improving mood and increasing energy that, in turn, can be channeled into a productive activity that increases self-esteem. Researchers have suggested that antidepressant medication, given alone or in combination with a psychological treatment, may be effective; however, further research is needed (Walker, Hansen, et al., 2014). When depression is severe, recurrent, or experienced in conjunction with psychotic symptoms, medication is indicated before psychotherapy (Pignone et al., 2002). Antidepressants have been found to be useful in treating depression in patients with cancer (Cope et al., 2017; NCCN, 2017).

The antidepressant medication chosen should be determined by assessing what side effects might be most beneficial or least antagonizing (see Table 17-1). For example, some have sedative side effects that might assist in reducing insomnia. Others have properties that contribute to blocking neuropathic pain.

Tricyclic antidepressants, heterocyclic antidepressants, selective serotonin reuptake inhibitors (SSRIs), serotonin–norepinephrine reuptake inhibitors (SNRIs), and monoamine oxidase inhibitors (MAOIs) are the major groups of antidepressants. Each has advantages and disadvantages that must be considered before prescribing. Tricyclic antidepressants take four to six weeks to take effect. The side effects, however, can begin shortly after the patient begins taking them. Serotonin inhibitors are a newer category of antidepressants that seem to be tolerated well and have short-lived initial side effects. MAOIs must be used with caution because of strict dietary restrictions (e.g., foods with tyramine [beer, wine, chocolate, cheese, broad beans] can cause a fatal hypertensive crisis). However, these drugs can be useful with long-term depression that has been resistant to other types of antidepressants.

Another class of medications useful in treating depression is the psychostimulants (e.g., methylphenidate). This treatment has not been researched as thoroughly as antidepressants,

### Table 17-1. Side Effect Profiles of Antidepressants

| Category | Examples | Features |
|---|---|---|
| SSRIs | Fluoxetine<br>Paroxetine[a]<br>Sertraline[b]<br>Citalopram<br>Escitalopram | Fewer and milder side effects than older drugs, but more sexual problems may occur. Fewer drug interactions occur. |
| SNRIs | Duloxetine<br>Venlafaxine[a]<br>Desvenlafaxine<br>Levomilnacipran | Fewer sexual side effects occur than with SSRIs. |
| Tricyclics | Imipramine<br>Amitriptyline<br>Doxepin<br>Trimipramine<br>Desipramine<br>Protriptyline | Cause more side effects than newer drugs. Can be lethal in overdose; suicidality should be considered before prescribing. |
| Heterocyclics | Amoxapine<br>Maprotiline<br>Trazodone | Inhibit the nerve cell's ability to reuptake norepinephrine and serotonin. Side effects include constipation, dry mouth, and shakiness. Risk of overdose exists. |
| MAOIs | Tranylcypromine<br>Phenelzine<br>Isocarboxazid | Strict diet restriction is required because of potentially lethal interactions with foods with tyramine and some medications. |
| Atypical antidepressants | Trazodone<br>Mirtazapine[c] (tetracyclic)<br>Bupropion | Trazodone and mirtazapine are sedating; taken in evening. Mirtazapine may take less time to improve mood than other drugs. Bupropion is less likely to case weight gain and sexual problems than other drugs. |

[a] Nausea and vomiting common side effect

[b] Associated with diarrhea

[c] Associated with weight gain

MAOIs—monoamine oxidase inhibitors; SNRIs—serotonin–norepinephrine reuptake inhibitors; SSRIs—selective serotonin reuptake inhibitors

*Note.* Based on information from Sadock et al., 2015; Townsend, 2015.

but small studies indicate its usefulness for relieving fatigue, rapidly reducing symptoms, which could be very important in a severely inhibiting depression (Musselman, 2011).

Antidepressants need to be prescribed in adequate dosages and administered over the proper amount of time required for them to take effect. Depressed people might need encouragement to comply with the treatment regimen if they are feeling excessively hopeless and helpless. Medications should be reconsidered or augmented if no improvement has occurred after 12 weeks. Providers not educated in psychopharmacology risk undertreating patients who are depressed. With psychotherapy and psychopharmacologic interventions, evaluation of efficacy of treatment should be continuous.

## Assessment and Intervention for Suicide

Although all patients should be assessed for suicide risk, studies have shown that the risk is greater in patients with lung, pancreatic, head and neck, and gastrointestinal cancers (Anguiano, Mayer, Piven, & Rosenstein, 2012).

Higher suicide risk is also associated with recent diagnosis (Johnson, Garlow, Brawley, & Master, 2012) and advanced stage of the disease (Bill-Axelson et al., 2010). Suicide is a topic that nurses often are reluctant to address, partially because of cultural taboos and nurses' lack of confidence in exploring such an emotionally charged topic. Table 17-2 summarizes nurses' difficulties in responding to suicidal patients. Screening tools can help clinicians demonstrate concern about another person's behavior and exercise due diligence to foresee and prevent suicide (Muehlbauer, 2013). Clinicians meet the standard of care by

### Table 17-2. Nurses' Difficulties in Responding to Suicidal Patients

| Theme | Description | Recommendations |
|---|---|---|
| Values about suicide | Personal attitudes or values suggest suicide is bad, taboo, wrong, cowardly, or unacceptable. | Coaching and reflection to clarify value conflicts |
| Feelings of discomfort | Person feels fearful, worried, hopeless, inadequate, and unable to care for suicidal patients. | Education and consultation; awareness of common reactions; recognitions of intervention limitations; clarifications of expectations |
| Skill, knowledge, experience deficit | Skills, knowledge, and experience are unequal to assisting suicidal person. | Education; skill building |
| Prior experiences with suicide of family or close friend | Reactions and grief to a prior suicide of a family member pose barriers to coping with suicidal patients. | Grief counseling; clarification of personal and professional roles |
| Professional obligations and duties are onerous | Conflicts occur between what one should do as a caring professional and legal, medical, and ethical obligations. | Consultation and case consultation to clarify personal and professional expectations |

*Note.* From "Management of Suicidal Patients" (p. 563), by S.M. Valente in A.W. Burgess (Ed.), *Psychiatric Nursing: Promoting Mental Health*, 1997, Stamford, CT: Appleton and Lange. Copyright 1997 by Appleton and Lange. Adapted with permission.

showing adherence to the assessment, screening, treatment, and management strategies that a reasonably prudent clinician would exercise under similar circumstances (Leung et al., 2013). Commonly used screening tools include the Hopelessness Scale (Beck, Rush, Shaw, & Emery, 1979), Index of Potential Suicide (Zung, 1974), Reasons for Living Inventory (Edelstein et al., 2009), the Suicide Probability Scale (Cull & Gill, 1982), and the Suicide Risk Measure (Plutchik, van Praag, Conte, & Picard, 1989). The Schedule of Attitudes toward Hastened Death, a self-report that measures desire for death among terminally ill patients, is also useful (Rosenfeld et al., 2000).

Clues that a patient is thinking of suicide may be written, spoken, or behavioral. Written clues may be notes indicating "I'd be better off dead." An example of a verbal clue would be a patient saying, "I do not know; I am so tired of all this. I should just jump out of this window!" Behavioral clues might involve a near-miss overdose where the patient arranges for rescue or intentionally "forgetting" to take life-saving medications. Other clues may be subtler, such as jokes or offhand remarks that indicate giving up, lack of hope, or feelings of worthlessness. In an assessment, the nurse must ask directly about suicidal thoughts (e.g., "Have you been thinking at all about wanting to kill yourself?"). If the patient responds affirmatively, the nurse should use follow-up questions to determine the immediacy and lethality of the plans, as well as offer the patient a chance to vent about what has caused such desperation (e.g., "What has been going on that has made you feel like that is a good alternative?"; "Have you thought about how you would do it?"). If the patient has a specific method, the nurse needs to find out how realistic that plan is for follow-through. For example, if the patient imagines shooting him- or herself, the nurse should determine if the patient has access to a gun and bullets. If the patient is considering taking pills, their access to such pills should be elicited (e.g., "Have prescriptions for antidepressants or pain medications been filled?"). If a clear method is described, the nurse should continue to find out how intent the patient is on following through with the plan. If a lethal plan is in place with high intent and availability of the method, a psychiatric consultation should be obtained immediately. In the past, no-suicide contracts were popular. These involved a nurse or other healthcare professional making a pact with the patient to not carry out with the plan or to seek contact if feelings reached an overwhelming point. However, evidence shows no-suicide contracts to be ineffective as a preventive method. Although the research does not show the benefits of a contract in reducing suicide risk, it may be useful in assessment (Puskar & Urda, 2011). Within the context of a trusting and caring relationship, the fact of the contract may keep a person from self-harm. No guarantee exists, however, and clinicians must use their judgment to determine the person's ability to keep a contract. Manipulative or angry patients might not be able to follow a stated plan and may need other, more intensive precautions, such as a suicide watch. Inpatient psychiatric treatment might be indicated. A nurse should not feel entirely responsible for a suicidal patient. The nurse should seek agency resources, and a care plan should be developed with a team of caregivers (professionals and significant others) (see Figure 17-2).

Interventions also should include assisting patients in mobilizing their own support systems, which might be unused because of feelings of "being stuck" or an unwillingness to ask for help. Assisting patients to take action of any kind is immensely helpful in restoring a sense of control and mastery of the situation. When a patient feels hopeless, he or she may develop tunnel vision where only one or two unacceptable alternatives are seen. For instance, if the patient feels that nothing will resolve a depression, no alternatives appear viable. However, if the nurse talks about depression treatments that have been successful where people have gone on to live with joy and purpose, alternatives may suddenly be viable. A suicide hotline number or a list of people to call must be available to patients. Clinicians or nurses should clearly explain that suicide cannot be an automatic solution to the problem and that intervention to improve symptom relief, quality of life, and depression should be considered. Danger lies in patients who assume that no solution exists and that a request to die is rational. A patient's hopelessness can be spread to the caregivers unless they understand that the depression is not inevitable and can be lessened. See Table 17-3 for a summary of clinical guidelines for suicide.

A significant number of patients with cancer who decide to attempt suicide base their decision on a lack of relief from untenable physical symptoms (Dees, Vernooij-Dassen, Dekkers, Vissers, & van Weel, 2011). A major practice in patients with cancer is to incorporate ongoing

### Table 17-3. Clinical Guidelines for Suicide Assessment and Intervention

| Assessment Factors | Interventions |
|---|---|
| Individual risk factors:<br>• Age<br>• Ethnicity<br>• Relationship status (e.g., widowed, single)<br>• Gives away prized objects<br>• Says good-bye<br>• Makes plans for death<br>• Attempts suicide<br>• Experiences signs of depression/hopelessness<br>• Psychiatric diagnosis (e.g., major mood disorder, schizophrenia, alcoholism, borderline/antisocial personality)<br>• Diagnosis (e.g., head and neck, pancreatic, or gastrointestinal cancer; HIV)<br><br>Additional risk factors for older adults:<br>• Physical illness<br>• Family conflict<br>• Loneliness | Risk factors indicate a need for comprehensive assessment. Ask the patient about suicidal thoughts or ideas and plans. |
| Evaluate medications/treatment: Have any of these contributed to onset or increase of suicidal ideas? | If so, consult with the treatment team about alternative medications less likely to increase risk. |
| Screening tools:<br>• Beck Hopelessness Scale<br>• Index of Potential Suicide<br>• Reasons for Living Inventory<br>• Geriatric Suicide Ideation Scale<br>• Patient Health Questionnaire-9<br>• Hospital Anxiety and Depression Scale<br>• Zung Self-Rating Depression Scale<br>• Schedule of Attitudes toward Hastened Death | Monitor scores over time of screening tools used. |
| Ask the patient:<br>• Have you been thinking about taking your own life?<br>• Have these thoughts started in the past 12 months? If so, do you know what may have triggered them?<br>• Do you have them now?<br>• Tell me if you have a plan, method, or means.<br>• If you use this method, do you intend to die, or do you intend something else (e.g., rescue)? | Ask questions straightforwardly and nonjudgmentally. |

*(Continued on next page)*

### Table 17-3. Clinical Guidelines for Suicide Assessment and Intervention *(Continued)*

| Assessment Factors | Interventions |
|---|---|
| Rate lethality:<br>• Low lethality: Cutting or few (nonlethal) drugs<br>• Moderate lethality: Uncertainty about plan or rescue<br>• High lethality: Precise plan and poor rescue plan in next 24/48 hours. Needs immediate intervention (hospital, safety, remove method). Lethal method includes gun, knife, jumping, drowning, or carbon monoxide poisoning. | Inform and collaborate with healthcare team.<br>Plan intervention.<br>Intervene immediately. |
| Interventions | Encourage medications and supportive and complementary therapies.<br>Manage pain and symptoms. |
| Barriers to treatment | Increase staff vigilance.<br>Improve environmental safety.<br>Place patient near nurses' station.<br>Install safe bathroom fixtures.<br>Install screens to prevent jumping.<br>Remove access to sharp objects.<br>Improve documentation.<br>Remove access to lethal and other methods.<br>Reassess risk. |
| Protective factors | Support effective observation and clinical care.<br>Increase family, community, and chaplain support.<br>Teach problem solving, and nonviolent conflict resolution.<br>Teach stress management.<br>Instill hope.<br>Offer suicide hotline phone number. |

assessment and treatment directed at relief of physical symptoms so that quality of life can improve (Loggers et al., 2013). Referrals can be made to pain specialists, oncologists, palliative care, and hospice organizations (Dees et al., 2011). Incorporating emotional distress assessment with physical assessment can help identify patients at risk.

The Oregon Death With Dignity Act (DWDA) was enacted in 1997 to allow terminally ill patients to hasten death with prescribed medication. Cancer was the primary diagnosis of these patients (78.9%) in 2016. Most patients (88.7%) were on hospice and reported that loss of autonomy (89.5%), decreasing ability to participate in activities that made life enjoyable (89.5%), and loss of dignity (65.4%) were the primary causes of their wish to hasten death, rather than pain or other physical suffering (Oregon Public Health Division, 2017). In 2016, 204 people received lethal medication prescribed under DWDA, and 133 people died from ingesting the medication, including 19 who had received lethal prescriptions from prior years (Oregon Public Health Division, 2017). For many, this could indicate the request for medication might have been to feel the need for an option—the need to feel in control rather than an outright wish to die (see Chapter 27 for information on ethical issues).

Suicide might appear to be a good option when a person fears becoming a burden to others, especially if caregivers, loved ones, and even nurses have subtly or inadvertently communicated their tiredness and impatience. Sometimes called a "duty to die," patients may interpret the behavior of others to mean "everyone would be better off if I was dead." Patients must address feelings of being a burden. Family members might be in relationships that make clearly stating one's own thoughts and feelings difficult. Intervening with caregiver stress by providing emotional support, resources for help at home, or addressing financial constraints can provide much needed relief.

## Rational Suicide

Some might assume that verbalizing a wish to die represents a request for a "rational" suicide (Schramme, 2013). Suicide is "rational" when it is planned by someone with a realistic assessment of the situation and alternatives, unimpaired mental processes, and an understandable justification (e.g., terminal illness, intractable pain and suffering).

Suggestions for evaluation of rational suicide are described and summarized in Figure 17-3. These questions can help oncology nurses to begin the sensitive dialogue to determine what is behind a desire to die. Today's trend toward societal acceptance of suicide as a choice for the terminally ill also may be a factor. It is important to remember that suicides involving patients with cancer often are associated with undiagnosed and untreated depressions or confusional states and poorly managed pain (Dees et al., 2011). Suicide might be one of several options considered in an attempt to gain control of a seemingly uncontrollable situation (Blair, 2012; Dees et al., 2011).

Avoiding countertransference responses is important for professional caregivers. These responses occur when the healthcare professional's personal beliefs impede caregiving. Nurses have reported that countertransference responses can impede their assessments of, interventions for, and relationships with patients. For example, oncology nurses have reported that feelings about their own loved one's suicide have made it difficult for them to care for suicidal patients. Other nurses reported difficulty evaluating suicidal patients because of personal values that forbid suicide (Valente, 2011). Such responses might manifest in overidentifying with a suicidal patient and then reacting to the patient as one did in a personal experience. Nurses should be able to reflect on their personal reactions and make a clear boundary between that experience and that of the patient. A study of palliative care nurses found that openly listening to a request for euthanasia and taking it seriously assisted patients to talk about the reasons for their request and thus helped them gain relief from the fears and anxieties that had led them to that request (Dierckx de Casterlé, Verpoort, De Bal, & Gastmans, 2006). With separateness, yet empathy for patients' experiences, the nurse can keep a line of communication open and encourage patients to say what *they* are thinking and share what *they* are feeling.

# Evidence-Based Practice

Depression has been extensively studied. Evidence suggests that people with depression have poorer outcomes from their physical illness than their counterparts who are not depressed; therefore, effective assessment and treatment are essential (Zager & Yancy, 2011). Because it is known that physicians and nurses may not always detect depression, objective tools like the HADS, the Beck Depression Inventory, and the Hamilton Rating Scale should be incorporated in the assessment process. A history of depression is known to increase risk for recurrent depression (Blair, 2012). Likewise, a history of suicide attempts greatly increases the risk for subsequent attempts (Leung et al., 2013). This information is key for professionals to incorporate in a thorough psychosocial history and assessment as part of the cancer care treatment plan. Evidence of improved outcomes for depression treatment should be communicated to patients to promote more acceptance of these available therapies and interventions.

---

1. Is the patient making a request for help? Is it a request for help in committing suicide—either in obtaining the means for suicide or in carrying out the act? Is it a request for help in justifying the suicide to others? Is it a request for help in avoiding a suicide one has already decided to commit?
2. Why is the patient consulting a health professional?
3. What has kept the patient from attempting or committing suicide so far? Is it fear of death or fear of violent means of death that discourages such action?
4. Is the request for help in suicide a request for someone else to decide?
5. How stable and consistent with the patient's values is the request?
6. How far in the future would the suicide take place?
7. Are the medical and nonmedical facts cited in the request accurate? Specifically, is the diagnosis accurate? What confirmation of the diagnosis does he or she have? What about the prognosis? How secure is it? Has an independent second or third opinion been obtained? Does the patient accurately understand treatment options for future stages of terminal illness (e.g., pain control in terminal cancer)?
8. Is the suicide plan financially motivated?
9. Has the patient considered the effects of suicide on other people? Has the patient considered possible emotional trauma to survivors? What about the stigma associated with suicide?
10. Does the patient fear becoming a burden?
11. What cultural influences are shaping the patient's choice?
12. Are the patient's affairs in order?
13. Has the patient picked a method of committing suicide?
14. Would the patient be willing to tell others about the suicide plan? Would he or she be willing to confide the plan to friends?
15. Does the patient see suicide as the only way out? Does he or she have an alternative plan for coping with terminal illness, and, if so, how realistic is this plan?
16. Does the patient have a hopeless condition?
17. Has the patient made the decision to commit suicide without coercion from others?
18. Has the person demonstrated the use of a sound decision-making process (e.g., mentally competent, nonimpulsive consideration of alternatives, congruence between suicide and personal values, consideration of impact on others, consultation with significant others)?

**Figure 17-3. Questions That Help Clinicians to Evaluate Rational Suicide**

*Note.* From "Rational Suicide: How Can We Respond to a Request for Help?" by M.P. Battin, 1991, *Crisis, 12*, pp. 74–77. Copyright 1991 by Hogrefe and Huber Publishers. Adapted with permission.

## Case Study

Lynnette is a very active 66-year-old married Caucasian woman who was asymptomatic when diagnosed with ductal cancer in situ. She had surgery, and shortly afterward, a biopsy showed a more invasive type of breast cancer; additional surgery was advised. A more extensive mastectomy was performed followed by chemotherapy. Lynnette is moderately overweight but in good health. She has no history of malignancy in first-degree relatives. Although her parents are deceased, Lynnette has a married brother and cousins who live nearby. She has never smoked and has no more than two alcoholic drinks per week. She has no prior history of substance abuse or psychiatric disorders.

During treatment, Lynnette wanted to continue her tennis, golf, church participation, and volunteer activities at the museum, pet shelter, and free clinic. The nurse continuously assesses her levels of distress at each visit. During a 12-month follow-up appointment, Lynnette reports not feeling hungry and often does not eat. The nurse inquires about stress management, social support, symptoms, and feelings. Lynnette responds that she has been too tired to play tennis and golf but was thinking about going to the gym for a light workout. She describes her coping mechanisms as reading, listening to music, walking, and sleeping. Further probing by the nurse reveals more concerns.

According to NCCN recommendations, the nurse screens for distress and is prepared to recommend psychosocial resources for high distress or depressive symptoms. Further questions reveal symptoms of weight loss, anhedonia, sadness, insomnia, thoughts of death, and suicidal impulses. Lynnette describes her tendency to become isolated when she feels depressed. She complains that she does not want to tell her partner or family about her sadness, and she thinks her chemotherapy treatment is more trouble than it is worth. The nurse suspects that a major depressive episode and suicidal impulses might have been triggered by the breast cancer or chemotherapy. When asked about suicidal impulses, Lynnette reports that she has "often thought of ending it all." Her depressed symptoms do not seem to occur in relation to the chemotherapy.

Lynnette fears she will continue to be too tired to participate in her favorite activities and will burden her partner and family. She has difficulty concentrating and feels worthless. She tends to stay at home and read or watch television, thinking that this will help her feel better. Lynnette feels worried that she will not have the future she wanted.

## Discussion

The nurse who suspected that Lynnette was having a major depressive episode and suicidal impulses realized that breast cancer survivors have an increased risk of depressive disorders in the first year and for several years after treatment. She received her diagnosis after the nurse's in-depth assessment. Working collaboratively with Lynnette and her treatment team, the nurse set initial goals to prevent suicide, reduce depressive symptoms, and improve social support. Referrals were made to psychosocial resources (e.g., psychotherapy or counseling, support groups, nutrition support, pastoral counseling, exercise support). The nurse also explored whether Lynnette would be interested in considering aromatherapy, music therapy, massage, relaxation, and yoga as alternative methods to improve mood and well-being.

After the nurse explained that both cancer and depression were treatable and that depression can occur after breast cancer, Lynnette agreed to a psychiatric consultation. She described her tendency to become isolated when she felt sad and wanted to learn more about myths and treatment of depression. Lynnette agreed to try antidepressant medication, attend a support group, and consider pastoral counseling. She was interested in massage, relaxation, aromatherapy, and yoga to see if they would reduce her distress and increase her energy. Lynnette was willing to talk about her sadness and fears with her two best friends. She also wanted the nurse to explain more about depression and some of the nonpharmacologic treatments.

## Conclusion

Patients with cancer are more likely than the general population to become depressed and suicidal. Depression often is undetected or undertreated because of the assumption that it is normal following a diagnosis of cancer or that, to some healthcare professionals and loved ones, suicide might be a rational choice. Clinical depression in patients with cancer can be relieved with interventions, including psychotherapy, medications, education, and self-care skill attainment. The key is to determine which interventions are most appropriate for patients, depending on individual preferences and availability of services. Oncology nurses need to become adept in accurately identifying patients at risk for depression and suicide. They need to be aware of their own attitudes about suicide and depression so that they can be effective in listening, interviewing, supporting, and planning care.

## References

Akechi, T.I., Ietsugu, T., Sukigara, M., Okamura, H., Nakano, T., Akizuki, N., ... Uchitomi, Y. (2009). Symptom indicator of severity of depression in cancer patients: A comparison of the DSM IV criteria with alternative diagnostic criteria. *General Hospital Psychiatry, 31,* 225–232. doi:10.1016/j.genhosppsych.2008.12.004

American Psychiatric Association. (2013). *Diagnostic and statistical manual of mental disorders* (5th ed.). Washington, DC: Author.

Anguiano, L., Mayer, D.K., Piven, M.L., & Rosenstein, D. (2012). A literature review of suicide in cancer patients. *Cancer Nursing, 35,* E14–E26. doi:10.1097/NCC.0b013e31822fc76c

Beck, A.R., Rush, J., Shaw, B.F., & Emery, G. (Eds.). (1979). *Cognitive therapy of depression.* New York, NY: Guilford Press.

Bill-Axelson, A.G., Garmo, H., Lambe, M., Bratt, O., Adolfsson, J., Nyberg, U., ... Stattin, P. (2010). Suicide risk in men with prostate-specific antigen-detected early prostate cancer: A nationwide population-based cohort study from PCBaSe Sweden. *European Urology, 57,* 390–395. doi:10.1016/j.eururo.2009.10.035

Blair, E. (2012). Understanding depression: Awareness, assessment, and nursing intervention. *Clinical Journal of Oncology Nursing, 16,* 463–465. doi:10.1188/12.CJON.463-465

Cope, D.G., Coignet, H., Conley, S., Doherty, A., Drapek, L., Feldenzer, K., ... Walker, D.K. (2017). Putting Evidence Into Practice: Depression. Retrieved from https://www.ons.org/practice-resources/pep/depression

Cosci, F.F., Fava, G.A., & Sonino, N. (2015). Mood and anxiety disorders as early manifestations of medical illness: A systematic review. *Psychotherapy and Psychosomatics, 84,* 22–29. doi:10.1159/000367913

Cull, J., & Gill, W.S. (1982). *Suicide Probability Scale (SPS) manual.* Los Angeles, CA: Western Psychological Services.

Davis, M.P., & Goforth, H.W. (2014). Long-term and short-term effects of insomnia in cancer and effective interventions. *Cancer Journal, 20,* 330–344. doi:10.1097/PPO.0000000000000071

Dees, M.V.-D., Vernooij-Dassen, M.J., Dekkers, W.J., Vissers, K.C., & van Weel, C. (2011). 'Unbearable suffering': A qualitative study on the perspectives of patients who request assistance in dying. *Journal of Medical Ethics, 37,* 727–734. doi:10.1136/jme.2011.045492

Degner, L., Hack, T., O'Neil, J., & Kristjanson, L.J. (2003). A new approach to eliciting meaning in the context of breast cancer. *Cancer Nursing, 26,* 169–178. doi:10.1097/00002820-200306000-00001

Dierckx de Casterlé, B., Verpoort, C., De Bal, N., & Gastmans, C. (2006). Nurses views on their involvement in euthanasia: A qualitative study in Flanders (Belgium). *Journal of Medical Ethics, 32,* 187–192.

Edelstein, B.A., Heisel, M.J., McKee, D.R., Martin, R.R., Koven, L.P., Duberstein, P.R., & Britton, P.C. (2009). Development and psychometric evaluation of the Reasons for Living—Older Adults Scale: A suicide risk assessment inventory. *Gerontologist, 49,* 736–745. doi:10.1093/geront/gnp052

Given, B., & Given, C.S. (2012). Family and caregiver needs over the course of the cancer trajectory. *Journal of Supportive Oncology, 10,* 57–64. doi:10.1016/j.suponc.2011.10.003

Hack, T.C., Carlson, L., Butler, L., Degner, L.F., Jakulj, F., Pickles, T., ... Weir, L. (2011). Facilitating the implementation of empirically valid interventions in psychosocial oncology and supportive care. *Supportive Care in Cancer, 19,* 1097–1105. doi:10.1007/s00520-011-1159-z

Johnson, T.V., Garlow, S.J., Brawley, O.W., & Master, V.A. (2012). Peak window of suicides occurs within the first month of diagnosis: Implications for clinical oncology. *Psycho-Oncology, 21,* 351–356. doi:10.1002/pon.1905

Krebber, A.M.H., Buffart, L.M., Kleijn, G., Riepma, I.C., de Bree, R., Leemans, C.R., ... Verdonck-de Leeuw, I.M. (2014). Prevalence of depression in cancer patients: A meta-analysis of diagnostic interviews and self-report instruments. *Psycho-Oncology, 23,* 121–130. doi:10.1002/pon.3409

Leung, Y.L., Li, M., Devins, G., Zimmerman, C., Rydall, A., Lo, C., & Rodin, G. (2013). Routine screening for suicidal intention in patients with cancer. *Psycho-Oncology, 22,* 2537–2545. doi:10.1002/pon.3319

Lloyd-Williams, M., Shiels, C., & Dowrick, C. (2007). The development of the Brief Edinburgh Depression Scale (BEDS) to screen for depression in patients with advanced cancer. *Journal of Affective Disorders, 99,* 259–264. doi:10.1016/j.jad.2006.09.015

Loggers, E.T., Starks, H., Shannon-Dudley, M., Back, A.L., Appelbaum, F.S., & Stewart, F.M. (2013). Implementing a death with dignity program at a comprehensive cancer center. *New England Journal of Medicine, 368,* 1417–1424. doi:10.1056/NEJMsa1213398

Lovell, M., Phillips, J., Luckett, T., & Agar, M. (2015). Improving the system for managing cancer pain. *Internal Medicine Journal, 45,* 361–362. doi:10.1111/imj.12677

Manicavasagar, V., Perich, T.P., & Parker, G. (2012). Cognitive predictors of change in cognitive behaviour therapy and mindfulness-based cognitive therapy for depression. *Behavioural and Cognitive Psychotherapy, 40,* 227–232. doi:10.1017/S1352465811000634

Massie, M.J., Lloyd-Williams, M., Irving, G., & Miller, K. (2011). The prevalence of depression in people with cancer. In D.W. Kissane, M. Maj, & N. Sartorius (Eds.), *Depression and cancer* (pp. 1–36). West Sussex, United Kingdom: Wiley-Blackwell.

Mishra, S.I., Scherer, R.W., Snyder, C., Geigle, P.M., Berlanstein, D.R., & Topaloglu, O. (2012). Exercise interventions on health-related quality of life for people with cancer during active treatment. *Clinical Otolaryngology, 37,* 390–392. doi:10.1111/coa.12015

Muehlbauer, P. (2013). Screen for psychosocial distress in patients with cancer. *ONS Connect, 28,* 34.

Musselman, D.L. (2011). Biology of depression and cytokines in cancer. In D.W. Kissane, M. Maj, & N. Sartorius (Eds.), *Depression and cancer* (pp. 51–80). West Sussex, United Kingdom: Wiley-Blackwell.

NANDA International. (2015). *Nursing diagnoses: Definitions and classification, 2015–2017.* Philadelphia, PA: Author.

National Comprehensive Cancer Network. (2017). *NCCN Clinical Practice Guidelines in Oncology (NCCN Guidelines®): Distress management* [v.2.2017]. Retrieved from https://www.nccn.org/professionals/physician_gls/pdf/distress.pdf

Oregon Public Health Division. (2017). *Oregon death with dignity annual report: 2016 data summary.* (2017). Retrieved from http://www.oregon.gov/oha/PH/PROVIDERPARTNERRESOURCES/EVALUATIONRESEARCH/DEATHWITHDIGNITYACT/Documents/year19.pdf

Pignone, M.G., Gaynes, B.N., Rushton, J.L., Mulrow, C.D., Orleans, C.T., Whitener, B.L., ... Lohr, K.N. (2002). Screening for depression: Systematic evidence review. Retrieved from https://www.ahrq.gov/downloads/pub/prevent/pdfser/depser.pdf

Pinquart, M., & Duberstein, P.R. (2010). Depression and cancer mortality: A meta-analysis. *Psychological Medicine, 40,* 1797–1810. doi:10.1017/S0033291709992285

Plutchik, R., van Praag, H.M., Conte, H.R., & Picard, S. (1989). Correlates of suicide and violence risk. 1. The suicide risk measure. *Comprehensive Psychiatry, 30,* 296–302. doi:10.1016/0010-40X(89)90053-9

Puskar, K., & Urda, B. (2011). Examining the efficacy of no-suicide contracts in inpatient psychiatric settings: Implications for psychiatric nursing. *Issues in Mental Health Nursing, 32,* 785–788. doi:10.3109/01612840.2011.599476

Raingruber, B. (2011). The effectiveness of psychosocial interventions with cancer patients: An integrative review of the literature (2006–2011). *International Scholarly Research Notices,* Article ID 638218. doi:10.5402/2011/638218

Rodin, G. (2014). Effective treatment for depression in patients with cancer. *Lancet, 384,* 1076–1078. doi:10.1016/S0140-6736(14)61342-8

Rosenfeld, B., Breitbart, W., Galietta, M., Kaim, M., Funesti-Esch, J., Pessin, H., ... Brescia, R. (2000). The Schedule of Attitudes toward Hastened Death: Measuring desire for death in terminally ill cancer patients. *Cancer, 88,* 2868–2877. doi:10.1002/1097-0142(20000615)88:12<2868::AID-CNCR30>3.0.CO;2-K

Sadock, B.J., & Sadock, V.A. (2007). *Kaplan and Sadock's synopsis of psychiatry: Behavioral sciences/clinical psychiatry* (10th ed.). Philadelphia, PA: Lippincott Williams & Wilkins.

Sadock, B.J., Sadock, V.A., & Ruiz, P. (2015). *Kaplan and Sadock's synopsis of psychiatry: Behavioral sciences/clinical psychiatry* (11th ed.). Philadelphia, PA: Lippincott Williams & Wilkins.

Schramme, T. (2013). Rational suicide, assisted suicide, and indirect legal paternalism. *International Journal of Law and Psychiatry, 36,* 477–484. doi:10.1016/j.ijlp.2013.06.008

Sharma, M.H., & Haider, T. (2013). Yoga as an alternative and complementary treatment for cancer: A systematic review. *Journal of Evidence-Based Complementary and Alternative Medicine, 19,* 870–875. doi:10.1177/2156587212460046

Sharpe, M.W., Walker, J., Holm Hansen, C., Martin, P., Symeonides, S., Gourley, C., ... Murray, G. (2014). Integrated collaborative care for comorbid major depression in patients with cancer (SMaRT Oncology-2): A multicentre randomized controlled effectiveness trial. *Lancet, 384,* 1099–1108. doi:10.1016/S0140-6736(14)61231-9

Siu, A.L., & U.S. Preventive Services Task Force. (2016). Screening for depression in adults: U.S. Preventive Services Task Force recommendation statement. *JAMA, 315,* 380–387. doi:10.1001/jama.2015.18392

Smith, G., Jr. (2011). Refractory pain, existential suffering, and palliative care: Releasing an unbearable lightness of being. *Cornell Journal of Law and Public Policy, 20,* 469–532.

Townsend, M.C. (2015). *Psychiatric mental health nursing: Concepts of care in evidence-based practice* (8th ed.). Philadelphia, PA: F.A. Davis.

Valente, S. (2010). Oncology nurses' knowledge of suicide evaluation and prevention. *Cancer Nursing, 33,* 290–295. doi:10.1097/NCC.0b013e3181cc4f33

Valente, S. (2011). Nurses' psychosocial barriers to suicide risk management. *Nursing Research and Practice, 2011,* Article ID 65076. doi:10.1155/2011/650765

Walker, J.S., Hansen, C.H., Martin, P., Symeonides, S., Gourley, C., Wall, L., ... Sharpe, M. (2014). Integrated collaborative care for major depression comorbid with a poor prognosis cancer (SMaRT Oncology-3): A multicentre randomized controlled trial in patients with lung cancer. *Lancet Oncology, 15,* 1168–1176. doi:10.1016/S1470-2045(14)70343-2

Walker, J., Sawhney, A., Hansen, C.H., Ahmed, S., Martin, P., Symeonides, S.G., ... Sharpe, M. (2014). Treatment of depression in adults with cancer: A systematic review of randomized controlled trials. *Psychological Medicine, 44,* 897–907. doi:10.1017/S0033291713001372

Williams, M.L., & Payne, S. (2003). A qualitative study of clinical nurse specialists' views on depression in palliative care patients. *Palliative Medicine, 17,* 334–338. doi:10.1191/0269216303pm747oa

Yennurajalingam, S., Urbauer, D.L., Casper, K.L., Reyes-Gibby, C.C., Chacko, R., Poulter, V., & Bruera, E. (2011). Impact of a palliative care consultation team on cancer-related symptoms in advanced cancer patients referred to an outpatient supportive care clinic. *Journal of Pain and Symptom Management, 41,* 49–56. doi:10.1016/j.jpainsymman.2010.03.017

Zager, B., & Yancy, M. (2011). A call to improve practice concerning cultural sensitivity in advance directives: A review of the literature. *Worldviews on Evidence-Based Nursing, 8,* 202–211. doi:10.1111/j.1741-6787.2011.00222.x

Zung, W. (1974). Index of potential suicide (IPS): A rating scale for suicide prevention. In T. Beck, H. Resnick, & D. Lettieri (Eds.), *The prediction of suicide* (pp. 221–249). Bowie, MD: Charles Press.

# CHAPTER 18

# Distress

*Nancy Jo Bush, DNP, RN, MN, MA, AOCN®, FAAN*

> *Without mental health, there can be no true physical health.*
> —Brock Chisholm

The journey across the cancer trajectory often brings distress for patients and families. Distress has been defined as an "unpleasant emotional experience of a psychological (i.e., cognitive, behavioral, emotional), social and/or spiritual nature that may interfere with the ability to cope effectively with cancer, its physical symptoms, and its treatment" (National Comprehensive Cancer Network® [NCCN®], 2017, p. 2) and severe enough to interfere with daily function (Mitchell, 2015). The causes of distress are multifactorial, can occur anywhere along the cancer continuum (diagnosis, treatment, end of treatment, recurrence, and end-of-life care), and may change over time (Gao, Bennett, Stark, Murray, & Higginson, 2010). Distress can range from normal feelings of fear, vulnerability, and sadness, to more serious symptoms of depression and anxiety, panic, social isolation, and existential and spiritual crisis (NCCN, 2017). Research has found that patient distress is associated with reduced quality of life, poor response and adherence to treatment, poor self-management, higher healthcare costs, and higher mortality (Estes & Karten, 2014; Fann, Ell, & Sharpe, 2012; Gao et al., 2010). The term *adjustment disorder* is often used to describe distress in the literature. Adjustment disorders with anxiety and/or depressed mood constitute the majority of psychiatric diagnoses found in the patient population (Holland & Alici, 2010). At any one time, 30%–50% of patients with a recent cancer diagnosis have also been diagnosed with an adjustment disorder (Mitchell, 2015). It is estimated that one-third to one-half of patients receiving outpatient cancer care have symptoms of distress due to pain, fatigue, insomnia, and depression (Fann et al., 2012), which often appear in symptom clusters.

In 2008, the Health and Medicine Division of the National Academies of Sciences, Engineering, and Medicine (formerly the Institute of Medicine [IOM]) changed cancer care by releasing *Cancer Care for the Whole Patient: Meeting Psychosocial Health Needs*. It recommended that psychosocial services such as the identification of patient distress be integrated into routine cancer care (Adler & Page, 2008). The goal of psychosocial care is to maximize patients' quality of life, not just their quantity of life (Fann et al., 2012; Jacobsen & Wagner, 2012). Once patient needs are identified, it is vital to provide psychosocial services and interventions (pharmacologic and nonpharmacologic) to meet those needs in a coordinated and timely fashion (Fann et al., 2012). An interprofessional approach to psychosocial care is prudent, and screening for distress is inherent in the role of the oncology nurse (Fitch, 2011).

## Important Principles Related to Distress

*Distress* is not a clinical term that appears in the *Diagnostic and Statistical Manual of Mental Disorders (DSM-V)* but instead is a clinically significant criterion that represents several mood disorders (Carlson, Waller, & Mitchell, 2012). The term was chosen by NCCN (2016) for cancer screening, assessment, and care because it is less stigmatizing than terms such as *psychiatric, psychosocial,* or *emotional.* It is more useful than psychiatric terms such as *anxiety* or *depression* (Carlson et al., 2012), and it can be defined and easily measured by self-report (NCCN, 2016).

Standards of care for distress management have been developed by NCCN (2016) and other organizations (e.g., American College of Surgeons Commission on Cancer [ACoS CoC], American Society of Clinical Oncology, Canadian Association of Psychosocial Oncology, IOM, Oncology Nursing Society [ONS]) in recent years, supporting a greater number of patients receiving psychosocial support services (Jacobsen & Wagner, 2012). A report by IOM in 2008 outlined the deleterious effects of unmet psychosocial needs and named the beneficial effects of providing psychosocial services to patients in need (Adler & Page, 2008; Jacobsen & Wagner, 2012). The report mandated that organizations evaluating quality cancer care establish a provision for psychosocial services. NCCN's (2017) standards state that distress should be assessed and managed according to clinical practice guidelines. In addition, distress should be recognized, monitored, documented, and treated promptly at all stages of disease in all settings. The standards focus on an interprofessional approach, including disciplines such as certified chaplains and mental health professionals, along with cancer care professionals such as physicians, nurses, and social workers. The interprofessional team can identify and treat distress and incorporate educational and training programs to ensure that all healthcare professionals in cancer care obtain the knowledge and skills to assess and manage distress. ACoS CoC, an accrediting body of hospitals, sets new standards for patient-centered care that require the development and implementation of psychosocial distress screening and referral for psychosocial services (ACoS CoC, 2015; Jacobsen & Wagner, 2012). Distress has been given the title of the sixth vital sign by some to increase attention to it (Mitchell, 2015). Even so, Jacobsen and Wagner (2012) asserted concern that the wider community of oncology professionals is not cognizant of these initiatives for psychosocial care. In their review of the evolution of psychosocial oncology, Bultz and Johansen (2011) noted that a uniform model of program integration is lacking overall, resulting in challenges to the value of psychosocial aspects of care and the discipline itself.

## Distress in Patients With Cancer

Distress can occur anywhere along the cancer continuum. Diagnosis is often met with normal fears and feelings of vulnerability. The treatment phase unleashes its own set of emotional challenges, including normal anxiety. Physiological states such as pain and insomnia can also induce distress. At the end of treatment, what Mullan (1984) referred to as the "reentry phase," patients often express normal fears of being abandoned by the treatment team. At this time, concurrent fears of recurrence often begin to surface. Advances in cancer care have improved survival rates for patients, yet survivorship may translate into long-term effects from the disease and treatment. Symptoms such as pain, fatigue, anxiety, and depression are often reported as interfering with activities of daily living. This, in turn, negatively affects quality of life (NCCN, 2017). In addition, patients may have had a preexisting psychiatric disorder that was exacerbated by long-term effects or interferes with their ability to cope with the disease (NCCN, 2017).

Patients at increased risk for psychosocial distress and periods of increased vulnerability have been identified. Characteristics of these patients are outlined in Figure 18-1 and include ineffective coping skills, limited access to medical care, and others (NCCN, 2017). A history of prior psychiatric disorder or substance abuse increases the risk of distress and uncontrolled symptoms (e.g., pain). Cognitive impairment and comorbid illnesses can also increase distress and social issues (e.g., inadequate social support). Communication barriers also may increase the occurrence of distress. Research has identified that individuals with certain cancers, such as lung, brain, and pancreatic, are more likely to be distressed. These patients also are more likely to have poorer quality of life, disabilities, and ongoing unmet needs (Carlson et al., 2012). The prevalence of psychological distress is highest among patients with advanced disease and a poor prognosis (Holland & Alici, 2010). Unmet needs have been defined as a mismatch between the care that patients receive and the care that they perceive neces-

**Risk Factors for Distress**
- History of psychiatric disorder/substance abuse
- History of depression/suicide attempt
- Cognitive impairment
- Communication barriers
- Severe comorbid illnesses
- Ineffective coping
- Insomnia
- Social issues
- Family/caregiver conflicts
- Inadequate social support
- Living alone
- Financial problems
- Limited access to medical care
- Younger age
- Gender (female)
- History of abuse (physical, sexual)
- Other stressors
- Spiritual/religious concerns
- Uncontrolled symptoms (pain, fatigue)

**Points of Vulnerability**
- Finding a suspicious symptom
- Diagnostic workup
- Diagnosis
- Treatment
- Symptoms related to treatments
- End of treatment
- Transition to survivorship
- Medical follow-up and surveillance
- Recurrence/progression
- Advanced cancer
- End of life

**Figure 18-1. Psychosocial Distress Patient Characteristics**

*Note.* Adapted with permission from the NCCN Clinical Practice Guidelines in Oncology (NCCN Guidelines®) for Distress Management V.2.2016. © 2016 National Comprehensive Cancer Network, Inc. All rights reserved. The NCCN Guidelines® and illustrations herein may not be reproduced in any form for any purpose without the express written permission of NCCN. To view the most recent and complete version of the NCCN Guidelines, go online to NCCN.org. The NCCN Guidelines are a work in progress that may be refined as often as new significant data becomes available. NCCN makes no warranties of any kind whatsoever regarding their content, use or application and disclaims any responsibility for their application or use in any way.

sary to receive in order to achieve optimal well-being (Waller, Boyes, Carey, & Sanson-Fisher, 2015). Recent studies have demonstrated that unmet needs associated with distress often include psychological needs and are associated with being female, being socially disadvantaged, being younger, having poor social support, and not being in remission (Waller et al., 2015).

Periods of increased vulnerability for distress include any transitional stage along the cancer continuum, such as diagnosis, treatment, reentry, recurrence, and advancing cancer. The prediagnosis phase of finding a suspicious symptom begins what might be a rollercoaster ride of fear and apprehension of what the future holds. For some patients, distress, anxiety, and significant complications of pain and fatigue remain elevated months or years after initial diagnosis (Waller et al., 2015). In a grounded theory investigation of the perceptions of distress in women with ovarian cancer, although experiences differed, the findings supported a theory of "existential assault" across the cancer trajectory. For participants, distress was experienced largely within a psychological, psychosocial, and existential context (DellaRipa et al., 2015).

## Emergence of Psychosocial Care

The evolution of psychosocial oncology has occurred over the last 30 years (Bultz & Johansen, 2011). In 1999, NCCN released one of the first sets of practice guidelines for the psychosocial care of cancer survivors, including assessment and treatment of patient distress. Updated annually, these guidelines provide criteria for the assessment, management, and evaluation of distress (NCCN, 2016). IOM elevated the field of psychosocial care by providing an extensive review of the evidence linking psychosocial health needs with outcomes of patients with cancer (Adler & Page, 2008; Wagner & Pearman, 2015). In 2007, the American Psychosocial Oncology Society (APOS) developed quality indicators for psychosocial care, including documentation in the medical record that the patient's emotional well-being was assessed and that action was taken if a problem was identified (Jacobsen & Wagner, 2012).

ACoS CoC (2015) approved new standards in 2012 to promote patient-centered care that included requirements for psychosocial distress screening for hospital accreditation. This advanced psychosocial care from clinical practice guidelines to a required standard of care (Wagner & Pearman, 2015). Jacobsen and Wagner (2012) addressed the three major developments in recent years that will inevitably increase the number of patients who receive psychosocial care: (a) the formulation of standards of cancer care that include psychosocial care, (b) the development of clinical practice guidelines for psychosocial care of patients with cancer, and (c) the implementation of measurable indicators of the quality of psychosocial care in oncology settings. Other professional societies have identified the need for psychosocial care. A joint position statement from APOS, the Association of Oncology Social Work, and ONS (Pirl et al., 2015) endorsed the new standards by ACoS CoC on psychosocial distress screening, recognizing that screening will address the unmet psychosocial needs of patients with cancer and ultimately provide cancer care for the whole patient. It is yet to be seen how upcoming changes in healthcare will move psychosocial care into the future, and this may depend upon accreditation requirements and reimbursement for services (Wagner & Pearman, 2015). Regardless of healthcare implementation, identifying distress in patients with cancer has become a standard of quality cancer care.

## Distress as the Sixth Vital Sign

Seminal research studies over the past 10 years have identified that the distress of patients with cancer is complex, multidimensional, and prevalent; despite this, institutions were not committed to integrate routine cancer distress screening in clinical practice (Bultz, Loscalzo, & Holland, 2015). Naming distress as the sixth vital sign in 2004 was based upon years of psycho-oncology research supporting findings that patient distress had a direct impact on quality of life (Bultz et al., 2015). Two quality care standards were thus proclaimed by the International Psycho-Oncology Society in 2009 and stated that quality cancer care must include integration of psychosocial care into routine assessment and management and that distress should become a measurable domain after temperature, blood pressure, pulse, respiratory rate, and pain (Bultz et al., 2015). In 1999, the Joint Commission required screening and management of pain to become a standard in patient care (Bultz et al., 2015). This move provided for more accurate and timely assessment and management of patient pain, thus becoming a standard of care and serving as a model for distress as the sixth vital sign (Bultz & Carlson, 2005; Bultz et al., 2015). The burgeoning role of distress becoming the sixth vital sign requires that patient distress be monitored using standardized subjective measures and managed using evidence-based interventions (Bultz et al., 2015). For accreditation, ACoS CoC (2015) currently requires cancer care institutions to carry out distress screening on all patients with cancer.

## Screening for Distress

Although strong recommendations and accreditation agencies have endorsed distress screening, the actual routine practice of distress screening in cancer centers appears to be limited. Screening for patient distress in clinical oncology settings using clinical judgment or validated screening tools has been mixed. The effectiveness and acceptability of screening has brought forth much discussion and research (Mitchell, 2015). Three key variables are important for successful screening of distress: accuracy, acceptability, and quality follow-up (Mitchell, 2015). Screening should be viewed as a multistep process, initially using an accurate assessment tool acceptable to both clinician and patient. If distress is identified, appropriate, evidence-based interventions or referral should be carried out. A needs assessment should determine unresolved concerns that patients are experiencing to determine if further assistance is needed as well as the level of assistance required (Carlson et al., 2012). Screening should be carried out, monitored, and promptly treated at all stages of the cancer continuum to ensure quality patient care. Research has demonstrated that screening for distress alone is not sufficient to positively influence patient outcomes; adequate follow-up and referrals are essential to ensure quality psychosocial care (NCCN, 2016).

Clinical judgment of distress by clinicians using straightforward questions such as "How are you coping at the moment?" is generally seen as suboptimal versus structured tools that have been tested for psychometric properties (Mitchell, 2015; Vodermaier, Linden, & Siu, 2009). An advantage for using systematic screening for emotional distress is that it may ensure equal access to psychological services, whereas clinician or patient-initiated referrals may fail to identify and/or overlook patients most in need of support (Vodermaier et al., 2009). One such tool is the NCCN (2016) Distress Thermometer, which is used with or without a problem checklist of unmet needs. The Distress Thermometer is not a diagnostic tool but instead a screening tool in a multistep process to identify psychosocial needs (Tavernier, 2014).

The Distress Thermometer has gained popularity because of its ease of administration and acceptability in clinical practice (Ma et al., 2014; Tavernier, 2014). The thermometer component is a 0–10 scale, with 0 indicating no distress and 10 indicating extreme distress. Based upon NCCN (2016) recommendations, the cutoff value for mild distress is 4. A meta-analysis by Ma et al. (2014) supported the use of the Distress Thermometer for screening cancer-related distress and recommended (2010) the cutoff of 4 for patients at different stages of the cancer trajectory. A score of 4 or more may be indicative of moderate to high levels of distress, and further assessment is required. Mild distress may include commonly occurring symptoms of patients with cancer, such as fatigue, sleep disturbances, and cognitive dysfunction (Cohen & Bankston, 2011). Moderate distress may include adjustment disorders related to anxiety and difficulty coping with change and may also include dementia and delirium. Severe distress may include psychiatric disorders such as depression, anxiety, and post-traumatic stress disorder (Cohen & Bankston, 2011). In addition to the thermometer, NCCN (2016) created a problem checklist of physical concerns and practical problems that may influence patient distress. In the checklist, patients are asked to indicate if they have experienced the problem during the past week, including the day of screening. An area for the patient to identify "other" problems not mentioned is also on the checklist. The problem list aids the healthcare professional in identifying what resources (e.g., mental health, social work, chaplaincy) are needed for support.

A multidomain extension to the Distress Thermometer, called the Emotion Thermometer, was proposed by Mitchell, Baker-Glenn, Park, Granger, and Symonds (2010). This tool screens for the following emotions: distress, depression, anxiety, and anger. Other areas can be added, such as need for help, quality of life, and pain. Other tools that may screen for distress include the Psychological Distress Inventory, the Brief Symptom Inventory, and the Hopkins Symptom Checklist, but all need further research to support their evidence base for practice in oncology (Mitchell, 2015). The Patient-Reported Outcomes Measurement Information System is used to obtain self-reported information about an individual's physical and psychosocial function as well as social support and health-related quality of life (Bevans, Ross, & Cella, 2014). The Hospital Anxiety and Depression Scale has been validated in multiple cancer settings and can be used as a second-step assessment tool if distress is identified in the patient. Of interest is a review of the literature by Ziegler et al. (2011), which provided a systematic summary of validated self-report measures for identifying psychosocial distress at key junctures across the cancer trajectory. The study did not find one single measure to have evidence to support its use across all major points of the illness continuum; however, it identified different tools that were effective at different illness stages. It is important to note that the term *screening tool* often refers to short tests that can be sensitive to identify distressed patients but may lack the specificity to rule out those patients wrongly identified as distressed (false positives). Longer tests are often needed to reach reliability and validity but may carry high costs and allocation of staff and resources for administration and training (Vodermaier et al., 2009). Although some tools can be self-administered, screening for distress is seen as enhancing trust and building a therapeutic relationship when it directly involves the clinician (Mitchell, 2015). Besides identifying that a tool meets appropriate psychometric properties, another criterion is that it is culturally applicable to the patient population.

## Barriers to Screening

Barriers to screening for distress occur across a continuum of patient, clinician, and system barriers (Cohen & Bankston, 2011). It should never be assumed that distress associated with the cancer experience is inevitable. Often, the patients experiencing distress are the least likely to share their feelings with a professional; the inability to cope with cancer continues to carry a social and cultural stigma (Cohen & Bankston, 2011). Clinicians put up barriers to distress screening because of their lack of knowledge regarding psychosocial issues and their inability to handle them, poor communication skills and lack of training, and their focus on more objective measures that have verified patient outcomes (e.g., lab values) (Cohen & Bankston, 2011). Overall, barriers to adopting the Distress Thermometer in practice included time, concern about the increased demand for referrals, lack of knowledge about how to screen for and then manage distress, and no perceived benefit of screening (Tavernier, 2014). System barriers include the lack of staff training for assessment and diagnosis, reimbursement for psychosocial services, and communication and care coordination between professionals across settings (e.g., inpatient, outpatient, primary care) (Cohen & Bankston, 2011). In a study exploring the views of cancer professionals regarding accountability for the detection and management of emotional distress, many participants noted the importance of detection but were uncertain of their roles and responsibilities, often turning to the expert clinician (e.g., clinical nurse specialist) to be responsible for psychosocial assessment and management (Absolom et al., 2011).

Many barriers can be avoided by educating and training staff, carrying out routine screening, and providing guidelines for management and referral. Most importantly, it is recommended that distress screening be supported at an organizational level to address the unmet needs of patients. This includes not only psychosocial support but practical support as well with the treatment of physical issues such as pain, fatigue, and sleep disturbances (Carlson et al., 2013). A paucity of studies address the implementation of routine screening tools in the clinical setting (Carlson et al., 2013; Fitch, 2011). One such study carried out in ambulatory oncology was able to address barriers, outcomes, and benefits implementing the NCCN distress management guidelines (Hammelef, Friese, Breslin, Riba, & Schneider, 2014). Although the sample was small and not statistically significant, referrals for psychosocial services increased, and the timing of receipt of those services was decreased through use of a screening tool and guidelines. A dearth of research data are available on the effects of routine screening for distress on patient-reported outcomes in randomized controlled trials (Carlson et al., 2012). Current best practice examples for psychosocial screening were discussed by Clark et al. (2012) and include institutions such as the City of Hope National Medical Center and the Cancer Support Community.

## Nursing Care of Patients Experiencing Distress

### Assessment

Oncology nurses play a pivotal role in both identifying distress in patients experiencing cancer and following through to identify needed interventions (see Figure 18-2). Estes and Karten (2014) discussed the "therapeutic presence" of nurses as a framework for assessment of distress in patients. For patients with mild distress related to common physical and emotional sequelae of the disease and treatment (e.g., fatigue), most often these issues can be appropriately managed by the cancer care team (Vitek, Rosenzweig, & Strollings, 2007). For patients with undue anxiety or depressive symptoms, appropriate referral should be carried out. Assessment for distress should be done at major points of transition across the cancer trajectory, and reevaluation of distress symptoms is imperative (Vitek et al., 2007). Assessment should begin with a thorough health history that includes any psy-

## Assessment
- Recognize the signs and symptoms of distress.
- Validate patients' perceptions of the cancer experience.
- Assess for distress at major transition points along the cancer continuum.
- Differentiate between normal or expected distress responses and abnormal responses.
- Assess for previous psychiatric disorders (e.g., mood or adjustment disorders).
- Assess for underlying medical conditions (e.g., pain, sepsis, medications, cognitive disruptions, metabolic imbalances, hormonal imbalances) that may be contributing to distress symptoms.
- Assess for concurrent symptoms of depression, anxiety, delirium, or dementia.

## Nursing Diagnoses (NANDA International, 2015)
- Anxiety
- Ineffective coping
- Post-trauma syndrome
- Impaired mood regulation
- Fear

## *DSM-V* Diagnoses (American Psychiatric Association, 2013)
- Adjustment disorder with mixed anxiety and depressed mood
- Generalized anxiety disorder
- Major depressive disorder
- Delirium
- Panic disorder
- Specific phobia (blood-injection-injury type)
- Post-traumatic stress disorder
- Anxiety or depressive disorder due to another medical condition
- Substance/medication-induced anxiety disorder

## Expected Outcomes
- Patients will identify feelings associated with distress.
- Patients will identify causative factors for distress.
- Patients will problem solve and develop ways to recognize and control distress.
- Patients will participate in strategies to relieve distress (e.g., relaxation techniques) if appropriate.

## Interventions
- Provide a safe, supportive environment.
- Routinely carry out distress screening.
- Educate patients regarding the disease and treatment.
- Utilize an interprofessional approach.
- Answer questions, and provide time for patients to reflect.
- Encourage verbalization of fears and anxieties.
- Normalize feelings for patients at each crisis point of the disease continuum.
- Assess present and past coping mechanisms.
- Identify resources within the setting (e.g., social work, chaplaincy).
- Teach cognitive behavioral techniques to decrease distress (e.g., relaxation exercises, cognitive reframing).
- Provide positive reinforcement for adaptive coping strategies.
- Administer anxiolytic or antidepressant medications, and educate patients about their purpose and effects.
- Refer patients for psychiatric evaluation, if necessary.
- Provide supportive resources for patients' coping (e.g., refer to support groups).
- Evaluate patients' outcomes, and revise the plan of care, when appropriate.

**Figure 18-2. Plan of Care**

chiatric history and treatment. The physical examination should follow to determine if any underlying symptoms of disease and treatment (e.g., uncontrolled pain) are contributing to distress. It is not uncommon in cancer treatment for physical symptoms to be associated with distress. Accurate assessment of distress may be challenging, as symptoms of distress are often difficult to distinguish from disease symptoms and treatment side effects (Estes & Karten, 2014).

Assessment for mild to severe distress includes identifying the following emotions or behaviors: excessive fears or worries that interfere with coping or carrying out activities of daily living; feelings of sadness, despair, or hopelessness; difficulty concentrating; religious crises; or dysfunction in relationships (e.g., family issues) (Vitek et al., 2007). Underlying psychiatric disorders, such as generalized anxiety disorder, dementia, delirium, adjustment disorder, substance abuse, or personality disorder may underlie distressful emotions and behaviors (Vitek et al., 2007). Appropriate guidelines (e.g., NCCN) can provide guidance for treatment and referral. Identification of comorbid illnesses (e.g., diabetes) also is important, as stress is associated with chronic illness and may exacerbate patients' distress levels (Petty & Lester, 2014). Distress in older adult patients often presents as somatic symptoms, which can be attributed to the cancer or treatment and therefore missed during assessment (Cohen & Bankston, 2011). Few studies have focused on minorities or have identified how low socioeconomic status affects distress in patients with cancer; however, some studies have identified differences in coping strategies used by different ethnicities (Cohen & Bankston, 2011) (see Chapters 4 and 5 for information on culture and coping). Some evidence suggests that quality of life is compromised in ethnic minorities diagnosed with cancer compared to their Caucasian counterparts (Stanton, 2012). A recent study of cancer experiences and health-related quality of life among racial and ethnic minority survivors of young adult cancer revealed that race/ethnicity had a significant effect on emotional, but not physical, social, or spiritual, health-related quality of life (Munoz et al., 2016). These studies highlight the need to assess cultural background to tailor care among racial and ethnic minorities. Therefore, an important objective for routine screening is to meet the needs of *all* underserved populations, such as those with low income, ethnic minorities, and psychosocially distressed individuals (Carlson et al., 2012).

## Differential Diagnosis

In patients experiencing emotional distress, factors other than their psychological state need to be ruled out first. A differential diagnosis must rule out symptoms of disease and treatment that can cause distress (e.g., pain). Underlying metabolic imbalances and medications can also contribute to patient distress. Once medical conditions contributing to distress have been ruled out and treated, the nurse must then direct attention to psychosocial causes. For patients with mild distress, expected feelings (e.g., fear) should be normalized so that the patient can understand that distress is common at different transitions across the cancer continuum. Patients with moderate or severe distress could be experiencing mood or adjustment disorders (mixed anxiety and depressive symptoms) that demand immediate attention. Patients must be assessed for a range of psychiatric conditions that often exist in the oncology setting (Holland & Alici, 2011; Mehta & Roth, 2015), and safety of the patient and others becomes the priority. Patients experiencing mood and adjustment disorders can develop suicidal tendencies and may be a danger not only to themselves but also to others, making psychiatric consultation warranted (NCCN, 2016). Overall, it is important to remember that psychiatric disorders in the cancer setting usually are direct responses to the illness or treatment, whereas others may be preexisting psychiatric problems exacerbated by the illness

(Mehta & Roth, 2015). A thorough health history and physical examination can provide the needed information for a differential diagnosis.

## Interventions

Mild distress is often expected with a cancer diagnosis and treatment and can easily be handled by the specialized oncology team. Most often, when physical side effects are treated (e.g., insomnia), distress is decreased. Interventions for mild distress include carrying out education to inform patients of what to expect from treatment, using appropriate medications for symptom control, and using nonpharmacologic interventions such as relaxation techniques and guided imagery (Vitek et al., 2007).

Stanton (2012) discussed the results of randomized trials to support that interventions offered at reentry/survivorship can be effective. These interventions include cognitive behavioral strategies, stress management (e.g., relaxation and mindfulness), and psychoeducational approaches. Evidence has shown that interventions confer benefits in domains such as depressive symptoms, physical functioning, fatigue, fear of recurrence, sexual health, and quality of life. Other problems shown to be responsive to cognitive behavioral interventions include insomnia, post-traumatic stress symptoms, menopausal symptoms, and pain. In addition, interventions directed at monitoring cancer-related thoughts and emotions (e.g., fear of recurrence) and behaviors (e.g., strengthening coping skills, goal setting, problem solving) have also been shown to be effective in reducing distress and improving the overall quality of life among patients with cancer (Holland & Alici, 2010). Interventions also may include psychoeducational, pharmacologic, and supportive approaches as well as individual and group or family therapies (Clark et al., 2012). Stanton (2012) emphasized that an opportune time to offer psychosocial care to survivors are at the end of treatment completion and into survivorship, at follow-up appointments, and during cancer surveillance. These points in the cancer trajectory offer times for nurses and other team members to inquire about emotional well-being, provide psychosocial care, and offer referrals if needed. Interventions should be discussed collaboratively with patients, and any plan should address the management of physical health problems, and any psychological, social, and spiritual consequences of the cancer experience (Clark et al., 2012). Readministration of any screening tools used and reevaluation of interventions are vital in determining whether patients' levels of distress have improved or if an intervention needs to be modified or replaced (Clark et al., 2012). Documentation of interventions are of importance to demonstrate that psychosocial interventions have been carried out (Clark et al., 2012).

## Nursing Interventions for Distress

To ensure patient-centered care, ACoS CoC (2015) updated requirements for institutional accreditation. This included making psychosocial distress screening in all cancer programs a standard care of patients with cancer. This standard mandates that a process be implemented each year that ensures to "integrate and monitor onsite psychosocial distress screening and referral for the provision of psychosocial care" (p. 56). This standard also outlines the following processes that the interprofessional team can follow to meet this requirement (ACoS CoC, 2015):
- **Timing of screening:** All patients with cancer must be screened at least once at a "pivotal time" across the cancer continuum. Pivotal times include but are not limited to time of diagnosis, time of surgery or chemotherapy/radiation, or when the practitioner deems to be a time of greatest risk for distress. Nurses are in a prime position to evaluate pivotal

times of distress across cancer settings, and the patient may require more than one screening (e.g., at diagnosis and recurrence).
- **Method:** The mode of administration of the screening instrument may be chosen by the cancer committee. It is required that all staff administering the tool be formally trained, which includes administration, interpretation, assessment, treatment, or referral for treatment for the source of distress identified by the instrument.
- **Tools:** A valid and reliable screening tool may be chosen and approved by the cancer committee. Different tools are available and researched, including the Distress Thermometer (Mitchell, 2010; NCCN, 2016).
- **Assessment and referral:** Screening must be discussed with each patient face-to-face at the medical visit. If moderate or severe distress is evident, the practitioner must identify the source of distress (e.g., physical, psychological, social, spiritual, financial) and refer the patient appropriately on-site or off-site (e.g., psychiatrist) if needed.
- **Documentation:** To facilitate "integrated, high-quality care," the results of screening, referral, and follow-up must all be documented in the patient's medical record (ACoS CoC, 2015, p. 57). Records must also be kept regarding the number of patients screened, number of patients referred for distress, follow-up carried out, and where patients were referred (e.g., on-site, referral source).

As part of an accreditation process, ACoS CoC (2015) stated that a designated oncology nurse manager or leader uses standards and guidelines for evidence-based practice. Nurses are in a prime position to lead the interprofessional team in psychosocial distress screening. ACoS CoC (2015) recommended a "psychosocial services coordinator" position that can be filled by a "professional trained in the psychosocial aspects of cancer care" (p. 57). To achieve optimal outcomes, who but a seasoned and trained oncology nurse leader is better equipped to lead this charge (Brown, 2014)?

## Case Study

Bill is a 55-year-old African American man with a history of prostate cancer initially treated with prostatectomy five years prior. He is admitted to the outpatient oncology unit to be treated for metastatic disease. Recently, he has complained of nonstop back discomfort. After follow-up computed tomography scans, he is found to have bone metastases located mainly in his lower spine. Because of the risk of spinal cord compression, Bill is started on docetaxel and is concurrently treated with radiation therapy for pain control.

Upon taking a thorough health history, the admitting nurse identifies that Bill is a proud and hardworking man. He worked as a construction manager and was the breadwinner for his wife and two sons. Bill is tearful after being asked, "How are you feeling emotionally?" The nurse uses the Distress Thermometer to gauge Bill's emotional distress; he scores a 7. He expresses that his diagnosis five years ago has brought on major depression as he dealt with impotence and urinary incontinence. Bill has not sought psychiatric help because his primary care doctor placed him on an antidepressant that "seemed to help." Eventually, he weaned himself off the medication because he hated to be on drugs to help him cope. He states that although his urinary incontinence has resolved, he and his wife still struggle with their sexual relationship.

Currently, Bill is fearful of how the recent diagnosis will affect his work, as his job requires a physical presence. He is also distressed about how the recurrence of his disease will affect his family. His father died of prostate cancer, and Bill knows all too well that this knowledge was difficult not only for his wife but also his two young adult sons. He feels that although they are concerned about him, they are also concerned about their own welfare if something happens to him. The nurse probes into Bill's current emotional state. She first inquires about physical symptoms that could be causing distress and finds that Bill's pain level is a constant 5, with no alleviating factors. He "hates to take pills," so he is not on any pain medication, nor is he taking anything for his anxiety. Additionally, he is having difficulty sleeping due to his "nerves" and feels that he has been battling insomnia for weeks since his diagnosis. In a caring and supportive manner, the nurse inquires about Bill's feelings of sadness and fear. She asks how often he is feeling sad and if it is interfering with his activities of daily living or his occupational or social roles. Bill responds that he feels he cannot concentrate. He feels sad nearly every day, most of the day, and suffers from fatigue and the inability to concentrate. He expresses to the nurse that he fears that these same symptoms were what he experienced "years ago." The nurse responsibly asks if Bill has had any suicidal thoughts or tendencies, and he has not. He mostly is worried about what this recurrence means for his future health and longevity. The nurse assures Bill that the oncology team will be able to support his physical and psychosocial needs and that he is in a safe environment to talk about his feelings. She explains to him that she will speak with other members of the team and report back to him with an individualized care plan.

## Discussion

This case is an exemplar of competent nursing assessment in identifying patient distress. The nurse recognized that Bill expressed many psychosocial concerns, and she was able to focus her assessment on his immediate needs. By listening to his fears and reassuring him that he was in a safe place to talk about his feelings, the nurse remained present. The nurse was able to recognize that recurrent disease was a major turning point for Bill along the cancer trajectory. At this stage, she knew he had no hope for cure and that focus should be on quality of life. Bill's recurrent disease was going to affect him across many avenues of his life—his family relationships and his occupation of utmost concern. The nurse also understood that Bill had a previous episode of depression with his initial diagnosis, which put him at risk for a subsequent episode at recurrence. The fact that Bill's father died of prostate cancer was important, as this loss framed his current experience. When taking the health history, the nurse also focused on physiologic factors that may have been contributing to Bill's present distress. She identified pain, insomnia, and difficulty in sexual relations as also contributing to psychological distress.

Consultations with Bill's physician confirmed her findings. An interprofessional team meeting was called to present Bill's case to the nursing staff, physicians caring for Bill, the social worker, and the chaplain. An individualized care plan was set in motion. First, Bill was to be started on a long-acting pain medication to control his discomfort. He also was prescribed a sleeping aid to address his insomnia and an anxiolytic, if needed, for anxiety. The social worker agreed to work with Bill regarding his relationship with his wife and his concerns about how his young adult sons were responding to his illness. The chaplain had knowledge that Bill's father had died of prostate cancer and that at this stage of recurrent disease, he most likely would have existential issues; he confirmed that he would stop by and speak with Bill. Lastly, the psychiatric clinical nurse specialist was contacted to see Bill to follow up on his feelings of sadness and to assess for depression. The psychiatric liaison team was also called in and informed that a referral might be needed for medication and follow-up. Bill's distress was going to be met at an integral time of initial treatment for recurrent disease, and preventive measures were put in place to help him cope with his many fears and concerns, hopefully preventing a major depressive episode as had previously occurred. The nurse's assessment proved vital in calling forth the interprofessional team to help in Bill's case, and her unique ability to stay present in Bill's distress proved pivotal when identifying the necessary psychosocial resources needed for his care.

## Conclusion

Distress is a normal response to cancer and can occur along the major transitional points of care. Assessment and screening for distress is now the standard for quality patient care across all oncology settings. Although mild distress may be normal, it is still difficult for patients and should be addressed by the oncology support team. Both physiological and psychological factors contributing to distress need to be evaluated and treated to improve patient outcomes (e.g., adherence to treatment). Adjustment disorder is not uncommon in patients with cancer and is characterized by severe anxiety or depressive symptoms related to a life stressor that interferes with occupational and social functioning. Mehta and Roth (2015) warned that adjustment disorder may be the beginning stages of a more severe anxiety or depressive disorder, demanding regular psychosocial assessment and follow-up to clarify diagnosis. Other diagnoses contributing to moderate to severe stress include delirium and dementia (see Chapter 11 for information on delirium and dementia). Nurses caring for patients with cancer are in a unique position to identify distress because holistic care is inherent in the role of nursing. Nurses build therapeutic and trusting relationships with their patients, thus providing a safe place for patients to express their fears and emotions. Therefore, nurses play a vital role on the interprofessional psychosocial team and can lead the team in evidence-based practice.

## References

Absolom, K., Holch, P., Pini, S., Hill, K., Liu, A., Sharpe, M., … Velikova, G. (2011). The detection and management of emotional distress in cancer patients: The views of health-care professionals. *Psycho-Oncology, 20,* 601–608. doi:10.1002/pon.1916

Adler, N.E., & Page, A.E.K. (Eds.). (2008). *Cancer care for the whole patient: Meeting psychosocial health needs.* Washington, DC: National Academies Press.

American College of Surgeons Commission on Cancer. (2015). *Cancer program standards: Ensuring patient-centered care* (2016 ed.). Retrieved from https://www.facs.org/~/media/files/quality%20programs/cancer/coc/2016%20coc%20standards%20manual_interactive%20pdf.ashx

American Psychiatric Association. (2013). *Diagnostic and statistical manual of mental disorders* (5th ed.). Washington, DC: Author.

Bevans, M., Ross, A., & Cella, D. (2014). Patient-reported outcomes measurement information system (PROMIS): Efficient, standardized tools to measure self-reported health and quality of life. *Nursing Outlook, 62,* 339–345. doi:10.1016/j.outlook.2014.05.009

Brown, C.G. (2014). Screening and evidence-based interventions for distress in patients with cancer: Nurses must lead the way. *Clinical Journal of Oncology Nursing, 18*(Suppl. 1), 23–25. doi:10.1188/14.CJON.S1.23-25

Bultz, B.D., & Carlson, L.E. (2005). Emotional distress: The sixth vital sign in cancer care. *Journal of Clinical Oncology, 23,* 6440–6441. doi:10.1200/JCO.2005.02.3259

Bultz, B.D., & Johansen, C. (2011). Screening for distress, the 6th vital sign: Where are we, and where are we going? *Psycho-Oncology, 20,* 569–571. doi:10.1002/pon.1986

Bultz, B.D., Loscalzo, M.J., & Holland, J.C. (2015). Distress as the sixth vital sign: An emerging international symbol for improving psychosocial care. In J.C. Holland, W.S. Breitbart, P.N. Butow, P.B. Jacobsen, M.J. Loscalzo, & R. McCorkle (Eds.), *Psycho-oncology* (3rd ed., pp. 735–738). New York, NY: Oxford University Press.

Carlson, L.E., Waller, A., Groff, S.L., Giese-Davis, J., & Bultz, B.D. (2013). What goes up does not always come down: Patterns of distress, physical and psychosocial morbidity in people with cancer over a one year period. *Psycho-Oncology, 22,* 168–176. doi:10.1002/pon.2068

Carlson, L.E., Waller, A., & Mitchell, A.J. (2012). Screening for distress and unmet needs in patients with cancer: Review and recommendations. *Journal of Clinical Oncology, 30,* 1160–1177. doi:10.1200/JCO.2011.39.5509

Clark, P.G., Bolte, S., Buzaglo, J., Golant, M., Daratsos, L., & Loscalzo, M. (2012). From distress guidelines to developing models of psychosocial care: Current best practices. *Journal of Psychosocial Oncology, 30,* 694–714. doi:10.1080/07347332.2012.721488

Cohen, M.Z., & Bankston, S. (2011). Cancer-related distress. In C.H. Yarbro, D. Wujcik, & B.H. Gobel (Eds.), *Cancer nursing: Principles and practice* (7th ed., pp. 667–684). Burlington, MA: Jones & Bartlett Learning.

DellaRipa, J., Conlon, A., Lyon, D.E., Ameringer, S.A., Kelly, D.L., & Menzies, V. (2015). Perceptions of distress in women with ovarian cancer. *Oncology Nursing Forum, 42,* 292–300. doi:10.1188/15.ONF.292-300

Estes, J.M., & Karten, C. (2014). Nursing expertise and the evaluation of psychosocial distress in patients with cancer and survivors. *Clinical Journal of Oncology Nursing, 18,* 598–600. doi:10.1188/14.CJON.598-600

Fann, J.R., Ell, K., & Sharpe, M. (2012). Integrating psychosocial care into cancer services. *Journal of Clinical Oncology, 30,* 1178–1185. doi:10.1200/JCO.2011.39.7398

Fitch, M.I. (2011). Screening for distress: A role for oncology nursing. *Current Opinion in Oncology, 23,* 331–337. doi:10.1097/CCO.0b013e32834791a1

Gao, W., Bennett, M.I., Stark, D., Murray, S., & Higginson, I.J. (2010). Psychological distress in cancer from survivorship to end of life care: Prevalence, associated factors, and clinical implications. *European Journal of Cancer, 46,* 2036–2044. doi:10.1016/j.ejca.2010.03.033

Hammelef, K.J., Friese, C.R., Breslin, T.M., Riba, M., & Schneider, S.M. (2014). Implementing distress management guidelines in ambulatory oncology: A quality improvement project. *Clinical Journal of Oncology Nursing, 18,* 31–36. doi:10.1188/14.CJON.S1.31-36

Holland, J.C., & Alici, Y. (2010). Management of distress in cancer patients. *Journal of Supportive Oncology, 8,* 4–12.

Jacobsen, P.B., & Wagner, L.I. (2012). A new quality standard: The integration of psychosocial care into routine cancer care. *Journal of Clinical Oncology, 30,* 1154–1159. doi:10.1200/JCO.2011.39.5046

Ma, X., Zhang, J., Zhong, W., Shu, C., Wang, F., Wen, J., ... Liu, L. (2014). The diagnostic role of a short screening tool—The distress thermometer: A meta-analysis. *Supportive Care in Cancer, 22,* 1741–1755. doi:10.1007/s00520-014-2143-1

Mehta, R.D., & Roth, A.J. (2015). Psychiatric considerations in the oncology setting. *CA: A Cancer Journal for Clinicians, 65,* 300–314. doi:10.3322/caac.21285

Mitchell, A.J. (2010). Short screening tools for cancer-related distress: A review and diagnostic validity meta-analysis. *Journal of the National Comprehensive Cancer Network, 8,* 487–495.

Mitchell, A.J. (2015). Screening and assessment for distress. In J.C. Holland, W.S. Breitbart, P.N. Butow, P.B. Jacobsen, M.J. Loscalzo, & R. McCorkle (Eds.), *Psycho-oncology* (3rd ed., pp. 384–395). New York, NY: Oxford University Press.

Mitchell, A.J., Baker-Glenn, E.A., Park, B., Granger, L., & Symonds, P. (2010). Can the Distress Thermometer be improved by additional mood domains? Part II. What is the optimal combination of Emotion Thermometers? *Psycho-Oncology, 19,* 134–140. doi:10.1002/pon.1557

Mullan, F. (1984). Re-entry: The educational needs of the cancer survivor. *Health Education Quarterly, 10,* 88–94.

Munoz, A.R., Kaiser, K., Yanez, B., Victorson, D., Garcia, S.F., Snyder, M.A., & Salsman, J.M. (2016). Cancer experiences and health-related quality of life among racial and ethnic survivors of young adult cancer: A mixed methods study. *Supportive Care in Cancer, 24,* 4861–4870. doi:10.1007/s00520-016-3340-x

NANDA International. (2015). *Nursing diagnoses: Definitions and classification, 2015–2017.* Philadelphia, PA: Author.

National Comprehensive Cancer Network. (2017). *NCCN Clinical Practice Guidelines in Oncology (NCCN Guidelines®): Distress management* [v.2.2017]. Retrieved from http://www.nccn.org/professionals/physician_gls/pdf/distress.pdf

Petty, L., & Lester, J. (2014). Distress screening in chronic disease: Essential for cancer survivors. *Journal of the Advanced Practitioner in Oncology, 5,* 107–114.

Pirl, W.F., Braun, I.M., Deshields, T.L., Fann, J.R., Fulcher, C.D., Greer, J.A., ... Bardwell, W.A. (2015). Implementing screening for distress: The joint position statement from the American Psychosocial Oncology Society, Association of Oncology Social Work, and Oncology Nursing Society. Retrieved from https://www.ons.org/advocacy-policy/positions/practice/distress-screening

Stanton, A.L. (2012). What happens now? Psychosocial care for cancer survivors after medical treatment completion. *Journal of Clinical Oncology, 30,* 1215–1220. doi:10.1200/JCO.2011.39.7406

Tavernier, S.S. (2014). Translating research on the distress thermometer into practice. *Clinical Journal of Oncology Nursing, 18*(Suppl. 1), 26–30. doi:10.1188/14.CJON.S1.26-30

Vitek, L., Rosenzweig, M.Q., & Strollings, S. (2007). Distress in patients with cancer: Definition, assessment, and suggested interventions. *Clinical Journal of Oncology Nursing, 11,* 413–418. doi:10.1188/07.CJON.413-418

Vodermaier, A., Linden, W., & Siu, C. (2009). Screening for emotional distress in cancer patients: A systematic review of assessment instruments. *Journal of the National Cancer Institute, 101,* 1464–1488. doi:10.1093/jnci/djp336

Wagner, L.I., & Pearman, T. (2015). Changes in U.S. policy: Psychosocial care as an integral component of cancer care delivery. In J.C. Holland, W.S. Breitbart, P.N. Butow, P.B. Jacobsen, M.J. Loscalzo, & R. McCorkle (Eds.), *Psycho-oncology* (3rd ed., pp. 729–734). New York, NY: Oxford University Press.

Waller, A., Boyes, A., Carey, M., & Sanson-Fisher, R. (2015). Screening and assessment for unmet needs. In J.C. Holland, W.S. Breitbart, P.N. Butow, P.B. Jacobsen, M.J. Loscalzo, & R. McCorkle (Eds.), *Psycho-oncology* (3rd ed., pp. 369–383). New York, NY: Oxford University Press.

Ziegler, L., Hill, K., Neilly, L., Bennett, M.I., Higginson, I.J., Murray, S.A., & Stark, D. (2011). Identifying psychological distress at key stages of the cancer illness trajectory: A systematic review of validated self-report measures. *Journal of Pain and Symptom Management, 41,* 619–636. doi:10.1016/j.painsymman.2010.06.024

CHAPTER 19

# Grief

*Katherine Brown-Saltzman, RN, MA*

> *Give sorrow words; the grief that does not speak*
> *Whispers the o'er fraught heart and bids it break.*
>
> —William Shakespeare

Patti, a 50-year-old woman diagnosed with acute myeloid leukemia, had failed traditional therapy and had undergone a bone marrow transplant. She had a normal course with manageable complications (an infection and significant pain from mouth sores). Patti had coped well with minimal supportive therapy from the social worker and daily visits from her family. Because she recovered quickly, discharge was timely and preparations were made for her homecoming. She remained home for only four days and was readmitted with severe nausea and dehydration. Her spouse, Chris, reported that, just two days after her return home, their eldest grandchild had been killed in an accidental shooting. In the hospital, Patti became more despondent. She experienced increased nausea, refused food, and began to vomit. She became weak and did not leave her hospital bed except to use the commode. Chris was fearful of the change he was witnessing in his normally strong wife. He reported that she occasionally was tearful, yet she expressed the wish not to talk about her grandson's death and seemed to become progressively more withdrawn. Chris felt helpless and expressed concern that Patti would not be able to "fight" and become well. A research nurse who knew the patient well referred her to the clinical nurse specialist for support after observing the increasing depression.

## Bereavement and Grief

To be bereaved is to be deprived of something ruthlessly (especially hope or joy) or to make desolate through loss. The etymology of the word comes from the German roots of the word that means "to rob" or "to seize by violence" ("Bereaved," n.d.). In personal terms, that translates as robbed of a loved one and of all the future hopes and plans for and with that loved one. Does the bereaved person even recognize how grief-filled he or she has become? Bereaved children lose not only a family member but also their surviving parent or parents, who are changed by sorrow and may become emotionally inaccessible. The patient who is dying also experiences many losses, and anticipatory grief evokes the loss of oneself and all that one knows and loves. Bereavement often is seen as the process of grief, most frequently related to loss through death or, as Lindemann (1944) noted, even the threat of death. Grief, as described by Corr and Doka (1994), is simply the reaction to loss. In oncology, healthcare professionals are familiar with losses that may occur throughout the trajectory of illness: amputation, colostomy, infertility, loss of hair, loss of appetite and normal sense of taste, a forfeiture of energy, loss of cognitive sharpness, and loss of sexual intimacy. Rando (2000) recognized these losses in anticipatory mourning of dying patients.

As patients come to know nurses, they may share stories of significant personal losses. Examples could be a significant other who left after the diagnosis, a marriage that fell apart because of the added pressures of illness, old wounds from a long-ago divorce that now are intensified, or the job or school left, even if only temporarily. Losing a sense of normalcy and innocence ("I will never be worry-free again. I will always wonder if it is coming back.") may have the greatest impact on a person. Nurses' roles in working with the bereaved are to develop a basic understanding of the grief process, to acquire assessment skills that enable them to delineate normal and complicated grief, and to discover potential interventions and referrals.

Many times, grief leaves healthcare professionals feeling helpless and uncomfortable. Remaining present in the face of such sorrow is not easy. Nurses may wonder about saying the right thing or that somehow the patients' feelings of grief were accentuated through a clumsy comment. Gaining knowledge about the grief process, nurses become more competent to care for patients with cancer and their families. This also assists nurses in understanding their own (and other healthcare team members') responses to patients' deaths.

Freud established that the task of grieving is a process of disconnecting from the one who has died; essentially, it is a process of decathexis and then a gradual reattachment to another (Strachey, 1961). Most theories of grief are based on this premise. In the 1940s, the Cocoanut Grove nightclub fire in Boston, Massachusetts, allowed Lindemann (1944) to study the survivors and describe grief reactions that lasted six to eight weeks. As a result of this work, a crisis intervention model of caring for the bereaved emerged that focused on the intensity of acute grief. The length of the experience of acute grief has been studied. Even though most individuals experience uncomplicated grief and resolve their grief within six months to two years after the loss, the process of grieving is individual and differs in intensity and duration (Maciejewski, Zhang, Block, & Prigerson, 2007; Sveen, Eilegård, Steineck, & Kreicbergs, 2014). Maciejewski et al. (2007) found an average peaking of grief indicators occurring at six months, thereby advocating evaluation for those who continued to score above average beyond that span. The participants in that study were younger and therefore may have been more resilient. Some have described grief as a lifelong process during which adjustments occur on anniversaries and during major life events. Edelman (1995) described a woman's lifetime grief over her mother: "The intervals between grief responses lengthen over time, but her longing never disappears. It always hovers at the edge of her awareness, ready to surface at any time" (p. 24). The Committee for the Study of Health Consequences of the Stress of Bereavement, formed by the Health and Medicine Division of the National Academies of Sciences, Engineering, and Medicine (formerly the Institute of Medicine) to study the impact of grief on health, found that a normal grief process may be lengthy for some individuals (Osterweis, Solomon, & Green, 1984). They noted that it is not the length of time per se that distinguishes normal from abnormal grief but the quality and quantity of reactions over time. People have come to understand another dimension of grief since the events of September 11, 2001. The issues of complicated and traumatic grief have been powerful, not only for the bereaved families and the survivors, but also for the whole country, as it went from disbelief, to anger, to despair and depression, and then finally to an attempt to find meaning and healing.

## Theoretical Tasks of Grief

Kübler-Ross (1969) was one of the early professionals to articulate the process of death and dying. Her concept of stages of dying established the expectation that a grieving person moved from denial, to anger, to bargaining, to depression, and, finally, to acceptance. This work opened doors to understanding the process, but it is now understood in a less rigid context. Patients can skip a stage or pass in and out of stages. Whether it is the work of the dying or the grief work of the living, it is a process.

Based on his studies of widows, Parkes (1986) described five aspects of grief. Alarm reflects the physiologic response. This is a state of high arousal with components of the fight or flight mechanism and irritability. In the area of research on stress responses, a growing body of literature exists related to the neurochemical and immune response to bereavement. Searching involves spontaneous "pangs" of grief that come over the bereaved. The pangs are described as episodes of severe anxiety and psychological pain and most often are expressed with sighing and weeping. These episodes are most intense in the first 5–14 days and then gradually lessen. Memories of the loss stimulate these episodes. Pining, a persistent and obtrusive wish for the person who is gone, also occurs. Parkes interpreted this as the need to search for the lost person. Searching contraindicates one's rational knowledge of death and can include restless movement, thoughts preoccupied by the deceased, a preconscious recognition that "sets" the bereaved to anticipate and "see" the dead person, actual scanning of the environment for the person, and a loss of concentration. At times, the bereaved may describe seeing, hearing, or calling out to the deceased. Mitigation is another aspect of the process. Behaviors used to lessen the pain include feeling comfort in sensing the presence of the dead person, talking or praying (either while awake or asleep) to the dead person with the belief that he or she hears, denying the loss, and turning away from thoughts about the dead person. Increasing activity, returning to work, putting away the deceased person's possessions, and leaving the area or home for a period of time are other methods of mitigation. An attempt also is made to make sense of the loss; Parkes saw this as a way of restoring what is lost by fitting its absence into some fundamental pattern.

Anger and guilt also are components of the bereavement process. Parkes (1986) found that anger was greatest in the first month and almost always occurred sometime during the first year. Maciejewski et al. (2007) found that anger peaked at five months. Anger and aggression may be focused at the dead person for "leaving," at God, or at the healthcare team for not saving the deceased. At times, anger and irritability were directed to those most near, even themselves. Those with the greatest anger became the most socially isolated. Guilt over some aspect of their relationship with the deceased was associated with complicated grief. The bereaved had difficulty relinquishing the deceased.

Finally, Parkes (1986) described gaining a new identity. An example of this is a widow in his study describing a sense of waking up and living again a year after her husband's death. The Committee for the Study of Health Consequences of the Stress of Bereavement described the culmination of a healthy bereavement process as including recovery of lost functions (including investment in current life, hopefulness, and the capacity to experience gratification), adaptation to new roles and status, and completion of acute grieving (Osterweis et al., 1984). Figure 19-1 presents a summary of additional grief theorists.

| Bowlby's Phases | Worden's Tasks | Rando's Processes for Complicated Mourning |
|---|---|---|
| 1. Begins with numbing with potential disturbances or anguish/anger<br>2. One of searching and longing for the deceased person<br>3. Disorganization and despair<br>4. Reorganization | 1. Accept the reality of the loss.<br>2. Experience the pain of the grief.<br>3. Adjust to an environment in which the deceased is missing.<br>4. Withdraw emotional energy from the deceased, and reinvest it in another relationship. | 1. Recognize the loss; acknowledge and understand the death.<br>2. React to, experience, and express the separation and pain; be aware of and grieve secondary losses.<br>3. Recollect thoughts about the deceased, remember him or her realistically, and revive feelings for him or her.<br>4. Relinquish old attachments to the deceased.<br>5. Readjust and adapt to new ways of being without the deceased while maintaining memories, and form a new identity.<br>6. Reinvest. |

**Figure 19-1. Additional Theoretical Perspectives of Grief**

*Note.* Based on information from Bowlby, 1980; Rando, 1993; Worden, 1991.

# Children and Bereavement

Nurses may feel stretched beyond their capabilities when helping a child to face death. In addition to feeling intimidated by the developmental issues, nurses may respond like society, with overwhelming sadness for the child. Still, nurses often will be the ones at the bedside when a crisis occurs and the "specialists" are not available. In the most recent statistics, more than 1.2 million children were receiving social security benefits in 2004 because of parental death (Tamborini, Cupito, & Shoffner, 2011). This gives perspective on the prevalence of children who have lost parents. Nurses who normally care for adults may be called upon to help with the patient's child or grandchild.

In a classic study, Nagy (1948) interviewed hundreds of Hungarian children and found that, prior to age 5, they viewed death as a separation that was reversible. Between the ages of 5 and 9, the children viewed death as personified (i.e., viewed as something that could be outrun). By the time the children had reached age 10, they had developed a mature, cognitive concept of death as something final and universal. American researchers have not been able to replicate these findings in regard to the personification of death. They attribute this to cultural differences. In fact, Koocher (1974) found that children avoided abstraction when describing death and relied on specific details. He attributed this to an attempt to "control" death. In questioning children, Koocher found that those in the preoperational stage (7 years of age and younger) described death as being reversible.

Children's initial reaction to death often is shock and sadness, but they quickly return to seemingly inappropriate laughter or activity. In reality, their suffering may take many forms. Bowlby (1969) showed that mourning begins at six months as the infant separates from the mother. Furman (1964) determined that children aged 2–3 are capable of comprehending the meaning of death. Like adults, children can somatize grief reactions with headaches and stomach pains and by imitating symptoms of the family member who has died. They also are likely to develop enuresis, separation anxieties, and phobias. As children grow and face new developmental challenges, they may reexperience the loss in new ways.

Helping a child to cope with death is a complex process. A good approach is to begin early and give the child some warning about the impending death. Nurses can make suggestions to help parents know how and what to tell a child and offer guidelines on what the child can do in the hospital room. Regardless of the child's age, he or she should be prepared for how the family member will look or act. This will help the child to anticipate and cope. If a visit is not possible because of distance or the child's fear, the parent can suggest that the child send drawings, letters, videos, or simple gifts. This can help the child to be present and say good-bye, even from afar. The child will long remember these offerings or a chance to talk. Allowing a child to help with the patient's care, where appropriate, also can ease some anxiety. Suggesting that the parent break up the visit with a special trip to the hospital cafeteria, museum, or a nearby park can make the experience more tolerable for the child. The institution's resources, such as child life specialists or pediatric unit nurses, also can be called on for help. Resources for children often are available at hospices and on the Internet, which has exploded with bereavement information. Bereavement centers that accommodate children may go beyond the traditional support group and offer a camp experience that normalizes grief (Bachman, 2013; Clute & Kobayashi, 2013; McClatchey & Wimmer, 2012). The American Cancer Society's "I Count, Too" is a support program for children and adolescents that assists them in dealing with the impact of the disease and sometimes aids in bereavement. Such programs may be available in the community. Being available to answer questions and respond to children's fears as well as helping them to understand the normalcy of family members' tears, anger, or sadness are important interventions. Nurses can consider writing a memory letter for a child. If a nurse has worked closely with the family member who has died, documenting the relationship, the characteristics of the person, and things he or she might have said about the child can provide a keepsake to later be cherished. See Figure 19-2 for additional suggestions. Nurses can turn to the literature to increase their understanding of children's needs during the terminal illness. When the child's loved one dies, not only will this direct them in responding to the child, but it will also help them guide the surviving adults in how to support the child (Christ & Christ, 2006; Laing & Moules, 2015).

---

- Use simple and truthful answers and questions.
- Use direct language; use the words "death" and "died."
- Discuss religious and spiritual beliefs in simple terms, but avoid omnipresent language, such as "God took your uncle to heaven to be with Him." This could create fear for the child of being taken. Although it may be comforting to envision a family member who has died now in heaven, endowing that person with the ability to see all the child does may leave the child feeling shadowed. This could be frightening and create guilt for the child when he or she does something wrong.
- Do not compare death to sleep, which also can create fears and sleep disturbances.
- Help the child to understand adult responses to loss.
- Give the child the whole picture that people heal and are not always engulfed by grief.
- Assess the child's belief that he or she is in some way responsible for the death and provide reassurance.
- Prepare the child for what he or she will see during the dying process, the funeral, or other rituals. Encourage the child's participation, if appropriate.
- Consider creating a memory book that allows the child to express emotions and document memories using drawings, pictures, collages, poems, etc.
- Encourage referrals for additional support.

**Figure 19-2. Ways to Help Children to Cope With Grief**

## Cultural Issues

Although guidelines and manuals are helpful in assisting healthcare professionals to understand death and grief practices, one cannot possibly know all the beliefs, customs, and nuances of individual families and sects. Asking for more information from the family and patient will help to unlock cultural complexities. Setting aside value judgments and acknowledging that the world can be viewed from many perspectives are important (Brown-Saltzman, 1995). The following story demonstrates the difficulty of sorting out the larger cultural issues and the individual interpretation and experience of those issues.

A young Filipino woman with a brain tumor died after a long and difficult course of chemotherapy and radiation. Her family had not been able to acknowledge her impending death until the very last moment, believing that a miracle would save her. Moments after the patient's death, the grandmother, who had remained at her bedside throughout the illness, asked to be left alone with the body. When the nurse returned, she found that the young girl's wrist had been slashed. Shocked by the site and the blood, the nurse ran from the room to call a security guard. After a great deal of confusion, they asked the grandmother what she had done. Through an interpreter, she shared that she had cut her granddaughter to let the blood flow out so that she could be sure that the patient was dead. The grandmother was afraid that her granddaughter would be buried alive and suffer as a friend of the family had. What appeared to be a bizarre act at first was, in fact, a last desperate act of love. Still, the staff viewed it as a desecration of the body. Although this is not a Filipino death tradition, one sees that the grandmother's long ago experience in her homeland left her wary of healthcare professionals' abilities to accurately determine death. Had the healthcare team been able to reassure the grandmother that they had reliable ways to determine death (e.g., a heart monitor, electroencephalogram), this incident might have been avoided. Even though healthcare professionals could barely comprehend this woman's action, showing understanding and compassion for her in that moment and acknowledging her fears and concerns while withholding judgment facilitated healing.

Another aspect to consider in working with other cultures is the immigration experience. Often, immigrants have come from war-torn countries and may have experienced the deaths of family and friends or, possibly worse yet, have family members who are missing. They may have experienced torture and abuses. Even if they emigrated from a peaceful country out of a desire for improved life or simply for adventure, many immigrants have endured multiple losses along the way (e.g., loss of daily contact with family and friends, traditions, language, changes in way of life or profession). Experiencing a new loss may awaken past losses and increase sadness and isolation, as well as complicate the grief process.

Cultural differences can also surface when addressing prolonged grief disorder (PGD) (see section on Complicated Grief). Goldsmith, Morrison, Vanderwerker, and Prigerson (2008) noted that African Americans may have higher levels of PGD. Laurie and Neimeyer (2008) made the following observations of this group: homicide was more often the cause of death, the connection with the dead was sustained longer, use of services was less frequent, and increased religious coping was reported.

Older adults may be at greater risk when it comes to bereavement, although the research is conflicting (Areán & Reynolds, 2005; Stroebe & Schut, 2001; Traylor, Hayslip, Kaminski, & York, 2003). One must avoid ageist stereotyping but at the same time be cognizant of the many factors affecting bereaved older adults, especially multiple losses. For example, those entering residential care experience potential loss of identity, control, spontaneity, and the right to take risks (Thompson, 2002). Older adults are at risk for disenfranchised grief, a loss that is not given full acknowledgment. This can be from a loss that may be viewed by some as stigmatized (e.g., suicide), insignificant (e.g., the loss of pet), unacknowledged (e.g., divorce), or prolonged (e.g., dementia) (Doka, 2002). The griever is excluded from expected bereavement support because others are unable to appreciate the impact of the loss. In addition, the many losses in aging can be considered "normal" and therefore lose their significance.

Within the healthcare environment, professionals must take on the responsibility of honoring other cultures. Witnessing the suffering of grief reactions stirs discomfort in every human soul and is barely tolerable, even when it is familiar to one's culture. When observing a reaction foreign to one's experience, professional fear and anxiety may increase. Clements et al. (2003) encouraged professionals to honor adaptive coping of individual cultures so that patients and families have permission to express grief according to their cultural norms. The challenge is to discover norms for every culture and individual.

# Completion of Case Study

To reflect Patti's case, one sees that this patient was in a state of numbness and more than likely was still experiencing alarm. In fact, she had not even allowed herself to cry or express emotion over her grandson's death. This reaction may be in keeping with Patti's personality, but it also may reflect her extreme vulnerability and fragility caused by all that she has been through. Her own health is still precarious. This becomes a delicate balance, as it takes emotional, physical, and spiritual energy to grieve, and sometimes the grief process is halted because of extreme situations (e.g., too many losses in a relatively short period of time).

During the initial interview with the clinical nurse specialist, Patti appeared drawn and exhibited little energy. She responded to questions with simple answers. Her affect was flat and distant. When her grandson's death was acknowledged, she fought back tears, she became shaky, and her mouth trembled. The magnitude of the grief was acknowledged. Gently, the nurse used reflective statements to describe a grief response: "You have been through a terrible loss, an overwhelming loss. I can see the pain of it in you, the sorrow." With the grief recognized, tears began to fall; Patti could not answer with words, but only nodded. The nurse took her hand, and Patti responded by holding tightly. The nurse continued, "It makes no sense. He was so young. We cannot make sense of such an accident, and yet we ask why, over and over again." These words and the nurse's empathy touched the deep hurt, and the patient began to sob. Even as these tears flowed, she fought to maintain some control; the sobs caught in her throat. The nurse acknowledged how overwhelming grief can feel when it spills from us seemingly out of control and assured her that it would not become uncontainable. Patti seemed reassured, and when the nurse offered to hold her, the sobs came without restraint. After being held and crying for some time, Patti began to talk and verbalize her contained grief. In between sighs, she described the feeling that she was going crazy, spiraling out of control. Now Patti could tell the story, how no one even told her the first day that he died because relatives were fearful that it would be too much for her. She had been too ill to attend the funeral, and she talked about how unreal the death seemed and how she woke each morning to the horror and knowledge, "He's dead!" When asked what had helped to get her through hard things in her life, she shook her head and responded, "I've always been strong. I just put one foot in front of another—Patti had a stiff upper lip. My family has always depended upon me. I have never fallen apart." "And now you are feeling like you are falling apart?" "Yes! Yes! I am very frightened." The nurse reflected, "You have been through so much. Losing your grandson has been the last straw. You came to this news already having lost so much." The tears began to fall again. The nurse continued, "First, you found out you had leukemia and you felt you lost your health and sense of well-being, the normalcy of life. You underwent treatment, hoping for a remission and cure, yet relapse brought another loss. Then you came in for a bone marrow transplant and, even though you gained this new life, it is as though you had to die first. You became incredibly vulnerable."

The patient nodded as the tears continued and she began to acknowledge the many losses. "Look at my skin. I look like an old woman. I never dreamed I would be so ill. I lost all of my strength. I am not the woman I was. I wonder over and over why I did this to myself." The nurse responded, "All of this, and now you lose your grandson. Of course you have fallen apart. How could it be otherwise? And sometimes you must wonder, 'Why him, why did he die, why not me?'" Now, the unmentionable has been said. Patti's eyes meet the nurse's gaze and she nods over and over. The tears pour out again. "I begged God to go back and take me instead. I feel guilty that my life was spared and his taken." The nurse held her hands and offered silent comfort. At last the nurse spoke, "I do not understand why. I am only grateful that you have been able to share these tears today. It is the only way that I know that your grief will heal—to share it with another."

The nurse then asked about spiritual beliefs. With downcast eyes, Patti replied that she was a Christian. Asked if she felt that God had abandoned her, she once again began to cry and confirmed the feeling. "I keep wondering over and over what I did to be punished so much." "Was there anything you could have done that would deserve such suffering?" the nurse asked. "No, no," Patti replied. She then summarized her worst sins in life: divorcing a husband who had been unfaithful and taking life for granted. She affirmed to herself that these were not worthy of such punishment. "Then sometimes I think I am being tested, and I think, 'God, I cannot take anymore.'" "Do you pray? Do you talk to God?" the nurse questioned. "I have not been able to since my grandson died" was her reply. The nurse then shared, "Lots of people are unable to pray when they are so burdened or so angry. Sometimes, it helps to have another pray for you." "I am angry, but how can I be angry at God?" The nurse shared a past experience. "An ill child taught me once that if God was as great as we thought He was, then He could handle our anger. I sometimes think that all God asks of us is to be in relationship with Him, and sometimes that means letting Him know when we've had it." "Yes, yes," she affirmed. The nurse then offered to pray for Patti, and she replied appreciatively, "Please." The nurse placed her hands on the patient's shoulders and a silent prayer was offered, ending with an audible prayer that the patient be brought comfort and the grandson blessed. The heaviness in the room changed; the sorrow, of course, was immense, but having been shared, it now was altered.

The nurse continued to see the patient daily for support. On the next visit, Patti told the nurse, "You saved my life yesterday. I was on the edge, and you helped me beyond words."

# Care of the Grieving Individual

## Assessment

The grief assessment is integrated into the conversation with the patient and is never simply a checklist. A nurse who sits with a form hurriedly checking off answers will come away with a very different picture of a patient than one who gathers information through conversations with the patient over time. If the patient is hospitalized and severely ill, issues such as sleep disturbance, appetite, and depression will be difficult to sort out in terms of what is a physical complication and what is caused by grief.

Each response to assessment questions brings the building of trust, a potential for teaching, and a therapeutic response and intervention. The family or patient is asked to tell what happened. So often in the past, they have abbreviated or edited their story to accommodate what family or friends can tolerate, but the nurse's openness allows for the outpouring of details and difficult aspects of the narrative.

The assessment includes not only what is relayed verbally by the patient but also other cues (e.g., trembling of the mouth, a change in breathing, sighing, tightening of the face as the individual attempts to contain the emotion). The nurse conducts the assessment gently without probing questions. The assessment is part of the process of building a trusting relationship. Imagine the difference if the nurse in the case study had entered the room saying, "Patti, I understand you lost your grandson while you were home. I am sorry. How did he die? Did you attend the funeral? How do you feel about this? Are you sleeping at night? How is your appetite?" Rather, the assessment should be intertwined with nurturing and comforting actions, soothing touch, a gentle voice, the impression that one has all the time in the world, and an intense sense of presence and compassion. Awareness of how the bereaved individual is caring for him- or herself physically also is important. Research has demonstrated a change in the immune response during periods of grief. For example, suppressed neutrophil superoxide production and raised cortisol have been observed in grieving people (Khanfer, Lord, & Phillips, 2011) as well as altered antibody titers (Phillips et al., 2006). Schultze-Florey et al. (2012) found increased inflammatory markers in bereaved spouses who had a genetic predisposition. In one study, a group of bereaved individuals participated in disclosure writing. Those who found heightened meaning over the course of the intervention showed increases in natural killer cell cytotoxicity (Bower, Kemeny, Taylor, & Fahey, 2003). In general, relaxation techniques have been found to reduce the effects of stress on the immune system (Buckley et al., 2012; Marketon & Glasser, 2008); however, they have limited effectiveness in reducing the compromised immune system in bereavement, with the exception of interventions in those with sustained sleep alteration. Future research will open doors to further understanding the physiologic response of grief.

Red flags, such as the passing comment "I sometimes wish I were dead," need direct and immediate assessment. Although this response is not uncommon, the patient's tendency toward suicide needs to be assessed. Szanto et al. (2002) found that older adults bereaved with high levels of complicated grief symptoms and depression were more likely to express suicidal ideation. In addition, those bereaved who had a history of suicide attempts tended to express more ideation than other bereaved older adults. Peteet, Maytal, and Rokni (2010) described contingent suicidal ideation, which can occur during anticipatory grief, when a family member insinuates either being unable to live without the dying loved one or actually voices the will to end their life when the patient dies. Although the relative is not the identified patient, the healthcare team has an obligation of careful assessment and psychiatric intervention where needed. If the nurse has established a relationship, simply asking, "Have you ever considered taking your own life?" will provide a good first step. If the response is positive, assess whether the relative has thought through a plan and have a strategy for intervention (see Chapter 17).

## Differential Diagnosis

Grief sometimes can be confused with depression, especially when the mourning period seems to extend beyond expected time frames. Although the fourth edition of the *Diagnostic and Statistical Manual of Mental Disorders (DSM)* categorized a major depressive disorder when the symptoms continue two months after the loss (American Psychiatric Association [APA], 2000), that exclusion has since been removed in the fifth edition *(DSM-V)* (APA, 2013). Although controversial, the *DSM-V* determined that it would not include the prolonged grief diagnosis (Bryant, 2014). Healthcare professionals are wary about medicalizing grief. Without the *DSM-V* diagnosis in place, concerns exist that those with prolonged grief will not receive adequate interventions, and that little research will be funded. Depression is characterized by feelings of worthlessness and low self-esteem. With grief, the individual's sadness is related more to the death and loss, and a tendency exists for the symptoms to vary in intensity. Individuals with a history of depression who lose a loved one may be more at risk for depression overlaying the grief (Zisook, Paulus, Schuchter, & Judd, 1997). Zisook, Shuchter, Sledge, Paulus, and Judd (1994) found that only 24% of those diagnosed with depression following the death of a spouse were being pharmacologically treated. This demonstrates real concerns about minimizing the potential consequences of depression, such as chronicity, suicide, and social isolation. Guldin, Vedsted, Zachariae, Olesen, and Jensen (2012) found that 15% of the bereaved caregivers experienced depression following their loss at moderate to severe levels, and only half of those accessed services.

## Interventions

Just as assessment is ongoing, interventions begin with the first contact with the individual and continue with each interaction. The telling of the story begins the healing. Being sensitive to what the person is expressing is essential. Teaching about normal grief occurs throughout the interaction. Again, handing the patient a list of normal grief reactions would not have the same effect. The important thing is the reassurance that someone understands an experience that the individual may be unable to put into words. This is not as simple as saying to a patient or family, "I know how you feel." When the nurse in the case study says, "It makes no sense. He was so young. We cannot make sense of such an accident, and yet we ask why, over and over again," she may be intuitively in touch with the patient's feelings and the experience of listening to many grieving families over time. Or, she may be completely wrong and the patient responds, "No, I do not feel that way. I trust in God. He knows what He is doing." This is the risk the nurse takes in being authentic with the patient, of learning from each new situation and letting it evolve, knowing that sometimes he or she will take the wrong fork in the road and have to retrace their steps back to the patient. Nevertheless, nurses still can educate patients about normal grief and relieve and reassure them. By giving the person permission to grieve, nurses may be contradicting the cultural "voice" that calls the bereaved to be strong. Nurses encourage the patients to voice their feelings. Interactions should allow the patient to "come up for air" after a particularly intense moment or when there are tears by providing quiet time and a slower pace. Periodically, nurses can ask less weighted questions and even use humor appropriately at times. This helps the patient to feel a sense of containment. This subtle change in the therapeutic flow teaches the patient that one can tap into what seems overwhelming and remain in control and secure. Nurses also can pace themselves. They are able to scan their own bodies and wonder if they are taking in too much of the patient's pain. Where are they holding the tension—in the shoulders, the face, or the back? Are they feeling pity or compassion? A deep breath at the appropriate moment will model a helpful coping mechanism for the patient. See Figure 19-3 for specific interventions used in the case study and Figure 19-4 for a plan of care.

Rabow, Hauser, and Adams (2004) encouraged physicians to become aware not only of caregiver burdens at the end of life (e.g., mental and physical health risks, financial and emotional weights) but to become skilled in communicating, empathically supporting, and understanding grief, which will help influence the adjustment of the bereaved. Research has also

- Assisted the patient in writing a letter to her grandson, reflecting all she wished she had been able to tell him
- Provided the patient with a period of time when the healthcare team and family did not push her to fight, allowing her to grieve and "lick her own wounds"
- Prayed with the patient and referred her to chaplaincy for additional support
- Assisted her in calling her younger sister, the bone marrow donor, to tell her about the grandson's death (she had refused to have the family call the sister, as she did not want to burden her with yet another sadness). During this call, Patti came to realize how much she had missed her sister's support and that she had underestimated her baby sister's strength.
- Elicited a life review, both of her own and her grandson's (photographs helped with this process)
- Encouraged the playing of music as a way of bringing life into the sterile hospital room and decreasing the sense of isolation
- Planned and anticipated her needs for when she returned home—some type of memorial service or death ritual, a visit to the gravesite, and ongoing support

**Figure 19-3. Specific Interventions Used With Patti**

demonstrated that supportive follow-up phone calls and condolence letters to the bereaved make a positive impact (Kaunonen, Aalto, Tarkka, & Paunonen, 2000; Morris & Block, 2015).

# Complicated Grief

The Committee for the Study of Health Consequences of the Stress of Bereavement (Osterweis et al., 1984) reviewed a number of grief theories, beginning with Freud's psychoanalytic model, and described the factors contributing to complicated grief. This model incorporates interpersonal dynamics and examines (a) the role of the preexisting personality (those who are psychologically healthy will do better; they will not experience less pain, but they have the coping skills to process that psychic pain), (b) the activation of latent negative self-images (these dormant negative thoughts of oneself are resurrected with the death and lead individuals to view themselves as bad or incompetent and, in turn, complicate the grieving process), (c) ambivalent relationships (in which conflict has been high and feelings of affection conflict with hostility; in turn, the hostility may awaken after a death and leave the mourner with feelings of guilt), and (d) dependent relationships (in which the adult experiences intense anxiety and fear with separation; these feelings are based on a perceived lack of protection during separation in childhood).

Examples of complicated grief include prolonged grief, absent grief (i.e., no obvious reaction), depression, and use of self-destructive behaviors (e.g., suicide, alcohol or drug abuse). Excessive guilt, feelings of worthlessness, and unusual or protracted functional impairment would also be of concern. Post-traumatic stress disorder (PTSD) also can occur in response to a traumatic death or multiple traumas. Thomas, Hudson, Trauer, Remedios, and Clarke (2014) found a correlation between PTSD and complicated grief. Traumatic grief has been proposed as containing symptoms including numbness, disbelief, distrust, anger, and a sense of futility about the future (Nanni, Biancosino, & Grassi, 2014; Prigerson et al., 1999). Separation distress (longing and searching) has also been noted in complicated grief (Nanni et al., 2014; Prigerson et al., 1999). Tofthagen, Kip, Witt, and McMillan (2017) reported that oncology nurses can provide early interventions for complicated grief to facilitate effective treatment.

More recently, research has suggested that complicated grief be replaced by prolonged grief disorder (PGD) with consideration of inclusion in the *DSM-V* (Chiambretto, 2008;

### Assessment
- Description of the death in the patients' or families' own words (e.g., "Tell me what happened.")
- Concurrent stressors and past losses, both deaths and other losses, and reaction to anniversaries
- Affective responses (e.g., anger, sadness, hopelessness, guilt, self-reproach, inability to concentrate, fear, anxiety)
- Somatic responses (e.g., sleep disturbances, poor appetite, headache, pain, weakness, symptoms similar to those of the person who died)
- Support systems (e.g., family, significant others, community)
- Financial concerns
- Past history of coping mechanisms and psychiatric history, particularly depression
- Suicidal tendencies
- Alcohol or drug abuse; increased use of tobacco
- Spiritual beliefs
- Cultural traditions
- Unusual experiences since the death

### Nursing Diagnoses (NANDA International, 2015)
- Hopelessness
- Risk for compromised human dignity
- Risk for loneliness
- Disturbed personal identity
- Risk for disturbed personal identity
- Stress overload
- Risk for post-traumatic syndrome
- Anxiety
- Compromised family coping
- Defensive coping
- Disabled family coping
- Ineffective coping
- Death anxiety
- Ineffective denial
- Grieving
- Complicated grieving
- Risk for complicated grieving
- Risk for compromised resilience
- Chronic sorrow
- Impaired individual resilience
- Stress overload
- Spiritual distress
- Risk for spiritual distress
- Risk for suicide
- Impaired comfort
- Readiness for enhanced comfort
- Social isolation

### *DSM-V* Diagnoses (American Psychiatric Association, 2013)
- Major depressive disorder
- Post-traumatic stress disorder

### Expected Outcomes
- Patients and/or families will begin the grief process within the context of their own cultural norms, spiritual practice, and family traditions.
- Patients and/or families will employ some beneficial coping mechanisms to support them through the bereavement process.
- Patients and/or families will seek support as needed.
- Patients and/or families will engage over time in life and other relationships.

**Figure 19-4. Plan of Care**

*(Continued on next page)*

**Interventions**
- Provide ongoing supportive listening.
- Elicit a life review when appropriate; photographs, journals, music, and art may be helpful.
- Provide patients and families with privacy.
- Encourage assessment of unfinished business, and assist patients and families in achieving intentions. Explore possible use of legacy work, and consider writing of letters or cards for future distribution.
- Respect and encourage use of cultural practices.
- Encourage attending to spiritual needs; offering spiritual support and referrals, as appropriate.
- Describe normal grief and what to expect. Inform that grief is an individual process with different time ranges. Help them appreciate people's inappropriate expectations that they "get over it quickly" and give them guidance as to how to handle poor responses from others.
- Integrate touch, holding, and presence, as appropriate.
- Recognize when silent presence is most important.
- Teach relaxation techniques, particularly breathing exercises, to reduce tension.
- Use guided imagery or meditation to create a safe haven or time out.
- Refer for appropriate support groups or psychiatric/psychological assistance, as needed. Explore concepts of resiliency.
- Encourage social support, increased contact, and connection.
- Discourage the use of alcohol and drugs to numb emotions.
- Promote healthy coping mechanisms, such as exercise, proper nutrition, and rest, that improve the immune system and help deal with grief and stress.
- Provide guidance on the use of alternative therapies, such as essential oils and massage, to assist in coping and comfort.

**Figure 19-4. Plan of Care *(Continued)***

Prigerson et al., 2009). Attachment concerns were particularly correlated with PGD, especially childhood separation anxiety (Prigerson et al., 2009).

Complicated grief and PGD are now frequently used interchangeably in the literature. The incidence of complicated grief is significant. One study found a rate of 40% for those who had cared for a family member with cancer in their home; however, clinicians underpredicted, noting only 21% of those cases (Guldin et al., 2012).

Complicated grief occurs more frequently with particular types of deaths and with certain characteristics of the bereaved (see Figure 19-5). One might think the chance for traumatic death in oncology would be limited, but this is not always the case. Death of a patient by hemorrhage, a witnessed resuscitation, or even extensive side effects that distort the person beyond recognition (e.g., graft-versus-host disease) might easily be categorized as traumatic. A related bone marrow donor whose family member dies is at particular risk for feeling a sense of responsibility for the death and deserves special attention.

**Form of Death**
- Traumatic death
- Sudden death
- Death of an organ or bone marrow transplant recipient
- Death by suicide or homicide
- Prolonged illness
- Death of a child
- Prolonged suffering or pain at end of life

**Characteristics of the Bereaved**
- Ambivalent or dependent relationship
- Multiple losses
- History of depression or mental illness
- History of drug or alcohol abuse

**Figure 19-5. Situations With Potential for Complicated Grief**

Osterweis et al. (1984) noted that bereavement might exacerbate a pattern of negative thoughts that could intensify or prolong grief in individuals with a premorbid tendency to see themselves and the world in a negative light. These individuals are at risk for avoiding the painful experience of grief because any thought of the deceased leads to heightened anxiety.

The family caregiver experiences a double loss after the death of the loved one. He or she may have been so absorbed in the patient's care that, ironically, a more intense attachment develops. After caring for a dying spouse, a widow may describe a different kind of intimacy: "You know, I never knew so much about his body before." After death, the time-consuming role of physical and supportive caring is lost. Without immediate pressing responsibilities, the caregiver wakes up in the morning with a loss of purpose. This may leave him or her feeling more empty and alone.

At the other extreme is premature detachment. In a prolonged dying process, the family may no longer be able to maintain the intense involvement with the patient. Exhausted by the caring and the suffering, they already have grieved and now find themselves wishing that death would come. Very often, this will create feelings of guilt either immediately or after the death. Helping families to understand that these feelings are normal and exploring ways for them to care for themselves and still maintain contact with the patient are important. Rando (1993) suggested that anything that the family can do to support the patient's coping, assist with life review, and maintain the balance of the patient's autonomy in the face of increasing dependency will, in turn, support healthy grieving.

# Anticipatory Grief

Rando (1997) has extensively researched and written about anticipatory grief, which, in a sense, might be called "preventive grief." Although her definition is expansive, it is worth quoting, as it encapsulates the process so well. Anticipatory grief is "the process of mourning, coping, interaction, planning, and psychosocial reorganization that is stimulated and begun in part in response to the awareness of the impending loss of a loved one and the recognition of associated losses in the past, present, and future" (Rando, 1997, p. 35). Rando goes on to define the therapeutic aspects of this anticipation in which the family must "balance among the mutually conflicting demands of simultaneously holding on to, letting go of, and drawing closer to the dying patient" (p. 35). The patient, too, goes through this process in facing death. Nurses might have the greatest impact in this area in terms of preventive work because during this time, they can help patients and families resolve some issues that, if left unresolved, might later produce complicated mourning. One enters into an anticipatory phase when the realization of death has been reinforced by the progression of the illness and an awareness gradually surfaces. The patient who enters hospice, makes decisions about code status, or takes care of financial and legal issues is more likely to be in this process. Rarely, however, are all of the family members and the patient in the same place in the process. Some members, particularly those who are coping long distance, may need special or additional support at some time. Each family member may be at a different point in the grief process. Johansson and Grimby (2012) found that as family members prepared for the death of the patient, they experienced significant emotional stress and a need for programs to assist in coping with anticipatory grief.

Healthcare professionals also may have difficulty with anticipatory grief. For example, when physicians and nurses focus on an aggressive treatment plan for a patient who will die without a bone marrow transplant, balancing the anticipatory work with fighting for the patient's survival becomes very difficult. If a patient develops complications from the treatment and begins to deteriorate, everyone has difficulty shifting the focus. If the disease is cured, how can the patient be allowed to die from the treatment? Sometimes, the patient or the family realizes that death is near before the healthcare team. Nurses may perceive its nearness before the physician. One begins anticipating death while the other remains focused on the cure. As multiorgan system failure occurs, the family may receive conflicting information from different members of the healthcare team. A consulting physician may indicate that the patient's liver or kidney function is improving, but the whole picture still represents impending death. The family and patient are left in crisis, and the benefits of anticipatory grieving may be lost (Barry, Kasl, & Prigerson, 2002). Healthcare professionals have an obligation to be aware of their own vulnerability and how it is affecting the care they are providing (Otis-Green, 2011).

# Evidence-Based Practice

Although the literature is rich in topics related to bereavement, actual research that can affect practice is more limited (Forte, Hill, Pazder, & Feudtner, 2004). Some of the ongoing difficulties of research in bereavement are difference in age, relationship to the deceased, culture, and other confounding factors that make it difficult to transfer the results broadly. Additionally, a need clearly exists for further research in this area, especially in the arena of nursing assessment and interventions. One such study done by a sociologist gave nursing powerful data that may alter outcomes for the bereaved (Carr, 2003). In this classic research, a large prospective study of 250 widowed older adults assessed the elements of death that altered bereavement symptoms. Perception of a painful death correlated with increased levels of yearning, anxiety, and intrusive thoughts in the bereaved. At the same time, an increased positive interaction with the spouse near the time of death or being present at the time of death decreased anger and intrusive thoughts during bereavement (Carr, 2003). Grande, Farquhar, Barclay, and Todd (2004) found difficult bereavement in survivors whose loved one had severe symptoms. In exploring the effect of preparation for death, Barry et al. (2002) recognized that prognostic awareness of death greater than six months promoted a state of acceptance for the bereaved. Complicated grief symptoms in family caregivers have been demonstrated prior to the loss (Garrido & Prigerson, 2014; Nanni et al., 2014).

Thomas et al. (2014) found that loved ones exhibited signs of PGD, even prior to the patient's death. Assessment risk factors, including spousal caregiving, schedule affected by caregiving, poor family functioning, decreased optimism, and greater dependency, were predictive at 6 and 13 months in the bereavement trajectory (Thomas et al., 2014). Surrogate decision makers who chose prolongation of life over a focus on comfort experienced higher levels of grief and complicated grief in bereavement (Lovell, Smith, & Kannis-Dymand, 2015). Based on these studies, nurses can integrate six interventions into preventive bereavement care:
1. Improve pain management.
2. Encourage skillful prognostication and truth telling (Barry et al., 2002).
3. When appropriate, obtain a timely do-not-resuscitate order, which is predicted to improve mental health in bereaved family members from before and after loss (Garrido & Prigerson, 2014).
4. Increase interaction prior to death between the patient and spouse (e.g., privacy, increased support) and amplify efforts to have the spouse present, when possible, at the time of death.

5. Screen for PGD in caregivers during the palliative care period and again at 6 and 13 months following the patient's death (when delayed onset may occur) (Thomas et al., 2014).
6. For caregivers with PGD symptoms, refer early for support (Thomas et al., 2014). Mental health services tend to be underutilized for those with PGD, and further efforts need to be enlisted for this group (Lichtenthal et al., 2011).

A study by Traylor et al. (2003) was primarily focused on parental loss and assessment of the relationship between grief and family systems. Three characteristics within families demonstrated less intense grief over time: affect (the ability to express emotions), communication of those feelings, and cohesion, which provides social support and refocused attachments. This study could enhance nursing's assessment of families at risk for more problematic grief reactions and those in need of additional support.

Christakis and Iwashyna's (2003) study encouraged nurses to suggest referrals to hospice not only for the dying patient but also for the bereaved spouse for support. This large retrospective study looked at bereavement survival in older adults and found that those who had hospice care provided for their spouse had lower death rates following the loss. This was particularly true in females, where the statistical significance was nearly equivalent to other health benefits, such as diet and exercise.

Another study of bereaved husbands and daughters of patients with breast cancer found that the older individuals experienced less grief (Bernard & Guarnaccia, 2003). The daughters in this study experienced more symptoms of depression and anxiety than the husbands. Careful assessment of families as a whole may help to reveal the different aspects of stress that a family death can cause and its ensuing effect on bereavement.

Additionally, nurses might consider Warner, Metcalf, and King's (2001) study regarding the use of benzodiazepines. This double-blind study demonstrated that the appropriate use of diazepam had no negative or positive effect on bereavement distress. Although a small study, it reminded nurses that grief is not in itself pathology that needs to be pharmacologically treated. Further research needs to be done in this area.

Gündel, O'Connor, Littrell, Fort, and Lane (2003) used magnetic resonance imaging to determine the neuroanatomy of grief. The activation of grief response in the brain was greatest when both a picture of the deceased was used in conjunction with grief-related words. Moderate responses were seen when those stimulants were used individually. This work also may help to find the underlying neuroanatomy of Bowlby's (1980) "attachment behavioral system," the theory that we experience attachment behavior as infants, which is played out in adulthood. This protective structure to attach and avoid prolonged separation is the antithesis of grief, the greatest separation humans experience. This work reminds us that the grief response is truly physiologic and may provide further insights into bereavement in the future. A great need exists for research in the area of bereavement. Even fundamental treatments such as antidepressants in those with prolonged grief are done without the needed randomized controlled studies essential to good practice (Bui, Nadel-Vicens, & Simon, 2012).

# When Death Approaches

As death approaches, the nurse's role becomes focused on providing comfort to the patient and family, preparing the family for what to expect, and anticipating and dealing with conflicts and crises (see Figure 19-6).

- Determine what the patient's and family's wishes are, and encourage their fulfillment where possible (e.g., a pet visit, funeral plans).
- Assess cultural or religious traditions, and provide for a flexible environment.
- Educate family members about physiologic aspects of death to increase their comfort (many may never have been present at a death).
- Encourage family participation in providing comfort measures to assist in alleviating their sense of helplessness (e.g., the family that is assisting the patient to eat can be encouraged to use teaspoons of diluted juice and ultimately to just give mouth care).
- Offer gestures of comfort (e.g., a cup of tea, a private phone).
- Explore symbolic language and the use of music.

**Figure 19-6. Interventions for Patients Who Are Close to Death**

When death appears to be near but is being prolonged by some unfinished business or because the patient believes the family is not ready, it has become common to coach families to grant permission for the dying person to "let go." This permission granting, however, can be confused with "pushing" the patient. When working with families, a key role is to help them understand that death, like birth, has its own timetable. The nurse can be a role model for appropriate behavior.

Symbolic language, from the patient, the family, and the professional, can be used to facilitate communication during this transition from life to death. Kelley and Callanan (1992) wrote about how dying patients often use special communication with themes that include travel or a need for change. Their words may seem like confusion or delirium but actually may be an attempt to communicate on a different level. Family and caregivers may be more comfortable using less direct language as a way to filter their pain. The metaphor is a way of speaking indirectly; its gentle nature allows one to hear the meaning and understand it. For example, the patient who is dying may speak of taking a trip, going home, or simply state "I need to get out of here" rather than speaking directly about death. The use of guided imagery can be a way to use metaphor and can be most helpful for patients during the transition of dying. An example of this follows.

The nurse spoke softly to the dying patient and began to describe the image of a flowing river, using a vivid description of the water. The river was depicted as coming to an obstacle that forced it to split and now create two paths. The imagery continued, describing the choice journey—to go against the current, or trust the flow and allow the river to carry one away. Symbolic language was used to help the patient to visualize alternatives and achieve some peace in whatever choice was made.

# Unusual Experiences

Unusual experiences of the bereaved in which individuals feel they have contact with the deceased often are discounted as dreams or a form of hallucinations (Rosenblatt, 1983). LaGrand (1997) coined the phrase "after-death communication" as spontaneous contact by the deceased loved one or the experiencing of the deceased by the mourner. This phenomenon is only now being addressed in the literature (Kwilecki, 2011). The actual incidence of these occurrences is not certain; however, they probably occur more frequently than some might think. Therapeutic effects of these experiences include affirmation of the death, completion of unfinished business, a sense that the dead person is all right, or a reduction in the bereaved person's suffering.

When bereaved people are asked directly about the topic, it is remarkable how often they will acknowledge strange experiences or coincidences. The following are accounts of unusual experiences:

- A nurse awoke suddenly in the night. She looked at the clock and felt her mother's presence. The phone rang, and she was told that her mother had died unexpectedly, at the exact time that she awakened.
- After her husband's death, one woman reported being so burdened that she kept forgetting to purchase bird seed, a task her husband had always taken care of. Each time she thought of it, she felt the need to continue the practice as he would have, but each day, distracted, she returned forgetting the seed. One day, she came home to find the counter where they kept messages and bills disheveled. Puzzled, she looked around, wondering if someone had been there. Her eye then caught sight of a miniature decorative bird cage that normally hung in the window but was now under the counter. A pen was wrapped around the wire hanger. Amazed, the woman believed her husband had found a way to communicate with her. She bought the birdseed and felt very comforted by this event.
- A nurse awoke one morning aware that she had had a strange dream that she could not remember. Later that day, a memory of the dream spontaneously returned. In the dream, she was at work and passed a deceased patient wearing a lab coat. She was startled and confused that he was alive. He smiled radiantly at her, and she asked, "Robert, how are you?" He replied, "I'm well," again with a tremendous smile. The nurse had only two brief interactions with this very sick patient before he died. In one conversation, the patient was so ill that he only shared a few words and never smiled; the other was the day he died, when he was barely responsive. She had entered the room, supported the wife, spoken with him about the dignity he carried and how he would carry that even as he died, and then prayed with the patient and his wife. Within moments, the patient died. The day of the dream, the nurse was scheduled to have a bereavement visit with the wife, and she dismissed it as unconscious processing for the anticipated visit. During the bereavement meeting, the wife mentioned that she thought about bringing a picture of her deceased husband and said, "I just wanted you to see his smile." The mention of the smile stirred the memory of the dream, and the nurse felt compelled to share it with the wife. The wife, moved by the dream, stated, "That is exactly how Robert would have responded to your question. That is what he always answered." When the nurse commented about being puzzled about the lab coat, the wife responded, "He was a researcher; he lived in a white lab coat!" This became a great comfort to the wife, who took it as a message from her husband that he was all right, something she had repeatedly hoped for but had feared was not true.

These experiences can be easily dismissed but may warrant continued exploration.

Morse's (1990, 1996) research on near-death experiences with children led to unusual and unexplainable scenarios in which children were able to describe events in other areas of the hospital or in their own homes while they were being resuscitated in the hospital. Morse suggested that sharing this near-death research might help other families to cope with anticipatory grieving and, ultimately, in bereavement. Families are reluctant to share these unusual stories for fear of being labeled crazy, especially given the feelings of loss of control related to the grief process. More research needs to be conducted in this area. Dr. Eben Alexander (2012), a neurosurgeon who experienced coma and near death, wrote a best-selling book, *Proof of Heaven*, about his experience and the difficulty of melding hard science and what we cannot explain. In a *New York Times* interview, he was quoted as saying, "Our spirit is not dependent on the brain or body. It is eternal, and no one has one sentence worth of hard evidence that it is not." (Kaufman, 2012, p. C1). Nurses should encourage the sharing of unusual events without passing judgment, dismissing them, or labeling them as hallucinations.

## Ethical Obligations

In the case study, Patti had become vulnerable, and her vulnerability as a patient called nurses to a level of commitment to respond. A nurse who sees a bereaved patient, who is present at the time of death, or is working with patients with cancer who are facing many levels of grief is beckoned to be present and engaged. This experience is encountered in a pivotal scene in the biographical adventure movie *Wild*. A young female protagonist comes to the hospital to find her ill mother's bed empty. Without the anchoring of her mother and overwhelmed with grief, the protagonist falls into substance abuse and begins exploiting her body. One wonders if things might have been different had the nurse who informed her of her mother's death responded more skillfully and compassionately. This is a practice that integrates ethics and calls us to a moral response; it demands that we consider the outcomes of our actions or the absence of a response. For the bereaved in the midst of forced detachment from one who has been loved, all the issues of attachment become paramount. In Michael Trout's work (2015) with attunement, he transferred the critical element of parent–child bonding, the act of being seen—to healthcare professionals in the act of connection and engagement. This ethical responsibility recognizes the necessity of beneficence and engagement; it recognizes, above all, the harm of indifference, whether in the sick patient or those grieving. Beyond nurses' individual duty, moving the agenda of bereavement forward within their institutions and communities is yet another level of obligation. Professional detachment is sometimes taught in schools of nursing, and frequently, the grief curriculum is lean. In clinical practice, however, we hear the need for guidance in empathic responses and more knowledge about bereavement. Curriculum should be addressed, and skillful mentoring should be in place for new graduate nurses. Despite national guidelines for palliative cancer care that include bereavement support for patients' families, one is hard pressed to find robust programs (National Comprehensive Cancer Network®, 2017; O'Connor, Abbott, & Demmer, 2009; Payne, 2004). Fully understanding the impact of grief and the potential for healing could include the following: the establishment of interventions that standardize practice; grief assessment and grief counseling for families while in the hospital, particularly in the intensive care units; child life specialist interventions when children are involved; chaplains with clinical pastoral education training; the development of bereavement packets and follow-up services; and the ongoing education of professionals (Granek, Mazzotta, Tozer, & Krzyzanowska, 2012; Morris & Block, 2015; Post et al., 2014). From a justice perspective, healthcare professionals also must ask if bereavement services are developed in an equitable way, especially given the poor mental health resources. Can low-income individuals access care, and is the institution's or hospital's bereavement care sensitive to the many cultures that might need services (Holtslander, 2008)?

# Professional Grief

The oncology nurse, in whatever setting he or she works, frequently establishes powerful and intimate bonds with patients. When a patient dies, the nurse faces the difficult task of mourning that loss regardless of the nature of the relationship (e.g., close, ambivalent, hostile) or the number of times he or she has experienced a death. The oncology nurse does not become immune to grief over time. Occasionally, the death of a particularly close patient results in an expression of grief that has been "saved up" from many deaths.

Slaby (1988) addressed the issue of dealing with death when he described the caregiver's task: "Those who care for patients with cancer must either directly confront their own mortality or expend psychic energy to mollify the intensity of the reality to allow for some reconciliation with the idea of death" (p. 139). As often is the case, oncology nurses reflect on the gifts the work brings. Living on the edge with others enhances one's appreciation of life. Still, the emotional work, grief, and its ensuing emotions need attention.

Saunders and Valente (1994) surveyed nurses attending bereavement workshops. They found that nurses reported coping well with "good" deaths. They defined those as deaths in which symptoms were managed, the nurse felt he or she gave the best care possible, the patient came to some resolution, and the death did not violate a natural order (i.e., the patient was not a child or young adult). Conversely, when the death was not considered "good" or the nurse was not present at the time of death, the grief was characterized as painful, complicated, distressing, or difficult.

In Western culture, anger is an emotion that is poorly tolerated; yet, anger is not an uncommon response to ongoing exposure to death and grief (Rueth & Hall, 1999). Slaby (1988) described anger in caregivers as a natural response to many demands that become increasingly difficult to fill and, if sustained, a contributing factor in burnout. Through interviewing oncology nurses, Watts, Botti, and Hunter (2010) found that they expressed anger toward patients and medical staff and also encountered anger from patients and their families. The anger can be magnified if one feels responsible for not curing the patient, not eliminating symptoms, or even worsening the symptoms because of the side effects of treatment. Anger can be passed back and forth between the patient/family and the healthcare team. Nurses working with patients with advanced cancer may hold themselves in the role of the "good" nurse who never has "bad" feelings. This can lead to a tremendous sense of isolation (Vachon, Lyall, & Freeman, 1978). Simply acknowledging anger can go a long way in helping to understand the secondary depression and guilt that it can create. Hill (1989) described the burdens aptly: "Will this be the time when I am truly depleted . . . that I must make a change because I can no longer care for my patients and can barely care for myself . . . when I barely managed to restrain myself from snapping at people who were trying to make appropriate referrals and when I used all my resources to walk through hospital room doors to see sick, sorrowful people one more time" (p. 146). Kutner and Kilbourn (2009) encouraged facing grief, finding meaning, and working toward a "good" death for patients that will assist physicians in coping with the challenges of caring for the dying and coping with loss. In oncology nursing, Perry's (2008) small study of exemplary nurses revealed how they circumvented compassion fatigue through "moments" of connection and the creation of moments of significance and energy. Feldstein and Gemma (1995) studied 50 professional oncology nurses using the Grief Experience Inventory to assess differences between those who remained in their positions and those who left. Both groups had high scores for despair, social isolation, and somatization. Those who remained in their positions scored low on loss of control and death anxiety, while those who left had low levels of anger/hostility, loss of control, and death anxiety. Of even greater interest was the high percentage who had experienced a death in their immediate family within the last year (31% of those who stayed and 37% of those who left). In both groups, spouses and close friends were used more frequently than colleagues for support. More studies like these are needed to give a greater insight into the complexity of professional grief and its impact.

## Self-Care

No single correct way exists to care for oneself. Support groups can help, and any way of reducing the isolation of feelings will make a difference. A monthly self-assessment regarding how many deaths have occurred and the toll taken can be useful. Addressing other areas of stress in one's life (e.g., lack of sleep or exercise, too many commitments) is helpful. The cumulative effect may have the greatest impact, generating grief overload (Vachon, 1998). Acknowledge limitations, and learn and use appropriate boundaries about how involved to become. The literature is rich in the significance of pairing engagement with detachment in this work (Carmack, 1997; Rittman, Rivera, Sutphin, & Godown, 1997). Be aware of signs when colleagues are stepping beyond their roles as professionals. Assess participation in life-affirming beliefs and actions (e.g., sexuality, spirituality, laughter, play, creativity). Clinics and units might consider ceremonies and programs that serve to acknowledge and discharge the cumulative grief of families and professionals (Burke & Gerraughty, 1994; Coolican & Pearce, 1995; Lewis, 1999; Medland, Howard-Ruben, & Whitaker, 2004; Morris & Block, 2015). Follow-up programs as simple as sending a bereavement card or as complex as telephone contact can be helpful for families and the staff (Kaunonen et al., 2000). Some institutions have a service that remembers those who have died; this is very common in hospice. Staff members at times resist attending such programs, not wanting to face the full measure of grief during an annual remembrance. Yet, these programs can function as catharses that allow them to begin again. Self-care, which is included in the American Nurses Association's (2015) *Code of Ethics for Nurses*, is especially important for those who care for the dying (Wakefield, 2000; Zerbe & Steinberg, 2000). New graduates in oncology nursing are at high risk for leaving the field if they are not mentored well in both the care of the dying and grief (Caton & Klemm, 2006). Fortunately, the need to address the emotional burdens of accumulative grief are being recognized throughout the oncology literature, and knowledge of self-care and programs addressing compassion fatigue and grief are demonstrating the power of prevention (Altounji, Morgan, Grover, Daldumyan, & Secola, 2013; Bush & Boyle, 2012; Fetter, 2012; Hildebrandt, 2012; Houck, 2014; Potter et al., 2013; Rice, Bennett, & Billingsley, 2014; Sanchez-Reilly et al., 2013; Shinbara & Olson, 2010). Whatever action is taken, the key is to initiate some action on individual, managerial, and institutional levels to acknowledge and cope with professional grief.

# Conclusion

In a culture that traditionally has been phobic about death, best-sellers have embraced the subject and hospices have been mainstreamed. Still, many families have never been at a bedside during the dying process. Bereavement care does not begin after the death but, in a preventive sense, in the many events leading up to the death. Nurses have an obligation to care for the bereaved, whether it is making sure that a child's needs are attended to, listening to a dying patient's grief, assisting families in communication, teaching families about the physiologic aspects of the dying process, making a call to the family or sending a card, or facilitating a bereavement support group. Nurses hold the opportunity to transform. The term *transform* comes from the Latin *trans*, meaning "across and beyond." When the nurse takes on the challenge of helping to heal grief, he or she impacts not only the individual but also all who are touched by the experience. The nurse changes the bereaved by helping them across the suffering, first and foremost by hearing the words, the moans, the ache, the breaking of the heart. This act of compassion begins the long journey back to wellness, when bittersweet memories bring the tears and the joy of who the person was and always will be in the lives of the bereaved.

# References

Alexander, E. (2012). *Proof of heaven*. New York, NY: Simon and Schuster.
Altounji, D., Morgan, H., Grover, M., Daldumyan, S., & Secola, R. (2013). A self-care retreat for pediatric hematology oncology nurses. *Journal of Pediatric Oncology Nursing, 30,* 18–23. doi:10.1177/1043454212461951
American Nurses Association. (2015). *Code of ethics for nurses*. Washington, DC: Author.
American Psychiatric Association. (2000). *Diagnostic and statistical manual of mental disorders* (4th ed.). Washington, DC: Author.
American Psychiatric Association. (2013). *Diagnostic and statistical manual of mental disorders* (5th ed.). Washington, DC: Author.
Areán, P.A., & Reynolds, C.F., III. (2005). The impact of psychosocial factors on late-life depression. *Biological Psychiatry, 58,* 277–282. doi:10.1016/j.biopsych.2005.03.037
Bachman, B. (2013). The development of a sustainable, community-supported children's bereavement camp. *Omega, 67,* 21–35. doi:10.2190/OM.67.1-2.c
Barry, L.C., Kasl, S.V., & Prigerson, H.G. (2002). Psychiatric disorders among bereaved persons: The role of perceived circumstances of death and preparedness for death. *American Journal of Geriatric Psychiatry, 10,* 447–457. doi:10.1097/00019442-200207000-00011
Bereaved. (n.d.). In *Merriam-Webster's online dictionary*. Retrieved from https://www.merriam-webster.com/dictionary/bereaved
Bernard, L.L., & Guarnaccia, C.A. (2003). Two models of caregiver strain and bereavement adjustment: A comparison of husband and daughter caregivers of breast cancer hospice patients. *Gerontologist, 43,* 808–816. doi:10.1093/geront/43.6.808
Bower, J.E., Kemeny, M.E., Taylor, S.E., & Fahey, J.L. (2003). Finding positive meaning and its association with natural killer cell cytotoxicity among participants in a bereavement-related disclosure intervention. *Annals Behavioral Medicine, 25,* 146–155.
Bowlby, J. (1969). Childhood mourning and its implications for psychiatry. *American Journal of Psychiatry, 118,* 481–498.
Bowlby, J. (1980). *Attachment and loss*. New York, NY: Basic Books.
Brown-Saltzman, K.A. (1995). Multicultural perspectives in palliative care. *Quality of Life: A Nursing Challenge, 3,* 41–47.
Bryant, R.A. (2014). Prolonged grief: Where to after *Diagnostic and Statistical Manual of Mental Disorders*, 5th edition? *Current Opinion in Psychiatry, 27,* 21–26. doi:10.1097/YCO.0000000000000031
Buckley, T., Sunari, D., Marshall, A., Bartrop, R., McKinley, S., & Tofler, G. (2012). Physiological correlates of bereavement and the impact of bereavement interventions. *Dialogues in Clinical Neuroscience, 14,* 129–139.
Bui, E., Nadal-Vicens, M., & Simon, N.M. (2012). Pharmacological approaches to the treatment of complicated grief: Rationale and a brief review of the literature. *Dialogues in Clinical Neuroscience, 14,* 149–157.
Burke, C., & Gerraughty, S.M. (1994). An oncology unit's initiation of a bereavement support program. *Oncology Nursing Forum, 21,* 1675–1680.
Bush, N.J., & Boyle, D. (2012). *Self-healing through reflection: A workbook for nurses*. Pittsburgh, PA: Hygeia Media.
Carmack, B. (1997). Balancing engagement and detachment in caregiving. *Image: The Journal of Nursing Scholarship, 29,* 139–144. doi:10.1111/j.1547-5069.1997.tb01546.x
Carr, D. (2003). A "good death" for whom? Quality of spouse's death and psychological distress among older widowed persons. *Journal of Health and Social Behavior, 44,* 215–232. doi:10.2307/1519809
Caton, A.P., & Klemm, P. (2006). Introduction of novice oncology nurses to end-of-life care. *Clinical Journal of Oncology Nursing, 10,* 604–608. doi:10.1188/06.CJON.604-608
Chiambretto, P. (2008). Prolonged grief disorder: Towards a new diagnostic category. *Giornale Italiano di Medicina del Lavoro ed Ergonomia, 30*(Suppl. B), B40–B46.
Christ, G.H., & Christ, A.E. (2006). Current approaches to helping children cope with a parent's terminal illness. *CA: A Cancer Journal for Clinicians, 56,* 197–212. doi:10.3322/canjclin.56.4.197
Christakis, N.A., & Iwashyna, T.J. (2003). The health impact of health care on families: A matched cohort study of hospice use by decedents and mortality outcomes in surviving, widowed spouses. *Social Science and Medicine, 57,* 465–475. doi:10.1016/S0277-9536(02)00370-2
Clements, P.T., Vigil, G.J., Manno, M.S., Henry, G.C., Wilks, J., Sarthak, D., ... & Foster, W. (2003). Cultural perspectives of death, grief, and bereavement. *Journal of Psychosocial Nursing, 41,* 18–26. doi:10.3928/0279-3695-20030701-12
Clute, M.A., & Kobayashi, R. (2013). Are children's grief camps effective? *Journal of Social Work in End-of-life and Palliative Care, 9,* 43–57. doi:10.1080/15524256.2013.758927

Coolican, M.B., & Pearce, T. (1995). Aftercare bereavement program. *Critical Care Nursing Clinics of North America, 7,* 519–527.

Corr, C.A., & Doka, K.J. (1994). Current models of death, dying and bereavement. *Critical Care Nursing Clinics of North America, 6,* 545–552.

Doka, K.J. (2002). *Disenfranchised grief: New directions, challenges, and strategies for practice.* Champaign, IL: Research Press.

Edelman, H. (1995). *Motherless daughters: The legacy of loss.* Reading, MA: Addison-Wesley.

Feldstein, M.A., & Gemma, P.B. (1995). Oncology nurses and chronic compounded grief. *Cancer Nursing, 18,* 228–236. doi:10.1097/00002820-199506000-00008

Fetter, K.L. (2012). We grieve too: One inpatient oncology unit's interventions for recognizing and combating compassion fatigue. *Clinical Journal of Oncology Nursing, 16,* 559–561. doi:10.1188/12.CJON.559-561

Forte, A.L., Hill, M., Pazder, R., & Feudtner, C. (2004). Bereavement care interventions: A systematic review. *BMC Palliative Care, 3,* 3–17. doi:10.1186/1472-684X-3-3

Furman, R. (1964). Death and the young child. *Psychoanalytic Study of the Child, 19,* 321–333.

Garrido, M.M., & Prigerson, H.G. (2014). The end-of-life experience: Modifiable predictors of caregivers' bereavement adjustment. *Cancer, 120,* 918–925. doi:10.1002/cncr.28495

Goldsmith, B., Morrison, R.S., Vanderwerker, L.C., & Prigerson, H.G. (2008). Elevated rates of prolonged grief disorder in African Americans. *Death Studies, 32,* 352–365. doi:10.1080/07481180801929012

Grande, G.E., Farquhar, M.C., Barclay, S.I.G., & Todd, C.J. (2004). Caregiver bereavement outcome: Relationship with hospice at home, satisfaction with care, and home death. *Journal of Palliative Care, 20,* 69–77.

Granek, L., Mazzotta, P., Tozer, R., & Krzyzanowska, M.K. (2012). What do oncologists want? Suggestions from oncologists on how their institutions can support them in dealing with patient loss. *Supportive Care in Cancer, 20,* 2627–2632. doi:10.1007/s00520-012-1528-2

Guldin, M.-B., Vedsted, P., Zachariae, R., Olesen, F., & Jensen, A.B. (2012). Complicated grief and need for professional support in family caregivers of cancer patients in palliative care: A longitudinal cohort study. *Supportive Care in Cancer, 20,* 1679–1685. doi:10.1007/s00520-011-1260-3

Gündel, H., O'Connor, M.-F., Littrell, L., Fort, C., & Lane, R.D. (2003). Functional neuroanatomy of grief: An fMRI study. *American Journal of Psychiatry, 160,* 1946–1953. doi:10.1176/appi.ajp.160.11.1946

Hildebrandt, L. (2012). Providing grief resolution as an oncology nurse retention strategy: A literature review. *Clinical Journal of Oncology Nursing, 16,* 601–606. doi:10.1188/12.CJON.601-606

Hill, H.L. (1989). To fill a heart: Oncology over the long haul. *Journal of Psychosocial Oncology, 7,* 145–152. doi:10.1300/J077v07n03_10

Holtslander, L.F. (2008). Caring for bereaved caregivers: Analyzing the context of care. *Clinical Journal of Oncology Nursing, 12,* 501–506. doi:10.1188/08.CJON.501-506

Houck, D. (2014). Helping nurses cope with grief and compassion fatigue: An educational intervention. *Clinical Journal of Oncology Nursing, 18,* 454–458. doi:10.1188/14.CJON.454-458

Johansson, Å.K., & Grimby, A. (2012). Anticipatory grief among close relatives of patients in hospice and palliative wards. *American Journal of Hospice and Palliative Medicine, 29,* 134–138. doi:10.1177/1049909111409021

Kaufman, L. (2012). Readers join doctor's journey to the afterworld's gates. *The New York Times.* Retrieved from http://www.nytimes.com/2012/11/26/books/dr-eben-alexanders-tells-of-near-death-in-proof-of-heaven.html?

Kaunonen, M., Aalto, P., Tarkka, M.-T., & Paunonen, M. (2000). Oncology ward nurses' perspectives of family grief and a supportive telephone call after death of a significant other. *Cancer Nursing, 23,* 314–324. doi:10.1097/00002820-200008000-00010

Kelley, P., & Callanan, M. (1992). *Final gifts: Understanding the special awareness, needs, and communication of the dying.* New York, NY: Poseidon Press.

Khanfer, R., Lord, J.M., & Phillips, A.C. (2011). Neutrophil function and cortisol: DHEAS ratio in bereaved older adults. *Brain, Behavior, and Immunity, 25,* 1182–1186. doi:10.1016/j.bbi.2011.03.008

Koocher, G. (1974). Talking with children about death. *American Journal of Orthopsychiatry, 44,* 404–411. doi:10.1111/j.1939-0025.1974.tb00893.x

Kübler-Ross, E. (1969). *On death and dying.* New York, NY: Macmillan.

Kutner, J.S., & Kilbourn, K.M. (2009). Bereavement: Addressing challenges faced by advanced cancer patients, their caregivers, and their physicians. *Primary Care, 36,* 825–844. doi:10.1016/j.pop.2009.07.004

Kwilecki, S. (2011). Ghosts, meaning, and faith: After-death communications in bereavement narratives. *Death Studies, 35,* 219–243. doi:10.1080/07481187.2010.511424

LaGrand, L.E. (1997). *Understanding after-death communication in the lives of the bereaved.* Paper presented at the International Conference on Grief and Bereavement in Contemporary Society, Washington, DC.

Laing, C.M., & Moules, N.J. (2015). Children's cancer camps: A way to understand grief differently. *Omega, 70,* 436–453. doi:10.1177/0030222815572605

Laurie, A., & Neimeyer, R.A. (2008). African Americans in bereavement: Grief as a function of ethnicity. *Omega, 57,* 173–193. doi:10.2190/OM.57.2.d

Lewis, A.E. (1999). Reducing burnout: Development of an oncology staff bereavement program. *Oncology Nursing Forum, 26,* 1065–1069.

Lichtenthal, W.G., Nilsson, M., Kissane, D.W., Breitbart, W., Kacel, E., Jones, E.C., & Prigerson, H.G. (2011). Underutilization of mental health services among bereaved caregivers with prolonged grief disorder. *Psychiatry Services Journal, 62,* 1225–1229. doi:10.1176/appi.ps.62.10.1225

Lindemann, E. (1944). Symptomatology and management of acute grief. *American Journal of Psychiatry, 101,* 141–148. doi:10.1176/ajp.101.2.141

Lovell, G.P., Smith, T., & Kannis-Dymand, L. (2015). Surrogate end-of-life care decision makers' postbereavement grief and guilt responses. *Death Studies, 39,* 647–653. doi:10.1080/07481187.2015.1047062

Maciejewski, P.K., Zhang, B., Block, S.D., & Prigerson, H.G. (2007). An empirical examination of the stage theory of grief. *JAMA, 297,* 716–723. doi:10.1001/jama.297.7.716

Marketon, J.I.W., & Glaser, R. (2008). Stress hormones and immune function. *Cellular Immunology, 252,* 16–26. doi:10.1016/j.cellimm.2007.09.006

McClatchey, I.S., & Wimmer, J.S. (2012). Healing components of a bereavement camp: Children and adolescents give voice to their experiences. *Omega, 65,* 11–32. doi:10.2190/OM.65.1.b

Medland, J., Howard-Ruben, J., & Whitaker, E. (2004). Fostering psychosocial wellness in oncology nurses: Addressing burnout and social support in the workplace. *Oncology Nursing Forum, 31,* 47–54. doi:10.1188/04.ONF.47-54

Morris, S.E., & Block, S.D. (2015). Adding value to palliative care services: The development of an institutional bereavement program. *Journal of Palliative Medicine, 18,* 915–922. doi:10.1089/jpm.2015.0080

Morse, M. (1990). *Closer to the light: Learning from the near-death experiences of children: Amazing revelations of what it feels like to die.* New York, NY: Ivy Books.

Morse, M. (1996). *Parting visions: Uses and meanings of pre-death, psychic, and spiritual experiences.* New York, NY: HarperCollins.

Nagy, M. (1948). The child's theories concerning death. *Journal of Genetic Psychology, 73,* 327. doi:10.1080/08856559.1948.10533458

NANDA International. (2015). *Nursing diagnoses: Definitions and classification, 2015–2017.* Philadelphia, PA: Author.

Nanni, M.G., Biancosino, B., & Grassi, L. (2014). Pre-loss symptoms related to risk of complicated grief in caregivers of terminally ill cancer patients. *Journal of Affective Disorders, 160,* 87–91. doi:10.1016/j.jad.2013.12.023

National Comprehensive Cancer Network. (2017). *NCCN Clinical Practice Guidelines in Oncology (NCCN Guidelines®): Palliative care* [v.2.2017]. Retrieved from http://www.nccn.org/professionals/physician_gls/pdf/palliative.pdf

O'Connor, M., Abbott, J.-A., & Demmer, C. (2009). A comparison of bereavement services provided in hospice and palliative care settings in Australia, the UK, and the USA. *Progress in Palliative Care, 17,* 69–74. doi:10.1179/0906992609X392240

Osterweis, M., Solomon, F., & Green, M. (Eds.). (1984). *Bereavement: Reactions, consequences, and care.* Washington, DC: National Academies Press.

Otis-Green, S. (2011). Embracing the existential invitation to examine care at the end of life. In S.H. Qualls & J.E. Kasl-Godley (Eds.), *End-of-life issues, grief, and bereavement: What clinicians need to know* (pp. 310–324). Hoboken, NJ: John Wiley & Sons.

Parkes, C.M. (1986). *Bereavement: Studies of grief in adult life* (2nd ed.). London, England: Penguin Books.

Payne, S. (2004). Overview. In S. Payne, J. Seymour, & C. Ingleton (Eds.), *Palliative care nursing: Principles and evidence for practice* (pp. 435–461). Berkshire, United Kingdom: Open University Press.

Perry, B. (2008). Why exemplary oncology nurses seem to avoid compassion fatigue. *Canadian Oncology Nursing Journal, 18,* 87–99. doi:10.5737/1181912x1828792

Peteet, J.R., Maytal, G., & Rokni, H. (2010). Unimaginable loss: Contingent suicidal ideation in family members of oncology patients. *Psychosomatics, 51,* 166–170. doi:10.1176/appi.psy.51.2.166

Phillips, A.C., Carroll, D., Burns, V.E., Ring, D., Macleod, J., & Drayson, M. (2006). Bereavement and marriage are associated with antibody response to influenza vaccination in the elderly. *Brain, Behavior, and Immunity, 20,* 279–289. doi:10.1016/j.bbi.2005.08.003

Post, S.G., Ng, L.E., Fischel, J.E., Bennett, M., Bily, L., Chandran, L., ... Roess, M.W. (2014). Routine, empathic and compassionate patient care: Definitions, development, obstacles, education and beneficiaries. *Journal of Evaluation in Clinical Practice, 20,* 872–880. doi:10.1111/jep.12243

Potter, P., Deshields, T., Berger, J.A., Clarke, M., Olsen, S., & Chen, L. (2013). Evaluation of a compassion fatigue resiliency program for oncology nurses. *Oncology Nursing Forum, 40,* 180–187. doi:10.1188/13.ONF.180-187

Prigerson, H.G., Horowitz, M.J., Jacobs, S.C., Parkes, C.M., Aslan, M., Goodkin, K., ... Maciejewski, P.K. (2009). Prolonged grief disorder: Psychometric validation of criteria proposed for *DSM–V* and *ICD-11. PLOS Medicine, 6,* 1–12. doi:10.1371/journal.pmed.1000121

Prigerson, H.G., Shear, M.K., Jacobs, S.C., Reynolds, C.F., III, Maciejewski, P.K., Davidson, J.R., ... Zisook, S. (1999). Consensus criteria for traumatic grief. *British Journal of Psychiatry, 174,* 67–73. doi:10.1192/bjp.174.1.67

Rabow, J.W., Hauser, J.M., & Adams, J. (2004). Supporting family caregivers at the end of life. *JAMA, 291,* 483–491. doi:10.1001/jama.291.4.483

Rando, T.A. (1993). *Treatment of complicated mourning.* Champaign, IL: Research Press.

Rando, T.A. (1997). Living and learning the reality of a loved one's dying: Traumatic stress and cognitive process in anticipatory grief. In K.J. Doka & J. Davidson (Eds.), *Living with grief when illness is prolonged* (pp. 33–50). Washington, DC: Hospice Foundation of America.

Rando, T.A. (2000). *Clinical dimensions of anticipatory mourning.* Champaign, IL: Research Press.

Rice, K.L., Bennett, M.J., & Billingsley, L. (2014). Using second life to facilitate peer storytelling for grieving oncology nurses. *Ochsner Journal, 14,* 551–562.

Rittman, M., Rivera, J., Sutphin, L., & Godown, I. (1997). Phenomenological study of nurses caring for dying patients. *Cancer Nursing, 20,* 115–119. doi:10.1097/00002820-199704000-00006

Rosenblatt, P.C. (1983). *Bitter, bitter tears: Nineteenth-century diarists and twentieth-century grief theories.* Minneapolis, MN: University of Minneapolis Press.

Rueth, T.W., & Hall, S.E. (1999). Dealing with the anger and hostility of those who grieve. *American Journal of Hospice and Palliative Care, 16,* 743–746. doi:10.1177/104990919901600613

Sanchez-Reilly, S., Morrison, L.J., Carey, E., Bernacki, R., O'Neill, L., Kapo, J., ... Thomas Jde, L. (2013). Caring for oneself to care for others: Physicians and their self-care. *Journal of Supportive Oncology, 11,* 75–81. doi:10.12788/j.suponc.0003

Saunders, J.M., & Valente, S.M. (1994). Nurse's grief. *Cancer Nursing, 17,* 318–325. doi:10.1097/00002820-199408000-00004

Schultze-Florey, C.R., Martínez Maza, O., Magpantay, L., Breen, E.C., Irwin, M.R., Gündel, H., & O'Connor, M.F. (2012). When grief makes you sick: Bereavement induced systemic inflammation is a question of genotype. *Brain, Behavior, and Immunity, 26,* 1066–1071. doi:10.1016/j.bbi.2012.06.009

Shinbara, C.G., & Olson, L. (2010). When nurses grieve: Spirituality's role in coping. *Journal of Christian Nursing, 27,* 32–37. doi:10.1097/01.CNJ.0000365989.87518.60

Slaby, A.E. (1988). Cancer's impact on caregivers. *Advances in Psychosomatic Medicine, 18,* 135–153. doi:10.1159/000415781

Strachey, J. (Ed.). (1961). *The standard edition of the complete works of Sigmund Freud.* London, England: Hogarth Press.

Stroebe, W., & Schut, H. (2001). Risk factors in bereavement outcome: A methodological and empirical review. In M.S. Stroebe, R.O. Hansson, W. Stroebe, & H. Schut (Eds.), *Handbook of bereavement research: Consequences, coping and care.* Washington, DC: American Psychological Association.

Sveen, J., Eilegård, A., Steineck, G., & Kreicbergs, U. (2014). They still grieve—A nationwide follow-up of young adults 2–9 years after losing a sibling to cancer. *Psycho-Oncology, 23,* 658–664. doi:10.1002/pon.3463

Szanto, K., Gildengers, A., Mulsant, B.H., Brown, G., Alexopoulos, G.S., & Reynolds, C.F., III. (2002). Identification of suicidal ideation and prevention of suicidal behaviour in the elderly. *Drugs and Aging, 19,* 11–24. doi:10.2165/00002512-200219010-00002

Tamborini, C.R., Cupito, E., & Shoffner, D. (2011). A profile of Social Security child beneficiaries and their families: Sociodemographic and economic characteristics. *Social Security Bulletin, 71,* 2011.

Thomas, K., Hudson, P., Trauer, T., Remedios, C., & Clarke, D. (2014). Risk factors for developing prolonged grief during bereavement in family carers of cancer patients in palliative care: A longitudinal study. *Journal of Pain and Symptom Management, 47,* 531–541. doi:10.1016/j.jpainsymman.2013.05.022

Thompson, S. (2002). Older people. In N. Thompson (Ed.), *Loss and grief: A guide for human services practitioners* (pp. 162–173). New York, NY: Palgrave.

Tofthagen, C.S., Kip, K., Witt, A., & McMillan, S.C. (2017). Complicated grief. *Clinical Journal of Oncology Nursing, 21,* 331–337. doi:10.1188/17.CJON.331-337

Traylor, E.S., Hayslip, B., Kaminski, P.L., & York, C. (2003). Relationships between grief and family system characteristics: A cross lagged longitudinal analysis. *Death Studies, 27,* 575–601. doi:10.1080/07481180302897

Trout, M. (2015, March). *Is attunement an ethical issue?* Paper presented at the Ethics of Caring National Nursing Ethics Conference, Los Angeles, CA.

Vachon, M. (1998). Caring for the caregiver in oncology and palliative care. *Seminars in Oncology Nursing, 14,* 152–157. doi:10.1016/S0749-2081(98)80021-1

Vachon, M.L., Lyall, W.A., & Freeman, S.J. (1978). Measurement and management of stress in health professionals working with advanced cancer patients. *Death Education, 1,* 365–375. doi:10.1080/07481187808252911

Wakefield, A. (2000). Nurses' responses to death and dying: A need for relentless self-care. *International Journal of Palliative Nursing, 6,* 245–251. doi:10.12968/ijpn.2000.6.5.8926

Warner, J., Metcalfe, C., & King, M. (2001). Evaluating the use of benzodiazepines following recent bereavement. *British Journal of Psychiatry, 178,* 36–41. doi:10.1192/bjp.178.1.36

Watts, R., Botti, M., & Hunter, M. (2010). Nurses' perspectives on the care provided to cancer patients. *Cancer Nursing, 33,* E1–E8. doi:10.1097/NCC.0b013e3181b5575a

Worden, J.W. (1991). *Grief counseling and grief therapy: A handbook for the mental health practitioner.* New York, NY: Springer.

Zerbe, K.J., & Steinberg, D.L. (2000). Coming to terms with grief and loss. Can skills for dealing with bereavement be learned? *Postgrad Medicine, 108,* 97–98, 101–104, 106. doi:10.3810/pgm.2000.11.1292

Zisook, S., Paulus, M., Shuchter, S.R., & Judd, L.L. (1997). The many faces of depression following spousal bereavement. *Journal of Affective Disorders, 45,* 85–95.

Zisook, S., Shuchter, S.R., Sledge, P.A., Paulus, M., & Judd, L.L. (1994). The spectrum of depressive phenomena after spousal bereavement. *Journal of Clinical Psychiatry, 55,* 29–36.

CHAPTER 20

# Guilt

*Rebecca Crane-Okada, PhD, RN, CNS, AOCN®*

> *The pangs of conscience are better than floggings.*
>
> —The Talmud

Guilt is defined as "the state of one who has committed an offense especially consciously" ("Guilt," n.d.). Medically speaking, guilt is defined as "morbid self-reproach often manifest in marked preoccupation with the moral correctness of one's behavior" ("Guilt," n.d.). It is a feeling that usually involves self-criticism and results from an internal conflict with one's conscience. One's conscience creates a sense of what is right and wrong and a compulsion to do what is right. The teachings of childhood, which are influenced by religious, cultural, and social norms, usually determine the boundaries of an individual's conscience. Mothers frequently have been accused of using guilt to manipulate their children. A request for correct behavior is accompanied by a statement geared toward generating guilt (e.g., "You know how much I worry when you . . . ."; "After all I have done for you, the least you could do is . . . ."). The guilt can be intended as punishment for past digressions as well as an inducement for future correct behavior. Often, these efforts at controlling behavior through guilt are done at a semiconscious level. The parent may say the words out of habit or experience and may not realize what is being said.

Guilt has been a component of many religions in an effort to control behavior. Feelings of guilt are so unpleasant that many will not commit a prohibited behavior, or if they do, they will feel so overwhelmed by guilt that they will never do the behavior again. As a shaper of filial, moral, and ethical behavior, guilt arguably may have value. However, the role of guilt in relation to cancer often is counterproductive.

Coping with a life-threatening yet often chronic disease is a unique experience for most people. Many individuals search for the "expected" or "accepted" behavior in this situation and believe that certain behaviors might not be "correct." If the "incorrect" somehow occurs, guilt frequently follows. In most cases, the problem is that no absolute right or wrong exists. If the purpose of guilt is to prevent the occurrence of "wrong" behavior and promote "right" behavior, the resulting feelings of guilt experienced by patients with cancer, their families, and healthcare professionals often are entirely unwarranted. This guilt then becomes an additional yet unnecessary source of emotional stress in an already highly stressful situation.

## The Nature of Guilt in Cancer

The seriousness of a cancer diagnosis and its ramifications naturally cause patients and families to ask "Why?" and examine personal behaviors and circumstances to find an answer. Potential sources of patients' guilt are almost limitless and include beliefs that they caused their cancer, delayed the diagnosis, chose the wrong treatment, did not adhere to their treatment plan, or survived when others have not. Researchers have found that levels of self-blame and guilt at the time of diagnosis, although unrelated to concurrent psychological distress, were significantly predictive of psychological distress four months later (Bennett, Compas, Beckjord, & Glinder, 2005; Malcarne, Compas, Epping-Jordan, & Howell, 1995). Self-blame and guilt also may be sources of long-term psychological distress (Aguado Loi et al., 2013; Daley et al., 2010; Friedman et al., 2010; Lobchuk, Murdoch, McClement, & McPherson, 2008; Posluszny et al., 2016). Spousal guilt has been shown to be related to quality of life, hope, and self-efficacy in caregivers of women with breast cancer (Duggleby et al., 2015). Guilt and self-blame may positively or negatively influence cancer prevention and long-term follow-up by cancer survivors (Lebel et al., 2013). Based on such research, as well as on clinical observation, it is not difficult to conclude that self-blame and guilt can be ongoing and significant sources of distress for people dealing with cancer. The guilt can take many forms (see Figure 20-1). The goal of cancer care providers is to assist those dealing with cancer to understand and eliminate their feelings of guilt whenever possible.

## Sources of Guilt

### Hero Myth

Perhaps the most pervasive and insidious source of guilt in patients with cancer stems from what Gray and Doan (1990) characterized as the "Hero Myth." This notion compares an individual's battle with cancer to the mythical warrior hero who overcomes the devouring monster after a series of trials and immense suffering. According to popular belief, the Hero Myth involves beating cancer through a psychological transformation that includes becoming a more effective, more expressive, more loving, more positive, and more coura-

---

**Conscience**—The consciousness of the right or wrong of one's own actions or motives.
**Guilt**—A painful feeling of self-reproach resulting from a belief that one has done something wrong.
**Hero Myth**—A popular cultural belief that patients have the power and ability to both cause their cancer and to cure themselves using psychological interventions.
**Justified guilt**—Feelings of guilt that arise when an incorrect behavior has led to a forewarned result (e.g., smoking and lung cancer). The patient/family and healthcare personnel may believe that the guilt is warranted.
**Positive attitude**—The belief that one or more options are available to deal with a problem and that at least one of these options will be successful. Positive attitude often is incorrectly interpreted as the absence of negative feelings.
**Self-blame**—To hold oneself responsible for something. Although sometimes used interchangeably with guilt, self-blame may or may not be accompanied by feelings of guilt.
**Survivor guilt**—The ironic feelings of guilt held by some patients who survive their cancer when others they know have died.

**Figure 20-1. Glossary of Terms**

geous person. Two basic assumptions underlie this myth in dealing with cancer: (a) Cancer is caused at least partly by psychological factors, and (b) progression of the disease is affected by these same factors. The implication is that controlling or fixing these problems can lead to a cure. Popular books such as *Getting Well Again* (Simonton, Matthews-Simonton, & Creighton, 1978), *Love, Medicine, and Miracles* (Siegel, 1986), and *Radical Remission: Surviving Cancer Against All Odds* (Turner, 2014) have expounded on the Hero Myth (Block, 2009; Servan-Schreiber, 2009). However, these books also offer ways of coping that help individuals take control of their lives in ways that can be life-giving on many levels.

Many patients with cancer feel a sense of guilt or self-blame for psychological problems and behavioral choices. For example, they may conjecture that they have a "cancer personality," meaning they have too much stress in their lives, did not eat well, drink too much, did not exercise enough, etc. Sometimes, more tangible problems may be related to the development of cancer, such as having had a great deal of sun exposure without adequate skin protection, chronic poor dietary habits, chronic stress, or a smoking problem. One or more of these psychological and behavioral factors may play a role in the development of the cancer. However, to be guilty, the person should know for a fact that the problem or behavior was contributory to the development of the cancer but then allow the problem or behavior to continue anyway. In the case of a genetic predisposition, this would mean being unable to reverse the heritable transmission but able to take action to reduce cancer risk by therapeutic intervention. For most people, however, guilt is not a rational approach. Many factors lead to the development of cancer. Although the association of tobacco use and incidence of oral and lung cancers is now well established, scientists more recently have identified the association of sunburns suffered as children to malignant melanoma later in life, the possible role of certain dietary factors and obesity with some types of cancer, and the role of viral exposure to some cancers. The degree to which these psychological problems and behavioral actions contribute to cancer is only partially understood. The relationship of stress to cancer remains a prominent area of research and yet elusive in a cause and effect relationship (Antoni, 2013; Lutgendorf & Andersen, 2015). Research has yet to explain why some people experience severe stress and yet do not develop cancer or other illnesses. A meta-analysis by Chida, Hamer, Wardle, and Steptoe (2008) suggested an adverse effect of stress-related psychosocial factors on cancer incidence and survival. If guilt or self-blame leads to depression and subsequent suppression of the immune system, then psychotherapeutic interventions to address these issues might positively affect risk of recurrence and long-term survival (Barrera & Spiegel, 2014). Psychoanalytic theories that cancer occurs or spreads because of some deep-seated desire for self-punishment or feeling of unworthiness have never been supported or substantiated. These issues should be explained logically and carefully to patients who admit to feeling guilt for causing their cancer and to family members who may be blaming patients for developing cancer.

The second assumption of the Hero Myth is that controlling factors that contribute to the development of cancer must therefore influence the course of the disease, even to a cure (Malcarne et al., 1995). Common sense and current research indicate that, at a minimum, patients can take actions that may improve their quality of life, reduce the risk of recurrence, and improve survival. Such activities include eating a better diet, maintaining a healthy weight, engaging in physical activity, managing stress, and enhancing coping abilities (Antoni, 2013; Mustafa, Carson-Stevens, Gillespie, & Edwards, 2013; Pekmezi & Demark-Wahnefried, 2011). Documented cases of spontaneous remission have occurred after patients embarked on these positive lifestyle changes and began showing and sharing their emotions (Turner, 2014).

Patients who assume more personal responsibility for their health and well-being after a diagnosis of cancer may experience benefits; however, it is important not to assume that changes in diet, stress, and coping alone, no matter how dramatic, are sufficient to cure cancer. Some comprehensive treatment models encourage such positive changes as an important adjunct to enhance the body's ability to respond to or endure standard medical treatment (e.g., surgery, chemotherapy, radiation therapy). Encouraging patients to take personal responsibility is a two-edged sword. Such tasks may give patients a sense of control and hopefulness. Conversely, patients may feel tremendous pressure to comply and may feel guilty when unable to on a regular basis. If the disease progresses or recurs, they may feel additional self-blame and guilt. Offering support to promote overall physical, emotional, spiritual, and social well-being with no guarantees; encouraging slow but steady lifestyle changes; and permitting occasional guilt-free lapses in the regimen might result in beneficial changes without ensuing guilt (Fawzy et al., 1990). Making sure patients and caregivers learn to recognize and experience emotions and communicate emotional needs and issues can lead to biopsychosocial/spiritual support through cancer treatment, survivorship, or end-of-life care.

The relationship of feelings to overall health is not well understood. A positive attitude comprises believing that options are available to address one's problems and that one or more of those options will be successful. Having a positive attitude does not mean that one will never feel or express a negative emotion. The diagnosis and treatment of cancer bring a whole range of painful emotions, such as anxiety, depression, anger, sadness, hopelessness, helplessness, lack of control, and guilt. When patients try to be "emotionally up" and happy all the time (i.e., what they view as having a positive attitude) or, in contrast, try to distance themselves from their feelings and experiences, guilt may ensue.

Patients who first acknowledge that they have these negative emotions, accept them as normal given the situation, and then appropriately express them seem to have much better quality of life, and, in some cases, their reactions may positively influence the course of their disease (Barrera & Spiegel, 2014; Fawzy et al., 1993; Spiegel, Bloom, Kraemer, & Gottheil, 1989).

People generally accept that thoughts and feelings kept bottled inside will serve as major stressors that can affect emotional state and may negatively affect the immune system and health outcomes (Chopra, 1989; Dossey & Keegan, 2013). Expressing these same thoughts and feelings will "put them on the outside" where they can no longer hurt as much. Having negative feelings toward cancer and finding ways of appropriately expressing them should never be a source of guilt for patients. Oncology healthcare professionals can do a great deal to help patients with cancer and their families to understand this.

## Justified Guilt

The concept that guilt might somehow be justified is suggested by the fact that a strong association exists between some factors and the development of cancer. For at least 50 years, smoking has been known to cause lung (and now other) cancers. For the person who chooses to smoke and subsequently develops lung cancer, guilt and self-blame may be all consuming. In an assessment of guilt and shame in patients with non-small cell lung cancer, a belief that the individual caused their own cancer was correlated with higher levels of guilt, shame, anxiety, and depression (LoConte, Else-Quest, Eickhoff, Hyde, & Schiller, 2008). Interestingly, in cases where such a patient continues to smoke, the guiding philosophy of interventions to get the patient to cease this harmful behavior has often relied on guilt. For instance, asking patients, "How can you possibly keep smoking when you can hardly breathe? You know that you are just making things worse, and all that passive smoke is harming your family" may not be the appropriate approach. Because the behavior (i.e., smoking) already has led to dire consequences (i.e., cancer), interventions for this population should be geared toward fostering self-forgiveness and moving beyond guilt. Although the message "smoking causes cancer" has decreased smoking rates, it has led to the stigmatization of smokers. This has led to feelings of guilt and censure and concealment of smoking from family members and healthcare professionals (Shin et al., 2014). For religious reasons, some patients may express the belief that their cancer diagnosis is justified punishment for their life choices or behaviors. Although counter to most beliefs and conventional wisdom, evaluation by appropriate expertise, as well as support that respects religious beliefs are critical.

## Diagnosis and Treatment

Patients who express guilt over delaying diagnosis, not initiating treatment soon enough, or not adhering with treatment recommendations require special assessment to uncover the reasons for their behavior. These reasons may include knowledge deficits, lack of understanding, an avoidant coping style, fear, denial, cultural, or something as practical as the inability to pay for medical care. If patients fail to understand their behavior, helping them to gain insight is the first step of intervention and long-term change. Addressing the specific issue is the next step. Letting go of the guilt and self-blame and moving on to a more health-promoting behavior is the ultimate goal.

One particularly sensitive issue is guilt if the cancer recurs, perhaps from choosing a treatment path against medical advice or not choosing healthy coping strategies or lifestyle behaviors. Perhaps the patient believes that he or she chose the wrong treatment, or perhaps no adjuvant treatment was chosen after surgery when initially offered. If the treatment was a standard medical option, reviewing any valid reasons for making the original choice, as well as current options, may be helpful. Reiterating that no cancer treatment comes with a guarantee also may help to alleviate guilt. If an alternative treatment was selected in place of standard therapy, the patient may need help in reviewing why he or she chose that option in the first place. Offering support that they most likely made the best decision with the information they had at the time may be helpful. Education about current standard treatments may need to be repeated, and the patient may need to be encouraged to try standard therapy in conjunction with other options. Disparaging remarks about alternative therapy choices or any manner of "I told you so" will only foster more guilt and might damage the patient–provider relationship. Caregivers need to be supported in a similar way, as they may carry their own feelings of guilt about their role in the outcome. As previously stated, the goal is to remove the feelings of guilt and to move on. This process is accomplished either by helping the patient to understand that the guilt is unwarranted or by fostering self-forgiveness.

## Survivor Guilt

Although not a common theme among patients with cancer, the issue of survivor guilt exists (Lebel et al., 2013; Posluszny et al., 2016). In essence, survivor guilt refers to those patients who are cured but are having difficulty understanding why they were spared when similar patients died. Exploring patients' feelings of self-esteem and pointing out their value and worth may be helpful. Ironically, these individuals may find themselves asking the question "Why me?" when they got the cancer and when they survived. In both instances, the only answer may be "Why not me?" Caregivers, parents, and siblings may also be asking "Why them and not me?" The "why" question can never be satisfactorily answered by anyone. Weaver (2014) suggested caregivers offer grace.

## Transmission Guilt

One of the most confusing sources of guilt relates to cancer inheritance. A number of cancers, including breast, colon, and ovarian, occur in families. Even without a strong family history, those who develop cancer are often concerned that they may be passing on an increased risk to their children. In the presence of a strong family history, the availability of genetic testing has now broadened the number of families who face often complex discussions about cancer risk, inheritance, and risk reduction measures. Guilt at passing on a genetic mutation that increases offspring's chances of developing cancer is not uncommon. Lerman, Croyle, Tercyak, and Hamann (2002) noted that healthcare providers would soon be encountering the complex psychological issues faced by individuals at risk for these diseases, and recent research has borne this out (Fisher et al., 2014; van Oostrom et al., 2007). Genetic counseling in these individuals should include ways to deal with feelings about transmission guilt and short- and long-term issues. Being prepared to address these healthcare issues can assist a family to grow in a healthy yet watchful manner.

Researchers have found that mothers who took the drug diethylstilbestrol (DES) between 1943 and 1971 to prevent miscarriages have an increased lifetime risk of breast cancer (Saunders, 1988). Further, their daughters have been found to have, among other anatomic and functional reproductive tract problems, an increased risk of clear-cell adenocarcinoma, a rare form of vaginal and cervical cancer. Male offspring of DES mothers also have reproductive problems and may have an increased risk of testicular cancer. Many of these mothers feel a sense of guilt for having caused these potentially life-threatening problems for their children. They need to be reminded that the reason they took DES was to preserve life and bring it into this world. If this issue has impaired the relationship between a mother and her daughter or son, referral to family therapy is indicated.

## Family Member Guilt

### Children

Siblings of children with cancer face a set of unique problems that can generate guilt. The healthy children in the family may experience difficult role changes, such as becoming babysitters or caretakers for the ill child or even cooks and housekeepers. They may find themselves shifted from place to place while their parents attend to the sick child during hospitalization. Plans often cannot be made or frequently are changed because of the uncertainty of the illness. Discipline and affection may be erratically and unevenly meted out between the sick child and the siblings. The healthy children may feel neglected, lonely, and unsupported while simultaneously feeling overprotected by parents who are now oversensitive and fearful for the safety of all their children (Bluebond-Langner, 1989). The healthy children may love the sick child, but the emergence of feelings of anger, resentment, and jealousy is understandable. Unfortunately, these feelings may lead to feelings of guilt (Alderfer et al., 2010). In addition, healthy children may have a fantasy about having caused the sick child's illness, perhaps having wished the sick child ill or inflicted with some injury during play or a fight. Finally, these children often feel guilty for surviving when their sibling has died. In some tragic cases, the parent who has lost a favorite child may foster this feeling. These feelings of guilt may persist for an extended period of time (Ahomäki et al., 2015).

Children, both healthy and sick, often do not receive the full information about the ill sibling's condition and, in an effort by the parents to protect them in some way, may receive misinformation. Parents conceptualize the reasons for their child's cancer in different ways, as they struggle to make sense of what is going on (Matteo & Pierluigi, 2008). An approach of nondisclosure, however, often exacerbates a bad situation.

The sick child, while dealing with all of the other emotions inherent in fighting a life-threatening disease, may feel anger at the healthy siblings and friends who do not have to go through this experience and subsequently feel guilt for thinking bad things about them. A sense of guilt may develop if the sick child thinks that the illness is punishment for some previous bad behavior, real or imagined.

Most children in a family triad have a much better grasp of the seriousness of what is going on than adults believe. Children may gather information by listening on phone extensions, intentionally eavesdropping behind closed doors, inadvertently overhearing snippets of conversation, sensing "emotional vibes" of the adults around them, or hearing rumors from their peers. This behavior in itself may generate guilt. Parents rarely sense all of the issues, juggle all of their responsibilities, and fully attend to the needs of both their sick and healthy children. In fact, parents may also be experiencing guilt when, in retrospect, they blame themselves for symptoms that were not recognized or taken seriously by healthcare providers (Evans, Wakefield, McLoone, & Cohn, 2015).

The healthcare team can foster an atmosphere of openness and communication among all family members, providing them with accurate information and emotional support. Nurses also can help parents by coaching them about warning signs of stress and potential guilt in their children, including changes in behavior such as being more withdrawn, angry, or acting out. Counseling may be warranted to assist all parties to understand, accept, and deal with these complex situations. The consequences of guilt or self-blame surrounding the cancer diagnosis have unknown effects on long-term coping of survivors, parents, and siblings (Ahomäki et al., 2015; Rosenberg et al., 2015; Yang, Sheng, Chen, & Hung, 2015).

## Adults

Guilt may be a cardinal feature of the caregiving experience (Spillers, Wellisch, Kim, Matthews, & Baker, 2008). Some family members are quick to label any concern about their own stress as self-pity and feel guilty about not being focused entirely on the patient. In contrast to this self-generated guilt, some patients induce guilt to get family members to stay with them and focus on their needs to the exclusion of the rest of the family (Vess, Moreland, Schwebel, & Kraut, 1988). Both patients and family members may need help in gaining insight into their behaviors. Everyone should understand and acknowledge that numerous needs exist in this situation (Spillers et al., 2008). Although the patient requires attention and support, the family caregivers must attend to their own needs as well as to those of the rest of the family to keep the family unit as intact as possible during this difficult time. Interventions directed to the caregiver and the patient concurrently may have benefit (Chambers et al., 2014) (see Figure 20-2).

Parents are as subject to feelings of guilt as children. They may feel guilty about not being available enough for both the healthy siblings and the ill child. They may feel guilty that they could not save the ill child. They may feel guilty for having passed on a genetic predisposition to the cancer (Fisher et al., 2014; van Oostrom et al., 2007). The patient and family members may think that the patient's illness is a burden and then feel guilty about having these thoughts. They may view this burden as financial, physical, and emotional. Recognizing that the patient did not deliberately develop cancer and is powerless to change the situation does little to lessen these guilty feelings. Again, the way to overcome this guilt is for both patients and family members to acknowledge these emotions, accept them as normal

---

**Assessment**
- Determine presence and degree of guilt or self-blame.
- Systematically evaluate for the presence of guilt or self-blame in patients with cancer by exploring, as appropriate, attributions of cause (e.g., "What do you think contributed to the development of your cancer?").
- Recognize spontaneous phrases that might indicate guilt (e.g., "This is my fault!"; "I caused my cancer"; "This is why I got cancer.").
- Differentiate between patients' beliefs that contributing factors for cancer development existed and their actual feelings of guilt.
- Determine the knowledge level of patients and family members regarding technical and social issues that might lead to the development of guilt (e.g., cancer development, Hero Myth, positive attitude).
- Discuss with patients and family members religious and cultural beliefs that might be influencing their feelings of guilt; determine how congruent their beliefs are with the stated belief or culture.
- Determine the impact of feelings of guilt on patients' overall affective state and treatment adherence.

**Nursing Diagnoses** (NANDA International, 2015)
- Ineffective coping
- Anxiety
- Deficient knowledge

***DSM-V* Diagnoses** (American Psychiatric Association, 2013)
- Adjustment disorder
- Major depression

**Expected Outcomes**
- Patients and family members will describe accurate technical knowledge about the relevant issues.
- Patients and family members will demonstrate understanding of the role of contributing social factors to the development of feelings of guilt or self-blame.
- Patients and family members will have a greater understanding of the role of their religious and cultural beliefs in the development of feelings of guilt.
- Patients and family members will express relief from feelings of guilt.

**Interventions**
- Provide appropriate information about whatever issue is related to guilt (e.g., cancer recurrence, genetics).
- Provide information about social factors contributing to guilt (e.g., Hero Myth, positive attitude).
- Discuss the effect of patients' belief systems (i.e., religious and cultural factors) in the development of feelings of guilt or self-blame; use insight, education, and reframing to assuage feelings of guilt without disparaging patients' beliefs.
- Allow patients to express and clarify perceptions of what has happened leading to a diagnosis of cancer.
- Consider psychiatric consultation for psychotherapy and pharmacologic management for patients whose feelings of guilt or self-blame are seriously affecting their emotional state or interfering with treatment adherence.
- Include family members in educational sessions and discussions whenever possible.
- Have separate discussions with family members, if necessary, to help them to understand the role that they may be playing in the development or maintenance of feelings of guilt; provide reassurance that they should not feel guilt for their behavior if it was based on their level of knowledge and best intentions at the time.

---

**Figure 20-2. Plan of Care**

and commonplace, and then work toward minimizing the effects of the illness on the family. Family members need to keep life as routine as possible and continue to participate in pleasurable activities. In most cases, both patients and family members feel less burden and guilt when family members attend to their own needs (Vess et al., 1988).

Family members may feel guilty for not having insisted that the adult patient be diagnosed earlier or for not getting a second opinion (Weaver, 2014). Guilt may stem from anger at the patient for not following these suggestions or from the belief that the patient caused the cancer (e.g., smoked for years). Healthcare professionals can help tremendously by pointing out that these kinds of feelings serve no beneficial purpose and by encouraging family members to let them go (Welch-McCaffrey, 1988).

Family members who are struggling to care for a dying relative may feel tremendous guilt if the patient is in pain. The poorer the health of the patient, the greater the caregiver guilt (Spillers et al., 2008). Healthcare professionals need to do everything possible to help the patient to achieve a level of comfort while being particularly cognizant of family members' levels of frustration and fear. Planned respites from the caregiving experience can help to rejuvenate exhausted caregivers and mitigate the burden of continuous care and high levels of negative emotions.

Family members often feel a sense of relief after a patient has died. This feeling is particularly common when the illness has been prolonged and difficult. Although it is a completely natural and understandable feeling, many family members subsequently feel guilty. Nurses should reassure family members that being glad the ordeal is over does not mean that they are glad the patient is gone from their lives. Whatever kind and caring behaviors they displayed while the patient was alive should be enumerated and praised. Reassuring the family that the deceased is now free from pain and that he or she was grateful for the care the family provided can support families experiencing these feelings.

## Healthcare Providers and Guilt

Healthcare providers working with patients with cancer have their own unique sources of guilt. Many healthcare professionals, especially nurses, often feel guilty for subjecting patients to painful, intrusive, and debilitating treatments, as well as for not intervening sooner or with a certain action. These guilty feelings intensify when the likelihood of the treatment resulting in cure is very low. The most intense feelings of guilt occur when patients die despite the best efforts of the healthcare team. Frequently, staff member guilt is related to denial of feelings of loss when treatment does not turn out as planned. Guilt is just one of many responses to caring for patients with cancer and their family members (Davis, Lind, & Sorensen, 2013; Granek, Bartels, Scheinemann, Labrecque, & Barrera, 2015). Remen (1996) cautioned healthcare providers that it is not possible to be immersed in suffering and loss daily and not be touched by it. She relates denial of these feelings to burnout.

Healthcare providers need to remember that they did not cause the cancer, and their care may have offered patients and family members some hope and a fighting chance. Healthcare providers also need to recognize that they are not omnipotent, and no one expects them to be all-powerful. Setting appropriate goals for each patient is helpful in preventing a sense of failure and guilt from developing. When a patient's remaining time is very clearly limited, switching the goal from cure or prolongation of life to assisting in a calm death is critical. This process may involve symptom control (including good pain management) and helping the patient and family to finish their instrumental business (e.g., wills, funeral preferences) and their emotional business (e.g., resolution of family conflicts). Allowing the patient the opportunity for verbal exploration of existential issues, such as beliefs in God and an afterlife and the meaning of one's life, is the final step in facilitating a calm death. Any nurse who has done all this for the patient will still feel sadness and loss but also a sense of satisfaction in a job well done.

## Case Study

Judy, a 54-year-old widow, underwent a lumpectomy followed by radiation for node-negative invasive ductal carcinoma six years ago. At that time, she had been advised to see a genetic counselor and did so. She was tested for a possible mutation associated with breast cancer. The subsequent result showed no mutation. She recently was diagnosed with a 1.2 cm contralateral breast cancer, and underwent a lumpectomy and sentinel lymph node biopsy, which was negative. Overall prognostic factors associated with the cancer led to the recommendation that she have adjuvant chemotherapy followed by radiation and estrogen blocking therapy.

At her first chemotherapy session, Judy begins crying and states, "This is all my fault. I cannot put my children through this again. I do not want to do this chemotherapy. Maybe it would be better if I just take my chances without it." Discussions with Judy regarding these statements reveal that she believes her first cancer was a result of the stress of her husband's death. She knows that having a positive attitude about life is important but has found that doing so has been impossible after suddenly losing her spouse of 23 years. She relates how depressed she had been at the time and how she was diagnosed with breast cancer six months later. Judy states that her three children provided a great deal of emotional support at the time of her first surgery. Afterward, they gave her many self-help books on how to survive cancer. They told her that they already had lost a father and that they simply could not stand losing a mother.

After the first surgery, Judy dutifully read everything that had been given to her and embarked on a course of self-improvement. She began eating a low-fat diet, started walking every day, lost weight, and began performing daily meditation with positive affirmations. Judy stated that she had kept this regimen up fairly well for about three years and then became more relaxed. Six months earlier, her twin sister died. Judy was devastated by this second major loss and again was unable to maintain a positive attitude. She now believes that her cancer has come back because she failed to stay on her health regimen and because of her inability to think positively. She feels especially bad for putting her children through this all again.

Over the next two cycles of chemotherapy, staff members discuss with Judy the concepts involved in having a positive attitude and the Hero Myth. She begins to understand that she is not responsible for causing either of her cancers. Judy is assured that the feelings of sadness and grief she is experiencing over the deaths of her husband and sister are part of a normal course of bereavement and have nothing to do with lacking a positive attitude.

At one point, Judy reported that she had been unable to convey this information clearly to her children. She feels that they still believe she is responsible for her cancer's return and are upset when she talks about it. Again, Judy states how guilty she feels about upsetting her children. A family conference is called. During the conference, her three children are very receptive to the information presented and are horrified to realize that they had inadvertently been contributing to their mother's sense of guilt and overall stress. They assure her that they are not blaming her and are just trying to do everything they can to ensure her survival and to feel as if they are doing something to help. They tell her that they are grateful that they can return some of the care and attention she has lavished on them for so many years. The staff reassures the children that they should not feel guilty for their behavior. They agree to attend a psychoeducational support group as a family to learn more about these issues.

### Discussion

The staff realized that Judy's belief system and subsequent guilt were seriously influencing her emotional or affective state. There was indication that this could affect her treatment adherence and, more seriously, contribute to suicidal ideation. Her strong support system had become a source of additional distress because of misinformation and miscommunication. Her depression and desire not to upset them inhibited her ability to understand and communicate information to her family members. A family conference was necessary to relay factual information to all concerned and to foster better communication and understanding between Judy and her children. This conference was considered very successful, but the staff realized that lifelong patterns of communication and belief systems could not be easily changed. The family, therefore, was referred to a psychoeducational support group offered by the hospital that would provide additional opportunities to gather information and reinforce effective coping skills.

## Conclusion

Guilt is a negative emotion stemming from the belief that one has done something wrong. In relation to cancer, feelings of guilt rarely, if ever, serve a useful purpose and frequently are a source of additional emotional stress in an already stressful situation. Patients, families, and the healthcare staff may feel guilt. Children and adults may suffer equally. The causes of guilt surrounding cancer may include things that were done or not done, thoughts or feelings that have occurred or the absence of these thoughts or feelings, and things said or left unspoken. These causes of guilt may be real or imagined. Healthcare professionals need to assess the presence of guilt in their patients and explore its sources. If reasons for guilt are unwarranted, misconceptions and misunderstandings need to be clarified. If the source of guilt seems real and justified, patients need help in letting go and moving on to a more effective coping behavior. For staff members suffering from guilt, the administration needs to provide whatever support and therapeutic assistance necessary to help them cope.

*The author would like to acknowledge Nancy W. Fawzy, RN, DNSc, and Phyllis Gorney Cooper, RN, MN, for their contributions to this chapter from the previous edition of this book.*

## References

Aguado Loi, C.X., Baldwin, J.A., McDermott, R.J., McMillan, S., Martinez Tyson, D., Yampolskaya, S., & Vandeweerd, C. (2013). Risk factors associated with increased depressive symptoms among Latinas diagnosed with breast cancer within 5 years of survivorship. *Psycho-Oncology, 22,* 2779–2788. doi:10.1002/pon.3357

Ahomäki, R., Gunn, M.E., Madanat-Harjuoja, L.M., Matomäki, J., Malila, N., & Lahteenmäki, P.M. (2015). Late psychiatric morbidity in survivors of cancer at a young age: A nationwide registry-based study. *International Journal of Cancer, 13,* 183–192. doi:10.1002/ijc.29371

Alderfer, M.A., Long, K.A., Lown, E.A., Marsland, A.L., Ostrowski, N.L., Hock, J.M., & Ewing, L.J. (2010). Psychosocial adjustment of siblings of children with cancer: A systematic review. *Psycho-Oncology, 19,* 789–805. doi:10.1002/pon.1638

American Psychiatric Association. (2013). *Diagnostic and statistical manual of mental disorders* (5th ed.). Washington, DC: Author.

Antoni, M.H. (2013). Psychosocial intervention effects on adaptation, disease course and biobehavioral processes in cancer. *Brain, Behavior, and Immunity, 30*(Suppl.), S88–S98. doi:10.1016/j.bbi.2012.05.009

Barrera, I., & Spiegel, D. (2014). Review of psychotherapeutic interventions on depression in cancer patients and their impact on disease progression. *International Review of Psychiatry, 26,* 31–43. doi:10.3109/09540261.2013.864259

Bennett, K.K., Compas, B.E., Beckjord, E., & Glinder, J.G. (2005). Self-blame and distress among women with newly diagnosed breast cancer. *Journal of Behavioral Medicine, 28,* 313–323. doi:10.1007/s10865-005-9000-0

Block, K. (2009). *Life over cancer: The block center program for integrative cancer treatment.* New York, NY: Random House.

Bluebond-Langner, M. (1989). Worlds of dying children and their well siblings. *Death Studies, 13,* 1–16. doi:10.1080/07481188908252274

Chambers, S.K., Girgis, A., Occhipinti, S., Hutchison, S., Turner, J., McDowell, M., ... Dunn, J.C. (2014). A randomized trial comparing two low-intensity psychological interventions for distressed patients with cancer and their caregivers [Online exclusive]. *Oncology Nursing Forum, 41,* E256–E266. doi:10.1188/14.ONF.E256-E266

Chida, Y., Hamer, M., Wardle, J., & Steptoe, A. (2008). Do stress-related psychosocial factors contribute to cancer incidence and survival? *Nature Clinical Practice Oncology, 5,* 466–475. doi:10.1038/ncponc1134

Chopra, D. (1989). *Quantum healing.* New York, NY: Random House.

Daley, E.M., Perrin, K.M., McDermott, R.J., Vamos, C.A., Rayko, H.L., Packing-Ebuen, J.L., ... McFarlane, M. (2010). The psychosocial burden of HPV: A mixed-method study of knowledge, attitudes and behaviors among HPV+ women. *Journal of Health Psychology, 15,* 279–290. doi:10.1177/1359105309351249

Davis, S., Lind, B.K., & Sorensen, C. (2013). A comparison of burnout among oncology nurses working in adult and pediatric inpatient and outpatient settings [Online exclusive]. *Oncology Nursing Forum, 40,* E303–E311. doi:10.1188/13.ONF.E303-E311

Dossey, B.M., & Keegan, L. (2013). *Holistic nursing: A handbook for practice* (6th ed.). Burlington, MA: Jones & Bartlett Learning.

Duggleby, W., Thomas, J., Montford, K.S., Thomas, R., Nekolaichuk, C., Ghosh, S., ... Tonkin, K. (2015). Transitions of male partners of women with breast cancer: Hope, guilt, and quality of life. *Oncology Nursing Forum, 42,* 134–141. doi:10.1188/15.ONF.134-141

Evans, N.T., Wakefield, C.E., McLoone, J.K., & Cohn, R.J. (2015). Familial diagnostic experiences in paediatric oncology. *British Journal of Cancer, 112,* 20–23. doi:10.1038/bjc.2014.516

Fawzy, F.I., Cousins, N., Fawzy, N.W., Kemeny, M.E., Elashoff, R., & Morton, D.L. (1990). A structured psychiatric intervention for cancer patients: I. Changes over time in methods of coping and affective distress. *Archives of General Psychiatry, 47,* 720–725. doi:10.1001/archpsyc.1990.01810200028004

Fawzy, F.I., Fawzy, N.W., Hyun, C.S., Elashoff, R., Guthrie, D., Fahey, J.L., & Morton, D.L. (1993). Malignant melanoma: Effects of an early structured psychiatric intervention, coping, and affective state on recurrence and survival 6 years later. *Archives of General Psychiatry, 50,* 681–689. doi:10.1001/archpsyc.1993.01820210015002

Fisher, C.L., Maloney, E., Glogowski, E., Hurley, K., Edgerson, S., Lichtenthal, W.G., ... Bylund, C. (2014). Talking about familial breast cancer risk: Topics and strategies to enhance mother–daughter interactions. *Qualitative Health Research, 24,* 517–535. doi:10.1177/1049732314524638

Friedman, L.C., Barber, C.R., Chang, J., Tham, Y.L., Kalidas, M., Rimawi, M.F., ... Elledge, R. (2010). Self-blame, self-forgiveness, and spirituality in breast cancer survivors in a public sector setting. *Journal of Cancer Education, 25,* 343–348. doi:10.1007/s13187-010-0048-3

Granek, L., Bartels, U., Scheinemann, K., Labrecque, M., & Barrera, M. (2015). Grief reactions and impact of patient death on pediatric oncologists. *Pediatric Blood and Cancer, 62,* 134–142. doi:10.1002/pbc.25228

Gray, R.E., & Doan, B.D. (1990). Heroic self-healing and cancer: Clinical issues for the health professions. *Journal of Palliative Care, 6,* 32–41.

Guilt. (n.d.). In *Merriam-Webster online dictionary.* Retrieved from http://www.merriam-webster.com/dictionary/guilt

Lebel, S., Feldstain, A., McCallum, M., Beattie, S., Irish, J., Bezjak, A., & Devins, G.M. (2013). Do behavioural self-blame and stigma predict positive health changes in survivors of lung or head and neck cancers? *Psychology and Health, 28,* 1066–1081. doi:10.1080/08870446.2013.781602

Lerman, C., Croyle, R.T., Tercyak, K.P., & Hamann, H. (2002). Genetic testing: Psychosocial aspects and implications. *Journal of Consulting and Clinical Psychology, 70,* 784–797. doi:10.1037/0022-006X.70.3.784

Lobchuk, M.M., Murdoch, T., McClement, S.E., & McPherson, C. (2008). A dyadic affair: Who is to blame for causing and controlling the patient's lung cancer? *Cancer Nursing, 31,* 435–443. doi:10.1097/01.NCC.0000339253.68324.19

LoConte, N.K., Else-Quest, N.M., Eickhoff, J., Hyde, J., & Schiller, J.H. (2008). Assessment of guilt and shame in patients with non-small-cell lung cancer compared with patients with breast and prostate cancer. *Clinical Lung Cancer, 9,* 171–178. doi:10.3816/CLC.2008.n.026

Lutgendorf, S.K., & Andersen, B.L. (2015). Biobehavioral approaches to cancer progression and survival: Mechanisms and interventions. *American Psychology, 70,* 186–197. doi:10.1037/a0035730

Malcarne, V.L., Compas, B.E., Epping-Jordan, J.E., & Howell, D.C. (1995). Cognitive factors in adjustment to cancer: Attributions of self-blame and perceptions of control. *Journal of Behavioral Medicine, 18,* 401–417. doi:10.1007/BF01904771

Matteo, B., & Pierluigi, B. (2008). Descriptive survey about causes of illness given by the parents of children with cancer. *European Journal of Oncology Nursing, 12,* 134–141. doi:10.1016/j.ejon.2007.08.003

Mustafa, M., Carson-Stevens, A., Gillespie, D., & Edwards, A.G. (2013). Psychological interventions for women with metastatic breast cancer. *Cochrane Database of Systematic Reviews, 2013*(6). doi:10.1002/14651858.CD004253.pub4

NANDA International. (2015). *Nursing diagnoses: Definitions and classification, 2015–2017.* Philadelphia, PA: Author.

Pekmezi, D.W., & Demark-Wahnefried, W. (2011). Updated evidence in support of diet and exercise interventions in cancer survivors. *Acta Oncologica, 50,* 167–178. doi:10.3109/0284186X.2010.529822

Posluszny, D.M., Dew, M.A., Beckjord, E., Bovbjerg, D.H., Schmidt, J.E., Low, C.A., ... Rechis, R. (2016). Existential challenges experienced by lymphoma survivors: Results from the 2010 Livestrong Survey. *Journal of Health Psychology, 21,* 2357–2366. doi:10.1177/1359105315576352

Remen, R. (1996). *Kitchen table wisdom.* New York, NY: Riverhead Books.

Rosenberg, A.R., Postier, A., Osenga, K., Kreicbergs, U., Neville, B., Dussel, V., & Wolfe, J. (2015). Long-term psychosocial outcomes among bereaved siblings of children with cancer. *Journal of Pain and Symptom Management, 49,* 55–65. doi:10.1016/j.jpainsymman.2014.05.006

Saunders, E.J. (1988). Physical and psychological problems associated with exposure to diethylstilbestrol (DES). *Hospital and Community Psychiatry, 39,* 73–77. doi:10.1176/ps.39.1.73

Servan-Schreiber, D. (2009). *Anticancer: A new way of life.* New York, NY: Viking.

Shin, D.W., Park, J.H., Kim, S.Y., Park, E.W., Yang, H.K., Ahn, E., ... Seo, H.G. (2014). Guilt, censure, and concealment of active smoking status among cancer patients and family members after diagnosis: A nationwide study. *Psycho-Oncology, 23,* 585–591. doi:10.1002/pon.3460

Siegel, B. (1986). *Love, medicine, and miracles: Lessons learned about self-healing from a surgeon's experience with exceptional patients.* New York, NY: Harper & Row.

Simonton, C.O., Matthews-Simonton, S., & Creighton, J. (1978). *Getting well again: A step-by-step, self-help guide to overcoming cancer for patients and their families.* New York, NY: St. Martin's Press.

Spiegel, D., Bloom, J., Kraemer, H., & Gottheil, E. (1989). Effect of psychosocial treatment on survival of patients with metastatic breast cancer. *Lancet, 2,* 888–891. doi:10.1016/S0140-6736(89)91551-1

Spillers, R.L., Wellisch, D.K., Kim, Y., Matthews, B.A., & Baker, F. (2008). Family caregivers and guilt in the context of cancer care. *Psychosomatics, 49,* 511–519. doi:10.1176/appi.psy.49.6.511

Turner, K.A. (2014). *Radical remission: Surviving cancer against all odds.* New York, NY: HarperCollins.

van Oostrom, I., Meijers-Heijboer, H., Duivenvoorden, H.J., Bröcker-Vriends, A.H., van Asperen, C.J., Sijmons, R.H., ... Tibben, A. (2007). A prospective study of the impact of genetic susceptibility testing for BRCA1/2 or HNPCC on family relationships. *Psycho-Oncology, 16,* 320–328. doi:10.1002/pon.1062

Vess, J.D., Moreland, J.R., Schwebel, A.I., & Kraut, E. (1988). Psychosocial needs of cancer patients: Learning from patients and their spouses. *Journal of Psychosocial Oncology, 6,* 31–51.

Weaver, M.S. (2014). Know guilt. *Journal of Clinical Oncology, 32,* 699–700. doi:10.1200/JCO.2013.54.4627

Welch-McCaffrey, D. (1988). Family issues in cancer care: Current dilemmas and future directions. *Journal of Psychosocial Oncology, 6,* 199–211.

Yang, H.-C., Mu, P.-F., Sheng, C.-C., Chen, Y.-W., & Hung, G.-Y. (2015). A systematic review of the experiences of siblings of children with cancer. *Cancer Nursing, 39,* E12–E21. doi:10.1097/NCC.0000000000000258

# CHAPTER 21

# Powerlessness

*Linda M. Gorman, RN, MN, PMHCNS-BC, CHPN, FPCN*

> *Do not go gentle into that good night,*
> *Old age should burn and rave at close of day;*
> *Rage, rage against the dying of the light.*
>
> —Dylan Thomas

An important part of the human experience is the extent to which people feel able to obtain good outcomes and avoid undesirable situations as a result of their own efforts. A sense of personal control is associated with a variety of positive outcomes for emotional well-being, confidence, and self-esteem. Power allows people to control outcomes, with respect to both the environment and the self. This control is considered to be a fundamental human need (Fast, Gruenfeld, Sivanathan, & Galinsky, 2009; Yang, Jin, He, Fan, & Zhu, 2015).

Powerlessness is a lived experience of lack of control over a situation with the perception that one's own actions do not significantly affect an outcome (Doenges, Moorhouse, & Murr, 2013). This perception contributes to overall general dissatisfaction, of being trapped in a negative situation, and emotional suffering (Carpenito-Moyet, 2010). Powerlessness is also associated with vulnerability and uncertainty. Patients' vulnerability puts them in a position in which they feel useless and inferior and must show a great deal of humility (Lavoie, Blondeau, & Picard-Morin, 2011; Sand, Strang, & Milberg, 2008). These effects emphasize the usefulness of perceived control and its opposite, lack of control or powerlessness, in understanding reactions to a traumatic situation, such as receiving a cancer diagnosis. Powerlessness is sometimes referred to as loss of control as well as helplessness.

Research studies on perceptions of control are based on social learning theory and learned helplessness. Rotter (1966) developed the notion of internal–external locus of control to measure how much an individual believes that outcomes depend on their own actions or on circumstances outside the individual's control. Powerlessness is not exactly synonymous with locus of control. Locus of control is a stable personality trait rather than situationally driven (Carpenito-Moyet, 2010). However, appreciation of this concept can assist nurses in understanding why some patients actively participate in their care, while others are passive or seem apathetic. For example, according to locus of control theory, a patient with internal locus of control believes that a treatment outcome can be affected by active involvement, such as performing regular exercise, reading literature about the diagnosis, and learning assertiveness skills. A person with external locus of control believes that treatment outcomes are outside of personal control and attributes outcomes to others' actions or to fate. Internally controlled people usually are more self-motivated, whereas externally controlled people usually need others to motivate them (see Figure 21-1).

Seligman (1975) further explained that people feel helpless and become depressed when they cannot identify a connection between what they do and the outcomes they experience.

Conversely, if they can see a connection between their behavior or choices and results or outcomes, individuals will feel that what they do can make a difference. Bandura (1977) found that people will change their behavior if they believe they can perform the desired action and that it will result in the desired outcome (e.g., "When I stop smoking, my chances of avoiding lung cancer will improve.").

The feelings of pride and freedom gained from autonomy provide an invaluable sense of well-being. In contrast, chronic powerlessness is associated with ineffective coping, including vulnerability, dependence, and depression and anxiety (Lavoie et al., 2011; Sand et al., 2008). Powerlessness is triggered by losses. Each new loss can promote a sense of powerlessness over one's life and contribute to anxiety (Corradi, 2007). Experiencing multiple losses can exacerbate powerlessness, as the person may feel that he or she is losing anchors that help maintain stability.

Powerlessness can be confused with hopelessness. A hopeless person sees no solution to problems or no way to achieve what is desired, even if the individual has control. However, Duggleby et al. (2015) found that loss of hope resulted in feelings of helplessness, lack of control, and distress in spouses of patients with breast cancer. In powerlessness, the person may see an alternative but is unable to do anything about it because of the perception of lack of control. Prolonged powerlessness may lead to hopelessness (Carpenito-Moyet, 2010).

Powerlessness has been studied extensively in relation to poverty and marginalized groups who view society as powerful and the individual as having limited impact (Mumtaz, Salway, Bhatti, & McIntyre, 2014; Zarowsky, Haddad, & Nguyen, 2013). Past experiences of powerlessness may predispose individuals to assume that they will have no impact on achieving a goal to improve their lives (e.g., finishing school, getting away from bad influences). It is also evident in abuse victims who feel powerless to get away from their abuser even though the opportunity is present (Townsend, 2015).

| External | Internal |
|---|---|
| • Talks of fate or luck being needed to control illness<br>• Has less interest in educational materials and self-monitoring programs<br>• Looks to family or healthcare professionals to make decisions and plan treatment<br>• Looks to others for motivation and encouragement<br>• Needs to be repeatedly prodded to follow through on making appointments or to complete self-monitoring<br>• May respond to rewards | • Expresses belief that one can actively control the course of the illness<br>• Actively seeks information about the illness<br>• Participates in self-care strategies, such as exercise programs and self-help groups<br>• Does not need prodding or reminding to follow through with self-monitoring<br>• Looks at how one's behavior can affect treatment |

**Figure 21-1. Assessment of External and Internal Locus of Control**

*Note.* Based on information from Carpenito-Moyet, 2010; Rotter, 1966.

Feeling powerlessness is uncomfortable for individuals. People often will make efforts to take some type of control to counteract this discomfort. How effective these efforts are may contribute to the extent of dysfunction that the feeling of powerlessness produces. Some dysfunctional responses can include venting anger in an effort to forcibly take control. This often results in more frustration as others react to the patient's anger.

## Powerlessness and Age-Specific Considerations

Young children usually are externally controlled; that is, they see their parents and teachers as responsible for determining outcomes. However, they can be taught internal control as they learn more independence and coping skills. Hospitalized children often experience powerlessness. Loss of control increases the perception of the threat and affects the child's coping skills (Algren, 2006). Interventions can be directed at manipulating the environment to provide opportunities for children to make choices and gain mastery over their illness experience through play activities. Play minimizes stress and provides a temporary way to gain some control (Algren, 2006). Providing a routine similar to one at home is a way to give the child a sense of control of the environment. Use of play also helps promote control, as the child can act out emotions in a safe way (Carpenito-Moyet, 2010).

Older adults are at high risk for powerlessness because as they age, they experience many more changes and losses (e.g., loss of role responsibilities, independence, income, health, friends) that are out of their control (Garrison, 2000). Aging is associated with multiple losses, potential deterioration in physical health, and changes in environment. The older adult may experience more powerlessness when put into the sick role. This leads to having to accept others taking control. The patient also has been viewed by others as having less ability to handle their own life, which leads to more loss of control. Normal changes from aging can result in feelings of powerlessness. Patients with a more external locus of control may accept those changes more easily. Increased dependence on caregivers can lead to an increase in perceived loss of control. Also, feelings of alienation and boredom, especially in institutionalized older adults, have a high correlation with powerlessness (Mor, Allen, & Malin, 1994).

## Powerlessness and Illness

Any disease process, whether acute or chronic, can cause or contribute to a perceived sense of powerlessness. Illness generally requires a person to accept a certain amount of dependence, whether that be on healthcare professionals and/or family. This dependence contributes to feeling powerless and can add to several behavioral responses.

Inability to perform usual activities, dietary restrictions, progressive immobility, or mental deterioration resulting from advancing disease or side effects of treatments may lead to feelings of powerlessness and vulnerability. Individuals forced to give up usual activities, even temporarily, may feel a sense of loss of control. They can begin to believe in the inevitability of deterioration or death. Powerlessness is a feeling that all people will experience to varying degrees when dealing with illness. Realizing that a disease, such as arthritis or diabetes, will never be cured and will always be a part of their lifestyle can cause some to feel helpless. For many, some aspect of the disease process (e.g., the psychological effects of hospitalization, fear of disapproval or isolation by family or friends, increased financial burden related to the illness) contributes to losing control over one's life and creates vulnerability and loss of confidence in personal abilities.

A certain amount of powerlessness is expected in many healthcare contacts. Exposure to new people, environments and procedures, as well as unfamiliar language all contribute to a sense that one is in a foreign land where usual sense of control is no longer present. The healthcare system itself can induce a sense of powerlessness and frustration (Sundeen, 2001). Patients with mental illness particularly are vulnerable to a sense of powerlessness (Fitzsimons & Fuller, 2002). Sheridan et al. (2015) found that a lack of engagement with the clinician for patients with chronic illness intensified this sense of powerlessness.

When patients accept a certain amount of powerlessness upon entering the healthcare system, it can be adaptive to getting the help they need. Being asked to undress in front of a stranger, hearing foreign terminology, and exposing oneself to discomfort (e.g., blood drawing) all require a certain amount of giving control to others for the sake of completing the goal of getting needed medical attention.

Feeling powerless can contribute to delay in seeking medical care. Nymark, Mattiasson, Henriksson, and Kiessling (2014) found that the time from symptoms to decision to seek medical care in acute myocardial infarction is associated with a sense of powerlessness brought on by the symptoms. This powerlessness was a factor in the decision to seek medical care.

## Powerlessness and Cancer

A diagnosis of cancer brings an individual's normal life to a halt. After receiving a cancer diagnosis, an individual's focus is on the illness, which pervades all thoughts and paralyzes the individual, demands attention, and creates anxiety, pain, and uncertainty. Cancer is often seen as a silent predator moving through the body without any awareness by the individual. Uncertainty has a constant presence from diagnosis through survivorship. Living with uncertainty contributes to a sense of powerlessness over the disease (Harpham, 2015).

From diagnosis to survivorship, patients anticipate the return of the disease after their treatment has been completed. This chronic uncertainty of health status during and after cancer treatment can be a significant psychological burden (Thewes et al., 2012). Patients living in fear of recurrence feel powerless over their disease. The anxiety from this fear can create tremendous distress and affect quality of life for cancer survivors. Patients need to develop strategies to challenge this fear, such as incorporating preventive health measures in their daily routines.

Facing cancer means having to let go of some valued aspects of one's life—at least initially and often temporarily—as the patient's life is interrupted and taken over by cancer and its treatment. This could mean letting go of one's head of hair, role as primary caregiver of a child, a long-planned trip, or returning to school. Each aspect of life that one must give up even temporarily can result in feeling powerless and vulnerable (Harpham, 2015).

Because many patients with cancer will go on to live long lives, more attention is being paid to the survivor journey. Pollin and Golant (1994), who described commonly experienced fears related to long-term illness, cited the fear of losing control as the most common fear that patients experienced. Patients with long-term illnesses such as cancer must make decisions and navigate a course through an experience they did not choose, and over which they have no control, toward an uncertain future that defies prediction.

Different aspects of the symptoms and treatment can contribute to powerlessness. For example, some patients can resist accepting analgesics, especially opioids, for fear of loss of more control (Rydahl-Hansen, 2013). Fearing that one is not in control of personal feelings while on opioids can be a factor in refusing analgesics in order to stay more alert. Side effects of cancer treatment, such as nausea and diarrhea, can come on suddenly and unexpectedly, contributing to a patient's sense of having no control.

Family members of patients with cancer also experience powerlessness. The inability to rescue a loved one from a serious diagnosis and potential suffering can create tremendous distress for family members. The sense of powerlessness can contribute to anxiety and depression as well as an effort to take control of the situation, no matter how irrational. Seeing a loved one distressed and suffering from the illness and treatment and being unable to contribute to improvements make a difficult situation that much worse. This can reinforce powerlessness that has already been initiated by the disease and prognosis. Zahlis and Lewis (2010) found that spouses of patients with breast cancer often experienced stress and frustration at being unable to fix their newfound life circumstances and reported being overwhelmed and unprepared for the challenges of caregiving.

Facing the end of life is the ultimate powerlessness. Despite all of us knowing that we will die, the reality of a terminal prognosis is often incomprehensible. People may react with ways to maintain some control over their lives. As the disease progresses, individuals are less able to control many aspects of daily life, such as self-care, taking care of family members, and meeting obligations. Facing these struggles may stir up feelings of loss of control over life and lead to distress. Some individuals may challenge this powerlessness with fighting to maintain power of some aspects of their lives. This can create challenges for family and oncology professionals who are trying to provide help. Others may withdraw and give in to the inevitable. Loss of control and autonomy are often cited as the primary reasons to pursue assisted suicide (Oregon Death With Dignity Act, 2017).

## Evidence-Based Practice

Limited research exists in the area of powerlessness as it relates to illness, but some small studies give a perspective on its impact. Braga and da Cruz (2003) interviewed postoperative cardiac surgery patients about their experience of powerlessness. They found that powerlessness most frequently was associated with verbal expression of having no control or influence over a situation, doubts about planning future objectives, and expression of doubts about role performance. Ryan, Hassell, Dawes, and Kendall (2003) identified factors that influence whether patients felt they had control over their rheumatoid arthritis. Factors that contributed to a greater sense of control included reduction of physical symptoms, matching of social support with perceived need, the provision of information, and the nature of the clinical consultations. These studies support the importance of many nursing interventions to enhance patients' sense of control over their illness. Sand et al. (2008) found that unexpected exposure to suffering resulted in existential loneliness and hopelessness. This study also found that their study population of patients with cancer sometimes denied feeling powerless but still gave descriptions of powerlessness. Being ignored, loneliness, and exacerbated symptoms such as pain, dyspnea, and incontinence increased the sense of powerlessness.

Lavoie et al. (2011) found that maintaining a sense of autonomy enabled palliative care patients to maintain control in their lives and, consequently, their personal identities. Kogan, Dumas, and Cohen (2013) found that family caregivers experienced increased powerlessness and were disenfranchised from their role when the patient was noncompliant with medical treatment.

## Nursing Care of Patients Experiencing Powerlessness

### Assessment

Because powerlessness is a subjective state, nurses must validate any inferences about patients' feelings of their experience. Nurses must assess each individual to determine their usual level of control and decision making and past experiences with powerlessness (Carpenito-Moyet, 2010). Whether the individual has an internal or external locus of control also contributes to their choices and reactions.

The major characteristics of powerlessness are overt or covert expressions of dissatisfaction, such as anger or apathy, over the inability to control a situation (e.g., diagnosis of cancer, poor prognosis, treatment complications, loss of job because of the illness) that is negatively affecting the patient's goals, future, and lifestyle. Other characteristics of powerlessness include depression, acting out or violent behaviors, apathy and resignation, passivity, dissatisfaction with dependence on others, as well as inability to problem solve, make decisions, or seek information. They may describe a sense of alienation. The person may defer decision making to others or generally avoid participating in them. Passivity can be demonstrated by lack of participation in care or decision making when the opportunity arises (Townsend, 2011). Anxiety and depression can contribute to powerlessness. Nurses should recognize that some patients' behaviors may be an attempt to regain power in a relationship or of the situation. These can include anger and lack of flexibility. Signs of powerlessness can include angry outbursts directed at seemingly safe sources, such as family or the nurse.

Once nurses determine that a patient is feeling powerless, they should try to identify factors that may be contributing to the perception of loss of control. Asking questions about usual patterns of coping with uncontrollable events and previous experiences with illness will provide that information. In addition, asking how the patient makes decisions and what their roles and responsibilities are will help nurses to assess potential problems the patient may be having with adjusting to the diagnosis or future treatment plans. Nurses need to pay special attention to the patient's information-seeking behaviors and motivation for involvement in treatment decision making. Emotional reactions to new information are important to note and discuss with the patient and family. Identifying the patient's tendency in locus of control can give important information. Asking questions about how the person has coped with situations in the past can give this information. Viewing how the person approaches a new problem can give this information as well.

### Differential Diagnosis

Powerlessness can be associated with hopelessness as well as denial. The use of denial temporarily may produce a sense of control, enabling the patient to be more functional. When the patient begins to think about the causes or consequences of the illness (i.e., when denial begins to break down or decrease), feelings of powerlessness may emerge or increase. It may be difficult to differentiate hopelessness and denial from powerlessness in some patients. Anxiety needs to be examined as a potential diagnosis because powerlessness can be caused by or result in it. A sense of no control over one's life can also be part of depression symptoms and contribute to suicidal ideation.

## Interventions

When initially intervening with patients who are feeling powerless, nurses should use a supportive, accepting approach to interview patients and family members about past crises and illness experiences. If patients are demonstrating pain or anxiety, these problems should be further assessed and reduced before expecting them to pay attention to new information or try new coping skills (see Figure 21-2).

Most interventions for powerlessness are focused in two key areas: addressing lack of knowledge and providing opportunities to control decisions and goals. Helping patients to understand their roles in new situations has been associated with empowerment and sense of control (Gaucher & Payot, 2011). Nurses can identify factors that their patients can control. This can be accomplished by providing education and information on what to expect with illness, treatment, and patient care. Providing a supportive environment to ask questions and participate in care will enhance the individual's sense of active involvement in the treatment plan. This includes confirming patients' understanding of the illness and treatment. Patients and their families can be involved in the treatment plan by learning self-management strategies; this also can provide a sense of control over what is happening. Incorporating exercise, reporting body temperature, and implementing ways to reduce infection are examples of how nurses can promote involvement and enhance a sense of control and participation in the plan.

Determining patients' readiness to participate in the treatment plan and decision making is important. Provide opportunities for participation in small steps.

Support groups and social media provide opportunities to share concerns and learn how others have gained a sense of power over the illness. Seeking out information on the Internet is often the first thing people do when they hear about their illness. Patients should be encouraged to share this information with their nurse so that any misinformation can be corrected. Group support can enhance a sense of empowerment, as one sees how others have adapted to a diagnosis. This can include virtual support groups on the Internet.

Facing cancer often means letting go of some aspects of life. Reinforcing how the person can retain some control by making a conscious decision to let go of losses can be a recurring theme throughout treatment. Harpham (2015) noted that letting go will make patients' lives better, rather than persistently focusing on the way things were before cancer. The control individuals retain by deciding to let go of some aspects of life during cancer treatment can be empowering. Nurses should reinforce that letting something go is not giving up (Harpham, 2015). A grieving process is involved in letting go of areas of life during cancer treatment (e.g., taking a leave of absence from work, less visits with grandchildren because of infection risk). However, helping patients to move on to identify the choices available (e.g., more time to take care of themselves and alternate ways to stay in touch with grandchildren) will empower them. Maintaining some autonomy during treatment will enhance individuals' sense of control and self-esteem.

A sense of control can be enhanced by participating in the treatment plan and incorporating preventive measures, such as good nutrition and more exercise. By getting more involved in treatment strategies, patients can feel like they are more than just a passive recipient of interventions. This includes finding ways to promote autonomy (Lavoie et al., 2011).

Anger often is an emotional reaction to powerlessness. As a way to regain control, patients may try to force themselves into achieving the unattainable. The emotional release is important to support, but patients will need support to move on from this state rather than dwell on frustration. Nurses often need to be able to tolerate the anger, which often can include projection of anger onto the healthcare team. Venting anger at a nurse for a late medication may represent the frustration of a prolonged hospital stay. Recognizing this can help nurses provide supportive interventions rather than becoming defensive.

## Assessment
- Recognize the types of powerlessness and differences in individual locus of control.
- Reassess patients' levels of powerlessness at different stages of the illness continuum (e.g., at diagnosis, during different treatments or hospitalizations, at time of recurrence).
- Consider patients' past coping behaviors related to uncontrollable events, especially illness.
- Differentiate among denial, hopelessness, and powerlessness.
- Determine patients' ability to use new information and motivation to change sense of control.
- Identify other people or events that can assist in reducing patients' feeling of powerlessness.

## Nursing Diagnoses (NANDA International, 2015)
- Powerlessness
- Deficient knowledge
- Hopelessness
- Ineffective coping

## *DSM-V* Diagnoses (American Psychiatric Association, 2013)
- Adjustment disorder with anxiety or depression
- Major depression

## Expected Outcomes
- Patients will identify factors that they can control or influence.
- Patients will make decisions regarding care, treatment, and future.
- Patients will verbalize a realistic ability to control/influence situations and outcomes.
- Patients will select and use alternative methods for increasing sense of control in illness-related situations.

## Interventions
- Provide effective communication regarding all procedures, rules, and options relevant to patients and families.
- Provide an opportunity for patients to express feelings.
- Allow time to answer questions; encourage patients and families to write down questions. If possible, plan specific meeting times with patients and family members.
- Keep patients and families informed about the schedule, changes, treatments, and results; anticipate questions/interests, and offer information.
- If pain or anxiety is a contributing factor, provide assessment and appropriate interventions (e.g., relaxation, deep breathing, prescribed medication).
- Provide consistent staffing and opportunities for family members to identify with selected nurses; keep promises, and follow through on agreed-upon care.
- While being realistic, identify positive changes in patients' conditions.
- Acknowledge patients' usual response style (e.g., internal or external locus of control); be sensitive to cultural differences.
- Provide as many opportunities as possible for patients to control decisions; assist patients to identify controllable factors and to accept what cannot be changed.
- Allow patients and families to participate in care; keep needed items within reach.
- Increase decision-making opportunities for patients as their condition progresses.
- Emphasize what patients can do; set short-term, achievable goals.
- Use encouragement, and reward small gains/achievements (e.g., walked five more feet, ate two more bites).
- Provide information about the illness and treatment plan.
- Identify strengths and assets.
- Promote problem solving.
- Challenge negative thinking.
- Avoid reinforcing negative thinking.
- Assist patients in identifying power from other sources (e.g., support groups, chaplain, prayer, food, pets, special rituals).
- When feelings of powerlessness decrease, evaluate with patients and family members what strategies have been effective, and discuss how they will manage feelings of powerlessness in the future.

**Figure 21-2. Plan of Care**

# Clinicians' Experience of Powerlessness

Oncology nurses can experience powerlessness and a sense of helplessness in the clinical setting, especially when faced with patients who have few options to prolong life or reduce suffering. The feeling of helplessness in the face of suffering is an unavoidable experience for clinicians who work with serious illness (Back, Rushton, Kaszniak, & Halifax, 2015). Common reactions to this helplessness include numbness, lethargy, and disengagement.

Back et al. (2015) made the following suggestion to address clinician helplessness: Recognize it, embrace your first reaction, nourish yourself, embody constructive engagement, and weave a new response. Recognizing these signs early can help nurses to develop different strategies to remain engaged with their patients and still care for themselves.

## Case Study

Joseph is an 80-year-old man with stage IV lung cancer. He has been on targeted therapy for the last year, and his cancer remained stable with no progression for that year. Joseph had been CEO of a construction company until his retirement 10 years prior. He was known as a problem solver who others turned to when they needed help. When Joseph was originally diagnosed with lung cancer, he had been very positive and hopeful for a cure. He had interviewed multiple oncologists and read extensively on options before agreeing to a treatment plan. He began developing more serious side effects from the targeted therapy in recent months, leading to a reduction in dose.

On his latest scans, it is noted that the lung cancer started advancing again. When the oncologist and oncology nurse practitioner inform Joseph, his wife, and son about the progression, the patient becomes very agitated and angry. He yells at the nurse practitioner (NP), "You promised these drugs would work!" He informs the doctor he would be finding another "more competent" replacement. He looks distraught and becomes tearful but refuses any comfort from his family. After several minutes, he composes himself and walks out of the consultation. The NP follows him out of the office, and the patient becomes more agitated, yelling at her that she should be working in another field because she is inadequate in this one. His wife and son are left to get more information from the doctor about the possible treatment options.

The patient takes a cab home by himself and researches alternative treatments for lung cancer on the Internet. He makes some inquiries about clinical trials. By the time his family returns home, Joseph is relaxed and confident again.

### Discussion

Joseph was someone who expected to be in control of new situations. He participated in all decisions and felt that he made good decisions in the treatment plan chosen for his cancer. He was faced with disease progression that was probably related to dose reduction of the targeted therapy. The side effects were beyond his control. Joseph became overwhelmed with a sense of powerlessness and saw his disease as getting out of his control. To control the panic, he returned to an approach that worked for him in the past—vent his anger and then identify some action to take charge again.

When Joseph's family returned home, they informed him of the options presented by the oncologist. Joseph was then able to realize that he still had options for treatment that he could discuss with his oncologist, including clinical trials. He met with the NP individually and apologized for his outburst. The NP encouraged him to identify more ways he could maintain control in his life during his treatment to help him face future challenges.

## Conclusion

Similar to denial and hopelessness, feelings of powerlessness and behaviors and thoughts indicative of perceived loss of control in the face of life-threatening illness tend to surface at the most stressful points in the cancer experience, including when first diagnosed, at the time of metastases or recurrence, and when facing end-stage disease. Having moderate to strong feelings of powerlessness at these times is appropriate and should not be considered abnormal. However, if patients or family members continue to experience such a level of loss of control that adaptive behaviors such as information seeking or decision making are impeded, then healthcare professionals must assess the factors contributing to the ongoing perception of loss of control. Prolonged powerlessness may lead to hopelessness and depression that may, in turn, negatively affect cancer treatment and outcomes.

Staff can use three types of control to assist patients dealing with feelings of powerlessness: behavioral, cognitive, and decisional. Regardless of patients' preferred locus of control, interventions supporting small gains or achievements in dealing with their illness or small efforts to accept what is not controllable may ameliorate the negative effects of powerlessness in the cancer experience.

## References

Algren, C.L. (2006). Family centered care of children during illness and hospitalization. In M.J. Hockenberry & D. Wilson (Eds.), *Wong's nursing care of infants and children* (8th ed., pp. 1046–1082). St. Louis, MO: Elsevier Mosby.

American Psychiatric Association. (2013). *Diagnostic and statistical manual of mental disorders* (5th ed.). Washington, DC: Author.

Back, A.L., Rushton, C.H., Kaszniak, A.W., & Halifax, J.S. (2015). "Why are we doing this?" Clinician helplessness in the face of suffering. *Journal of Palliative Medicine, 18*, 26–30. doi:10.1089/jpm.2014.0115

Bandura, A. (1977). Self-efficacy: Toward a unifying theory of behavioral change. *Psychological Review, 84*, 191–215. doi:10.1037/0033-295X.84.2.191

Braga, C.G., & da Cruz, A. (2003). The powerlessness psycho-social response in the postoperative period in cardiac surgery patients. *Revista da Escola de Enfermagem da USP, 37*, 26–35.

Carpenito-Moyet, L.J. (2010). *Nursing diagnosis: Application to clinical practice* (13th ed.). Philadelphia, PA: Lippincott Williams & Wilkins.

Corradi, R.B. (2007). Turning passive into active: A building block of ego and fundamental mechanism of defense. *Journal of the American Academy of Psychoanalysis and Dynamic Psychiatry, 35*, 393–416. doi:10.1521/jaap.2007.35.3.393

Doenges, M.E., Moorhouse, M.F., & Murr, A.C. (2013). *Nursing diagnosis manual: Planning, individualizing, and documenting client care* (4th ed.). Philadelphia, PA: F.A. Davis.

Duggleby, W., Montford, K., Thomas, R., Nekolaichuk, C., Ghosh, S., Cumming, C., & Tonkin, K. (2015). Transitions of male partners of women with breast cancer: Hope, guilt, and quality of life. *Oncology Nursing Forum, 42*, 134–141. doi:10.1188/15.ONF.134-141

Fast, N.J., Gruenfeld, D.H., Sivanathan, N., & Galinsky, A.D. (2009). Illusory control: A generative force behind power's far-reaching effects. *Psychological Science, 20,* 502–508. doi:10.1111/j.1467-9280.2009.02311.x

Fitzsimons, S., & Fuller, R. (2002). Empowerment and its implications for clinical practice in mental health: A review. *Journal of Mental Health, 11,* 481–499. doi:10.1080/09638230020023

Garrison, T.M. (2000). Chronic illness and rehabilitation. In A.G. Lueckenotte (Ed.), *Gerontologic nursing* (2nd ed., pp. 348–369). St. Louis, MO: Mosby.

Gaucher, N., & Payot, A. (2011). From powerlessness to empowerment: Mothers expect more than information from the prenatal consultation for preterm labour. *Paediatrics and Child Health, 16,* 638–642.

Harpham, W.S. (2015). The medicine of "letting it go." *Oncology Times, 37*(6), 49. doi:10.1097/01.COT.0000462871.28832.17

Kogan, N.R., Dumas, M., & Cohen, S.R. (2013). The extra burdens patients in denial impose on their family caregivers. *Palliative and Supportive Care, 11,* 91–99. doi:10.1017/S1478951512000491

Lavoie, M., Blondeau, D., & Picard-Morin, J. (2011). The autonomy experience of patients in palliative care. *Journal of Hospice and Palliative Nursing, 13,* 47–53. doi:10.1097/NJH.0b013e318202425c

Mor, V., Allen, S., & Malin, M. (1994). The psychosocial impact of cancer on older versus younger patients and their families. *Cancer, 74*(Suppl. 7), 2118–2127. doi:10.1002/1097-0142(19941001)74:7+<2118::AID-CNCR2820741720>3.0.CO;2-N

Mumtaz, Z., Salway, S., Bhatti, A., & McIntyre, L. (2014). Addressing invisibility, inferiority, and powerlessness to achieve gains in maternal health for ultra-poor women. *Lancet, 383,* 1095–1097. doi:10.1016/S0140-6736(13)61646-3

NANDA International. (2015). *Nursing diagnoses: Definitions and classification, 2015–2017.* Philadelphia, PA: Author.

Nymark, C., Mattiasson, A.-C., Henriksson, P., & Kiessling, A. (2014). Emotions delay care-seeking in patients with an acute myocardial infarction. *European Journal of Cardiovascular Nursing, 13,* 41–47. doi:10.1177/1474515113475953

Oregon Public Health Division. (2017). Oregon Death With Dignity Act, 2016. Retrieved from http://www.oregon.gov/oha/PH/PROVIDERPARTNERRESOURCES/EVALUATIONRESEARCH/DEATHWITHDIGNITYACT/Documents/year19.pdf

Pollin, I., & Golant, S. (1994). *Taking charge: Overcoming the challenges of long-term illness.* New York, NY: Times Books.

Rotter, J.B. (1966). Generalized expectations for internal versus external control of reinforcement. *Psychological Monographs, 80,* 1–28. doi:10.1037/h0092976

Ryan, S., Hassell, A., Dawes, P., & Kendall, S. (2003). Perceptions of control in patients with rheumatoid arthritis. *Nursing Times, 99,* 36–38.

Rydahl-Hansen, S. (2013). Conditions that are significant for advanced cancer patients' coping with their suffering—As experienced by relatives. *Journal of Psychosocial Oncology, 31,* 334–355. doi:10.1080/07347332.2013.778933

Sand, L., Strang, P., & Milberg, A. (2008). Dying cancer patients' experiences of powerlessness and helplessness. *Supportive Care in Cancer, 6,* 853–862. doi:10.1007/s00520-007-0359-z

Seligman, M.E. (1975). *Helplessness: On depression, development, and death.* San Francisco, CA: W.H. Freeman.

Sheridan, N.F., Kenealy, T.W., Kidd, J.D., Schmidt-Busby, J.I., Hand, J.E., Raphael, D.L., ... Rea, H.H. (2015). Patients' engagement in primary care: Powerlessness and compounding jeopardy. A qualitative study. *Health Expectations, 18,* 32–43. doi:10.1111/hex.12006

Sundeen, S.J. (2001). Psychiatric rehabilitation. In G.W. Stuart & M.T. Laraia (Eds.), *Principles and practice of psychiatric nursing* (7th ed., pp. 246–264). St. Louis, MO: Mosby.

Thewes, B., Butow, P., Zachariae, R., Christensen, S., Simard, S., & Gotay, C. (2012). Fear of cancer recurrence: A systematic literature review of self-report measures. *Psycho-Oncology, 21,* 571–587. doi:10.1002/pon.2070

Townsend, M.C. (2011). *Nursing diagnosis in psychiatric nursing: Care plans and psychotropic medications* (8th ed.). Philadelphia, PA: F.A. Davis.

Townsend, M.C. (2015). *Psychiatric mental health nursing: Concepts of care* (8th ed.). Philadelphia, PA: F.A. Davis.

Yang, W., Jin, S., He, S., Fan, Q., & Zhu, Y. (2015). The impact of power on humanity: Self-dehumanization in powerlessness. *PLOS ONE, 10.* doi:10.1371/journal.pone.0125721

Zahlis, E.H., & Lewis, F.E. (2010). Coming to grips with breast cancer: The spouse's experience with his wife's first six months. *Journal of Psychosocial Oncology, 28,* 79–97. doi:10.1080/07347330903438974

Zarowsky, C., Haddad, S., & Nguyen, V.K. (2013). Beyond 'vulnerable groups': Contexts and dynamics of vulnerability. *Global Health Promotion, 20*(Suppl. 1), 3–9. doi:10.1177/1757975912470062

# SECTION IV

# Psychosocial Interventions

Chapter 22. Crisis Intervention

Chapter 23. Interpersonal and Therapeutic Skills Inherent in Oncology Nursing

Chapter 24. Substance Abuse and Addiction

Chapter 25. Therapeutic Modalities in Psychosocial Care

CHAPTER 22

# Crisis Intervention

*Sharon Van Fleet, MS, RN, PMHCNS-BC*

> *If you aren't in over your head, how do you know how tall you are?*
>
> —T.S. Eliot

A crisis is an event that threatens one's equilibrium, challenging usual coping mechanisms (Aguilera, 1998). Aguilera's classic model of crisis intervention specifies three balancing factors that determine whether a crisis occurs: the individual's perception of the event, the situational supports available, and the individual's coping mechanisms. When one has a realistic perception of the event, has adequate supports available, and uses effective coping mechanisms, equilibrium is maintained. When one or more of these factors are absent, disequilibrium results and a crisis occurs. Figure 22-1 illustrates the development of a crisis. Crisis intervention aims to reduce distress, return one's equilibrium, prevent further trauma, and, ideally, promote psychological growth (King, 2012). Crisis intervention has been identified by Hudacek (2008) as one of the seven dimensions of caring defining nursing practice. Thus, developing skills to assist patients and families is an important role for oncology nurses (Chase, 2013). Roberts and Ottens's (2005) Seven-Stage Crisis Intervention Model is a useful approach in acute situations and illnesses such as cancer. The model emphasizes performing an assessment, establishing the relationship, addressing feelings and emotions, identifying problems and solutions, forming a plan, and performing follow-up. This model is used as a guide in this chapter.

## Crisis Assessment

### The Patient

Patients in a crisis are unable to effectively reduce their distress with characteristic coping strategies and are often more amenable to assistance than they would be otherwise (King, 2012). During a crisis or a potential crisis, nurses must assess and quickly intervene. Varcarolis (2013) highlighted the importance of assessing three key areas: perceptions held by the person about the crisis event, the support systems available to the person, and the person's coping skills.

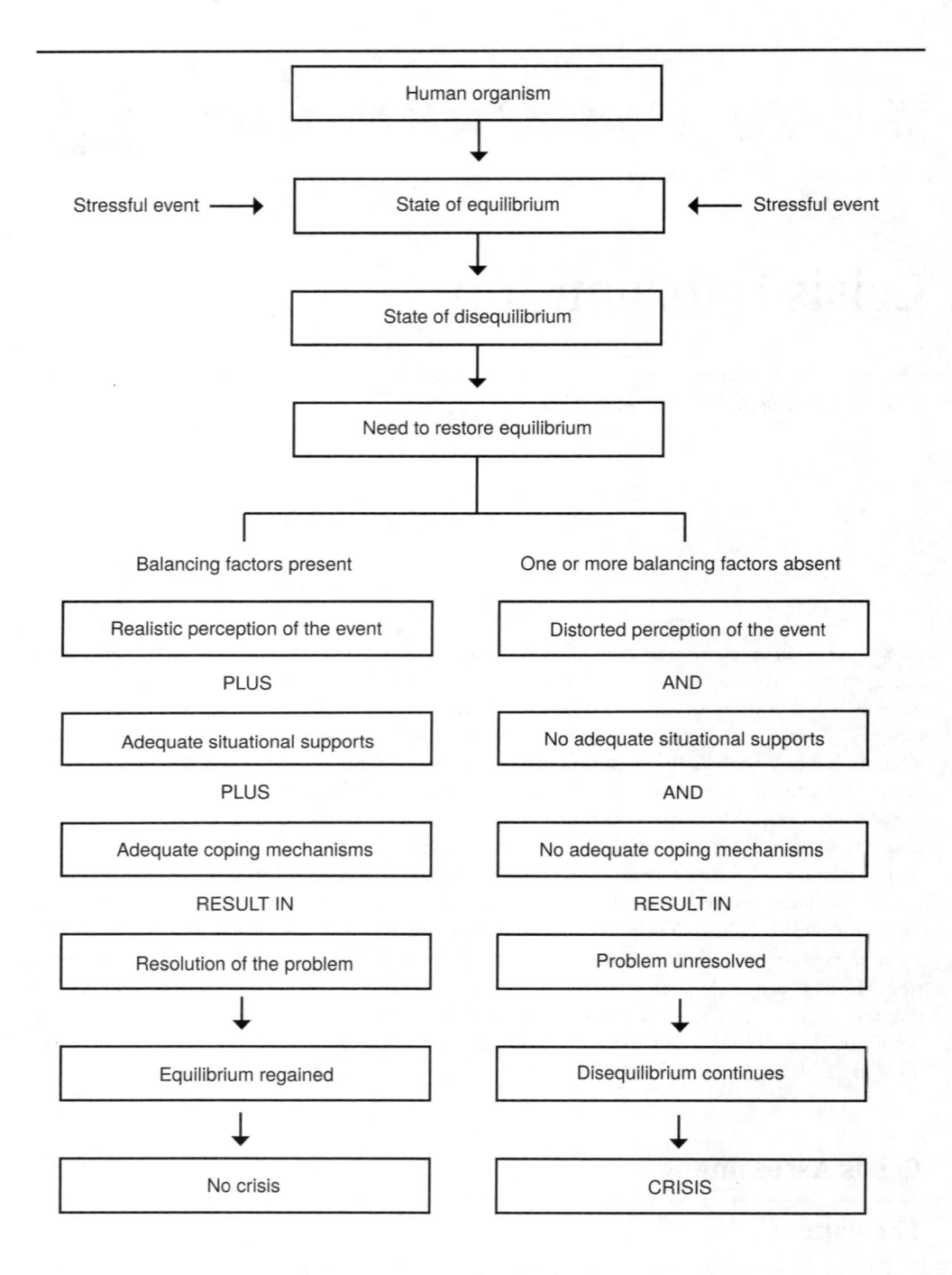

```
                        Human organism
                             │
                             ▼
Stressful event ──▶   State of equilibrium   ◀── Stressful event
                             │
                             ▼
                     State of disequilibrium
                             │
                             ▼
                   Need to restore equilibrium
                             │
              ┌──────────────┴──────────────┐
     Balancing factors present      One or more balancing factors absent

   Realistic perception of the event    Distorted perception of the event
                PLUS                                 AND
   Adequate situational supports        No adequate situational supports
                PLUS                                 AND
   Adequate coping mechanisms           No adequate coping mechanisms
              RESULT IN                           RESULT IN
   Resolution of the problem            Problem unresolved
                 │                                   │
                 ▼                                   ▼
   Equilibrium regained                 Disequilibrium continues
                 │                                   │
                 ▼                                   ▼
           No crisis                              CRISIS
```

**Figure 22-1. Crisis Intervention Model**

*Note.* From *Crisis Intervention: Theory and Methodology* (8th ed., p. 33), by D.C. Aguilera, 1998, St. Louis, MO: Elsevier Mosby. Copyright 1998 by Elsevier Mosby. Reprinted with permission.

Perceptions of the crisis event can be assessed by asking the patient questions concerning how they perceived their lives prior to the event, the impact the event has had on their lives, and how they view their future as a result of the event (Varcarolis, 2013). Essentially, this line of questioning focuses on the meaning of the event for individuals. Many factors influence how a person perceives and adjusts to a situation, including the existence of multiple stressors and losses, the impact of the illness, the presence of pain and/or other distressing symptoms, and history of psychiatric illness and/or substance abuse (King, 2012). Obtaining the patient's report regarding the events precipitating the crisis is helpful (Townsend, 2015). In addition, it is important to assess the patient's views of their strengths and areas for growth. Nurses also must assess the patient's understanding of the illness and current medical status, determining whether he or she possess any realistic understanding of the situation and being careful in challenging any misperception (Townsend, 2015).

Available support systems can be determined by asking about the patient's living situation and social network (Varcarolis, 2013): Who do they trust? Who do they go to for help? Do they have a spiritual belief system that sustains them through difficulties?

Coping skills can be evaluated through questioning the patient about what they do for relief of tension or anxiety (Varcarolis, 2013). What has helped them through past challenges? It is critical to assess the patient for suicide risk. Maladaptive reactions to crisis include extended or excessive episodes of anxiety, hopelessness, helplessness, and impaired functioning (King, 2012). Nurses should watch for signs such as disorganized behavior, agitation, deterioration in self-care and activities, social withdrawal, and suicidal thinking and behavior (King, 2012; Townsend, 2015). Nurses also must consider the person's affective response, if the response is typical of an individual in this situation, and if it is interfering with the person's functioning to the extent that referral to a mental health professional might be warranted. The use of psychoactive medications and substances is another important area for assessment (Townsend, 2015). Figure 22-2 lists questions for assessing individual coping mechanisms and perceptions.

---

- "How are you? How are things going?"
- "What are your concerns?"
- "What are your expectations from your cancer treatment?"
- "How well are you managing with your symptoms?"
- "How is your illness affecting your mood? Your life? Your relationships?"
- "What is the hardest part of your situation?"
- "What have you tried so far to help you cope? What happened?"
- "What do you usually do when you are stressed?"
- "What has helped in the past with lessening your stress? Have you tried this recently? If so, what happened? If it is not working now, why do you think that is?"
- "What do you find most helpful in managing your situation now? What is not working well for you?"
- "What is your support system? Is it enough? If not, what keeps you from getting the help you want or need?"
- "What is the likelihood that you will be able to get the help or support you need?"
- "How has illness affected your life? How has it affected your relationships and the people closest to you?"
- "What do you think you need?"
- "What do you need from your team? How can we help you?"
- "Where's your hope at this time? When you think about your future, what do you see?"
- "How does your faith (or spirituality) affect your ability to cope? What beliefs or practices do you find helpful? How can your care providers support your efforts?"
- "What strengths do you have that can help you?"

**Figure 22-2. Sample Questions for Assessing Individuals in Crisis**

*Note.* Based on information from Goldsmith et al., 2013; Taylor, 2014; Townsend, 2015; van Servellen, 2009; Varcarolis, 2011.

Per the American College of Surgeons Commission on Cancer (2015), distress screening is now an accreditation standard for all cancer centers. The screening guidelines from the National Comprehensive Cancer Network® (NCCN®, 2017) offer a patient-rated distress measurement scale and a problem checklist to identify specific potential sources of distress, but other screening options exist (Bidstrup, Johansen, & Mitchell, 2011) (see Chapter 18).

## The Family

Family assessment and intervention is essential, because a crisis involves and affects the family, whose response, in turn, affects the patient and their outcome (Northouse, 2012; Northouse, Katapodi, Song, Zhang, & Mood, 2010). Figure 22-3 outlines questions that nurses can use to help guide family assessment. The approach used to assess individuals also may be used to organize the assessment of the functioning of individual family members. Nurses must recognize the necessary interdependence in patient and family caregiver relationships (Northouse, 2012). Slaikeu (1990) described four tasks of crisis resolution with families. One task is for the family to physically survive the crisis as well as manage financially without developing additional illness. The second task is to manage feelings and the resultant effects on individual members, family life, other generations of family members, and social networks. The third task is cognitive mastery of the crisis. Nurses assess family norms and values and how families manage boundaries, power, and alignments. The final task is making the necessary interpersonal and behavioral adjustments precipitated by the crisis. Determining how family roles and relationships have changed since the crisis can provide important information. Nurses can help to determine what additional changes are needed in family functioning to help with adaptation to the crisis.

## Cultural and Other Assessment Factors

Many cultural factors impact the response to illness (Grendell, 2012a). Cultural influences significantly affect patients' and families' perceptions of events, the responses to be consid-

---

- "Which family members are closest? Who else has close ties? Who has conflicted relationships?"
- "What information do you need? What else do you think you need?"
- "What are the problems the family is facing right now?"
- "How often does the family talk about problems?"
- "What is the hardest part of this situation?"
- "What stressors has the family experienced in the past? What did you learn from the experience that you might be able to use now? What is your family doing to manage the stress?"
- "What has helped your family manage stress in the past?"
- "What needs to change in how family members are managing the situation?"
- "To whom do you look for support? Do family members have support outside the family? Is that support enough?"
- "How has the illness affected relationships inside the family? Outside the family?"
- "Which family member is most distressed?"
- "What are family members doing to take care of themselves?"
- "How much emotional stress do you experience while providing care?"
- "How does your family make decisions?"
- "For what are you hoping? How do you see your future?"

**Figure 22-3. Sample Questions for Assessing Families in Crisis**

*Note.* Based on information from Chase, 2013; Goldsmith et al., 2013; Hendricks-Ferguson, 2000; Northouse, 2012; Taylor, 2014; Townsend, 2015; van Servellen, 2009; Varcarolis, 2011.

ered appropriate following the events, and the decision-making process used in responding to events. Awareness of these influences is very important (Huang, Yates, & Prior, 2009). Although conventional crisis intervention theory has been promoted throughout the world, it is important to remember that the patient and family will perceive and respond to the crisis through the lens of their own culture. Any therapeutic approach must incorporate patients' and families' uniqueness, and the process from assessment through intervention must involve an appreciation of all cultures (Miller, 2011). Factors to consider include health beliefs, spirituality, experiences, community, value systems, and sources of authority and guidance (Grendell, 2012a). Differences also appear to exist in the types of services sought by members of different ethnic groups (Fiszer, Dolbeault, Sultan, & Brédart, 2014). Emphasizing strengths and positive coping skills rather than deficits is especially important in working with diverse cultures and has been an increasing trend in crisis intervention (Greene & Lee, 2015) (see Chapter 5 on culture).

Given the complexity of many crises, nurses may have difficulty determining when a situation exceeds their abilities. Nursing intervention may be appropriate for circumstances involving minimal levels of distress. Referrals to other professionals are generally recommended for moderate or severe distress (Sheldon, Harris, & Arcieri, 2012). NCCN distress management guidelines provide direction for typical distress symptoms generally amenable to nonspecialist monitoring, as well as management and direction regarding when referrals are recommended (NCCN, 2017). Changes in mood, behavior, or thinking require further assessment and possible intervention (Sheldon et al., 2012).

## Interventions

### Establishing Rapport and Developing the Relationship

Crisis intervention is primarily a reality-based, problem-solving approach that invloves the provision of information and support (King, 2012; Townsend, 2015). One of the initial goals of this intervention is the development of a rapport and a collaborative relationship (King, 2012). Establishing a calm atmosphere conducive to the development of an empathic, accepting, supportive, respectful, and trusting relationship is essential for the nurse who joins patients and families in problem solving with a focus on reality (King, 2012; Townsend, 2015). Patients and families must have the opportunity to express concerns, and the need to feel accepted, heard, understood, and supported. Nurses can offer validation of their responses to the crisis and may assist in gently revising distorted perceptions and identifying options available for resolving the crisis (King, 2012; Townsend, 2015). Although hope is an essential element, nurses should be aware of the risk of closing off communication if patients feel forced into assuming a particular outlook (Tod, Warnock, & Allmark, 2011). Generally, given the anxiety inherent in crisis situations, nurses need to take an active role (Varcarolis, 2011), and safety is the first priority (Roberts & Ottens, 2005; Tod et al., 2011), especially in situations involving serious risk to physical or mental well-being. Nurses should gather information in a direct, straightforward manner, focusing on the current situation (Varcarolis, 2011). Figure 22-4 lists basic principles of crisis intervention.

### Dealing With Feelings and Emotions

Crisis intervention often involves reframing events that may impact feelings and emotions. Anxiety created by the crisis can be reduced as reframing aids in problem solving.

- The individual's and family's perception of the event and the meaning attributed to the event are key factors in determining whether a crisis exists.
- Each patient and crisis situation is unique, but situations are similar.
- The focus remains on problem solving around the crisis and the precipitating events.
- Immediate intervention is the focus. Crises are usually not emergent but require prompt action.
- The nurse takes an active, directive, problem-solving stance, but the decision regarding the solution remains with the patient.
- The nurse reinforces patient and family strengths and resources and facilitates the use of available support systems.
- The nurse communicates patience, hope, self-confidence, and knowledge and uses therapeutic communication strategies.
- The more severe the crisis, the more directive the nurse must be.
- The nurse helps the patient and family to identify previous means of successful coping and possible strategies to help solve the current problem.
- The nurse allows opportunities for identification and expression of feelings.
- The nurse provides opportunities for the patient and family to learn skills to help with future crises.
- Crises usually are self-limiting, but intervention can prevent sequelae and increase the likelihood of optimal resolution.

**Figure 22-4. Principles of Crisis Intervention**

*Note.* Based on information from Aguilera, 1998; Hendricks-Ferguson, 2000; King, 2012; Roberts & Ottens, 2005; Townsend, 2015; van Servellen, 2009; Varcarolis, 2011.

Nurses must use caution to avoid discouraging expression of feelings (Tod et al., 2011). Nurses sometimes attempt to limit their own distress by discouraging patients from crying. Crying may serve as a therapeutic catharsis (Williams, 2014), and by avoiding prematurely ending the patient's expression of intense feeling, nurses can offer support. Although expression of some negative emotions should be supported, nurses must avoid reinforcing those maladaptive reactions (Townsend, 2015). Anxiety needs to be reduced before effective communication and problem solving can occur. Mild anxiety is essential for learning, but moderate anxiety can limit functioning. Anxiety at severe levels alters perception and attention. Motor activity, as well as cognitive and emotional expression, may be helpful to reduce anxiety. When anxiety reaches panic levels, nurses need to be more directive. An active approach provides essential structure and creates a secure atmosphere while communicating an expectation that the crisis will be resolved. Despite the need for an active approach, nurses need to avoid the urge to offer advice or a solution. Unless safety is at risk, they should instead assist patients in exploring several solutions (McDonald, 2012).

## Identifying Problems and Solutions, Formulating a Plan, and Performing Follow-Up

Once the initial phase of shock has subsided and patients are sufficiently calm to participate in discussion, nurses can assist patients in reviewing thoughts, feelings, and concerns for the purpose of problem identification (van Servellen, 2009). Nurses should help patients and families by reviewing the issues related to the crisis and asking about strategies used to cope in the past. The specific meaning of the crisis event is explored (Roberts & Ottens, 2005), as well as the event's effect on goals, expectations, and assumptions. Nurses can offer information and suggest alternatives to enable patients and families to plan appropriate actions. The assessment approach taken initially can be useful for problem identification, planning, and follow-up. Patients' perceptions of an initial event can be addressed in terms of what they and their families can do differently to help change preceptions. Patients and families can be assisted by seeing if and how their social support systems might be optimized. Finally, coping skills can be enhanced in various ways so that distress can be lessened, and the crisis can be viewed more adaptively.

Nurses assist patients and families in discussing goals and how they wish to achieve them (Roberts & Ottens, 2005). A strategy is adaptive if it helps one to function, effectively solve problems, and prevent significant emotional deterioration. A person's strengths should be actively sought and used to enhance resilience (King, 2012; Roberts & Ottens, 2005). Nurses can offer empathy while communicating confidence that the distress will lessen. Anxiety exceeding mild levels interferes with relationships; family and friends may need assistance in maintaining interactions with the patient and each other that are as close to normal as possible.

Nurses need to listen for cues regarding concerns, seek specific concrete details, and help to break concerns into manageable components for discussion, ultimately assisting in prioritizing problems. Nurses should avoid prematurely confronting irrational beliefs and errors or distortions in thinking (which are very common during a crisis). Rather, the focus should be on addressing irrational beliefs and distortions sensitively and generally by addressing them more indirectly through further questioning and using strategies such as reframing or "playing devil's advocate" (Roberts & Ottens, 2005).

Hendricks-Ferguson (2000) emphasized the role of nurses along the entire crisis intervention process in continuing to clarify issues, assessing the impact of stressors on coping, and assessing current coping strategies. The author also noted the importance of nurses reviewing the adjustments and goals achieved, as well as planning for future crises.

## Cancer as a Crisis

Whereas a crisis generally is thought to be short term and self-limited, cancer can precipitate intermittent crises throughout the illness trajectory, from diagnosis to survivorship, depending on the situation and the individual's vulnerability. NCCN (2017) distress guidelines call for screening initially, when clinically indicated, and at each change in disease status. Linden, MacKenzie, Rnic, Marshall, and Vodermaier (2015) highlighted the need for repeated assessments. Intervention is needed and can be most helpful at points when new coping strategies may be required.

### Diagnosis

Diagnosis engenders a variety of emotional responses, including a sense of detachment, fear, anxiety, anger, and helplessness (Grendell, 2012b). Several necessary tasks emerge during diagnosis, including accepting dependency, establishing and understanding the treatment, accepting the diagnosis, making decisions, and establishing new routines. Patients require information to begin making needed treatment decisions, and nurses serve as a resource, remembering that information may need repetition. Anxiety is very common (Smith, Hyde, & Stanford, 2014) and can precipitate denial and/or treatment interference. Information regarding typical emotional responses and validation of feelings can reduce anxiety. Referrals for other sources of information and assistance, such as a support group, may be appropriate.

## Treatment

In planning for initial treatment, patients and families require information about the specific malignancy, prognosis, treatment goals, treatment options and side effects, diagnostic tests, activity limitations, interpersonal relationships, and the availability of support groups and other resources (Meropol et al., 2013; Tariman, Doorenbos, Schepp, Singhal, & Berry, 2014). Patients fear treatment side effects, pain, body image changes, and death (Puts et al., 2015). Some may fear abandonment by family and friends. Issues such as major depression or severe anxiety should prompt referral for psychiatric consultation. Nurses may attempt to intervene in situations where, for example, a patient expresses an interest in postponing or avoiding treatment. In this case, they could explore concerns, provide pertinent information, correct misunderstandings, assist with problem solving, and facilitate access to resources.

## Remission and Survivorship

During the adaptation phase, patients and families attempt to return to some level of their previous lifestyles and find many challenges, including experiencing differences between patients and family members in adjustment (van Servellen, 2009). At this time, support from others may decline, despite a possibly increased need for assistance. When treatment concludes, patients often experience the loss of a safety net and may continue to experience significant distress (Stanton, 2012). Patients and families require information and proactive intervention to enhance the potential for positive adaptation. If distress becomes moderate or severe, thus interfering with functioning, assessment by a psychiatric specialist is specified in current standards (Sheldon et al., 2012).

## Recurrence/New Primary

Recurrence often requires different strategies because physical problems often affect problem solving (van Servellen, 2009), and anxiety is usually increased. Shock and disbelief are common responses, along with anxiety and depressive symptoms (Schapira, 2010). Fear of additional loss, increased dependency, and uncontrollable pain may develop. The threat of death frequently is greater after recurrence, and acknowledging this can promote discussion. Feelings of failure and guilt, as well as concerns regarding impact on family, may surface (Ekwall, 2007). Hope can be sustained through person-centered strategies demonstrating regard, avoiding abandonment, and attending to dignity and comfort (Schapira, 2010). Maladaptive reactions involving significant distress, behavior changes, or suicidal ideation necessitate a psychiatric referral, as is the case at any point along the trajectory.

## Advanced and Terminal Illness

Facing advancing and terminal illness represents a crisis period for many patients and families. When palliative care becomes the focus, nurses have much to offer to assist patients and families with adjustment. Goldsmith, Ferrell, Wittenberg-Lyles, and Ragan (2013) reviewed the nurse's role in helping a patient with advanced cancer. Some of these roles include preparing the patient and family members for the future according to their needs and preferences, discussion and clarification of goals and needs, along with the exploration of the distress experienced. The increased loss associated with advanced disease can overwhelm and itself precipitate crisis (van Servellen, 2009). In a study, van Servellen (2009) stressed the importance of encouraging discussion of all emotions experienced by patients and families despite some reactions seeming typical and expected. Reassurance that patients and family members will have access to information and support is essential. Goldsmith et al. (2013) suggested that nurses ask questions such as "How can we help you live in the best way possible?" and "What makes life worthwhile?"

Given the fact that the degree and nature of the response in a crisis is often disproportionate to expectations in a particular situation, nurses must anticipate a variety of potential reactions. They must also expect that patients and family members will not grieve in a parallel manner (van Servellen, 2009). This discrepancy can create conflict because changes that some family members make may be incompatible with those made by the patient or others.

The nurse's role with a dying patient involves supporting family members by enabling them to be present with the dying person and emphasizing the importance of their presence (Williams, Bailey, Woodby, Wittich, & Burgio, 2013). Nurses can assist family members by encouraging them to view the situation according to the dying person's preferences. Family members need concrete information about what to expect in the final days, and nurses must be prepared to repeat this information.

## Interventions at the Patient's Death

Experiencing the death of a loved one may precipitate a crisis for some survivors. Focusing on concrete items, such as helping to make phone calls or ensuring that a family member is not left alone and will not have to drive home alone, can be important interventions during a crisis. It is important to recognize, however, that some people may prefer private time alone with the patient after he or she dies (Fortinash, 2012). Nurses must assess the family members' ability to adjust to the loss. Using the crisis intervention model can be helpful during acute grief. Questions about how the loss is experienced, the adequacy of social support, coping behaviors, and history of loss can elicit useful information. Caregiver characteristics predicting complicated mourning include female gender and lack of support (Chiu, 2010), as well as fewer years of education and the presence of baseline depressive symptoms (Allen, Haley, Small, Schonwetter, & McMillan, 2013). Younger age at death also appears to be a predictor for complicated grief. Bereaved individuals at greater risk may need additional intervention, including phone calls and referrals (see Chapter 19 for information on grief and bereavement).

# Evaluation of Interventions Across All Phases of Cancer

Generally, successful resolution of a crisis is apparent through reduced distress and improved coping. When usual coping mechanisms are working adequately again and the problem seems surmountable, the crisis can be considered resolved. Nurses can make referrals to address remaining concerns (Townsend, 2015).

## Evidence-Based Practice

In the past decade, investigators have continued to evaluate the use of nurse-led intervention against distress in patients and caregivers. Studies have investigated the impact of nursing intervention on coping, mostly involving the provision of support and information. Typically, studied interventions were offered as part of planned, programmatic support and not as crisis intervention per se. Chambers et al. (2014) determined that a single-session psychoeducation/stress management intervention offered by nurses via telephone and aided at home by self-management materials held promise in reducing distress and enhancing adjustment. Such an intervention could be offered as part of a tiered approach, where patients requiring more intensive assistance could have access to mental health professionals (Chambers et al., 2014). Meneses et al. (2007) found quality of life improved following a nurse-led psychoeducational intervention in cancer survivors. Additional research has employed specially trained oncology nurses to provide problem-focused counseling to address the social, psychological, and physical effects of disease and treatment. One example of such work is seen in a study by van der Muelen et al. (2013), where researchers noted significantly lower depressive symptoms in patients receiving a nurse-led, problem-focused intervention in conjunction with regular follow-up visits. Galway et al. (2012) tentatively concluded that nurse-led efforts offering information and support may be helpful with newly diagnosed patients, noting that the state of current evidence limited the ability to form a solid conclusion.

Strategies using multimedia as part of nurse-initiated interventions are being studied. Oh and Kim (2010) investigated the effects of a two-week psychoeducational intervention for patients receiving adjuvant therapy. The intervention used an instructional CD-ROM, along with telephone counseling provided by a doctorate-prepared nurse researcher. Increased self-care activity and "fighting spirit" were noted in the intervention group compared with controls. More recent research has explored the use of palliative care and oncology clinical nurse specialists (Clark et al., 2015).

Some evidence suggests that screening results in some positive effects on patient–clinician communication and in the use and timeliness of referrals (Carlson, Waller, & Mitchell, 2012). Other experts, however, have questioned the feasibility of routine distress screening (Absolom et al., 2011; Bidstrup et al., 2011; Howell, Hack, Green, & Fitch, 2014; Mitchell, Lord, Slattery, Grainger, & Symonds, 2012; Thombs & Coyne, 2013). Furthermore, numerous barriers and issues related to routine distress screening performed by nurses have been identified (Chen & Raingruber, 2014; Mitchell et al., 2012). Others have emphasized the need for nurses to have additional training in order to provide quality routine psychosocial care (Absolom et al., 2011; Gosselin, Crane-Okada, Irwin, Tringali, & Wenzel, 2011; Stadelmaier, Duguey-Cachet, Saada, & Quintard, 2014; Wittenberg-Lyles, Goldsmith, & Ferrell, 2013). It also is difficult to find quality evidence supporting the provision of psychosocial crisis intervention by staff-level oncology nurses. More research needs to be conducted on the training needed to provide effective crisis intervention. Given the reality that many of the interventions with established effectiveness exist outside the scope of the oncology nurse, nurses can suggest strategies to explore and, most importantly, offer referrals (Fulcher, Kim, Smith, & Sherner, 2014).

# Conclusion

Nurses in all oncology settings will encounter patients and families experiencing the crisis of cancer. Crises will occur across all phases of the cancer continuum. Nurses must recognize the various crises that patients and families face and how they can effectively intervene, within their scope and ability, to assist with a successful resolution and restoration of equilibrium.

*The author would like to gratefully acknowledge Deborah Lawless, MALS, who eagerly assisted with article retrieval and offered input into search strategies.*

# References

Absolom, K., Holch, P., Pini, S., Hill, K., Liu, A., Sharpe, M., ... Velikova, G. (2011). The detection and management of emotional distress in cancer patients: The views of healthcare professionals. *Psycho-Oncology, 20,* 601–608. doi:10.1002/pon.1916

Aguilera, D.C. (1998). *Crisis intervention: Theory and methodology* (8th ed.). St. Louis, MO: Mosby.

Allen, J.Y., Haley, W.E., Small, B.J., Schonwetter, R.S., & McMillan, S.C. (2013). Bereavement among hospice caregivers of cancer patients one year following loss: Predictors of grief, complicated grief, and symptoms of depression. *Journal of Palliative Medicine, 16,* 745–751. doi:10.1089/jpm.2012.0450

American College of Surgeons Commission on Cancer. (2015). *Cancer program standards: Ensuring patient-centered care* (2016 ed.). Retrieved from https://www.facs.org/~/media/files/quality%20programs/cancer/coc/2016%20coc%20standards%20manual_interactive%20pdf.ashx

Bidstrup, P.E., Johansen, C., & Mitchell, A.J. (2011). Screening for cancer-related distress: Summary of evidence from tools to programmes. *Acta Oncologica, 50,* 194–204. doi:10.3109/0284186X.2010.533192

Carlson, L.E., Waller, A., & Mitchell, A.J. (2012). Screening for distress and unmet needs in patients with cancer: Review and recommendations. *Journal of Clinical Oncology, 30,* 1160–1177. doi:10.1200/JCO.2011.39.5509

Chambers, S.K., Girgis, A., Occhipinti, S., Hutchison, S., Turner, J., McDowell, M., ... Dunn, J.C. (2014). A randomized trial comparing two low-intensity psychological interventions for distressed patients with cancer and their caregivers [Online exclusive]. *Oncology Nursing Forum, 41,* E256–E266. doi:10.1188/14.ONF.E256-E266

Chase, E. (2013). Crisis intervention for nurses. *Clinical Journal of Oncology Nursing, 17,* 337–339. doi:10.1188/13.CJON.337-339

Chen, C.H., & Raingruber, B. (2014). Educational needs of inpatient oncology nurses in providing psychosocial care [Online exclusive]. *Clinical Journal of Oncology Nursing, 18,* E1–E5. doi:10.1188/14.CJON.E1-E5

Chiu, Y.-W. (2010). Determinants of complicated grief in caregivers who cared for terminal cancer patients. *Supportive Care in Cancer, 18,* 1321–1327. doi:10.1007/s00520-009-0756-6

Clark, J.E., Aitken, S., Watson, N., McVey, J., Helbert, J., Wraith, A., ... Catesby, S. (2015). Training oncology and palliative care clinical nurse specialists in psychological skills: Evaluation of a pilot study. *Palliative and Supportive Care, 13,* 537–542. doi:10.1017/S1478951513000163

Ekwall, E. (2007). Recurrence of ovarian cancer—Living in limbo. *Cancer Nursing, 30,* 270–277. doi:10.1097/01.NCC.0000281729.10362.3a

Fiszer, C., Dolbeault, S., Sultan, S., & Brédart, A. (2014). Prevalence, intensity, and predictors of the supportive care needs of women diagnosed with breast cancer: A systematic review. *Psycho-Oncology, 23,* 361–374. doi:10.1002/pon.3432

Fortinash, K.M. (2012). Grief: In loss and death. In K.M. Fortinash & P.A. Holoday Worret (Eds.), *Psychiatric mental health nursing* (5th ed., pp. 640–659). St. Louis, MO: Elsevier Mosby.

Fulcher, C.D., Kim, H.-J., Smith, P.R., & Sherner, T.L. (2014). Putting evidence into practice: Evidence-based interventions for depression. *Clinical Journal of Oncology Nursing, 18*(Suppl. 6), 26–37. doi:10.1188/14.CJON.S3.26-37

Galway, K., Black, A., Cantwell, M., Cardwell, C.R., Mills, M., & Donnelly, M. (2012). Psychosocial interventions to improve quality of life and emotional well-being for recently diagnosed cancer patients. *Cochrane Database of Systematic Reviews, 2012*(11). doi:10.1002/14651858.CD007064.pub2

Goldsmith, J., Ferrell, B., Wittenberg-Lyles, E., & Ragan, S.L. (2013). Palliative care communication in oncology nursing. *Clinical Journal of Oncology Nursing, 17,* 163–167. doi:10.1188/13.CJON.163-167

Gosselin, T.K., Crane-Okada, R., Irwin, M., Tringali, C., & Wenzel, J. (2011). Measuring oncology nurses' psychosocial care practices and needs: Results of an Oncology Nursing Society psychosocial survey. *Oncology Nursing Forum, 38,* 729–737. doi:10.1188/11.ONF.729-737

Greene, G.J., & Lee, M.-Y. (2015). How to work with clients' strengths in crisis intervention: A solution-focused approach. In K.R. Yeager & A.R. Roberts (Eds.), *Crisis intervention handbook: Assessment, treatment and research* (4th ed., pp. 69–98). New York, NY: Oxford University Press.

Grendell, R.N. (2012a). Culture, ethnicity, and spirituality. In K.M. Fortinash & P.A. Holoday Worret (Eds.), *Psychiatric mental health nursing* (5th ed., pp. 140–183). St. Louis, MO: Elsevier Mosby.

Grendell, R.N. (2012b). Mental and emotional responses to medical illness. In K.M. Fortinash & P.A. Holoday Worret (Eds.), *Psychiatric mental health nursing* (5th ed., pp. 660–676). St. Louis, MO: Elsevier Mosby.

Hendricks-Ferguson, V.L. (2000). Crisis intervention strategies when caring for families of children with cancer. *Journal of Pediatric Oncology Nursing, 17,* 3–11. doi:10.1177/104345420001700102

Howell, D., Hack, T.F., Green, E., & Fitch, M. (2014). Cancer distress screening data: Translating knowledge into clinical action for a quality response. *Palliative and Supportive Care, 12,* 39–51. doi:10.1017/S1478951513000382

Huang, Y.-L., Yates, P., & Prior, D. (2009). Accommodating the diverse cultural needs of cancer patients and their families in palliative care. *Cancer Nursing, 32,* E12–E21. doi:10.1097/01.NCC.0000343370.16894.b7

Hudacek, S.S. (2008). Dimensions of caring: A qualitative analysis of nurses' stories. *Journal of Nursing Education, 47,* 124–129. doi:10.3928/01484834-20080301-04

King, D.E. (2012). Crisis: Theory and intervention. In K.M. Fortinash & P.A. Holoday Worret (Eds.), *Psychiatric mental health nursing* (5th ed., pp. 481–501). St. Louis, MO: Elsevier Mosby.

Linden, W., MacKenzie, R., Rnic, K., Marshall, C., & Vodermaier, A. (2015). Emotional adjustment over 1 year post-diagnosis in patients with cancer: Understanding and predicting adjustment trajectories. *Supportive Care in Cancer, 23,* 1391–1399. doi:10.1007/s00520-014-2492-9

McDonald, S.F. (2012). Therapeutic communication: Interviews and interventions. In K.M. Fortinash & P.A. Holoday Worret (Eds.), *Psychiatric mental health nursing* (5th ed., pp. 59–86). St. Louis, MO: Elsevier Mosby.

Meneses, K.D., McNees, P., Loerzel, V.W., Su, X., Zhang, Y., & Hassey, L.A. (2007). Transition from treatment to survivorship: Effects of a psychoeducational intervention on quality of life in breast cancer survivors. *Oncology Nursing Forum, 34,* 1007–1016. doi:10.1188/07.ONF.1007-1016

Meropol, N.J., Egleston, B.L., Buzaglo, J.S., Balshem, A., Benson, A.B., III, Cegala, D.J., ... Weinfurt, K.P. (2013). A web-based communication aid for patients with cancer: The CONNECT Study. *Cancer, 119,* 1437–1445. doi:10.1002/cncr.27874

Miller, G. (2011). *Fundamentals of crisis counseling.* Hoboken, NJ: John Wiley & Sons.

Mitchell, A.J., Lord, K., Slattery, J., Grainger, L., & Symonds, P. (2012). How feasible is implementation of distress screening by cancer clinicians in routine clinical care? *Cancer, 118,* 6260–6269. doi:10.1002/cncr.27648

National Comprehensive Cancer Network. (2017). *NCCN Clinical Practice Guidelines in Oncology (NCCN Guidelines®): Distress management* [v.2.2017]. Retrieved from https://www.nccn.org/professionals/physician_gls/pdf/distress.pdf

Northouse, L.L. (2012). Helping patients and their family caregivers cope with cancer. *Oncology Nursing Forum, 39,* 500–506. doi:10.1188/12.ONF.500-506

Northouse, L.L., Katapodi, M.C., Song, L., Zhang, L., & Mood, D.W. (2010). Interventions with family caregivers of cancer patients: Meta-analysis of randomized trials. *CA: A Cancer Journal for Clinicians, 60,* 317–339. doi:10.3322/caac.20081

Oh, P.J., & Kim, S.H. (2010). Effects of a brief psychosocial intervention in patients with cancer receiving adjuvant therapy [Online exclusive]. *Oncology Nursing Forum, 37,* E98–E104. doi:10.1188/10.ONF.E98-E104

Puts, M.T., Tapscott, B., Fitch, M., Howell, D., Monette, J., Wan-Chow-Wah, D., ... Alibhai, S.M. (2015). A systematic review of factors influencing older adults' decision to accept or decline cancer treatment. *Cancer Treatment Reviews, 41,* 197–215. doi:10.1016/j.ctrv.2014.12.010

Roberts, A.R., & Ottens, A.J. (2005). The seven-stage crisis intervention model: A road map to goal attainment, problem solving, and crisis resolution. *Brief Treatment and Crisis Intervention, 5,* 329–339. doi:10.1093/brief-treatment/mhi030

Schapira, L. (2010). Dealing with cancer recurrence. In D.W. Kissane, B.D. Bultz, P.M. Butow, & I.G. Finlay (Eds.), *Handbook of communication in oncology and patient care* (pp. 191–201). New York, NY: Oxford University Press.

Sheldon, L.K., Harris, D., & Arcieri, C. (2012). Psychosocial concerns in cancer care: The role of the oncology nurse. *Clinical Journal of Oncology Nursing, 16,* 316–319. doi:10.1188/12.CJON.316-319

Slaikeu, K.A. (Ed.). (1990). *Crisis intervention: A handbook for practice and research* (2nd ed.). Upper Saddle River, NJ: Pearson Education.

Smith, A., Hyde, Y.M., & Stanford, D. (2014). Supportive care needs of cancer patients: A literature review. *Palliative and Supportive Care, 13,* 1013–1017. doi:10.1017/S1478951514000959

Stadelmaier, N., Duguey-Cachet, O., Saada, Y., & Quintard, B. (2014). The Basic Documentation for Psycho-Oncology (PO-Bado): An innovative tool to combine screening for psychological distress and patient support at cancer diagnosis. *Psycho-Oncology, 23,* 307–314. doi:10.1002/pon.3421

Stanton, A.L. (2012). What happens now? Psychosocial care for cancer survivors after medical treatment completion. *Journal of Clinical Oncology, 30,* 1215–1220. doi:10.1200/JCO.2011.39.7406

Tariman, J.D., Doorenbos, A., Schepp, K.G., Singhal, S., & Berry, D.L. (2014). Information needs priorities in patients diagnosed with cancer: A systematic review. *Journal of Advanced Practice in Oncology, 2014,* 115–122.

Taylor, E. (2014). Spiritual distress. In C.H. Yarbro, D. Wujcik, & B.H. Gobel (Eds.), *Cancer symptom management* (4th ed., pp. 683–697). Burlington, MA: Jones & Bartlett Learning.

Thombs, B.D., & Coyne, J.C. (2013). Moving forward by moving back: Re-assessing guidelines for cancer distress screening. *Journal of Psychosomatic Research, 75,* 20–22. doi:10.1016/j.jpsychores.2013.05.002

Tod, A., Warnock, C., & Allmark, P. (2011). A critique of positive thinking for patients with cancer. *Nursing Standard, 25*(39), 43–47. doi:10.7748/ns.25.39.43.s50

Townsend, M.C. (2015). *Psychiatric mental health nursing: Concepts of care in evidence-based practice* (8th ed.). Philadelphia, PA: F.A. Davis.

van der Meulen, I.C., May, A.M., Ros, W.J., Oosterom, M., Hordijk, G.-J., Koole, R., & de Leeuw, J.R. (2013). One-year effect of a nurse-led psychosocial intervention on depressive symptoms in patients with head and neck cancer: A randomized controlled trial. *Oncologist, 18,* 336–344. doi:10.1634/theoncologist.2012-0299

van Servellen, G. (Ed.). (2009). *Communication skills for the health care professional* (2nd ed.). Boston, MA: Jones & Bartlett Learning.

Varcarolis, E.M. (2011). *Manual of psychiatric nursing care planning: Assessment guides, diagnoses, and psychopharmacology* (4th ed.). St. Louis, MO: Elsevier Saunders.

Varcarolis, E.M. (2013). *Essentials of psychiatric-mental health nursing: A communication approach to evidence-based care* (2nd ed. revised reprint). St. Louis, MO: Elseiver Saunders.

Williams, A. (2014). Therapeutic communication in mental health nursing. In S. Walker (Ed.), *Engagement and therapeutic communication in mental health nursing* (pp. 5–22). London, England: Sage Publications.

Williams, B.R., Bailey, F.A., Woodby, L.L., Wittich, A.R., & Burgio, K.L. (2013). "A room full of chairs around his bed": Being present at the death of a loved one in Veterans Affairs Medical Centers. *Omega, 66,* 231–263. doi:10.2190/OM.66.3.c

Wittenberg-Lyles, E., Goldsmith, J., & Ferrell, B. (2013). Oncology nurse communication barriers to patient-centered care. *Clinical Journal of Oncology Nursing, 17,* 152–158. doi:10.1188/13.CJON.152-158

CHAPTER 23

# Interpersonal and Therapeutic Skills Inherent in Oncology Nursing

*Kathryn E. Pearson, RN, CNS, MN, AOCN®*

> *I did not hear the words you said. Instead, I heard the love.*
>
> —Joan Walsh Anglund

As patients and families experience the myriad of emotional challenges along the continuum of cancer care, nurses frequently face feelings of being inadequately prepared to respond in a skilled and supportive manner (Helft, Chamness, Colin, & Ulrich, 2011). Nurses also may become overwhelmed by the anxiety, fears, uncertainties, grief, anger, and depression that patients and families experience. Nurses who are uncomfortable responding to patients' and families' emotional behaviors are at risk for causing more harm by escalating the intensity of the situation or by avoiding and withdrawing from needed interventions (Helft et al., 2011). It is generally recognized that ineffective communication skills may contribute to patient and family feelings of distress, uncertainty, and dissatisfaction with care (Uitterhoeve, Bensing, Grol, deMulder, & van Achterberg, 2010). In contrast, psychosocially skilled oncology nurses are recognized as being instrumental in assisting patients and families to achieve a sense of control and well-being during times of stress. Positive patient outcomes from therapeutic communication and relationships with patients may include improved decision making and quality of life and increased levels of satisfaction with health care (Arnold, 2016a; Fukui, Ogawa, & Yamagishi, 2011).

Oncology patients, particularly those with advanced disease, have special expectations of nurses that include understanding, empathy, and support (Winterburn & Wilkinson, 2011). Most often, patients consider the nurse to be the primary communication link to the healthcare system, ultimately impacting their treatment and survival (Winterburn & Wilkinson, 2011). Communication skills training programs have been developed for nurses (Fukui et al., 2011; Moore, Rivera Mercado, Grez Artigues, & Lawrie, 2013; Winterburn & Wilkinson, 2011; Goldsmith, Ferrell, Wittenberg-Lyles, & Ragan, 2013) and may be effective in improving both patient and nurse outcomes. In a randomized controlled trial, Wilkinson, Perry, Blanchard, and Linsell (2008) demonstrated the effectiveness of communication skills training in cancer and palliative care; however, further research is needed to strengthen the evidence supporting the effects of different training strategies on outcomes (Moore et al., 2013). When educated in appropriate interpersonal and social skills, nurses may be prepared to provide the needed emotional support for patients and families (Winterburn & Wilkinson, 2011; Wittenberg-Lyles et al., 2013). These communication skills include recognition of the individual's uniqueness, attentive listening and mindful presence, reflection, and supportive problem solving. The ultimate goal of professional communication is to facilitate a trusting nurse–patient relationship.

## Cultural Competence and Communication

In any communication and relationship, oncology nurses first must take into account the social, cultural, and ethnic background of patients and families and be aware of how these belief systems will influence their response to health and illness. The Health and Medicine Division of the National Academies of Sciences, Engineering, and Medicine (formerly the Institute of Medicine [IOM]) asserted that ineffective communication among minority populations in the United States resulted in unequal care and health outcomes (IOM, 2002). Cultural competence is applying a set of cultural behaviors and attitudes that enable the professional to effectively communicate and establish relationships in cross cultural situations (Arnold, 2016b). To be culturally sensitive, professionals must be open to different cultural beliefs and values, always incorporating the patient's cultural beliefs and values into their care (Arnold, 2016b). Transcultural caring relationships, such as that between nurse and patient, often reflect that patients' perceptions of the nurse–patient relationship can be equally as important as the language used in communicating (Arnold, 2016b); therefore, communication is both verbal and nonverbal (behavioral). Second, caring for patients and family members when they are confronting life-changing and life-threatening illness will challenge nurses' own belief systems and emotions (Arnold, 2016b). This is especially true in circumstances where cultural, language, or healthcare settings contribute to patients and families feeling threatened, which compounds their fears and anxieties. To establish a trusting relationship, nurses must carry out evidence-based and culturally sensitive interventions to promote comfort and to provide psychosocial care in a safe environment and in a therapeutic manner. Figure 23-1 lists reasons why healthcare professionals may feel reluctant to act on cultural differences in patients. Building trust and rapport and being able to satisfy the patient's needs and expectations are a few of the basic requirements to delivering quality care in a multicultural setting (Thomas, Lounsberry, & Carlson, 2011).

- The fear of being construed as racist
- The fear that focusing on patient differences will overlook similarities
- The fear of promoting stereotypes
- The fear of making the interaction complex
- The fear of facing the uncomfortable realization that there may be multiple and equally valid approaches to life circumstances

**Figure 23-1. Reluctance to Act Upon Cultural Differences**

*Note.* Based on information from Thomas et al., 2011.

## Social Skills

Initiating professional interactions requires the use of basic social skills that are considered "good manners." This begins when the nurse offers a professional introduction and shows respect by explaining the nurse's role and purpose to patients. Simply approaching a patient and family in a nonthreatening manner will increase their comfort in the nurse's presence (Boggs, 2016a; Ross & Johansen, 2002). Nonverbal behaviors, such as a handshake, smile, and eye contact, reinforce spoken words. The physical environment should be adjusted to allow for privacy, comfort, and interpersonal space (Arnold, 2016a), and nurses should avoid separating themselves from patients by standing behind physical barriers, such as tables and desks. Skilled nurses adjust their verbal tone and behavior to suit the situation of each patient and family member. For example, if the nurse is aware that the patient has just received bad news, the nurse may adjust a normally cheery introduction to one conveying respect and empathy.

One's interpersonal skills (i.e., verbal and nonverbal communication) and attitude can positively or negatively influence how individuals treat others; self-reflection is an important prerequisite for effective client-centered communication (Arnold, 2016a). Interacting with patients in a sensitive, caring, and helpful manner may be challenging to nurses if personal emotional responses are triggered by patients' or families' behavior or by other environmental or personal factors (Arnold, 2016a; Royak-Schaler et al., 2006). By gaining insight into their own feelings, nurses are better equipped to choose the behavior appropriate to the situation and, therefore, act and respond professionally even if they may feel differently.

Ross and Johansen (2002) found in their qualitative study of psychosocial home visits to patients with colon cancer that nurses' attitudes toward patients were crucial to the outcome of interactions. Effective nurse–patient and nurse–family interactions resulted when patients and families were authentically viewed as fellow human beings and not merely as people experiencing a cancer diagnosis (Ross & Johansen, 2002). Being authentic requires nurses to recognize personal vulnerabilities, strengths, and limitations and to be able to engage with patients on a human, emotive level prior to engaging in cognitive, solution-oriented aspects of communication (Arnold, 2016a; McGilton, Irwin-Robinson, Boscart, & Spanjevic, 2006). Oncology nurses who are able to behave in a trustworthy, dependable manner are secure enough within themselves to establish professional boundaries and yet feel warmth, caring, fondness, interest, and respect toward patients. The result is a rewarding, professional relationship that is healing to patients and families (Arnold, 2016a).

Nurses must be aware of nonverbal language, which may lead to communicating conflicting messages. The nurse may communicate what is really thought or felt through nonverbal behaviors, which may conflict with what is communicated verbally. For example, a family member may be convinced that the patient's confused behavior is related to chemotherapy and be unable to accept that the patient is experiencing functional decline. The nurse may feel frustrated by the family member's denial but may attempt to explore the family's understanding in greater depth. The nurse may ask, "How do you think the confusion is caused by the chemotherapy?" At the same time, the nurse's deep sigh or perturbed expression after the question creates the conflicting message by nonverbally communicating frustration. Nonverbal communication style must take body language into account or the conscious or unconscious body positioning or actions of the communicator (Boggs, 2016b). Leaning forward communicates interest, facial expressions reflect emotion, eye contact shows interest, and gestures such as an affirmative nod also convey attention (Boggs, 2016b). As important, the nurse must also be attentive to the patient's nonverbal body cues. Figure 23-2 outlines personal beliefs, attitudes, and behaviors that can interfere with therapeutic communication and support.

- Discounting or devaluing emotional symptoms
- Believing that talking about sensitive issues with patients takes too much time
- Believing that talking about emotions (or becoming tearful) is detrimental for patients
- Believing that talking about death is taboo
- Believing that there is no hope
- Believing that anger is an unwarranted emotion that interferes with patient care
- Labeling (stereotyping) patients as:
  - Noncompliant
  - Lazy
  - Manipulative
  - Attention seeking
- Personalizing a patient's anger by becoming defensive or feeling out of control
- Overcompensating to be the "nice nurse"
- Giving false reassurance (e.g., saying "Do not worry" when you do not know what the patient is worried about)
- Changing the topic, ignoring cues, or making jokes (putting off patients' true concerns)
- Being judgmental
- Giving trite advice
- Lecturing
- Excessive questioning
- Ill-timed use of emotionally charged words and phrases
- Self-focusing behaviors
- Double-bind messages (conflicting verbal and nonverbal messages)
- Lacking confidence in own professional role and abilities

**Figure 23-2. Beliefs, Attitudes, and Behaviors That Interfere With Therapeutic Communication**

*Note.* Based on information from Frost et al., 1997; Heaven & Maguire, 1996; Lovejoy & Matteis, 1997; Maguire, 1985; Peterson, 1988; Smith & Hart, 1994; Wilkinson, 1991; Zamanzadeh et al., 2014.

From "Coping With Cancer: Patient Issues" (p. 9), by D.M. Sivesind and S. Paire in C.C. Burke (Ed.), *Psychosocial Dimensions of Oncology Nursing Care* (2nd ed.), 2009, Pittsburgh, PA: Oncology Nursing Society. Copyright 2009 by Oncology Nursing Society. Adapted with permission.

## Communication Skills

Communication skills that elicit information from patients and families are required to establish the psychosocial data upon which nursing diagnoses and interventions are based. Patient-centered communication is a respectful dialogue between nurses and patients aimed at learning about each patient as a "person" as the basis of care (Arnold, 2016a). Patient-centered communication requires nurses to differentiate between therapeutic and nontherapeutic communication techniques.

**Nontherapeutic communication:** A blocking style of communication is superficial and ignores the verbal and behavioral cues that may indicate areas of psychosocial distress in patients and family members. Behaviors that characterize a blocking style of communication include using closed-ended or leading questions, changing the focus of conversation prematurely, giving inappropriate advice, or using stereotypical comments. Closed-ended questions are those that elicit a yes/no response or a definitive answer (Arnold, 2016a) such as, "What was your level of fatigue after your last chemotherapy administration on the 0–10 scale?"

An early study aimed at investigating how nurses communicate with patients with cancer found that nurses who used blocking techniques tended to have less self-awareness, poor communication techniques, and poor relationships with colleagues (Wilkinson, 1991). Blocking communication techniques most often were used by nurses when patients disclosed feelings and interpreted that the nurses were uncomfortable with emotional distress. Conversely, nurses who were more comfortable confronting patient distress tended to employ a facilitative style of communication (Wilkinson, 1991). Zamanzadeh et al. (2014) reported similar findings in their study of factors that influence nurse communication on cancer wards in Iran.

Barriers exist in the clinical setting that also block effective communication. These include other demands on nursing staff and the limitations of time. "Being unsure of ways to proceed with patients in light of their hopes and concerns may lead to nurses using blocking behaviors, such as changing the subject or ignoring cues" (Baer & Weinstein, 2013, p. E47). It also is common for nurses to use defense mechanisms to protect themselves from patient distress due to a lack of confidence and training to address those emotions (Baer & Weinstein, 2013).

**Therapeutic communication:** Allowing patients and families to "story" the illness experience is an effective therapeutic tool that provides an opportunity to problem solve and find meaning in what is happening. Stories tell "who people are, where they've been, and where they are going" (Smith & Liehr, 2013, p. 225). People will tell their story when they believe the nurse is listening (Liehr, 2005). Back, Arnold, and Tulsky (2010) emphasized the need to establish patient–provider rapport in a clinical relationship, which includes giving each other undivided attention. Skilled nurses employ a facilitating communication style using open-ended questions, reflection, clarification, and empathy.

A variety of questioning techniques can facilitate the telling of the patient's story. Open-ended questions are intended to let the patient and family members answer in their own words without being influenced or "led" by the interviewer (Arnold, 2016a; Paice, 2002). Open-ended questions usually begin with "how," "why," "what," "where," "can you tell me about," and "in what way" (Arnold, 2016a). An example of an open-ended question is "How did you feel after your last chemotherapy administration?" In contrast to general open-ended questions that allow for a variety of answers, open-ended but focused questions are more directed such as, "How was the fatigue you experienced after your last chemotherapy administration?"

Circular questions focus on the interpersonal context in which the illness occurs (Kist, 2016) and are useful in therapeutic communication designed to help solve problems. Circular questioning leads to introspection, a deeper level of understanding, and, ultimately, behavior change (Kist, 2016). One might use a difference question, such as "What is the best and worst advice that you have received from family and friends after your diagnosis?" An example of a behavioral question is "In your opinion, which member of your family is the most affected by your cancer? In what way has this person been affected?" Hypothetical and future-oriented questions pose a "what-if" scenario that can be useful in problem solving (e.g., "If you were to tell your wife about your concerns regarding your cancer, what would she say and do?"). Triadic questions bring in the behaviors of a third party, such as "How do your wife's coworkers help to support her after her chemotherapy treatments?"

# Listening Skills

Effective communication between the nurse and patient begins with empathetic listening. "Active listening allows both communicators to offer presence and bear witness to one another in the telling of the client's story" (Arnold, 2016a, p. 80). Active listening is an interactive process in which the listener not only hears the words being said but also interprets and finds meaning within the attached attitudes and feelings (Arnold, 2016a; Stanley, 2002). Active listeners observe the tone of voice and nonverbal expressions in posture, gestures, and affect. Listening or "attending" behaviors communicate one's interest and respect. Attending behaviors include making eye contact, nodding, and making listening responses such as "yes," "OK," and "um-hum." Active listeners clarify meaning by asking questions such as "Are you saying that . . . ?" or ensure understanding by paraphrasing or summarizing what has been said (e.g., "Do you mean . . . ?"). Interpretation of nonverbal behaviors also should be acknowledged during communication, for instance, "You are clenching your fist. How are you feeling right now?" Restatements and reflections as frequent as every one to two minutes have been found to communicate support and interest as opposed to being detached (Rautalinko, 2013).

If patients or family members are rambling or giving too much information in an anxious or insistent manner, nurses can intervene by writing down major points to help them to focus and become more specific. With this technique, nurses confirm the points for accuracy by repeating, rephrasing, or summarizing the information. Another way to focus the communication is to ask for more information, examples, or details at key junctures, such as asking specifically how many episodes of vomiting the patient experienced after chemotherapy.

Touch is another response that active listeners can use. It has been identified as an important aspect of supportive communication that can convey concern and empathy. It can convey positive and negative reactions depending on the people involved (Townsend, 2015). However, patients' attitudes toward touch vary according to personal belief systems and cultures (Boggs, 2016b). Some patients see supportive touch as being comforting and empathic, whereas others may find that their space has been violated and find touch threatening (Hughes, 2009). Strategies to assess whether patients would welcome touch include asking their permission, taking cues from their body language, and being aware of the meaning of touch in diverse cultures.

Silence is a useful tool in giving patients time to gather thoughts to make a significant point. During quiet pauses, nurses remain silent but maintain attentive behaviors to preserve the interpersonal connection (Boggs, 2016b). Comfortable silences also convey concern, acceptance, and presence and support (Stanley, 2002). In our fast-paced communications, nurses often become uncomfortable with silence, yet this technique can be used therapeutically to provide patients time to think and reflect (Boggs, 2016b).

Patient expression of emotional or informational needs may be primarily communicated indirectly through cues. Cues are verbal or nonverbal hints related to patient concerns that are not being explicitly expressed. Cues may be present 1–30 times during a nurse–patient interaction (Uitterhoeve et al., 2009). One study found that when nurses responded to emotional cues, patient recall improved. Conversely, a distancing response reduced recall (Jansen et al., 2010).

The acronym EMPATHY has been used to assist clinicians in the assessment of nonverbal cues (Riess & Kraft-Todd, 2014). **E**ye contact is a signal of attention and engagement. **M**uscles of facial expression may convey strong emotions such as fear or anger. **P**osture can convey emotive responses independent of facial expressions such as submissiveness, defeat, or defiance. **A**ffect and **T**one of voice may further offer other cues such as fear, anxiety, disengagement, or confusion. **H**earing the whole patient requires that the clinician interpret nonverbal cues in the context of the patient's verbal communication. The acronym incorporates assessment of the clinician response (**Y**our response) as a crucial component in patient communication (Riess & Kraft-Todd, 2014). As previously discussed, nurses must be attentive to their own nonverbal cues in order to create a trusting relationship, avoid emotional leakage, and enhance patient outcomes such as patient satisfaction.

# Language Skills in Communication

Effective communication requires nurses to be aware of the language and communication styles that patients and families use (Boggs, 2016b; Wittenberg et al., 2013). Words and phrases commonly used in medical terminology frequently have different meanings in lay language, and medical jargon is often confusing to patients and families (Boggs, 2016b). Words such as *progressing* and *positive nodes* may hold different, the same, or opposite meanings to patients and family members (Fallowfield, Jenkins, & Beveridge, 2002). The word *tumor* may imply a benign process that is not cancer. Patients and families may interpret an *incurable* condition as one that is imminently life threatening. Staging classifications can be perceived as a step-wise process in which an unspoken stage V is interpreted as a death sentence. Therefore, patients diagnosed with stage III or IV cancers often inaccurately interpret that death is imminent. The use of *complete response* or *partial response* to treatment may imply cure to lay individuals unfamiliar with the terminology. Active listening and directed questioning will help nurses to verify how patients and families interpret medical information to avoid misunderstanding and unnecessary fears.

The cultural and ethnic interpretation of words, phrases, and communication styles also will influence how patients and families understand information regarding diagnosis, treatment, and prognosis. Education regarding the disease and treatment should be presented in a clear, concise, and understandable manner. Medical terminology must make sense to the patient and family in terms of their lay view of ill health and should acknowledge and respect the patient's experience and interpretation of their own condition (Helman, 2007). Helman identified a major criterion for successful communication as "reflexivity," a heightened sense of self-awareness. Health professionals communicate from their own perspective on health and illness, and these perspectives are personal, cultural, and professional. Therefore, unless one is aware of one's own beliefs, it will be difficult to understand and communicate with other people's beliefs and perspectives (Helman, 2007).

Many of the words and phrases used in oncology have multiple metaphors and myths attached that should be avoided (Hughes, 2009). To a layperson, the word *cancer* may imply a painful death sentence. The word *hospice* frequently is emotionally charged and may be perceived as giving up or abandonment. One should not avoid using correct words such as *cancer* but should explore the meaning of the word with patients and families to dispel myths and misconceptions. In describing the psychological responses of patients receiving a cancer diagnosis, Schofield et al. (2003) exemplified this point by concluding that higher patient satisfaction occurred among those patients when the word *cancer* was directly used to inform them of their diagnosis.

Words can positively or negatively influence how patients and families cope along the different phases of the cancer journey. An example is the word *victim*. Patients who are perceived or labeled as being victims are those who feel powerless in the face of the illness. To combat "victimization," the National Coalition for Cancer Survivorship described all people experiencing cancer as "survivors" (Donaldson, 2004). In using the word *survivor*, the perception is reframed to represent a person who is empowered and who can successfully cope with the challenges of cancer. It also implies active decision making and reflects hopefulness, not powerlessness (Mullan, 1996).

A point on the cancer continuum that demands expert counseling and communication skills is the emotional time of transition from active treatment to palliative care or hospice. To identify patients' interpretations of communication regarding ending active treatment, Friedrichsen, Strang, and Carlsson (2002) identified words and phrases that proved confusing for patients and families. Indirect warning words were evasive words from which patients had to decipher an implied message. Words such as *unfortunately* or other phrases of forewarning caused patients and family members to anticipate something unpleasant. Evasive, vague phrases, such as "You may have three months to five years," leave patients and families confused and anxious as to the actual meaning of the message (Friedrichsen et al., 2002).

Emotionally charged words and phrases elicit an emotional response above and beyond the original message. Phrases such as "There is nothing more to do" bring forth feelings of abandonment and fear (Friedrichsen et al., 2002), and patients may believe that even comfort measures such as pain medicine will be withdrawn. Studies across a variety of oncology settings have shown that patients do desire information regarding their cancer status (Baile & Parker, 2011).

In contrast, fortifying and supportive words communicate strength and confirmation. Examples include "We are going to help you with this" and "There are things that can be done to . . . ." The goal of supportive language is to communicate and present information in a positive manner that gives patients and families a measure of control and assures them that they will not be abandoned. Verbal confirmation of patients' and families' feelings, thoughts, and decisions through statements such as "This must be a difficult time for you" is supportive and helpful (Friedrichsen et al., 2002). Siminoff (2011) described the ethical implications of communication and asserted that for overall communication to be effective, the following four essential topics must be addressed in a straightforward manner: the rationale for any procedure, the risks involved, the potential benefits of a procedure, and available treatment alternatives.

## Humor as Communication

Nurses should not be reluctant to use humor as part of personalized and compassionate care (Dean & Major, 2008). When used appropriately, humor can lighten many situations and break down communication barriers. Johnson (2002) found that patients perceived stronger nurse–patient relationships when nurses used humor. Using humor can "test the waters" to see how the listener will receive sensitive topics or concerns. It also may be used to break away from a line of thought that is too painful to explore in the moment. Humor and laughter also have been found to be therapeutic in relieving stress. Humor can help to reframe perception. Despite the benefits, nurses must be sensitive to patients' and families' interpretations of humor and be cautioned that humor is used to laugh with and not at others (MacDonald, 2004).

Humor is a social concept and is defined by culture. What one finds humorous may not be humorous to another. Patient response to nurse humor may not be tolerated if the nurse has not first established a trusting relationship (Tanay, Roberts, & Ream, 2013). Additionally, it may take time for newly diagnosed patients to identify humor related to their situation (Johnson, 2002). Humor research has evaluated the value of humor for enabling communication, fostering relationships, easing tension, and managing emotions (Dean & Major, 2008). Other studies identify the inappropriate use of humor involving serious discussions and heightened anxiety (Dean & Major, 2008). Although the benefits and value of humor have been identified, evidence-guided humor-related interventions are in early development. It is an area ripe for nursing research (Christie & Moore, 2004).

# Communicating Bad News

Bad news often is couched in vague phrases in an effort to provide hope or to protect the messenger, but doing so robs patients and families of the information needed to understand the situation and interferes with decision making and problem solving (Baile & Parker, 2011). Using medical terminology also can be evasive if patients and families do not have a reference point by which to interpret meaning. For example, a statement such as "the tumor marker is going up" delivered in an ominous verbal tone and without accompanying explanation leaves patients and families without the information needed to accurately process the meaning or its implications. Researchers also have found that when benefits from treatment are discussed primarily in terms of statistics and probabilities, patients' and families' feelings of uncertainty increase (Mishel et al., 2002).

Robert Buckman's (1992) seminal book *How to Break Bad News: A Guide for Healthcare Professionals* outlined interventions appropriate for supporting both professionals and patients when they must discuss bad news. Later termed the SPIKES model (Baile et al., 2000; Buckman, 2005), these practical, step-by-step directions were designed to improve the outcomes of sensitive encounters so that the communication itself does not increase the distress of patients and family members on the receiving end of bad news (Baile & Parker, 2011; Fallowfield et al., 2002; Hauser & Makoul, 2011) (see Figure 23-3). The SPIKES model has been widely used in programs that teach communication skills with breaking bad news (Baer & Weinstein, 2013; Hauser & Makoul, 2011). The SPIKES model has been researched in clinical trials and has proven to be valid and reliable (Hauser & Makoul, 2011).

When the doctor leaves the room after disclosing bad news to a patient, the role of the oncology nurse often involves "picking up the pieces." The most supportive technique for nurses at this point may be to stand by quietly while patients and family members absorb the information (Higgins, 2002). They can then give support by answering questions, provid-

---

Step 1: Setting up the interview
- Rehearse mentally.
- Arrange for privacy.
- Involve significant others.
- Sit down.
- Make a connection with the patient (eye contact).
- Manage time constraints and interruptions.

Step 2: Assessing the patient's Perception.
- "What have you been told . . . ?"

Step 3: Obtaining the patient's Invitation
- How much information does the patient want?

Step 4: Giving Knowledge and information to the patient

Step 5: Addressing the patient's Emotions

Step 6: Strategy and Summary
- "What will we do now?"

**Figure 23-3. SPIKES Model**

*Note.* From "SPIKES—A Six-Step Protocol for Delivering Bad News: Application to the Patient With Cancer," by W.F. Baile, R. Buckman, R. Lenzi, G. Glober, E.A. Beale, and A.P. Kudelka, 2000, *Oncologist, 5,* pp. 305–308. Copyright 2000 by AlphaMed Press. Adapted with permission.

ing safety and privacy to handle emotions, and staying present. Depending on the ability of patients and family members to absorb the information or to identify which family members were present, it was found that the information frequently fell to nurses to repeat the SPIKES process (Higgins, 2002). The skills represented by the SPIKES model are understandable and easily practiced, allowing professionals to easily move away from using the model as a script to adapting the model as a flexible framework that can be used for sensitive interactions (Bauer & Weinstein, 2013; Hauser & Makoul, 2011).

## Communication to Support Shared Decision Making

Shared decision making has been defined as a partnership between health professionals and patients in which each individual contributes to decisions about treatment and care (Tattersall, 2011). Nurses are in a pivotal position to be a resource for patients and families as they search for solutions at stressful transition points, especially at the time of diagnosis, throughout treatment, and during end-of-life decision making. Keys to effective communication include mutual respect between patients and nurses, the sharing of intimate feelings in confidence, and reflection. As patients and families grapple with issues of quality of life, treatment options, and mortality, nurses should encourage them to consider available choices within the framework of their own beliefs, values, and life circumstances (Shannon-Dorcy & Wolf, 2003).

During the decision-making process, questions such as "Did you think about . . . ?" or "How did you reach that decision?" help and support patients and families to explore the issues (Shannon-Dorcy & Wolf, 2003). Additionally, nurses must be knowledgeable in order to respond to questions and ensure that patients have adequate, accurate, and thorough information to guide their decisions (Chelf et al., 2001; MacDonald, 2002; Shannon-Dorcy & Wolf, 2003). The more active patients are in their own decision making, the more information they require. Therefore, nurses must be able to recognize priority educational needs and provide information in a concise and clear manner. Early research by Chelf et al. (2001) identified the primary information areas that influence patients' decisions: the recommendations of healthcare providers, the potential for cure and recurrence, and information regarding symptoms and side effects. A recent study described that similar influences impacted collaborative and independent decision making in older adults with breast cancer (Harder, Ballinger, Langridge, Ring, & Fallowfield, 2013). Factors that facilitate shared decision making have been identified: the patient trusts the professional, the patient is prepared (knowledgeable about disease and treatment), and the patient is emotionally ready for the decision-making process (Tattersall, 2011).

Hope is essential throughout the cancer care continuum (Nail, 2001), but during decision-making processes, it is key that hope is not used in a coercive manner, nor should it be taken away. In situations where hope for a good long-term prognosis is unrealistic, nurses can help to refocus hope in terms of incremental steps in daily life (Shannon-Dorcy & Wolf, 2003) and quality of life as defined by patients and families. Professionals are concerned that hearing bad news will destroy the patient's hope, especially when discussing poor prognosis or end-of-life care (Baile & Parker, 2011). Protective factors to preserve hopefulness include making all current treatment options available and stating that the healthcare team will not abandon the patient (Baile & Parker, 2011).

Nurses' mediation and conflict management skills become critical when families and patients disagree about decisions (Zhang & Siminoff, 2003). Although patients and families may not bring up their distress over disagreements in decision making, sensitively asked questions such as "How do you each feel about this decision?" will give permission for patients and family members to acknowledge disagreement. This technique will allow for open discussions that can elucidate the concerns of each individual, clarify assumptions, identify problems, and work to find resolution to conflicts or disagreements (Kist, 2016). Acknowledging family roles in providing support and care to patients can decrease the risk of family members feeling helpless and out of control of their circumstances. Including families in the decision-making process opens channels of communication within the family, solidifying their support and understanding of the patients' experiences.

# Behavioral Therapeutic Techniques

Nurses can use several cognitive restructuring and behavioral techniques described in psychiatric nursing literature (Townsend, 2015) in daily interactions with patients to strengthen their coping and decision-making skills. The goals of these techniques are to increase patients' self-esteem, increase their sense of control, and modify thoughts that negatively affect them.

## Problem-Solving Skills

Problem solving occurs within the context of cognitive restructuring. As patients confront the stressors of the cancer experience, the mind appraises the internal feelings of threat and modifies internal and external choices to cope effectively. If patients are able to successfully solve problems and confront challenges associated with cancer and cancer treatment, these events become less threatening. Problem-solving interventions have been shown to help patients with self-management of symptoms (Lee, Chiou, Chang, & Hayter, 2010). Problem-solving steps include defining the problem, generating alternatives, choosing among the alternatives, and implementing possible solutions (Mishel et al., 2002). The nurse's role as educator, providing patients with information, resources, and alternatives, enhances problem-solving and communication skills. Cognitive reframing allows patients to interpret events as manageable, thereby reducing uncertainties as they encounter new stresses and challenges at different stages of the cancer continuum. For example, if a nurse explains to a patient the rationale behind taking pain medication around the clock, the fear commonly associated with the pain experience can be reframed by assisting the patient to be in control. Therefore, the nurse's role as a competent clinician, educator, and counselor can help patients to reframe the cancer experience as a challenging rather than a threatening event if mastery results in positive outcomes.

## Emotional Support

In addition to strengthening problem-solving skills, cognitive reframing can be used to strengthen and support coping mechanisms. Reframing provides a different, positive interpretation that helps to broaden the patient's perspective, accentuating the patient's strengths (Arnold, 2016a). Patients with cancer will react and cope according to their previous life experiences. Their perceptions or internal viewpoints will influence how they experience the situation. Nurses can assist patients and families in reframing their perceptions by offering insight into why they may be experiencing feelings such as fear, anxiety, and anger. Nurses also can help patients to apply another meaning to the event. For example, patients and families often interpret "Keep a good attitude" to mean "Do not feel sad or depressed." This creates an unrealistic emotional expectation, blocks communication, and creates a sense of failure for patients. Reframing the perception of keeping a good attitude to mean that patients try to maintain a positive, problem-solving approach to coping with the cancer separates the perception from the feelings being experienced. Nurses can then normalize expected feelings to the cancer experience (e.g., grief, loss).

Reframing gives patients the permission to share and address these feelings and explore effective ways in which to cope with them. This may include both problem-solving coping and emotion-focused coping, a balanced approach to adapting to the challenges confronting the patient. Maliski, Heilemann, and McCorkle (2002) found that providing specific information to newly diagnosed patients with prostate cancer and their spouses enabled them to reframe the appraisal of their cancer from a "death sentence" to a "good cancer" and increased their ability to problem solve, make decisions, and cope with the diagnosis.

## Thought-Stopping Techniques

Patients confronting cancer may find that they have ruminating thought processes grounded in uncertainty and fear. Unlike reviewing alternative solutions in the problem-solving process, these ruminations are circular and serve only to reinforce feelings of helplessness and fear. This may be especially true for patients who have a history of generalized anxiety disorder (see Chapter 14). Typically, individuals are unable to sleep or concentrate and constantly may worry about real or perceived threats. A thought-stopping technique may be useful to stop these repeated, unproductive thoughts. In thought stopping, individuals are taught to put up a mental stop sign to interrupt the thought cycles. For example, a patient is unable to sleep because of continued ruminations of self-blame related to having delayed seeking medical care. Teaching the patient to self-talk and carry out a mental "stop" to the repeated thought processes can provide distraction and help to interrupt the course.

Other interventions such as guided imagery and relaxation techniques also can be used to help patients to relax. Finally, nurses can help patients to learn to redirect their thoughts toward a more positive perspective and can encourage them to stop negative self-talk and replace it with positive self-talk with simple communication techniques (e.g., "I understand that you are upset with yourself because you are so tired from chemotherapy, but tell yourself how well you are doing to be setting your priorities and reaching out to your family for help."). If patients continue to experience overwhelming feelings that interfere with their ability to function, nurses should refer them to a mental health professional for support.

## Journaling

Journaling is a therapeutic tool that enables patients to externalize their internal experiences and emotions, taking a positive step toward active problem solving. Journaling techniques can vary between structured journaling (i.e., writing about reactions to certain feelings or events) and free-thought, free-floating journaling. Ullrich and Lutgendorf (2002) asserted that journaling to address both cognitive (factual) and emotional expression provides more personal growth and healing after traumatic events than a purely expressive style of journaling. For example, patients write about an actual experience and its meaning (e.g., finding a breast lump and the possibility that it is cancer) and then write about their emotional reaction to the event (e.g., fear). Milbury et al. (2014) conducted a randomized trial with 277 patients with renal cancer that explored the use of an expressive writing intervention. Their findings were suggestive of a reduction of cancer-related symptoms, including fatigue, which may be related to the early facilitation of cognitive processing through the expressive writing process.

Although journaling can be a sophisticated technique used by psychologists and counselors, it also can be a valuable technique for nurses to teach patients. Rancour and Brauer (2003) described the use of letter writing as a healing method to address altered body image in a patient with breast cancer. Sealy (2012) described how reflective journaling helped to uncover past emotional issues that impacted her during treatment and recovery from breast cancer. A method of journaling that frequently is used in outpatient clinics is journals that serve as day planners, side-effect monitoring tools, and self-care journals. In line with cognitive reframing, patients should include the positive aspects of their experience as well as the negative to gain beneficial insight from their journaling experience (Ullrich & Lutgendorf, 2002).

## Role-Play Techniques

Role-play techniques are another constructive tool that can help patients to build confidence in a desired behavior and help them explore useful alternatives of action. For example, a patient who is having difficulty asking the physician questions can safely role play strategies of asking the questions in different ways until a level of comfort is felt. Nurses can participate by providing feedback and by role playing different responses. Nurses can suggest that patients mentally play out different scenarios (e.g., "What would happen if . . . ?"). Participants can act out scenarios without restriction on how roles are to be played or interpreted. Through supporting or defending a behavior in role play, participants can become aware of other behaviors and their personal bias, experiencing a broader perspective on an issue or situation.

## Nurses' Responses to Patient and Family Emotions

The acting out of strong emotions by patients and families frequently elicits strong feelings in nurses. A sobbing or angry patient may trigger the desire to protect oneself by withdrawing from the patient or, conversely, prompt the nurse to become overly involved in the moment. Instead of withdrawing or participating in displays of emotion, nurses can maintain a professional stature by being calm and present. Helpful nurse responses include role modeling positive behaviors, using helpful communication skills, and actively listening (Stanley, 2002).

The ultimate challenge occurs when patients' or family members' anger is projected directly at the nurse (see Chapter 13). Frequently, the nurse's initial reaction is to feel personally attacked and withdraw or disengage from the situation in self-defense. Unfortunately, defensive behavior is more likely to increase the anger (Thomas, 2003). Figure 23-4 outlines interventions that can help to defuse anger. Simple strategies such as repeating phrases or stating "That must have been very upsetting" can be helpful (Philip & Kissane, 2011). Phrases used in the context of empathic engagement serve to not only acknowledge the distress but also to rename the anger as an alternative emotion (Philip & Kissane, 2011). The emotional reactions of patients and families can be very intense at transitional points in the cancer journey, when apprehension and fear of the unknown are heightened

- Remain calm, maintain calm body postures, and speak softly.
- Implement communication and listening skills to identify why patients are angry. Do not say "Calm down."
- Maintain respectful body language and eye contact. Do not stand or sit too close. Position oneself at an angle (nonconfrontive).
- Validate the complaint (e.g., "I can understand why you are upset.").
- Set limits on inappropriate anger expression, such as punching the wall.
- Avoid doing anything that can be perceived as controlling or dismissive.
- As the anger expression settles, use open-ended questions and problem-solving techniques to work toward resolution.
- Reassure patients that you are concerned and want to understand.
- Maintain one-on-one dialogue. Avoid temptation to involve two to three people in the immediate situation to avoid confusion.
- Teach patients how to communicate concerns in a more effective manner.

**Figure 23-4. Nursing Interventions to Defuse Anger in Patients**

*Note.* Based on information from Garnham, 2001; Sachs, 1999; Thomas, 2003.

(e.g., diagnosis, beginning and cessation of active treatment, recurrence, end of life). Many interventions are available to support nurses to effectively deal with patient and family emotions. How nurses respond will influence positively or negatively how the patients and families respond. First, nurses must be aware of their own feelings regarding what is happening to patients (e.g., is the nurse also grieving the impending death of the patient?). Second, nurses must be knowledgeable regarding the normal, expected emotional reactions to the cancer experience and be able to identify and differentiate these emotions from abnormal emotions that interfere with patients' ability to cope. Lastly, nurses must carry out self-care strategies to remain emotionally healthy and nourished to deal with the challenges of oncology nursing.

Philip and Kissane (2011) outlined strategies for responding and communicating with difficult emotions. Preparation for meeting with patients and families is crucial. Know the details of the diagnosis, treatment, and test results to be reported and make the time. Asking open-ended questions allows the narrative to unfold; listen attentively and develop a shared understanding of the experience. Providing symptom relief is vital for patients to be present in the communication. If anger persists, nurses should reframe and reconsider their approach. If behaviors present danger or disruption of care, nurses should consider setting limits to the expression of heightened emotions. Looking for support among other team members (i.e., social work) and involving experienced clinicians is helpful (Philip & Kissane, 2011).

# Nurses' Roles in Support Groups

Patients and families often seek out support and self-help groups (see Appendix) to find a place to share experiences and to obtain new knowledge from patients in similar situations. This helps to normalize and destigmatize individual emotions and counteracts feelings of isolation. Most group participants verbalize that involvement in a group gives them a community feeling and a safe place to expose feelings and affirm each other (Adamsen & Rasmussen, 2003). For many, groups offer inspiration by experiencing the courage of others, witnessing the motivation to fight, and being exposed to the role modeling of other patients with cancer. Some concerns may prevent healthcare professionals from recommending support groups, including patient exposure to misinformation or bias and the undermining of coping and satisfaction with decision making (Turner, 2011). Therefore, nurses can play an important role in investigating supportive services to ensure that groups are led by professionally trained individuals.

In addition to referring patients and families to support groups, nurses are qualified to participate directly in support groups as therapeutic leaders who create the group framework and identify the ground rules (e.g., confidentiality). In support groups, the nurse's role is that of an initiator, social networker, consultant, resource person, and catalyst (Adamsen & Rasmussen, 2003). Nurses promote the exchange of experience and offer guidance. Nurses as group leaders can make major contributions to psychoeducational groups by providing expert knowledge of treatment, side effects, nutrition, and disease processes. Regardless if the group is a psychoeducational group, a closed focus group, a self-help group, an open continuing group, or an Internet-based group, participation calls for emotional and intimate contact by the nurse therapist. Nurse facilitators and group members together establish a culture or social network that fosters closeness and reduces social isolation (Adamsen & Rasmussen, 2003). Additional responsibilities are to provide safety and support for participants to share their stories and articulate their feelings to provide validation for both (see Figure 23-5). A major goal of support groups is to promote and strengthen the coping skills of participants; the focus of therapeutic groups is not about the leader. However, nurses will gain a great deal of wisdom and insight from the intimate connection with group members. These valuable life lessons are gifts that most often are incorporated into nurses' personal attitudes and belief systems, further contributing to their expertise and knowledge as caring and compassionate professionals.

---

- Establish discussion guidelines at the beginning of the session, such as expectations of confidentiality, no side conversations, and respect of the dignity of others.
- The nurse's role is to facilitate: Do not monopolize the discussion. Nurses do not have to have all the answers.
- Use reflective listening and feedback skills to aid in mutual understanding.
  - Clarify by saying "Let's see if I understand" or "Are you saying . . . ?"
  - Rephrase for emphasis and reflection ("Did I hear you say . . . ?").
  - Framing: Summarize and explain how an idea may fit into a larger concept ("I think the larger issue the group has identified is . . . .").
  - Focus: "It seems that our attention is wandering . . . ."
  - Observe nonverbal behaviors within the group (e.g., facial expressions, body movements).
- Promote group cohesion and facilitate problem solving.
  - Give participants full credit for ideas. Promote active problem solving.
  - Use a conversational approach. Address participants by names.
  - Reinforce participant contributions. Use validating statements such as "Good point" or "I'm glad you raised that issue."
  - Use statements as a "bridge" to move the discussion ("Let's move on to . . . .").
  - Keep discussions from being monopolized by one or two people ("Thank you for your input, but . . . .").
  - Elicit responses from all participants by asking for their ideas/feelings ("Mr. X, how do you feel about that?").
  - Corroborate group response ("Is this consistent with how all of you are feeling?").
  - Respond to all input in a positive manner. Find something positive to say about all participant contributions, no matter how off target they may be.
  - Reaffirm individual input by referring back to what the person may have said or discussed earlier.

**Figure 23-5. Practical Tips for Group Facilitation**

*Note.* Based on information from National Center for Training, Support, and Technical Assistance, 2009.

## The Role of Oncology Nurses in Interprofessional Cancer Care

Nurses are strategic members of the oncology interprofessional team throughout the cancer care continuum (Rieger, 2002). The interprofessional team approach to cancer care can provide patients with access to comprehensive specialty care. However, incomplete or inadequate flow of information can lead to inconsistency in patient/family-centered communication. Nurses' skill in managing their intermediary role is crucial as team members work together to elevate the quality of care given (Wittenberg-Lyles et al., 2013). Communication training models, therefore, must include interprofessional communication in the program (Turner, 2011; Wittenberg-Lyles et al., 2013).

Interprofessional pathways have been developed to help define the different roles of team members to optimize psychosocial outcomes. The use of standardized psychosocial assessments is burgeoning (e.g., National Comprehensive Cancer Network® Distress Thermometer), setting a standard for oncology professionals to identify psychosocial problems and refer to appropriate interprofessional team members when necessary.

As a valuable team member, the nurse's role is to participate and support interprofessional care and carry out interprofessional referrals when needed. Nurses have a responsibility, along with team members, to monitor patient outcomes in psychosocial care, to create evidence-based practice, to evaluate cost-effective pathways that promote psychosocial interventions, and to help coordinate interprofessional team communication (Rieger, 2002).

The interprofessional team not only serves to bring rich resources to the complex problems presented by patients with cancer and their families but also serves to bring those same resources to support the team members themselves. Medland, Howard-Ruben, and Whitaker (2004) described using the resources of the interprofessional team to develop a "circle of care" retreat. The goal of this retreat was to create a community among nurses and team members to examine work stress, promote effective coping mechanisms, and reduce burnout among interprofessional team members. The Schwartz Center sponsors Schwartz Center Rounds, which are interprofessional forums that explore the patient–caregiver relationship in more than 350 hospitals nationwide. As a result of these rounds, healthcare professionals involved have expressed an enhanced sense of team building and community (Manning, Acker, Houseman, Pressman, & Goodman, 2008). The interprofessional team approach also decreases the risks of professional isolation and feelings of professional inadequacy by supporting and validating the challenges that each member faces when involved in meeting the complex needs of patients experiencing cancer. Team members can find comfort and safety to express their feelings in a supportive atmosphere. Oncology nurses must recognize that they are an integral part of the patient's team, which is made up of all the professionals who are involved in the care of the patient and their family. This includes members in settings from the hospital to outpatient and home care, including nurses and physicians, social workers, chaplains, and mental health professionals. Nurses must recognize all members who contribute to the psychosocial care of patients and family members as valuable resources to consult. This may include hospital volunteers or nurse aides who take part in patients' experience of care.

## Conclusion

Patients with cancer and their families emotionally respond to the experience of cancer in many different ways based on their own life experiences, belief systems, coping mechanisms, culture and ethnicity, and communication styles. Therefore, oncology nurses must be prepared for a myriad of emotional responses, many of which are not always evident and easy to assess (e.g., patients who display outwardly stoic behavior). The emotional pain of these patients may go unaddressed and unattended in contrast to the patients who demonstrate visible emotions and behaviors, such as tearfulness or anger. Through mastering professional communication skills and active listening techniques, oncology nurses can recognize cues to enhance patient and family communication, problem solving, and coping. Oncology nurses who are competent in interpersonal and therapeutic skills and skilled members of an interprofessional team are better equipped to provide holistic psychosocial care to patients and families.

# References

Adamsen, L., & Rasmussen, J.M. (2003). Exploring and encouraging through social interaction: A qualitative study of nurses participation in self-help groups for cancer patients. *Cancer Nursing, 26,* 28–36. doi:10.1097/00002820-200302000-00004

Arnold, E.C. (2016a). Developing therapeutic communication skills. In E.C. Arnold & K.U. Boggs (Eds.), *Interpersonal relationships: Professional communication skills for nurses* (7th ed., pp. 75–97). St. Louis, MO: Elsevier.

Arnold, E.C. (2016b). Intercultural communication. In E.C. Arnold & K.U. Boggs (Eds.), *Interpersonal relationships: Professional communication skills for nurses* (7th ed., pp. 113–135). St. Louis, MO: Elsevier.

Back, A., Arnold, R., & Tulsky, J. (2010). *Mastering communication with seriously ill patients: Balancing honesty with empathy and hope.* New York, NY: Cambridge University Press.

Baer, L., & Weinstein, E. (2013). Improving oncology nurses' communication skills for difficult conversations [Online exclusive]. *Clinical Journal of Oncology Nursing, 17,* E45–E51. doi:10.1188/13.CJON.E45-E51

Baile, W.F., Buckman, R., Lenzi, R., Glober, G., Beale, E.A., & Kudelka, A.P. (2000). SPIKES—A six-step protocol for delivering bad news: Application to the patient with cancer. *Oncologist, 5,* 302–311. doi:10.1634/theoncologist.5-4-302

Baile, W.F., & Parker, P.A. (2011). Breaking bad news. In D.W. Kissane, B.D. Bultz, P.M. Butow, & I.G. Finlay (Eds.), *Handbook of communication in oncology and palliative care* (pp. 101–112). New York, NY: Oxford University Press.

Boggs, K.U. (2016a). Professional guides for nursing communication. In E.C. Arnold & K.U. Boggs (Eds.), *Interpersonal relationships: Professional communication skills for nurses* (7th ed., pp. 22–39). St. Louis, MO: Elsevier.

Boggs, K.U. (2016b). Variation in communication styles. In E.C. Arnold & K.U. Boggs (Eds.), *Interpersonal relationships: Professional communication skills for nurses* (7th ed., pp. 99–112). St. Louis, MO: Elsevier.

Buckman, R.A. (1992). *How to break bad news: A guide for healthcare professionals.* Baltimore, MD: Johns Hopkins University Press.

Buckman, R.A. (2005). Breaking bad news: The S-P-I-K-E-S strategy. *Community Oncology, 2,* 138–142. doi:10.1016/S1548-5315(11)70867-1

Chelf, J.H., Agre, P., Axelrod, A., Cheney, L., Cole, D.D., Conrad, K., ... Weaver, C. (2001). Cancer-related patient education: An overview of the last decade of evaluation and research. *Oncology Nursing Forum, 28,* 1139–1147.

Christie, W., & Moore, C. (2004). The impact of humor on patients with cancer. *Clinical Journal of Oncology Nursing, 9,* 211–218. doi:10.1188/05.CJON.211-218

Dean, R.A.K., & Major, J.E. (2008). From critical care to comfort care: The sustaining value of humour. *Journal of Clinical Nursing, 17,* 1088–1095. doi:10.1111/j.1365-2702.2007.02090.x

Donaldson, S. (2004). Introduction. In B. Hoffman (Ed.), *A cancer survivor's almanac: Charting your journey* (3rd ed., pp. 1–2). Hoboken, NJ: John Wiley & Sons.

Fallowfield, L.J., Jenkins, V.A., & Beveridge, H.A. (2002). Truth may hurt but deceit hurts more: Communication in palliative care. *Palliative Medicine, 16,* 297–300. doi:10.1191/0269216302pm575oa

Friedrichsen, M.J., Strang, P.M., & Carlsson, M.E. (2002). Cancer patients' interpretations of verbal expressions when given information about ending cancer treatment. *Palliative Medicine, 16,* 323–330. doi:10.1191/0269216302pm543oa

Frost, M.H., Brueggen, C., & Mangan, M. (1997). Intervening with the psychosocial needs of patients and families: Perceived importance and skill level. *Cancer Nursing, 20,* 350–358. doi:10.1097/00002820-199710000-00006

Fukui, S., Ogawa, K., & Yamagishi, A. (2011). Effectiveness of communication skills training on the quality of life and satisfaction with healthcare professionals among newly diagnosed cancer patients: A preliminary study. *Psycho-Oncology, 20,* 1285–1291. doi:10.1002/pon.1840

Garnham, P. (2001). Understanding and dealing with anger, aggression and violence. *Nursing Standard, 16*(6), 37–42.

Goldsmith, J., Ferrell, B., Wittenberg-Lyles, E., & Ragan, S.L. (2013). Palliative care communication in oncology nursing. *Clinical Journal of Oncology Nursing, 17,* 163–167. doi:10.1188/13.CJON.163-167

Harder, H., Ballinger, R., Langridge, C., Ring, A., & Fallowfield, L.J. (2013). Adjuvant chemotherapy in elderly women with breast cancer: Patients' perspectives on information giving and decision making. *Psycho-Oncology, 22,* 2729–2735. doi:10.1002/pon3338

Hauser, J., & Makoul, G. (2011). Medical student training in communication skills. In D.W. Kissane, B.D. Bultz, P.M. Butow, & I.G. Finlay (Eds.), *Handbook of communication in oncology and palliative care* (pp. 75–85). New York, NY: Oxford University Press.

Heaven, C., & Maguire, P. (1996). Training hospice nurses to elicit patient concerns. *Journal of Advanced Nursing, 23,* 280–286. doi:10.1111/j.1365-2648.1996.tb02668.x

Helft, P., Chamness, A., Colin, T., & Ulrich, M. (2011). Oncology nurses' attitudes toward prognosis-related communication: A pilot mailed survey of Oncology Nursing Society members. *Oncology Nursing Forum, 38,* 468–474. doi:10.1188/11.ONF.468-474

Helman, C.G. (2007). *Culture, health and illness* (5th ed.). London, England: Hodder Arnold.

Higgins, D. (2002). Breaking bad news in cancer care part 2: Practical skills. *Professional Nurse, 17,* 670–671.

Hughes, M. (2009). Communication issues for oncology nurses at difficult times. In C.C. Burke (Ed.), *Psychosocial dimensions of oncology nursing care* (2nd ed., pp. 29–57). Pittsburgh, PA: Oncology Nursing Society.

Institute of Medicine. (2002). *Unequal treatment: What healthcare providers need to know about racial and ethnic disparities in healthcare.* Washington, DC: National Academies Press.

Jansen, J., van Weert, J., de Groot, J., van Dulmen, S., Heeren, T.J., & Bensing, J.M. (2010). Emotional and informational patient cues: The impact of nurses' responses on recall. *Patient Education and Counseling, 79,* 218–224. doi:10.1016/j.pec.2009.10.010

Johnson, P. (2002). The use of humor and its influences on spirituality and coping in breast cancer survivors. *Oncology Nursing Forum, 29,* 691–695. doi:10.1188/02.ONF.691-695

Kist, S. (2016). Communicating with families. In E.C. Arnold & K.U. Boggs (Eds.), *Interpersonal relationships: Professional communication skills for nurses* (7th ed., pp. 217–240). St. Louis, MO: Elsevier.

Lee, Y.-H., Chiou, P.-Y., Chang, P.-H., & Hayter, M. (2010). A systematic review of the effectiveness of problem-solving approaches towards symptom management in cancer care. *Journal of Clinical Nursing, 20,* 73–85. doi:10.1111/j.1365-2702.2010.03401.x

Liehr, P. (2005). Story theory for practice and research. In L. Williams, *Stories of oncology family caregiving.* Instructional session presented at the 30th Annual Congress of the Oncology Nursing Society, Orlando, FL.

Lovejoy, N., & Matteis, M. (1997). Cognitive-behavioral interventions to manage depression in patients with cancer: Research and theoretical initiatives. *Cancer Nursing, 20,* 155–167. doi:10.1097/00002820-199706000-00001

MacDonald, C.M. (2004). A chuckle a day keeps the doctor away: Therapeutic humor and laughter. *Journal of Psychosocial Nursing and Mental Health Services, 42*(3), 18–25.

MacDonald, D.J. (2002). Women's decisions regarding management of breast cancer risk. *MEDSURG Nursing, 11,* 183–186.

Maguire, P. (1985). Barriers to psychological care of the dying. *BMJ, 29,* 1711–1713. doi:10.1136/bmj.291.6510.1711

Maliski, S.L., Heilemann, M.V., & McCorkle, R. (2002). From "death sentence" to "good cancer": Couples' transformation of a prostate cancer diagnosis. *Nursing Research, 51,* 391–397. doi:10.1097/00006199-200211000-00007

Manning, C., Acker, M., Houseman, L., Pressman, E., & Goodman, I. (2008). *The Schwartz Center Rounds® evaluation report.* Retrieved from http://www.theschwartzcenter.org/media/PTXAAE65CHR5UU4.pdf

McGilton, K., Irwin-Robinson, H., Boscart, V., & Spanjevic, L. (2006). Communication enhancement: Nurse and patient satisfaction outcomes in a complex continuing care facility. *Journal of Advanced Nursing, 54,* 35–44. doi:10.1111/j.1365-2648.2006.03787.x

Medland, J., Howard-Ruben, J., & Whitaker, E. (2004). Fostering psychosocial wellness in oncology nurses: Addressing burnout and social support in the workplace. *Oncology Nursing Forum, 31,* 47–54. doi:10.1188/04.ONF.47-54

Milbury, K., Spelman, A., Wood, C., Matin, S., Tannir, N., Jonasch, E., ... Cohen, L. (2014). Randomized controlled trial of expressive writing for patients with renal cell carcinoma. *Journal of Clinical Oncology, 32,* 663–670. doi:10.1200/JCO.2013.50.3532

Mishel, M.H., Beylyea, M., Germino, B.B., Stewart, J.L., Bailey, D.E., Jr., Robertson, C., & Mohler, J. (2002). Helping patients with localized prostate carcinoma manage uncertainty and treatment side effects: Nurse-delivered psychoeducational intervention over the telephone. *Cancer, 94,* 1854–1866. doi:10.1002/cncr.10390

Moore, P.M., Rivera Mercado, S., Grez Artigues, M., & Lawrie, T.A. (2013). Communication skills training for healthcare professionals working with people who have cancer. *Cochrane Database of Systematic Reviews, 2013*(3). doi:10.1002/14651858.CD003751.pub3

Mullan, F. (1996). Survivorship: A powerful place. In B. Hoffman (Ed.), *A cancer survivor's almanac: Charting your journey* (pp. xvii–xix). Silver Spring, MD: National Coalition for Cancer Survivorship.

Nail, L.M. (2001). I'm coping as fast as I can: Psychosocial adjustment to cancer and cancer treatment. *Oncology Nursing Forum, 28,* 967–970.

National Center for Training, Support, and Technical Assistance. (2009). Working with groups: A group facilitation manual. Retrieved from http://www.proceedinc.com/_media/GroupFacilitationManual-COPYRIGHT.pdf

National Comprehensive Cancer Network. (2017). *NCCN Clinical Practice Guidelines in Oncology (NCCN Guidelines®): Distress management* [v.2.2017]. Retrieved from https://www.nccn.org/professionals/physician_gls/pdf/distress.pdf

Paice, J.A. (2002). Managing psychological conditions in palliative care: Dying need not mean enduring controllable anxiety, depression, or delirium. *American Journal of Nursing, 102*(11), 36–43. doi:10.1097/00000446-200211000-00023

Peterson, M. (1988). The norms and values held by three groups of nurses concerning psychosocial nursing practice. *International Journal of Nursing Studies, 25,* 85–103. doi:10.1016/0020-7489(88)90077-6

Philip, J., & Kissane, D. (2011). Responding to difficult emotions. In D.W. Kissane, B.D. Bultz, P.M. Butow, & I.G. Finlay (Eds.), *Handbook of communication in oncology and palliative care* (pp. 136–145). New York, NY: Oxford University Press.

Rancour, P., & Brauer, K. (2003). Use of letter writing as a means of integrating an altered body image: A case study. *Oncology Nursing Forum, 30,* 841–846. doi:10.1188/03.ONF.841-846

Rautalinko, E. (2013). Reflective listening and open-ended questions in counseling: Preferences moderated by social skills and cognitive ability. *Counseling and Psychotherapy Research, 13,* 24–31. doi:10.1080/14733145.2012.687387

Rieger, P. (2002). Collegiality. *Oncologist, 7*(Suppl. 2), 7. doi:10.1634/theoncologist.7-suppl_2-7

Riess, H., & Kraft-Todd, G. (2014). E.M.P.A.T.H.Y.: A tool to enhance nonverbal communication between clinicians and their patients. *Academic Medicine, 89,* 1108–1112. doi:10.1097/ACM.0000000000000287

Ross, L., & Johansen, C. (2002). Psychosocial home visits in cancer treatment. *Cancer Nursing, 25,* 350–357.

Royak-Schaler, R., Gadalla, S.M., Lemkau, J.P., Ross, D.D., Alexander, C., & Scott, D. (2006). Family perspectives on communication with healthcare providers during end-of-life cancer care. *Oncology Nursing Forum, 33,* 753–760. doi:10.1188/06.ONF.753-760

Schofield, P.E., Butow, P.N., Thompson, J.F., Tatersall, M.H.N., Beeney, L.J., & Dunn, S.M. (2003). Psychological responses of patients receiving a diagnosis of cancer. *Annals of Oncology, 14,* 48–56. doi:10.1093/annonc/mdg010

Sealy, P. (2012). Autoethnography: Reflective journaling and meditation to cope with life-threatening breast cancer. *Clinical Journal of Oncology Nursing, 16,* 38–41. doi:10.1188/12.CJON.38-41

Shannon-Dorcy, K., & Wolf, V. (2003). Decision making in the diagnosis and treatment of leukemia. *Seminars in Oncology Nursing, 19,* 142–149.

Siminoff, L.A. (2011). The ethics of communication in cancer and palliative care. In D.W. Kissane, B.D. Bultz, P.M. Butow, & I.G. Finlay (Eds.), *Handbook of communication in oncology and palliative care* (pp. 51–61). New York, NY: Oxford University Press.

Smith, M.E., & Hart, G. (1994). Nurses' response to patient anger: From disconnecting to connecting. *Journal of Advanced Nursing, 20,* 643–651. doi:10.1046/j.1365-2648.1994.20040643.x

Smith, M.J., & Liehr, P.R. (2013). Story theory. In M.J. Smith & P.R. Liehr (Eds.), *Middle range theory for nursing* (3rd ed., pp. 225–252). New York, NY: Springer.

Stanley, K. (2002). The healing power of presence: Respite from the fear of abandonment. *Oncology Nursing Forum, 29,* 935–940. doi:10.1188/02.ONF.935-940

Tanay, M.A., Roberts, J., & Ream, E. (2013). Humour in adult cancer care: A concept analysis. *Journal of Advanced Nursing, 69,* 2131–2140. doi:10.1111/jan.12059

Tattersall, M.H.N. (2011). Clinician perspectives on shared decision-making. In D.W. Kissane, B.D. Bultz, P.M. Butow, & I.G. Finlay (Eds.), *Handbook of communication in oncology and palliative care* (pp. 339–349). New York, NY: Oxford University Press.

Thomas, B.C., Lounsberry, J.J., & Carlson, L.E. (2011). Challenges in communicating with ethnically diverse populations. In D.W. Kissane, B.D. Bultz, P.M. Butow, & I.G. Finlay (Eds.), *Handbook of communication in oncology and palliative care* (pp. 375–387). New York, NY: Oxford University Press.

Thomas, S.P. (2003). Anger: The mismanaged emotion. *MEDSURG Nursing, 12,* 103–110.

Townsend, M.C. (2015). *Psychiatric mental health nursing.* Philadelphia, PA: F.A. Davis.

Turner, J. (2011). Working as a multidisciplinary team. In D.W. Kissane, B.D. Bultz, P.M. Butow, & I.G. Finlay (Eds.), *Handbook of communication in oncology and palliative care* (pp. 245–257). New York, NY: Oxford University Press.

Uitterhoeve, R., Bensing, J., Dilven, E., Donders, R., deMulder, P., & van Achterberg, T. (2009). Nurse–patient communication in cancer care: Does responding to patient's cues predict patient satisfaction with communication. *Psycho-Oncology, 18,* 1060–1068. doi:10.1002/pon.1434

Uitterhoeve, R., Bensing, J., Grol, R., deMulder, P., & van Achterberg, T. (2010). The effect of communication skills training on patient outcomes in cancer care: A systematic review of the literature. *European Journal of Cancer Care, 19,* 442–457. doi:10.1111/j.1365-2354.2009.01082.x

Ullrich, P.M., & Lutgendorf, S.K. (2002). Journaling about stressful events: Effects of cognitive processing and emotional expression. *Annals of Behavioral Medicine, 24,* 244–250. doi:10.1207/S15324796ABM2403_10

Wilkinson, S. (1991). Factors which influence how nurses communicate with cancer patients. *Journal of Advanced Nursing, 16,* 677–688. doi:10.1111/j.1365-2648.1991.tb01726.x

Wilkinson, S., Perry, R., Blanchard, K., & Linsell, L. (2008). Effectiveness of a three-day communication skills course in changing nurses' communication skills with cancer/palliative care patients: A randomized controlled trial. *Palliative Medicine, 22,* 365–375. doi:10.1177/0269216308090770

Winterburn, S., & Wilkinson, S. (2011). The challenges and rewards of communication skills training for oncology and palliative care nurses in the United Kingdom. In D.W. Kissane, B.D. Bultz, P.M. Butow, & I.G. Finlay (Eds.), *Handbook of communication in oncology and palliative care* (pp. 425–438). New York, NY: Oxford University Press.

Wittenberg-Lyles, E., Goldsmith, J., & Ferrell, B. (2013). Oncology nurse communication barriers to patient-centered care. *Clinical Journal of Oncology Nursing, 17,* 152–158. doi:10.1188/13.CJON.152-158

Zamanzadeh, V., Rassouli, M., Abbaszadeh, A., Nikanfar, A., Alavi-Majd, H., & Ghahramanian, A. (2014). Factors influencing communication between the patients with cancer and their nurses in oncology wards. *Indian Journal of Palliative Care, 20,* 12–20. doi:10.4103/0973-1075.125549

Zhang, A.Y., & Siminoff, L.A. (2003). The role of the family in treatment decision making by patients with cancer. *Oncology Nursing Forum, 30,* 1022–1028. doi:10.1188/03.ONF.1022-1028

CHAPTER 24

# Substance Abuse and Addiction

*Yu-Ping Chang, PhD, RN, FGSA, and Peggy Compton, RN, PhD, FAAN*

> *We don't choose to be addicted; what we choose to do is deny our pain.*
>
> —Anonymous

Substance abuse and addiction disorders are chronic diseases that can complicate the nursing care of patients with cancer in subtle yet challenging and important ways. They may affect patients' ability to comply with treatment protocols, affect physiologic responses to therapy and surgery, and complicate responses to pain management and the use of analgesia. Effective treatments for these diseases exist, and recovery brings improvements in multiple aspects of the individual's life. Substance abuse and addiction are not uncommon comorbidities in patients with cancer, and, at least in the case of alcohol and smoking, play a demonstrated role in the etiology of oncologic disease. Assessment for and management of addiction in patients with cancer are necessary to provide optimal nursing care.

## Epidemiology

Substance use disorders, more commonly referred to as substance abuse, substance dependence, or addiction, are not uncommon in the United States today and are therefore likely to be encountered in oncology nursing. The most prevalent cases are those associated with alcohol and nicotine use. According to the National Survey on Drug Use and Health (NSDUH), in 2013, approximately half (52.2%) of all Americans aged 12 or older reported having had at least one alcoholic drink in the past 30 days, with 6.6% meeting the criteria of alcohol use disorder (Substance Abuse and Mental Health Services Administration [SAMHSA], 2014). Furthermore, more than one-fifth (22.9%) of people aged 12 or older engaged in binge drinking (drinking five or more drinks on one occasion) at least once in the past 30 days, with another 6.3% reporting that they engaged in heavy drinking (five or more drinks on five or more occasions during the past 30 days) (SAMHSA, 2014).

In 2013, approximately 21.3% of the U.S. population (55.8 million) identified as being current cigarette smokers. Along with this number, 4.7% of people (12.4 million) smoked cigars,

3.4% (12.4 million) used smokeless tobacco, and 0.9 % (2.3 million) smoked tobacco in pipes (SAMHSA, 2014). Cigarette use among youth has been particularly concerning, as young cigarette smokers are more likely to use illicit drugs, with 53.9% reporting concurrent illicit drug use, as compared to only 6.1% in nonsmokers. Eighty-eight percent of adult daily smokers first smoked by the age of 18, and 99% had first smoked by the age of 26 (SAMHSA, 2014).

The use of illicit drugs is also prevalent in the United States. In 2013, an estimated 9.4% of Americans (24.6 million) aged 12 or older had used an illicit drug in the month prior to taking the SAMHSA survey (see Table 24-1). Although increasingly decriminalized, marijuana is by far the most commonly used "illicit" drug in the United States. It was used by 80% of those who identified as illicit drug users in 2013, representing 7.5% (19.8 million) of the population (SAMHSA, 2014). Following in prevalence is the nonmedical use of prescription drugs (i.e., pain relievers, tranquilizers, stimulants, or sedatives) by 2.5% Americans (6.5 million), with the majority (4.5 million) reporting nonmedical use of prescription pain relievers (SAMHSA, 2014). Illicit drug use is also associated with alcohol use. Among youths who were heavy drinkers, 67% also were current illicit drug users, whereas among nondrinkers, the rate was only 5.6% (SAMHSA, 2014).

With repeated use, some substance users will develop the neuropsychological disease of a "substance use disorder" described in the *Diagnostic and Statistical Manual of Mental Disorders (DSM-V)* (American Psychiatric Association [APA], 2013). The *DSM-V* conceptualizes substance abuse as a single disorder measured on a continuum of severity from mild to severe, determined by the number of diagnostic criteria met by an individual. Each specific substance is addressed as a separate use disorder, but all are characterized on the same overarching criteria. For example, mild substance use disorder in the *DSM-V* requires two to three symptoms from a list of 11 (see Figure 24-1) and is based on evidence of impaired control (e.g., inability to control use, continued use despite consequences), social impairment

### Table 24-1. Illicit Drug Use in the Past Month Among Individuals Aged 12 or Older

| Substance | Aged 12 or Older Number in Thousands | Percent | Aged 12 to 17 Number in Thousands | Percent | Aged 18 or Older Number in Thousands | Percent |
|---|---|---|---|---|---|---|
| All illicit drugs | 24,573 | 9.4 | 2,197 | 8.8 | 22,376 | 9.4 |
| Marijuana | 19,810 | 7.5 | 1,762 | 7.1 | 18,048 | 7.6 |
| Cocaine | 1,549 | 0.6 | 43 | 0.2 | 1,505 | 0.6 |
| Inhalants | 496 | 0.2 | 121 | 0.5 | 375 | 0.2 |
| Hallucinogens | 1,333 | 0.5 | 154 | 0.6 | 1,179 | 0.5 |
| Heroin | 289 | 0.1 | 13 | 0.1 | 277 | 0.1 |
| Nonmedical use of prescription-type drugs | 6,484 | 2.5 | 549 | 2.2 | 5,935 | 2.5 |
| Pain relievers | 4,521 | 1.7 | 425 | 1.7 | 4,096 | 1.7 |

Numbers and percentages do not sum to the illicit drug use estimate, as individuals may have used more than one illicit drug.

*Note.* Based on information from Substance Abuse and Mental Health Services Administration, 2014.

A problematic pattern of alcohol use leading to clinically significant impairment or distress, as manifested by at least two of the following, occurring within a 12-month period:
- Alcohol is often taken in larger amounts or over a longer period than was intended.
- There is a persistent desire or unsuccessful efforts to cut down or control alcohol use.
- A great deal of time is spent in activities necessary to obtain alcohol, use alcohol, or recover from its effect.
- Craving, or a strong desire or urge to use alcohol.
- Recurrent alcohol use resulting in a failure to fulfill major role obligations at work, school, or home
- Continued alcohol use despite having persistent or recurrent social or interpersonal problems caused or exacerbated by the effects of alcohol.
- Important social, occupational, or recreational activities are given up or reduced because of alcohol use.
- Recurrent alcohol use in situations in which it is physically hazardous.
- Alcohol use is continued despite knowledge of having a persistent or recurrent physical or psychological problem that is likely to have been caused or exacerbated by alcohol.
- Tolerance, as defined by either of the following:
  – A need for markedly increased amounts of alcohol to achieve intoxication or desired effect.
  – A markedly diminished effect with continued use of the same amount of alcohol.
- Withdrawal, as manifested by either of the following:
  – The characteristic withdrawal syndrome for alcohol.
  – Alcohol (or a closely related substance, such as a benzodiazepine) is taken to relieve or avoid withdrawal symptoms.

Mild: Presence of 2–3 symptoms
Moderate: Presence of 4–5 symptoms
Severe: Presence of 6 or more symptoms

**Figure 24-1. Diagnostic Criteria for Alcohol Use Disorder and Other Substance Abuse Disorders**

*Note.* From *Diagnostic and Statistical Manual of Mental Disorders* (5th ed., pp. 490–491), by American Psychiatric Association, 2013, Washington, DC: Author. Copyright 2013 by American Psychiatric Association. Reprinted with permission.

(e.g., failure to fulfill role obligations), risky use, and pharmacologic symptoms. An estimated 8.2% of Americans (21.6 million) aged 12 or older were diagnosed with a current substance use disorder in 2013, and approximately 20.3 million adults aged 18 or older had a substance use disorder in the past year, which translates to 8.5% of adults (SAMHSA, 2014).

Thus, at any one point in time, almost 1 out of 7 Americans (14.6%) meet the diagnostic criteria for substance use disorder, making it one of the most common chronic diseases in the United States (Kessler et al., 2005). Its impact on crime (e.g., domestic violence, child abuse) and health (e.g., organ impairment, infections, motor vehicle accidents) make it one of the most expensive diseases in this country, costing Americans more than $700 billion annually. This includes approximately $295 billion for tobacco ($130 billion in health care) (U.S. Department of Health and Human Services [U.S. DHHS], 2014), $224 billion for alcohol ($25 billion in health care) (Centers for Disease Control and Prevention, 2014), and $224 billion for illicit drugs ($11 billion in health care) (U.S. Department of Justice, 2011). These numbers do not fully describe consequences of substance abuse and addiction with respect to the suffering experienced by users and their families.

# Substance Use Disorders in Oncology Populations

The prevalence of substance use disorder in cancer populations is not well documented. For the purposes of this review, the term *substance abuse* will be used interchangeably with substance use disorder. A low rate of substance abuse was reported in early studies that found that less than 5% of patients with cancer had substance abuse disorders (Derogatis et al., 1983; Passik, Portenoy, & Ricketts, 1998). This low rate was likely due to underreporting and sample section biases. A single longitudinal observational cohort study using Surveillance, Epidemiology, and End Results–Medicare linked data from 2000 to 2009 found the prevalence of substance use disorder in men with advanced prostate cancer to be 10.6% (Chhatre, Metzger, Malkowicz, Woody, & Jayadevappa, 2014). One year following diagnosis, those patients with prostate cancer who had substance use disorder or drug-related psychoses had greater odds of inpatient hospitalizations, outpatient hospital visits, and emergency department visits; 60%–70% higher health costs; and higher hazard of all-cause mortality, compared to those without substance use disorders and/or psychoses (Chhatre et al., 2014).

Alcohol use disorders are prevalent but often go undiagnosed in patients with cancer. Recent studies showed that between 17% and 24% of patients with cancer screen positive for alcoholism (Dev et al., 2011; Jenkins, Schulz, Hanson, & Bruera, 2000; Parsons et al., 2008). In a chart review study of 598 patients with advanced cancers who completed the CAGE substance abuse screening tool (see Figure 24-2), 17% were screened as alcoholic; however, only 13% of those were identified as alcoholic before their palliative care consultation (Dev et al., 2011). Compared to CAGE-negative patients, alcoholic patients were more likely to be referred to the palliative consultation earlier; report more severe symptoms (e.g., pain, sleep, dyspnea, well-being, distress) at baseline referral; and were more frequently on opioids at baseline (referral) and follow-up (Parsons et al., 2008). Both CAGE-positive patients and patients with a history of tobacco use were more likely to receive potent opioids at the time of their palliative care consultation (Dev et al., 2011).

Two recent studies reported even higher rates of substance abuse in patients with cancer receiving opioid therapy (39% to 45%) (Anghelescu, Ehrentraut, & Faughnan, 2013; Barclay, Owens, & Blackhall, 2014). Using structured interviews and the Screener and Opioid Assessment for Patients with Pain–Revised (SOAPP-R), Anghelescu et al. (2013) found that 15 of 38 patients with cancer (39.5%) receiving chronic opioid therapy were at high-risk for aberrant opioid misuse. Using a chart review, Barclay et al. (2014) found that 43% of 114 patients with cancer receiving opioid treatment in a palliative care clinic were at medium to high risk for opioid abuse based on a self-reported opioid risk tool. Of those patients with available urine drug testing (UDT) results, 45.6% showed abnormal findings, including absence of prescribed medications and presence of illicit drugs (primarily marijuana) (Barclay et al., 2014). Younger age and a personal history of alcohol and illicit drug abuse were common risk factors associated with self-reported opioid misuse, while a positive family history of alcohol abuse and a personal history of illicit drug abuse were risk factors of abnormal UDT findings (Barclay et al., 2014). The risk factors identified in Barclay's study are similar to many other studies conducted in patients receiving opioid therapy for noncancer pain (Jamison & Edwards, 2013).

---

- Have you ever felt you could **C**ut down on your drinking (or drug use)?
- Have people **A**nnoyed you by criticizing your drinking (or drug use)?
- Have you ever felt bad or **G**uilty about your drinking (or drug use)?
- Have you ever had an **E**ye-opener first thing in the morning to steady your nerves or get rid of a hangover?

**Figure 24-2. The CAGE Questionnaire**

*Note.* Based on information from Ewing, 1984.

# Addictive Disease

As with all chronic diseases, addiction has multiple risk factors and a pathophysiologic basis. It can be diagnosed according to a well-described cluster of signs and symptoms, follows a predictable pattern of progression, and can be managed and treated with interventions of known efficacy. As with other diseases, its expression in the individual is unique and varied, and its negative effects protract onto psychological and social domains. Treatment approaches include pharmacotherapy, cognitive behavioral skills training, motivational interviewing, counseling, family therapy, group support, and lifestyle changes (Miller, Forcehimes, Zweben, & McLellan, 2011).

Not unlike Parkinson disease, schizophrenia, and depression, addiction is a disease of the brain. All drugs of abuse, including alcohol and nicotine, activate two key pathways in the brain, which are believed to underlie their "addictive" properties (see Figure 24-3). First, drugs and alcohol activate so-called "reward" pathways in subcortical areas extending from the ventral tegmental area to the nucleus accumbens, providing very reinforcing or pleasurable feelings. Next, this reward sets very strong memories that drive subsequent behaviors to repeat the rewarding experience. Over time, the drug-induced behaviors take

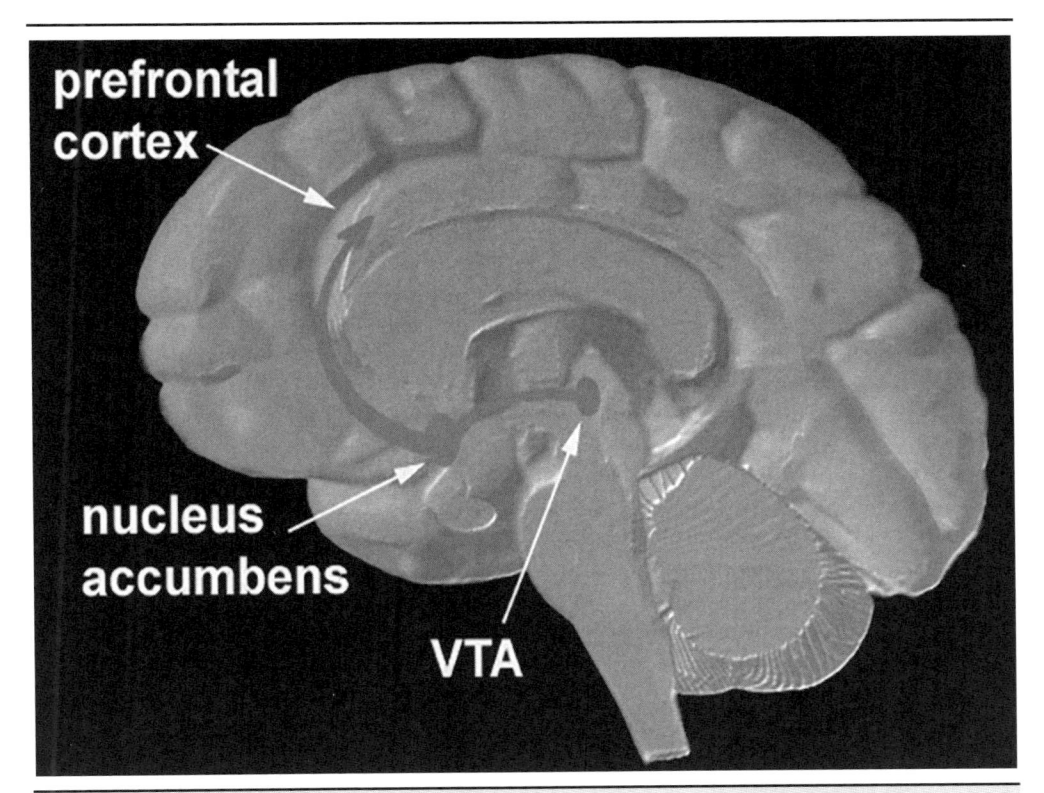

**Figure 24-3. Brain Pathways Involved in Addictive Disease (The Reward Pathway)**

VTA—ventral tegmental area

*Note.* From "The Neurobiology of Drug Addiction," by National Institute of Drug Abuse, 2007. Retrieved from http://www.drugabuse.gov/publications/teaching-packets/neurobiology-drug-addiction/section-ii-reward-pathway-addiction/3-reward-pathway.

over more volitional behaviors to become the predominant behavior state of the diseased individual, meeting the diagnostic criteria of a substance use disorder (Brick & Erickson, 2012).

The nature and course of addictive disease have been well characterized. Not uncommonly does the sufferer of addictive disease also suffer from a concurrent psychiatric illness or disorder. NSDUH data show that serious mental illness, which is defined as a diagnosable mental, behavioral, or emotional disorder meeting *DSM-V* criteria (APA, 2013), resulting in functional impairment that substantially interferes with or limits one or more major life activities, is strongly correlated with substance dependence or abuse (SAMHSA, 2014). Among adults with substance use disorder, 20.4% also had a serious mental illness in the past year. Conversely, 23.2% of adults with serious mental illness were dependent on or abused alcohol or illicit drugs, a rate almost three times higher than adults without serious mental illness. An estimated four million adults met the criteria for both serious mental illness and substance use disorder in 2014 (SAMHSA, 2014).

Addiction also is a familial disease. A family history of substance abuse, whether for alcohol or other prescribed or illicit drugs, is a risk factor for addictive disease in all clinical populations. Large surveys of adoptees and twins reared apart from their biologic family of origin indicate that heredity is a stronger predictor of alcoholism than is environment (Tyndale, 2003). Children of alcoholics and members of certain ethnic groups demonstrate patterned differences in their physiologic responses to alcohol (Evans & Levin, 2003). However, the importance of the family environment in predicting adult drug and alcohol dependence cannot be minimized. First exposure to a drug that might be only mildly rewarding in a neutral or comfortable environment becomes highly rewarding when the individual is experiencing significant or chronic stress—conditions that are more likely to be present in families experiencing alcoholism or addiction (Bjarnason et al., 2003).

With respect to the course of addictive disease, relapse is a relatively common occurrence, especially within the first 90 days of recovery or during times of undue stress (Bossert, Marchant, Calu, & Shaham, 2013; Everitt, 2014; Shalev, Erb, & Shaham, 2010). Too often considered a failure or an endpoint in the treatment of addictive disease, relapse reflects an exacerbation of a chronic disease or a disease state not under good control. In working with an addicted patient who has relapsed, the oncology nurse must try to minimize the extent of the relapse episode and help the patient to reframe it as a "slip" and a learning opportunity. If relapse is viewed as "part and parcel" of recovery as opposed to a treatment failure, positive outcomes are more likely (Witkiewitz & Marlatt, 2004).

Stress is a primary precipitator of relapse (Haass-Koffler & Bartlett, 2012; Schank, Ryabinin, Giardino, Ciccocioppo, & Heilig, 2012); strong psychological reliance on alcohol or drug use in addicted individuals functions to maintain behavior. As people become increasingly dependent on drugs and alcohol, their repertoire of adaptive coping responses to stress narrows, with drug use eventually becoming their primary coping mechanism. Drug- and alcohol-induced behaviors are extremely resistant to degradation and, unless the individual has developed alternate behaviors via coping strategies, supports, pharmacologic adjuncts, resources, or skills, drug and alcohol use will resume under stressful situations.

## Substances of Abuse as Carcinogens

The pathologic effects of abused substances on cells and body tissues play a role in inducing neoplastic changes. Best understood are the links between tobacco and alcohol abuse and cancer development. Little is known about carcinogenic effects of specific illicit drugs; however, a single recent study found a link between chronic marijuana use and lung cancer. In a 40-year cohort study in which 49,321 men aged 18–20 were followed, researchers found that using marijuana over 50 times throughout the study was associated with a two-fold risk of lung cancer (Callaghan, Allebeck, & Sidorchuck, 2013).

## Smoking and Cancer

Considerable evidence supports the strong link between tobacco use and lung cancer. Tobacco use also increases the risk for cancers of the mouth, lips, nose and sinuses, larynx, pharynx, esophagus, stomach, pancreas, kidney, bladder, uterus, cervix, colon/rectum, ovary (mucinous), and acute myeloid leukemia (American Cancer Society [ACS], 2014, 2017). Tobacco use accounts for at least 30% of all cancer deaths, causing 87% of lung cancer deaths in men and 70% of lung cancer deaths in women (ACS, 2014, 2017). Female smokers are 25.7 times more likely than female nonsmokers to develop lung cancer, and men smokers face 25 times the risk than men who never smoked (U.S. DHHS, 2014). Smoking contributes to cancer development by causing mutations in tumor suppressor genes and dominant oncogenes, impairing mucociliary clearance in the lungs, and decreasing immunologic response (Lee, Taneja, & Vassallo, 2012; Warren & Singh, 2013). Evidence supports that continued smoking increases the likelihood of a second cancer. Persons who initially presented with both smoking-related and non–smoking-related malignancy had increased risk of a second malignancy at the same site or another site if they continued to smoke (Gritz et al., 2006; Parsons, Daley, Begh, & Aveyard, 2010). Evidence is even stronger that continued smoking increases the risk of new primary cancers for up to 20 years after original diagnosis.

## Alcohol and Cancer

U.S. DHHS (2016) identified alcoholic beverages as a known human carcinogen. Considerable evidence suggests that increased alcohol consumption increased a person's risk of developing an alcohol-associated cancer. In 2009, it was estimated that 3.5% of all cancer deaths in the United States (about 19,500 deaths) were alcohol related (Nelson et al., 2013).

The strongest link between alcohol and cancer involves neoplasias of the upper digestive tract, including the esophagus, mouth, pharynx, larynx, liver, breast, colon, rectum, and pancreas (Boffetta & Hashibe, 2006). Chronic heavy drinkers have a higher incidence of esophageal cancer than that of the general population, and the risk increases with alcohol consumption. In fact, people who consume 50 or more grams of alcohol daily (approximately 3.5 or more drinks per day) have two to three times the risk of developing these cancers than nondrinkers (Baan et al., 2007).

Not surprisingly, alcohol consumption is an independent risk factor for and a primary cause of hepatocellular carcinoma (Grewal & Viswanathen, 2012). With respect to alcohol use and breast cancer, a meta-analysis of 53 studies (a total of 58,515 women with breast cancer) showed that women who consumed more than 45 grams of alcohol daily (approximately three drinks) had 1.5 times the risk of developing breast cancer than nondrinkers (Collaborative Group on Hormonal Factors in Breast Cancer, 2002). A slightly higher estimate of breast cancer was found in a study of 28,000 women with breast cancer in the United Kingdom, indicating that for every 10 grams of alcohol consumed daily (slightly less than one drink), the risk of breast cancer increased by 12% (Allen et al., 2009). Alcohol consumption is also associated with a modestly increased risk of cancers of the colon and rectum. A meta-analysis of 57 cohort and case-control studies showed that people who regularly consumed

50 or more grams of alcohol daily (approximately 3.5 drinks) had 1.5 times the risk of developing colorectal cancer as nondrinkers or occasional drinkers. As with breast cancers, for every 10 grams of alcohol consumed per day, the risk of colorectal cancer increases by 7% (Fedirko et al., 2011).

Although the actual mechanism by which alcohol increases cancer risk has not been fully understood, several potential explanations provide some understanding. Alcohol irritates the tissues of the mouth and throat, resulting in cellular injury, and in cellular repair processes, damaged cells may suffer DNA changes, resulting in neoplastic changes (Seitz & Stickel, 2007). Alcohol and its metabolites directly damage hepatocytes, leading to inflammation and scarring, again resulting in the potential DNA errors (Seitz & Stickel, 2007). Alcohol can lower the body's ability to absorb folate, and low folate levels have been shown to play a role in the risk of breast and colorectal cancers (Chen et al., 2014; Nan et al., 2013). This is worsened in heavy drinkers, who often do not get enough nutrients in their diet. Alcohol can raise the level of estrogen in the body, which affects the growth and development of breast tissue, potentially increasing the risk of breast cancer (Chen, Rosner, Hankinson, Colditz, & Willett, 2011).

In addition to its role as a primary carcinogen, alcohol may act as a cocarcinogen by enhancing the carcinogenic effects of other chemicals. This appears to explain why the combination of smoking and drinking is much more likely to cause cancers in the mouth or throat than either smoking or drinking alone. Alcohol may serve as a solvent in helping other carcinogens in tobacco to enter the cells lining the upper digestive tract more easily and make the mucosa more permeable for these carcinogens (Boffetta & Hashibe, 2006; Bosetti et al., 2002; Castellsagué et al., 1999; Hashibe et al., 2009). In humans, the risk for oral, tracheal, and esophageal cancers is 35 times greater for people who both smoke and drink than for people who neither smoke nor drink, supporting a cocarcinogenic interaction between alcohol- and tobacco-related carcinogens.

## Substance Abuse, Addiction, and Cancer Treatment

Ongoing use of tobacco, alcohol, and illicit drugs can interfere with the efficacy of therapies to treat cancer. Best described in the case of alcohol, pathophysiologic effects of abused substances and behavioral changes associated with addiction can thwart treatment effectiveness.

### Surgical Outcomes

Often, the treatment of oncologic disease includes surgical intervention. It is well-established that alcohol exerts chronic toxic effects on immune, cardiac, and hematopoietic function, and rates of postoperative morbidity and mortality resulting from infection, cardiopulmonary insufficiency, or bleeding disorders are two to five times greater in alcohol-dependent patients than in the general surgical population (de Wit, Goldberg, Hussein, & Neifeld, 2012; Genther & Gourin, 2012; Gili-Miner et al., 2014; Tønnesen & Kehlet, 1999; Tønnesen et al., 1992). Accordingly, alcoholics often require prolonged postoperative intensive care unit treatment and overall hospital stays (Gili-Miner et al., 2014) related to preoperative immune suppression, preoperative subclinical cardiomyopathy, and preoperative altered coagulation. Continued smoking is also related to increased rate of general complications after surgery (Khullar & Maa, 2012; Sharma et al., 2013). Smokers have slower postoperative wound healing because both nicotine and carbon monoxide cause vasoconstriction, inhibition of epithelization, and creation of cellular hypoxia (Khullar & Maa, 2012).

## Immunosuppressive Therapies

With respect to the effects of drugs and alcohol on the immune system, the effects of alcohol have been the most studied. Alcohol consumption has clearly been associated with suppression of the human immune system, which influences innate and adaptive immunity (Ippolito, Curtis, Choudhry, & Kovacs, 2013; Zhang, Bagby, Happel, Raasch, & Nelson, 2008). Common mechanisms by which alcohol alters the immune system include aberrant signal transduction pathways, excessive inflammation and oxidative stress, and defective epithelial barriers (Ippolito et al., 2013), rendering chronic alcohol abusers who are receiving immunosuppressive therapy more susceptible to various infections. Accumulating evidence has suggested a causal linkage between heavy drinking and some infectious diseases, including tuberculosis (Lönnroth, Williams, Stadlin, Jaramillo, & Dye, 2008; Rehm et al., 2009), hepatitis C viral infection in the liver (Siu, Foont, & Wands, 2009), HIV (Baliunas, Rehm, Irving, & Shuper, 2010; Shuper et al., 2010), and pneumonia (Samokhvalov, Irving, & Rehm, 2010).

All opioids, especially morphine, can alter or suppress the functionality of the various cell types of both innate and adaptive immunity (Roy et al., 2011), although it is difficult to rule out the effects of the drug-abusing lifestyle in human models. Some evidence supports that cannabinol suppresses T-cell function and cell-mediated immunity (Tashkin, Baldwin, Sarafian, Dubinett, & Roth, 2002). Beyond the scope of this chapter, people in a severely immunocompromised state as a result of their addictive disease will need carefully managed immunosuppressive cancer therapy.

## Radiation and Chemotherapy

Continued use of tobacco during radiation therapy for head and neck cancers is linked to poorer outcomes. Researchers found that 55% of patients who had quit smoking prior to treatment were still alive five years later, compared with 23% of those who continued to smoke. The poorer outcomes for persistent smokers were reported for both patients who had surgery prior to radiation therapy and patients who had radiation therapy alone (Chen, Chen, et al., 2011). It is debatable whether consumption of alcohol is safe during chemotherapy. The cancer type and stage, as well as the type of treatment, should be taken into consideration when deciding whether to drink alcohol during treatment. For example, many of the drugs used to treat cancer are metabolized through the liver, and alcohol could impair drug breakdown, thus increasing side effects. For patients who suffer from liver damage or are undergoing treatment for liver cancer, alcohol should be avoided completely. Mucositis, a common complication associated with head and neck radiation or many types of chemotherapy, is compounded by alcohol use. Nurses should discuss with their patients the use of alcohol during and/or immediately following chemotherapy treatment.

## Compliance With Cancer Treatment

The care plan of a patient receiving treatment for oncologic disease typically includes recommendations for adequate activity and rest, good nutrition and water intake, the adding of new medications to daily regimens, and the scheduling of multiple appointments with multiple specialists; all of these require new behavioral changes that the patient must integrate into their daily life. As previously described, the behavioral repertoire of the actively addicted patient is relatively narrow, and the patient may not have the ability to integrate new treatment-related behaviors into a substance-using lifestyle, may not take medications as scheduled, or may miss appointments. Drug and alcohol use may continue at the expense of adequate nutritional intake and restful sleep. Ongoing drug and alcohol addiction precludes optimal adherence to the cancer treatment plan, which ultimately results in poorer outcomes.

## Assessment for Substance Abuse and Addiction in Patients With Cancer

Clearly, the coexistence of a substance use disorder and cancer has a negative impact on therapeutic responses and health outcomes. Therefore, it is important to incorporate substance use screening and treatment into cancer care guidelines, and care coordination for both conditions. The first goal of assessment is to determine whether the patient has a history of substance abuse, and then to determine whether he or she is actively abusing, is in drug-free recovery, or is being medically maintained (e.g., methadone) in recovery. Several reliable and valid screening tools for substance abuse are available at www.integration.samhsa.gov/clinical-practice/screening-tools#drugs. Some are generic and used to screen for many types of substance use, while others are used to screen for abuse of specific substance (e.g., alcohol, tobacco). In terms of screening for opioid misuse, two of the most commonly used screening tools, SOAPP-R and the Current Opioid Misuse Measure, are available at www.painedu.org/soap.asp.

When taking a patient's substance use history, nurses should use a matter-of-fact approach and explain that drinking alcohol or using certain medications or drugs can influence responses to cancer medications and treatment. In addition to the medical history, questions regarding substance use patterns (e.g., onset, frequency, types, amounts, circumstances of use) and current use, including the last episode, should be explored. Family history of addiction, as well as problems indicative of a substance abuse disorder in legal, employment, and social domains, must be asked. In addition, nurses must inquire about psychiatric history, including prior treatment for addiction, depression, anxiety, and suicide attempts, as well as take note of obvious signs of intoxication or withdrawal. Other signs of chronic substance use, such as the medical sequelae of abuse (e.g., liver dysfunction, infection), can aid in identification of addicted patients.

With patients who are in remission (drug-free recovery), nurses should ask for how long and under what circumstances they have been drug or alcohol free. The primary substance of abuse should be noted as well as any current relationship with a support/recovery therapy group and/or sponsor. Patients' concerns about exposure to pain medications with abuse liability (opioids, marijuana) over the course of treatment should be explored. For patients who are taking methadone or buprenorphine for the treatment of opioid addiction, nurses should note the daily dose the patient receives and, with the patient's permission, initiate contact with the clinic provider to ensure continuity of care. Patients should be assured that pharmacologic therapy for the treatment of addiction will continue throughout cancer treatment and not interfere with the provision of adequate analgesia as needed.

One of the most difficult challenges for clinicians is identifying patients who are addicted and either in denial about the problem or do not want to disclose the behavior to healthcare personnel. Vague or inconsistent responses to specific questions about substance abuse should be explored. Red flags on history include first use at an early age (younger than age 15), trauma in higher frequency than expected, single-vehicle accidents, seizures with onset between ages 10 and 30, family history of addictive disease, sexual abuse as a child, prior history of addictive disease, and a psychiatric history. Laboratory markers, such as mean corpuscular volume, gamma-glutamyl transferase, and, increasingly, carbohydrate-deficient transferrin, provide evidence of the toxic effects of chronic alcohol abuse on body tissues and function but do not prove that the patient is physically dependent on alcohol (Helander, Péter, & Zheng, 2012). As noted, immunologic abnormalities may be noted in drug users.

One of the surest ways to determine whether a patient's social or recreational drug or alcohol use constitutes a disorder is to ask the patient to limit or curtail their use of the substance for a given period of time (e.g., limit intake of alcohol to one glass of wine per evening for two weeks). If patients find that they are unable to control their use, the presence of a substance use disorder should be considered.

## Approaches to Addiction Treatment in Patients With Cancer

The treatment of addictive disease is beyond the scope of oncology nursing practice, but the ongoing nature of the relationship between oncology nurses and patients provides an ideal therapeutic setting to support recovery efforts. Via assessment and case identification strategies, oncology nurses may initiate addiction treatment by referring patients for a formal evaluation. Many oncology groups and clinics have psychiatrist and psychologist affiliates to whom such referrals can be made; in other settings, referrals are made to community mental health centers or clinics. Twelve-step programs are readily available and can be recommended to all patients.

A diagnosis of cancer may be enough to motivate some individuals to enter drug or alcohol treatment, but this is not always the case. A powerful strategy that oncology nurses can use to prepare patients for drug treatment, as well as to support their efforts at recovery, is an interpersonal technique known as motivational interviewing (MI) (Miller & Rollnick, 2013). MI is a brief intervention technique designed to augment an individual's motivation to change problematic behaviors. Miller and Rollnick (2002) defined MI as a "client-centered, directive method for enhancing intrinsic motivation to change by exploring and resolving ambivalence" (p. 25). The method relies on nonconfrontational approaches, which ideally result in patients, rather than nurses, eliciting concerns about alcohol or drug use and expressing the need to reduce or cease substance intake. Miller and Rollnick (1991) described eight general motivational strategies:
- Giving advice
- Removing barriers
- Providing choice
- Decreasing desirability
- Practicing empathy
- Providing feedback
- Clarifying goals
- Active helping

The techniques central to MI are consistent with those demonstrated to be effective in brief intervention settings, making it an ideal intervention for the short and episodic patterns of care often characteristic of oncology nursing (Miller et al., 2011).

MI techniques take into account what is known about the stages of behavioral change (Prochaska & DiClemente, 1982). Acknowledging that people proceed through a predictable sequence of stages in achieving and maintaining a behavioral change, Miller and Rollnick (1991) conceptualized a "wheel of change" illustrating the steps individuals go through toward changing problematic drug or alcohol use. In this conceptualization, five stages are shown on the wheel, with a sixth, the precontemplation stage, lying outside the wheel as the entry point to change. The circular nature of these stages reflects the revolving nature of change and the fact that people typically have to go around the wheel multiple times (an average between four and seven times) before maintaining the change. Thus, relapse to alcohol or drug use is recognized as a distinct stage of change and not a failure to change; if approached appropriately, relapse can result in a renewed and refined change effort.

Nurses must understand that different nursing skills and interpersonal techniques are required at different stages of change (see Table 24-2); patients just beginning to accept that they may have a problem with alcohol intake (in the precontemplation or contemplation stages) require different motivational approaches than people engaging in activities to bring about change (action stage). If techniques appropriate for one stage are applied at another, the likely patient response is resistance to change, commonly interpreted as a "lack of motivation" (Miller & Rollnick, 1991). By recognizing where patients are with respect to changing their addictive behavior, oncology nurses can use interactions with patients as opportunities to enhance their motivation for change.

## Smoking Cessation

Specific to tobacco addiction, validated smoking cessation techniques, including behavioral strategies, pharmacotherapies (e.g., nicotine replacement), or combined pharmacologic–behavioral treatments, have proven to be cost-effective, accessible, and efficacious methods across different patient populations (Cahill, Stevens, Perera, & Lancaster, 2013; Cooley et al., 2012). However, few smoking intervention studies have been conducted with patients with cancer, as many have quit smoking at the time of diagnosis, and many have comorbidities that prevent enrollment in clinical trials (Martinez et al., 2009).

Nicotine replacement products include nicotine inhalers, polacrilex gums, lozenges, and patches and are designed to relieve nicotine withdrawal symptoms. Consideration of potential adverse effects is necessary prior to the initiation of these replacement products, especially for those patients who are pregnant or nursing, are younger than 18, have a cardiovascular disease (e.g., irregular heartbeat, hypertension), have current or a history of esophagitis or peptic ulcer disease, are using insulin for diabetes, or are taking prescription drugs for other conditions. Other pharmacologic treatments include agents targeting nicotine receptors (e.g., varenicline) and agents targeting neurotransmitters (e.g., bupropion hydrochloride) involved in the pathogenesis of nicotine withdrawal and craving (Benowitz, 2008). Fluoxetine hydrochloride also appears to be an effective treatment for smoking cessation. Both varenicline and bupropion hydrochloride may increase the risk of depression and other neuropsychiatric symptoms, including suicidal behaviors (Benowitz, 2008). If pharmacotherapy is chosen for smoking cessation, nurses should educate patients regarding possible side effects.

MI (Heckman, Egleston, & Hofmann, 2010; Hettema & Hendricks, 2010; Lai, Cahill, Qin, & Tang, 2010), cognitive behavioral therapy (Perkins, Conklin, & Levine, 2008), and acceptance and commitment therapy (Ruiz, 2010) are common counseling styles incor-

### Table 24-2. Motivational Tasks by Stages of Change

| Client Stage | Definition | Clinician's Motivational Tasks |
|---|---|---|
| Precontemplation | The entry stage to the process of change; the patient may not even recognize that their use of alcohol or drugs is problematic and thus is not considering a behavioral change. A patient in this stage needs information and feedback to be delivered in a nonconfrontational manner to raise their awareness of a problem and the possibility of change. | Raise doubt—Increase the client's perception of risks and problems with current behavior. |
| Contemplation | The first stage of change; the patient is willing to consider that their use of drugs or alcohol may constitute a problem and that changing this behavior may be necessary. Characterized by ambivalence. | Tip the balance—Evoke reasons to change and explain the risks of not changing; strengthen the client's self-efficacy for change of current behavior. |
| Determination | Occurs when the patient expresses a commitment to take action and decides to take steps to stop the problem behavior. May be transient, and, if not capitalized upon, the patient can slip back into the contemplation stage. | Help the client to determine the best course of action to take in seeking change. |
| Action | The agreed-upon change strategy is implemented, and the role of the clinician is to enhance or maintain the patient's sense of self-efficacy, praise accomplishments, and attribute successes to the capabilities of the patient. The action stage usually lasts three to six months with most addicted patients. | Help the client to take steps toward change. |
| Maintenance | Once the new behavior patterns initiated in the action stage become firmly established, the patient is described as having entered the maintenance stage. To maintain the change, the patient must adopt a new set of skills and behavior patterns, which are different from those needed to initiate a change. To be successful, these behaviors must include strategies to prevent relapse. | Help the client to identify and use strategies to prevent relapse. |
| Relapse | Relapses are normal and expected as individuals attempt to change a long-standing behavior to which they have multiple and powerful attachments. | Help the client to renew the processes of contemplation, determination, and action, without becoming stuck or demoralized because of relapse. |

*Note.* From *Motivational Interviewing: Preparing People to Change Addictive Behavior* (p. 18), by W.R. Miller and S. Rollnick, 1991, New York, NY: Guilford Press. Copyright 1991 by Guilford Press. Reprinted with permission.

porated into behavioral interventions (group or individual format) for smoking cessation. These behavioral interventions have proven to be effective alone and augmented when combined with pharmacotherapy (Cooley et al., 2012). Moreover, smoking cessation support via the Internet, telephone quitlines (e.g., 1-800-QUIT-NOW), or in person is also an effective approach (Helgason et al., 2004; Zhu et al., 2002), and telephone cessation support with medication is more effective than medication alone (Stead, Perera, & Lancaster, 2006). Although less tested, self-help groups (e.g., Nicotine Anonymous) for smoking cessation may benefit some individuals with tobacco use disorder (Glasser, 2010). ACS provides clear steps for quitting smoking, including making the decision to quit, setting a quit day, establishing a plan, dealing with withdrawal, and staying tobacco free (maintenance). Detailed information can be found at www.cancer.org.

## Management of Opioid Abuse and Addiction in Patients With Cancer Pain

For optimal cancer outcomes, as well as meaningful end-of-life experiences, well-treated addiction and recovery brings with it improved familial relationships, functionality, and psychological states. Adequate comfort without undue sedation is typically the goal of pain management. For patients with addictive disease and cancer, the use of potentially addicting drugs (e.g., marijuana, opioids) poses special consideration.

### Addiction and Pain

For more than 25 years, researchers have known that the parts of the brain that mediate pain and pleasure overlap neuroanatomically and neurophysiologically via endogenous opioids, suggesting that individuals who have altered opioid-related reward pathways from addictive disease may have altered pain pathways as well. In other words, the substance abuser's experience of pain is likely different from that of a nonabuser.

Evidence supports that the presence of addiction worsens the pain experience for patients. More than 20 years ago, Savage and Schofferman (1995) described a "syndrome of pain facilitation," in which discomfort is augmented by subtle withdrawal syndromes, intoxication or withdrawal-related sympathetic arousal or muscular tension, sleep disturbances, affective changes, or functional changes. Experimental pain data support decreased pain tolerance in males currently using opioids or cocaine as compared to patients in recovery and matched normal controls (Compton, 1994; Compton, Charuvastra, Kintaudi, & Ling, 2000). It appears that addictive disease decreases one's ability to endure discomfort.

In the case of opioid addiction, clear effects on pain systems and pain management are evident. With respect to the provision of opioid analgesics, the effect of analgesic tolerance must be considered. Patients who are actively abusing opioids or participating in a methadone or buprenorphine maintenance program will have some degree of pharmacokinetic and functional analgesic tolerance. The abused or prescribed opioid provides little, if any, pain relief, and patients typically need analgesic doses slightly higher than nonaddicted patients, in addition to their daily methadone or buprenorphine dose, to manage pain (Alford, Compton, & Samet, 2006). The definitions of key terminologies used in treating chronic pain with opioids are summarized in Table 24-3.

It appears that as tolerance for morphine (or other full μ-opioid agonists) develops in the absence of pain, as is the case for opioid addiction, an appreciable degree of opioid-induced hyperalgesia also develops. In other words, people with an opioid addiction are more sensitive to pain than they were prior to opioid exposure—a finding that has been repeatedly demonstrated in animal models and correlated with methadone and buprenorphine maintenance in humans. As theorized mechanisms of tolerance and opioid-induced hyperalgesia merge, what was previously defined as "analgesic tolerance" may become recognized as

## Table 24-3. Substance Abuse Terminology

| Term | Definition |
|---|---|
| Aberrant drug-related behavior | Taking a controlled substance medication in a manner that is not prescribed. Causes for this may include the following:<br>• Lack of understanding about how to appropriately take the opioid<br>• External pressures, such as to give to another person for their pain<br>• Chemical coping<br>• Pseudoaddiction<br>  – Physical tolerance and resultant inadequate pain control<br>  – Opioid-resistant pain<br>  – Opioid-induced hyperalgesia<br>  – Progression of pain generator or disease<br>• Addiction or substance use disorder (such as prescription opioid use disorder [POUD])<br>• Diversion<br>A behavior outside the boundaries of the agreed-on treatment plan, which is established as early as possible in the doctor–patient relationship. |
| Abuse | Misuse with consequences. The use of a substance to modify or control mood or state of mind in a manner that is illegal or harmful to oneself or others. Potentially harmful consequences include accidents or injuries, blackouts, legal problems, and sexual behavior that increases the risk of HIV infection. |
| Addiction | A primary, chronic, neurobiologic disease with genetic, psychosocial, and environmental factors influencing its development and manifestations. It is characterized by behaviors that include one or more of the following: impaired control over drug use, compulsive use, continued use despite harm, and craving. |
| Misuse | Taking a prescription for a reason or at a dose or frequency other than for which it was prescribed; this may or may not reflect POUD. Nonmedical use of a medication or for reasons other than prescribed (e.g., altering dosing or sharing medicines). Misuse does not refer to use for mind-altering purposes. |
| Opioid-induced hyperalgesia | A state of nociceptive sensitization caused by exposure to opioids. The condition is characterized by a paradoxical response, when a patient receiving opioids for the treatment of pain could become more sensitive to certain painful stimuli. The type of pain experienced might be the same as the underlying pain or might be different from the original underlying pain. |
| Physical dependence | A state of adaptation manifested by a drug class–specific withdrawal syndrome that can be produced by abrupt cessation, rapid dose reduction, decreasing blood level of the drug, and/or administration of an antagonist. |
| Pseudoaddiction | An iatrogenic syndrome of "addiction-like" behaviors in which the patient seeks opioids to relieve pain—such as seeking different doctors, self-adjusting the opioid dose, early refills of opioids—rather than to achieve pleasure or other non-pain–related effects. At times mistaken for true addiction, these behaviors tend to resolve, and function improves once analgesia is better addressed. Further defined as behavioral changes in patients that are similar to those in patients with opioid dependence or addiction but are secondary to inadequate pain control. |
| Substance use disorder (SUD) | A diagnosis of SUD is based on evidence of impaired control, social impairment, risky use, and pharmacologic criteria of the *Diagnostic and Statistical Manual of Mental Disorders*. SUD is categorized as mild, moderate, or severe to indicate the level of severity, determined by the number of diagnostic criteria met by an individual. |

*(Continued on next page)*

### Table 24-3. Substance Abuse Terminology *(Continued)*

| Term | Definition |
|---|---|
| Therapeutic dependence | Drug-seeking secondary to anxiety about having an adequate supply of medication. |
| Tolerance | A state of adaptation in which exposure to a drug induces changes that result in a diminution of one or more opioid effects over time. |

*Note.* From "Management of Chronic Pain With Chronic Opioid Therapy in Patients With Substance Use Disorders," by Y.-P. Chang and P. Compton, 2013, *Addiction Science and Clinical Practice, 8*, p. 2. Copyright 2013 by Chang and Compton. Adapted with permission.

hyperalgesia (Compton, Athanasos, & Elashoff, 2003; Compton et al., 2000; Compton, Charuvasta, & Ling, 2001). It is likely that the pain experienced by an opioid-dependent patient with cancer is worsened by such hyperalgesic states.

Thus, the presence of addiction might alter the pain experience of patients with cancer, and an untreated substance use disorder likely complicates the pain management. Adequate treatment of pain is critical, and effective opioid analgesia actually may protect patients from relapse. As previously mentioned, one of the best-known precipitators for relapse, regardless of the substance, is stress. Poorly or inadequately treated pain is a significant stressor that easily can lead the individual to seek relief or comfort with a substance previously paired with providing relief and comfort (Chang & Compton, 2013). Evidence supports that taking opioids while in moderate to severe pain actually may protect patients from some of their "addictive" qualities. Under conditions of acute pain, animals developed significantly less morphine analgesic tolerance and physical withdrawal symptoms (Vaccarino et al., 1993), and humans reported significantly less opioid reward or euphoria (Zacny et al., 1996) than in pain-free models. Taking opioids in the presence of pain may mitigate their addictive potential.

## Analgesic Drug Seeking in Patients With Cancer

Two classes of drugs with abuse liability are commonly used to treat the pain in patients suffering cancer pain: marijuana and opioids. Clinicians become concerned about the presence of a substance use disorder when patients appear to be "drug seeking" these psychoactive medications. Individuals seek and obtain analgesic drugs for myriad reasons, only one of which is because they are addicted. Although clear in the case of drugs that have no psychoactive effect (e.g., antibiotics, nonopioid analgesics), the distinction between appropriate drug seeking and addiction becomes less apparent when a patient seeks a drug with a known abuse potential. The confusion is compounded by the inability to objectively quantify the severity of pain, as can only be subjectively reported (Gianutsos, Safranek, & Huber, 2008).

Patients with pain may take what appear to be extraordinary steps to ensure adequate medication supply, which may, in fact, be appropriate responses to either under-relieved or well-relieved pain. In the case of the former, drug-seeking behaviors arise when a patient cannot obtain tolerable relief with the prescribed dose of analgesic and seeks alternate sources or increased doses, a phenomenon called "pseudoaddiction" (Weissman & Haddox, 1989). Alternatively, patients receiving good pain relief may drug-seek because they fear not the reemergence of pain and possibly the emergence of withdrawal symptoms. Rather than indicating addictive disease, such behaviors, called *therapeutic dependence* (Portenoy, 1994), are the efforts of an anxious patient trying to maintain a tolerable level of comfort. Unfortunately, clinicians too often view such behaviors as evidence of abuse or addiction in patients without considering that they may be seeking opioid analgesics for pain relief (Chang & Compton, 2013).

## Managing Cancer Pain in Substance Abusers

Managing pain with opioid therapy in patients with cancer with a history of substance abuse can be challenging. For the management of noncancer pain with opioids, guidelines for risk assessment and stratification in opioid therapy have been well developed, and pain clinicians are suggested to incorporate them into their practice (Chang & Compton, 2013; Oliver et al., 2012; U.S. Food and Drug Administration, 2012). However, few guidelines address the issue of substance abuse in oncology, palliative care, and hospice settings (Anghelescu et al., 2013). Just as for managing noncancer pain, patients receiving chronic opioid therapy should be assessed for risk factors of misuse and abuse, stratified into different levels of risk categories, and monitored during the course of therapy (Chang & Compton, 2013; Oliver et al., 2012). An interprofessional team approach comprising oncology and addiction medicine expertise is highly recommended (Passik & Theobald, 2000).

For patients with active addiction, it is critical to build trust and a therapeutic relationship. Oncology nurses are encouraged to openly acknowledge the patient's history of addiction and allow discussion on fears about how this may affect pain management and treatment by staff. Respect and believe the patient's report of pain, keeping in mind that a person with active addictive disease is likely to be less tolerant of pain than nonaddicted patients. Aggressively treat reports of pain; remember that provision of adequate analgesia in this population carries the additional benefit of averting relapse and, although not the priority during acute pain periods, makes the patient more receptive to addiction treatment interventions. If opioids will be self-administered, the treatment plan should be broadened to include an opioid treatment contract that enables careful monitoring of opiate use, including the use of a single provider, urine toxicology screens, and methods of obtaining rescue doses. Analgesic use and response should be carefully documented.

With respect to providing opioid analgesics to patients with a history of addictive disease, many principles are the same as with other patients (Chou et al., 2009). Clinicians are encouraged to choose long-acting opioids with gradual onset of action and administered around the clock. Patient-controlled analgesia should be considered; not only does it decrease total opioid requirements, but it also decreases drug-seeking behaviors and is not abused by substance abusers (Alford et al., 2006; Mehta & Langford, 2006). For patients who are physically dependent on opioids, alcohol, or sedative hypnotics, it is critical to provide long-acting substitute medications to prevent withdrawal. During opioid withdrawal, opioid-induced hyperalgesia is most pronounced; thus, patients will be very sensitive to pain (Compton et al., 2003). If substitution therapy is provided, monitor for emergence of withdrawal symptoms at least every four hours and treat aggressively and symptomatically. Remember that it is illegal to provide opioids to a known opioid addict for the treatment of addiction, unless a physician is specialty certified and has obtained a Drug Enforcement Administration waiver for the office-based prescription of buprenorphine. If pain improves, opioids should be tapered slowly to minimize the emergence of withdrawal symptoms. For patients who are methadone or buprenorphine maintained, continue their daily methadone dose for the treatment of the addictive disease and provide opioids for pain control as you would for any other patient, titrating to effect. It is helpful to maintain contact with the methadone clinic nurse and coordinate care as cancer treatments are instituted.

For patients in recovery, it also is very important to build trust. Openly acknowledge their history of addiction, and allow patients, families, and staff to discuss fears of relapse. Explain any intent to use opioids, marijuana, or other psychoactive medications, and respect patients' rights to decide whether to take these medications for pain relief. Reassure them that if they decide against opioid analgesia now, they can always opt for this treatment in the future.

During this stressful time, oncology nurses should broaden the treatment plan to support patients' recovery efforts and include their recovery program or sponsor in patients' care when possible. Stress relief interventions should be offered. Again, an addiction medicine specialist and the use of support groups (12-step programs or otherwise) may reinforce patients' recovery. Keep in mind that a relapse may occur during this stressful time period, but the goal of the oncology nurse is to minimize the extent of the lapse and get the patient back to the determination stage of the wheel of change.

## Education in Managing Substance Abuse for Oncology Clinicians

Managing chronic pain in substance abusers has historically been complicated by several factors, but perhaps less so in the context of oncologic or end-of-life care. Prescribing opioids to people with addiction has been restricted by a generalized "opiophobia" (Bennett & Carr, 2002; Morgan, 1989); regulatory sanctions for opioid prescribing practices; punitive moral and social views of addiction; and clinician concerns about being "duped" into providing an opioid to an addict. These concerns are less salient in the care of cancer, especially at the end of life. Oncology nurses must remember to consider an addicted patient like any other patient with a coexisting medical condition; specific interventions may have to be modified while still working toward the goal of providing adequate pain relief.

Although oncology clinicians often encounter patients with substance use disorder, they frequently have little training and are poorly prepared for managing substance abuse in their patients with cancer. No data on nursing knowledge have been reported, but a recent study surveyed palliative clinicians' educational preparation and training in managing patients with cancer with opioid misuse and their competence in caring for those patients (Childers & Arnold, 2012). The findings of this study showed that 58% of palliative care fellows reported less than four hours of training in managing opioid abuse in their fellowship, and 11% reported no training; 60% of fellows had less than four hours of education in their residency education, and 11% had no education. These clinicians also reported a low level of competence in caring for patients with high risk of addiction, and only 21% of clinicians were satisfied with their skills in treating pain and symptoms in patients with cancer with substance use disorders (Childers & Arnold, 2012). These findings suggested an urgent need to provide more education to clinicians in this area.

## Conclusion

Addiction is a chronic, relapsing disease that affects up to 10% of the general population and a somewhat higher number of patients with cancer. Untreated symptoms or exacerbations of the disease have health implications ranging from bleeding disorders to family violence and motor vehicle accidents. The effects of addiction complicate the course of cancer treatment in multiple domains, specifically with patients' ability to comply with prescribed regimens and to achieve good surgical or immunosuppressive therapeutic outcomes. For these reasons, oncology nurses must take a leadership role in assessing for and identifying addictive disease in patients with cancer and work to be a motivational force in patients' process of changing their addictive behavior. With an understanding that pain and addiction systems are interrelated, oncology nurses can provide aggressive and appropriate pain care to individuals with addictive disease in the manner most likely to control its symptoms.

# References

Alford, D.P., Compton, P., & Samet, J.H. (2006). Acute pain management for patients receiving maintenance methadone or buprenorphine therapy. *Annals of Internal Medicine, 144,* 127–134.

Allen, N.E., Beral, V., Casabonne, D., Kan, S.W., Reeves, G.K., Brown, A., & Green, J. (2009). Moderate alcohol intake and cancer incidence in women. *Journal of the National Cancer Institute, 101,* 296–305. doi:10.1093/jnci/djn514

American Cancer Society. (2014). *Cancer facts and figures 2014.* Retrieved from http://www.cancer.org/acs/groups/content/@research/documents/webcontent/acspc-042151.pdf

American Cancer Society. (2017). *Cancer facts and figures 2017.* Retrieved from https://www.cancer.org/content/dam/cancer-org/research/cancer-facts-and-statistics/annual-cancer-facts-and-figures/2017/cancer-facts-and-figures-2017.pdf

American Psychiatric Association. (2013). *Diagnostic and statistical manual of mental disorders* (5th ed.). Washington, DC: Author.

Anghelescu, D.L., Ehrentraut, J.H., & Faughnan, L.G. (2013). Opioid misuse and abuse: Risk assessment and management in patients with cancer pain. *Journal of the National Comprehensive Cancer Network, 11,* 1023–1031.

Baan, R., Straif, K., Grosse, Y., Secretan, B., El Ghissassi, F., Bouvard, V., ... Cogliano, V. (2007). Carcinogenicity of alcoholic beverages. *Lancet Oncology, 8,* 292–293. doi:10.1016/S1470-2045(07)70099-2

Baliunas, D., Rehm, J., Irving, H., & Shuper, P. (2010). Alcohol consumption and risk of incident human immunodeficiency virus infection: A meta-analysis. *International Journal of Public Health, 55,* 159–166. doi:10.1007/s00038-009-0095-x

Barclay, J.S., Owens, J.E., & Blackhall, L.J. (2014). Screening for substance abuse risk in cancer patients using the Opioid Risk Tool and urine drug screen. *Supportive Care in Cancer, 22,* 1883–1888. doi:10.1007/s00520-014-2167-6

Bennett, D.S., & Carr, D.B. (2002). Opiophobia as a barrier to the treatment of pain. *Journal of Pain and Palliative Care Pharmacotherapy, 16,* 105–109. doi:10.1080/J354v16n01_09

Benowitz, N.L. (2008). Neurobiology of nicotine addiction: Implications for smoking cessation treatment. *American Journal of Medicine, 121*(4 Suppl. 1), S3–S10. doi:10.1016/j.amjmed.2008.01.015

Bjarnason, T., Andersson, B., Choquet, M., Elekes, Z., Morgan, M., & Rapinett, G. (2003). Alcohol culture, family structure and adolescent alcohol use: Multilevel modeling of frequency of heavy drinking among 15–16 year old students in 11 European countries. *Journal of the Study of Alcohol, 64,* 200–208. doi:10.15288/jsa.2003.64.200

Boffetta, P., & Hashibe, M. (2006). Alcohol and cancer. *Lancet Oncology, 7,* 149–156. doi:10.1016/S1470-2045(06)70577-0

Bosetti, C., Gallus, S., Franceschi, S., Levi, F., Bertuzzi, M., Negri, E., ... La Vecchia, C. (2002). Cancer of the larynx in nonsmoking alcohol drinkers and in non-drinking tobacco smokers. *British Journal of Cancer, 87,* 516–518. doi:10.1038/sj.bjc.6600469

Bossert, J.M., Marchant, N.J., Calu, D.J., & Shaham, Y. (2013). The reinstatement model of drug relapse: Recent neurobiological findings, emerging research topics, and translational research. *Psychopharmacology, 229,* 453–476. doi:10.1007/s00213-013-3120-y

Brick, J., & Erickson, C. (2012). *Drugs, the brain, and behavior: The pharmacology of abuse and dependency* (2nd ed.). New York, NY: Routledge.

Cahill, K., Stevens, S., Perera, R., & Lancaster, T. (2013). Pharmacological interventions for smoking cessation: An overview and network meta-analysis. *Cochrane Database of Systematic Reviews, 2013*(5). doi:10.1002/14651858.CD009329.pub2

Callaghan, R.C., Allebeck, P., & Sidorchuk, A. (2013). Marijuana use and risk of lung cancer: A 40-year cohort study. *Cancer Causes and Control, 24,* 1811–1820. doi:10.1007/s10552-013-0259-0

Castellsagué, X., Muñoz, N., De Stefani, E., Victora, C.G., Castelletto, R., Rolón, P.A., & Quintana, M.J. (1999). Independent and joint effects of tobacco smoking and alcohol drinking on the risk of oesophageal cancer in men and women. *International Journal of Cancer, 82,* 657–664. doi:10.1002/(SICI)1097-0215(19990827)82:5<657::AID-IJC7>3.0.CO;2-C

Centers for Disease Control and Prevention. (2014). Excessive drinking costs U.S. $223.5 billion. Retrieved from https://www.cdc.gov/features/alcoholconsumption

Chang, Y.-P., & Compton, P. (2013). Management of chronic pain with chronic opioid therapy in patients with substance use disorders. *Addiction Science and Clinical Practice, 8,* 21. doi:10.1186/1940-0640-8-21

Chen, A.M., Chen, L.M., Vaughan, A., Sreeraman, R., Farwell, D.G., Luu, Q., ... Vijayakumar, S. (2011). Tobacco smoking during radiation therapy for head-and-neck cancer is associated with unfavorable outcome. *International Journal of Radiation, Oncology, and Biology Physics, 79,* 414–419. doi:10.1016/j.ijrobp.2009.10.050

Chen, P., Li, C., Li, X., Li, J., Chu, R., & Wang, H. (2014). Higher dietary folate intake reduces the breast cancer risk: A systematic review and meta-analysis. *British Journal of Cancer, 110,* 2327–2338. doi:10.1038/bjc.2014.155

Chen, W.Y., Rosner, B., Hankinson, S.E., Colditz, G.A., & Willett, W.C. (2011). Moderate alcohol consumption during adult life, drinking patterns, and breast cancer risk. *JAMA, 306,* 1884–1890. doi:10.1001/jama.2011.1590

Chhatre, S., Metzger, D.S., Malkowicz, S.B., Woody, G., & Jayadevappa, R. (2014). Substance use disorder and its effects on outcomes in men with advanced-stage prostate cancer. *Cancer, 120,* 3338–3345. doi:10.1002/cncr.28861

Childers, J.W., & Arnold, R.M. (2012). "I feel uncomfortable 'calling a patient out'": Educational needs of palliative medicine fellows in managing opioid misuse. *Journal of Pain and Symptom Management, 43,* 253–260. doi:10.1016/j.jpainsymman.2011.03.009

Chou, R., Fanciullo, G.J., Fine, P.G., Adler, J.A., Ballantyne, J.C., Davies, P., ... Miaskowski, C. (2009). Clinical guidelines for the use of chronic opioid therapy in chronic noncancer pain. *Journal of Pain, 10,* 113–130. doi:10.1016/j.jpain.2008.10.008

Collaborative Group on Hormonal Factors in Breast Cancer. (2002). Alcohol, tobacco and breast cancer—Collaborative reanalysis of individual data from 53 epidemiological studies, including 58,515 women with breast cancer and 95,067 women without the disease. *British Journal of Cancer, 87,* 1234–1245. doi:10.1038/sj.bjc.6600596

Compton, M. (1994). Cold-pressor pain tolerance in opiate and cocaine abusers: Correlates of drug type and use status. *Journal of Pain and Symptom Management, 9,* 462–473. doi:10.1016/0885-3924(94)90203-8

Compton, P., Athanasos, P., & Elashoff, D. (2003). Withdrawal hyperalgesia after acute opioid physical dependence in nonaddicted humans: A preliminary study. *Journal of Pain, 4,* 511–519. doi:10.1016/j.jpain.2003.08.003

Compton, P., Charuvastra, V.C., Kintaudi, K., & Ling, W. (2000). Pain responses in methadone-maintained opioid abusers. *Journal of Pain and Symptom Management, 20,* 237–245. doi:10.1016/S0885-3924(00)00191-3

Compton, P., Charuvastra, V.C., & Ling, W. (2001). Pain intolerance in opioid-maintained former opiate addicts: Effect of long-acting maintenance agent. *Drug and Alcohol Dependence, 63,* 139–146. doi:10.1016/S0376-8716(00)00200-3

Cooley, M.E., Wang, Q., Johnson, B.E., Catalano, P., Haddad, R.I., Bueno, R., & Emmons, K.M. (2012). Factors associated with smoking abstinence among smokers and recent-quitters with lung and head and neck cancer. *Lung Cancer, 76,* 144–149. doi:10.1016/j.lungcan.2011.10.005

de Wit, M., Goldberg, S., Hussein, E., & Neifeld, J.P. (2012). Health care–associated infections in surgical patients undergoing elective surgery: Are alcohol use disorders a risk factor? *Journal of the American College of Surgeons, 215,* 229–236. doi:10.1016/j.jamcollsurg.2012.04.015

Derogatis, L.R., Morrow, G.R., Fetting, J., Penman, D., Piasetsky, S., Schmale, A.M., ... Carnicke, C.L., Jr. (1983). The prevalence of psychiatric disorders among cancer patients. *JAMA, 249,* 751. doi:10.1001/jama.1983.03330300035030

Dev, R., Parsons, H.A., Palla, S., Palmer, J.L., Del Fabbro, E., & Bruera, E. (2011). Undocumented alcoholism and its correlation with tobacco and illegal drug use in advanced cancer patients. *Cancer, 117,* 4551–4556. doi:10.1002/cncr.26082

Evans, S.M., & Levin, F.R. (2003). Response to alcohol in females with a paternal history of alcoholism. *Psychopharmacology, 169,* 10–20. doi:10.1007/s00213-003-1474-2

Everitt, B.J. (2014). Neural and psychological mechanisms underlying compulsive drug seeking habits and drug memories—Indications for novel treatments of addiction. *European Journal of Neuroscience, 40,* 2163–2182. doi:10.1111/ejn.12644

Ewing, J.A. (1984). Detecting alcoholism: The CAGE questionnaire. *JAMA, 252,* 1905–1907. doi:10.1001/jama.1984.03350140051025

Fedirko, V., Tramacere, I., Bagnardi, V., Rota, M., Scotti, L., Islami, F., ... Jenab, M. (2011). Alcohol drinking and colorectal cancer risk: An overall and dose–response meta-analysis of published studies. *Annals of Oncology, 22,* 1958–1972. doi:10.1093/annonc/mdq653

Genther, D.J., & Gourin, C.G. (2012). The effect of alcohol abuse and alcohol withdrawal on short-term outcomes and cost of care after head and neck cancer surgery. *Laryngoscope, 122,* 1739–1747. doi:10.1002/lary.23348

Gianutsos, L.P., Safranek, S., & Huber, T. (2008). Clinical inquiries: Is there a well-tested tool to detect drug-seeking behaviors in chronic pain patients? *Journal of Family Practice, 57,* 609–610.

Gili-Miner, M., Béjar-Prado, L., Gili-Ortiz, E., Ramírez-Ramírez, G., López-Méndez, J., López-Millán, J.M., & Sharp, B. (2014). Alcohol use disorders among surgical patients: Unplanned 30-days readmissions, length of hospital stay, excessive costs and mortality. *Drug and Alcohol Dependence, 137,* 55–61. doi:10.1016/j.drugalcdep.2014.01.009

Glasser, I. (2010). Nicotine Anonymous may benefit nicotine-dependent individuals. *American Journal of Public Health, 100,* 196–197. doi:10.2105/AJPH.2009.181545

Grewal, P., & Viswanathen, V.A. (2012). Liver cancer and alcohol. *Clinics in Liver Disease, 16,* 839–850. doi:10.1016/j.cld.2012.08.011

Gritz, E.R., Fingeret, M.C., Vidrine, D.J., Lazev, A.B., Mehta, N.V., & Reece, G.P. (2006). Successes and failures of the teachable moment: Smoking cessation in cancer patients. *Cancer, 106,* 17–27. doi:10.1002/cncr.21598

Haass-Koffler, C.L., & Bartlett, S.E. (2012). Stress and addiction: Contribution of the corticotropin releasing factor (CRF) system in neuroplasticity. *Frontiers in Molecular Neuroscience, 5,* 91. doi:10.3389/fnmol.2012.00091

Hashibe, M., Brennan, P., Chuang, S.-C., Boccia, S., Castellsague, X., Chen, C., ... Boffetta, P. (2009). Interaction between tobacco and alcohol use and the risk of head and neck cancer: Pooled analysis in the International Head and Neck Cancer Epidemiology Consortium. *Cancer Epidemiology, Biomarkers and Prevention, 18,* 541–550. doi:10.1158/1055-9965.EPI-08-0347

Heckman, C.J., Egleston, B.L., & Hofmann, M.T. (2010). Efficacy of motivational interviewing for smoking cessation: A systematic review and meta-analysis. *Tobacco Control, 19,* 410–416. doi:10.1136/tc.2009.033175

Helander, A., Péter, O., & Zheng, Y. (2012). Monitoring of the alcohol biomarkers PEth, CDT and EtG/EtS in an outpatient treatment setting. *Alcohol and Alcoholism, 47,* 552–557. doi:10.1093/alcalc/ags065

Helgason, A.R., Tomson, T., Lund, K.E., Galanti, R., Ahnve, S., & Gilljam, H. (2004). Factors related to abstinence in a telephone helpline for smoking cessation. *European Journal of Public Health, 14,* 306–310. doi:10.1093/eurpub/14.3.306

Hettema, J.E., & Hendricks, P.S. (2010). Motivational interviewing for smoking cessation: A meta-analytic review. *Journal of Consulting and Clinical Psychology, 78,* 868–884. doi:10.1037/a0021498

Ippolito, J.A., Curtis, B.J., Choudhry, M.A., & Kovacs, E.J. (2013). Alcohol and immunology: Summary of the 2012 Alcohol and Immunology Research Interest Group (AIRIG) meeting. *Alcohol, 47,* 589–593. doi:10.1016/j.alcohol.2013.09.003

Jamison, R.N., & Edwards, R.R. (2013). Risk factor assessment for problematic use of opioids for chronic pain. *Clinical Neuropsychologist, 27,* 60–80. doi:10.1080/13854046.2012.715204

Jenkins, C.A., Schulz, M., Hanson, J., & Bruera, E. (2000). Demographic, symptom, and medication profiles of cancer patients seen by a palliative care consult team in a tertiary referral hospital. *Journal of Pain and Symptom Management, 19,* 174–184. doi:10.1016/S0885-3924(99)00154-2

Kessler, R.C., Berglund, P., Demler, O., Jin, R., Merikangas, K.R., & Walters, E.E. (2005). Lifetime prevalence and age-of-onset distributions of *DSM-IV* disorders in the National Comorbidity Survey Replication. *Archives of General Psychiatry, 62,* 593–602. doi:10.1001/archpsyc.62.6.593

Khullar, D., & Maa, J. (2012). The impact of smoking on surgical outcomes. *Journal of the American College of Surgeons, 215,* 418–426. doi:10.1016/j.jamcollsurg.2012.05.023

Lai, D.T., Cahill, K., Qin, Y., & Tang, J.L. (2010). Motivational interviewing for smoking cessation. *Cochrane Database of Systematic Reviews, 2010*(1). doi:10.1002/14651858.CD006936.pub2

Lee, J., Taneja, V., & Vassallo, R. (2012). Cigarette smoking and inflammation: Cellular and molecular mechanisms. *Journal of Dental Research, 91,* 142–149. doi:10.1177/0022034511421200

Lönnroth, K., Williams, B.G., Stadlin, S., Jaramillo, E., & Dye, C. (2008). Alcohol use as a risk factor for tuberculosis: A systematic review. *BMC Public Health, 8,* 289. doi:10.1186/1471-2458-8-289

Martinez, E., Tatum, K.L., Weber, D.M., Kuzla, N., Pendley, A., Campbell, K., ... Schnoll, R.A. (2009). Issues related to implementing a smoking cessation clinical trial for cancer patients. *Cancer Causes and Control, 20,* 97–104. doi:10.1007/s10552-008-9222-x

Mehta, V., & Langford, R.M. (2006). Acute pain management for opioid dependent patients. *Anaesthesia, 61,* 269–276. doi:10.1111/j.1365-2044.2005.04503.x

Miller, W.R., Forcehimes, A.A., Zweben, A., & McLellan, A.T. (2011). *Treating addiction: A guide for professionals.* New York, NY: Guilford Press.

Miller, W.R., & Rollnick, S. (1991). *Motivational interviewing: Preparing people to change addictive behavior.* New York, NY: Guilford Press.

Miller, W.R., & Rollnick, S. (2002). *Motivational interviewing: Preparing people for change* (2nd ed.). New York, NY: Guilford Press.

Miller, W.R., & Rollnick, S. (2013). *Motivational interviewing: Helping people for change* (3rd ed.). New York, NY: Guilford Press.

Morgan, J.P. (1989). American opiophobia: Customary underutilization of opioid analgesics. In C.S. Hill & W.S. Fields (Eds.), *Advances in pain research and therapy* (Vol. 11, pp. 181–189). New York, NY: Raven Press.

Nan, H., Lee, J.E., Rimm, E.B., Fuchs, C.S., Giovannucci, E.L., & Cho, E. (2013). Prospective study of alcohol consumption and the risk of colorectal cancer before and after folic acid fortification in the United States. *Annals of Epidemiology, 23,* 558–563. doi:10.1016/j.annepidem.2013.04.011

Nelson, D.E., Jarman, D.W., Rehm, J., Greenfield, T.K., Rey, G., Kerr, W.C., ... Naimi, T.S. (2013). Alcohol-attributable cancer deaths and years of potential life lost in the United States. *American Journal of Public Health, 103,* 641–648. doi:10.2105/AJPH.2012.301199

Oliver, J., Coggins, C., Compton, P., Hagan, S., Matteliano, D., Stanton, M., ... Turner, H.N. (2012) American Society for Pain Management nursing position statement: Pain management in patients with substance use disorders. *Pain Management Nursing, 13,* 169–183. doi:10.1016/j.pmn.2012.07.001

Parsons, A., Daley, A., Begh, R., & Aveyard, P. (2010). Influence of smoking cessation after diagnosis of early stage lung cancer on prognosis: Systematic review of observational studies with meta-analysis. *BMJ, 340,* b5569. doi:10.1136/bmj.b5569

Parsons, H.A., Delgado-Guay, M.O., El Osta, B., Chacko, R., Poulter, V., Palme, J.L., & Bruera, E. (2008). Alcoholism screening in patients with advanced cancer: Impact on symptom burden and opioid use. *Journal of Palliative Medicine, 11,* 964–968. doi:10.1089/jpm.2008.0037

Passik, S.D., Portenoy, R.K., & Ricketts, P.L. (1998). Substance abuse issues in cancer patients. Part 1: Prevalence and diagnosis. *Oncology, 12,* 517–521, 524.

Passik, S.D., & Theobald, D.E. (2000). Managing addiction in advanced cancer patients: Why bother? *Journal of Pain and Symptom Management, 19,* 229–234. doi:10.1016/s0885-3924(00)00109-3

Perkins, K.A., Conklin, C.A., & Levine, M.D. (2008). *Cognitive-behavioral therapy for smoking cessation: A practical guidebook to the most effective treatment.* New York, NY: Routledge.

Portenoy, R.K. (1994). Opioid therapy for chronic non-malignant pain: Current status. In H.L. Fields & J.C. Liebes-Kind (Eds.), *Progress in pain research and management* (pp. 247–287). Seattle, WA: IASP Press.

Prochaska, J.O., & DiClemente, C.C. (1982). Transtheoretical therapy: Toward a more integrative model of change. *Psychotherapy: Theory, Research and Practice, 19,* 276–288. doi:10.1037/h0088437

Rehm, J., Samokhvalov, A.V., Neuman, M.G., Room, R., Parry, C., Lönnroth, K., ... Popova, S. (2009). The association between alcohol use, alcohol use disorders and tuberculosis (TB): A systematic review. *BMC Public Health, 9,* 450. doi:10.1186/1471-2458-9-450

Roy, S., Ninkovic, J., Banerjee, S., Charbonneau, R., Das, S., Dutta, R., ... Meng, J. (2011). Opioid drug abuse and modulation of immune function: Consequences in the susceptibility to opportunistic infections. *Journal of Neuroimmune Pharmacology, 6,* 442–465. doi:10.1007/s11481-011-9292-5

Ruiz, F.J. (2010). A review of Acceptance and Commitment Therapy (ACT) empirical evidence: Correlational, experimental psychopathology, component and outcome. *International Journal of Psychology and Psychological Therapy, 10,* 125–162.

Samokhvalov, A.V., Irving, H.M., & Rehm, J. (2010). Alcohol consumption as a risk factor for pneumonia: A systematic review and meta-analysis. *Epidemiology and Infection, 138,* 1789–1795. doi:10.1017/S0950268810000774

Savage, S.R., & Schofferman, J. (1995). Pharmacological therapies of pain in drug and alcohol addictions. In N.S. Miller & M.S. Gold (Eds.), *Pharmacological therapies for drug and alcohol addiction* (pp. 373–409). New York, NY: Marcel Dekker.

Schank, J.R., Ryabinin, A.E., Giardino, W.J., Ciccocioppo, R., & Heilig, M. (2012). Stress-related neuropeptides and addictive behaviors: Beyond the usual suspects. *Neuron, 76,* 192–208. doi:10.1016/j.neuron.2012.09.026

Seitz, H.K., & Stickel, F. (2007). Molecular mechanisms of alcohol-mediated carcinogenesis. *Nature Reviews Cancer, 7,* 599–612. doi:10.1038/nrc2191

Shalev, U., Erb, S., & Shaham, Y. (2010). Role of CRF and other neuropeptides in stress-induced reinstatement of drug seeking. *Brain Research, 1314,* 15–28. doi:10.1016/j.brainres.2009.07.028

Sharma, A., Deeb, A.P., Iannuzzi, J.C., Rickles, A.S., Monson, J.R., & Fleming, F.J. (2013). Tobacco smoking and postoperative outcomes after colorectal surgery. *Annals of Surgery, 258,* 296–300. doi:10.1097/SLA.0b013e3182708cc5

Shuper, P.A., Neuman, M., Kanteres, F., Baliunas, D., Joharchi, N., & Rehm, J. (2010). Causal considerations on alcohol and HIV/AIDS: A systematic review. *Alcohol and Alcoholism, 45,* 159–166. doi:10.1093/alcalc/agp091

Siu, L., Foont, J., & Wands, J.R. (2009). Hepatitis C virus and alcohol. *Seminars in Liver Disease, 29,* 188–199. doi:10.1055/s-0029-1214374

Stead, L.F., Perera, R., & Lancaster, T. (2006). Telephone counselling for smoking cessation. *Cochrane Database of Systematic Reviews, 2006*(3). doi:10.1002/14651858.CD002850.pub2

Substance Abuse and Mental Health Services Administration. (2014). *Results from the 2013 National Survey on Drug Use and Health: Summary of national findings.* Retrieved from http://store.samhsa.gov/shin/content/NSDUH14-0904/NSDUH14-0904.pdf

Tashkin, D.R., Baldwin, G.C., Sarafian, T., Dubinett, S., & Roth, M.D. (2002). Respiratory and immunologic consequences of marijuana smoking. *Journal of Clinical Pharmacology, 42*(Suppl. 11), S71–S81. doi:10.1002/j.1552-4604.2002.tb06006.x

Tønnesen, H., & Kehlet, H. (1999). Preoperative alcoholism and postoperative morbidity. *British Journal of Surgery, 86,* 869–874. doi:10.1046/j.1365-2168.1999.01181.x

Tønnesen, H., Petersen, K.R., Højgaard, L., Stokholm, K.H., Nielsen, H.J., Knigge, U., & Kehlet, H. (1992). Postoperative morbidity among symptom-free alcohol misusers. *Lancet, 340,* 334–337.

Tyndale, R.F. (2003). Genetics of alcohol and tobacco use in humans. *Annals of Internal Medicine, 35,* 94–121. doi:10.1080/07853890310010014

U.S. Department of Health and Human Services. (2014). *The health consequences of smoking–50 years of progress: A report of the Surgeon General.* Retrieved from http://ash.org/wp-content/uploads/2014/01/full-report.pdf

U.S. Department of Health and Human Services. (2016). *Report on carcinogens* (14th ed.). Retrieved from https://ntp.niehs.nih.gov/pubhealth/roc/index-1.html

U.S. Department of Justice. (2011). *National drug threat assessment, 2011.* Retrieved from https://www.justice.gov/archive/ndic/pubs44/44849/44849p.pdf

U.S. Food and Drug Administration. (2012). Risk evaluation and mitigation strategy (REMS) for extended-release and long-acting opioid analgesics. Retrieved from http://www.fda.gov/drugs/drugsafety/informationbydrugclass/ucm163647.htm

Vaccarino, A.L., Marek, P., Kest, B., Ben-Eliyahu, S., Couret, L.C., Jr., Kao, B., & Liebeskind, J.C. (1993). Morphine fails to produce tolerance when administered in the presence of formalin pain in rats. *Brain Research, 627,* 287–290.

Warren, G.W., & Singh, AK. (2013). Nicotine and lung cancer. *Journal of Carcinogenesis, 12,* 1. doi:10.4103/1477-3163.106680

Weissman, D.E., & Haddox, D.J. (1989). Opioid pseudoaddiction—An iatrogenic syndrome. *Pain, 36,* 363–366. doi:10.1016/0304-3959(89)90097-3

Witkiewitz, K., & Marlatt, G.A. (2004). Relapse prevention for alcohol and drug problems: That was Zen, this is Tao. *American Psychologist, 59,* 224–235. doi:10.1037/0003-066X.59.4.224

Zacny, J.P., McKay, M.A., Toledano, A.Y., Marks, S., Young, C.J., Klock, P.A., & Apfelbaum, J.L. (1996). The effects of a cold-water immersion stressor on the reinforcing and subjective effects of fentanyl in healthy volunteers. *Drug and Alcohol Dependence, 42,* 133–142. doi:10.1016/0376-8716(96)01274-4

Zhang, P., Bagby, G.J., Happel, K.I., Raasch, C.E., & Nelson, S. (2008). Alcohol abuse, immunosuppression, and pulmonary infection. *Current Drug Abuse Reviews, 1,* 56–67. doi:10.2174/1874473710801010056

Zhu, S.-H., Anderson, C.M., Tedeschi, G.J., Rosbrook, B., Johnson, C.E., Byrd, M., & Gutiérrez-Terrell, E. (2002). Evidence of real-world effectiveness of a telephone quitline for smokers. *New England Journal of Medicine, 347,* 1087–1093. doi:10.1056/NEJMsa020660

CHAPTER 25

# Therapeutic Modalities in Psychosocial Care

*Linda M. Gorman, RN, MN, PMHCNS-BC, CHPN, FPCN*

> *We rise by lifting others.*
>
> —Robert Ingersoll

A variety of modalities are available to assist the patient coping with psychosocial distress. Supportive interventions, such as active listening skills, reframing, and empathy, are commonly used by oncology nurses. In addition, oncology nurses often are in the role of educators as well as leaders/co-leaders of support groups. These skills are essential in nursing practice for supporting patients with cancer (see Chapter 23 for information on therapeutic skills).

Fawzy and Fawzy (2011) identified the four most common forms of psychosocial interventions for medically ill patients as education, behavioral training, coping skills training, and supportive therapy. These interventions incorporate many nursing actions, including patient/family education, listening skills, emotional support, and incorporation of behavioral strategies to address patients' fears. Nurses may provide these psychosocial interventions as part of patient care, assisting with support groups and providing and coordinating patient education. Patients who require further intervention may benefit from a variety of approaches that necessitate additional training for the nurse as well as other professionals from the interprofessional team, including psychologists, psychiatrists, chaplains, social workers, and other therapists.

This chapter will review therapeutic modalities that are generally not part of basic nursing practice and emotional support. Many of these therapeutic interventions require some type of advanced training, specialty certification, and/or specific license. Oncology nurses need to be aware of these approaches to ensure that patients can obtain the resources and support needed. Knowledge of these interventions is important for oncology nurses who are in the position of identifying problems and implementing referrals and access to resources for patients and families. The recognition of the need for a variety of modalities to treat the psychosocial distress of patients with cancer has been emphasized since the Health and Medicine Division of the National Academies of Sciences, Engineering, and Medicine (formerly the Institute of Medicine) published its report on meeting psychosocial health needs (Adler & Page, 2008).

Although some of these modalities have limited research data, they remain useful approaches for some patients to attempt. Generally, risks to these therapies are limited. Some may involve a time commitment, costs, and access to specially trained professionals.

## Psychoeducation

Psychoeducation, also referred to as psychoeducational interventions, encompasses a broad range of activities that combine education with other interventions (e.g., counseling, emotional support). Psychoeducation was originally developed as part of comprehensive schizophrenia treatment incorporated within family therapy. Patients and their relatives were, by means of preliminary briefing concerning the illness, supposed to develop a fundamental understanding of the therapy and further be convinced to commit to more long-term involvement (Bäuml, Froböse, Kraemer, Rentrop, & Pitschel-Walz, 2006). Psychoeducation has grown in the past few years to incorporate education on a variety of psychiatric disorders for patients and their families. It is now recognized that patients and families need education on the factors contributing to distress and how to cope with the condition. Psychoeducational intervention may be delivered individually or in groups and may be tailored or standardized. It is formally included in psychiatric treatment today rather than the informal role it had in the past.

Psychoeducation has expanded to be an important part of cancer care (Oncology Nursing Society, n.d.). This type of intervention generally includes providing patients with information about the psychosocial effects of treatments, symptoms, resources, and services; training to provide care and respond to disease-related problems; and problem-solving strategies for coping with cancer. Many formats are used, including individual or group settings, multimedia, and Internet-based materials. Psychoeducation for patients with cancer and families can cover a broad spectrum. Some examples include understanding post-traumatic stress after diagnosis, understanding grief, and using techniques to improve communication with healthcare providers. Schou et al. (2014) found that psychoeducation groups for patients with cancer differed from support groups by providing more emphasis on health education, behavioral training, problem solving, self-control strategies, and stress management techniques. Their study found that psychoeducation was more effective than support groups in the short term to reduce depression and anxiety. Providing education encourages empowerment to better handle the stresses and distresses, as well as enhancing coping skills. Oncology nurses with specialized knowledge often provide psychoeducation.

Psychoeducation is used to help both patients and families (sometimes referred to as "informal caregivers"). Applebaum and Breitbart (2013) reviewed the literature and found that psychoeducation to informal caregivers of patients with cancer has positively affected their knowledge base and ability to provide care.

Integrative oncology programs often incorporate psychoeducation into treatment. It helps patients to improve both emotional and cognitive intelligence, thus enabling them to better negotiate cancer treatment systems (Garchinski, DiBiase, Wong, & Sagar, 2014).

## Counseling and Psychotherapy

### Counseling

The term *counseling* can have many meanings. Generally, a counselor is someone who listens to the client and reviews feelings related to difficulties experienced in life (Townsend, 2015). Counselors can have a variety of backgrounds and specialty training. Counseling often is used in a very broad sense in cancer care to describe a relationship with a patient to address specific concerns such as sexual, fertility, or nutrition issues. Generally, counseling is short term and appropriate for individuals who wish to focus on improving their problem-solving abilities and coping techniques. Unlike psychotherapy, deeper issues are usually not addressed in counseling. However, the difference between counseling and psychotherapy can be less clear and, in some cases, are used interchangeably (Strada & Sourkes, 2015).

## Psychotherapy

Psychotherapy is practiced by a clinician licensed to perform it and is based on a specific theoretical framework in which the clinician is trained. The American Psychological Association (APA) defines *psychotherapy* as "the informed and intentional application of clinical methods and interpersonal stances derived from established psychological principles for the purpose of assisting people to modify their behaviors, cognitions, emotions, and/or other personal characteristics in directions that the participants deem desirable" (Norcross, 1990, p. 218). Generally, all psychotherapy emphasizes the importance of the therapeutic alliance with the therapist. Psychotherapy of all types can be conducted in groups, among families and couples, and individually. The appropriate form of psychotherapy for patients with cancer needs to be evaluated by a psychology professional. The three most utilized psychotherapies for individuals and families are psychodynamic, cognitive behavioral, and supportive (expressive) (Strada & Sourkes, 2015).

### *Psychodynamic Therapy*

Psychodynamic therapy, or insight therapy, is a form of psychotherapy that focuses on unconscious processes manifested in current behavior. Self-awareness and understanding how the past influences current behavior are emphasized. Behaviors are analyzed and interpreted based on the assumption that the subsequent insight and the experiences in the therapeutic relationship can be transferred to the world outside the therapeutic setting (de Vries & Stiefel, 2014). A basic tenet of this therapy is that the past is repeating itself in the present in ways that create difficulty for patients. For example, disappointment in a current relationship may resonate with early problems with parents or siblings.

Psychodynamic psychotherapies rely on key theoretical concepts, including the following:

> the existence of an unconscious, which influences our thoughts, emotions, and behaviors; the impact of early development on later stages of life; the organization of the psyche by the ego, which has the capacity to reason and to anticipate; the id, which is a source of sexual and aggressive drives; and the superego, which contains theses drives by a guilty conscience; the protection of the individuals' equilibrium by (unconscious) defense mechanisms, such as rationalization, projection, or denial, which are triggered by threatening emotions or thoughts; and the observation, that unresolved issues of the patient are reenacted in the therapeutic setting. (de Vries & Stiefel, 2014, p. 125)

### *Psychoanalysis*

Psychoanalysis is a subset of psychodynamic therapy. It is a system of psychological theory and therapy that aims to treat mental disorders by investigating the interaction of conscious and unconscious elements in the mind and bringing repressed fears and conflicts into the conscious mind. Psychoanalysis is particularly associated with dream interpretation and attention to free association as well as analysis of the therapist–patient relationship. Psychoanalysis requires specialized training postdoctorally. Therapy is generally long term, though some shorter-term variations in the form of group and family and couple therapies have been developed (APA, n.d.).

## Cognitive Behavioral Therapy

Cognitive behavioral therapy (CBT) encompasses a broad range of psychological approaches that focus on the role of thoughts and behaviors in creating and maintaining psychological distress. The essential aim is to understand how people's cognitive distortions and subsequent irrational thinking adversely affect their ability to cope optimally with stressful life events and then to help identify distorted beliefs. Recognition of the influence of negative automatic thoughts is a key part of the therapy. Automatic reactions to repetitive stressors can create a cycle of anxiety and negative thinking. Learning ways to challenge these negative thoughts is key in this therapy. Therapists will assist their patients to identify these negative thoughts and how they influence behavior. Learning ways to challenge the negative thinking through techniques such as problem solving, reframing, and thought stopping can allow patients to develop new coping patterns. Physical sensations can also contribute to negative thought patterns. Pain and nausea, for example, can be exacerbated by negative thinking. Therapy helps people question whether their current view is accurate or helpful and then supports their exploration of alternatives. CBT has been found to be helpful for symptoms such as fatigue and insomnia.

CBT can be conducted in individual and group formats and is generally short term and structured. Behavioral therapies such as relaxation techniques can be incorporated to teach strategies to control negative thoughts. Individual and group cognitive therapy are being used with increasing frequency in the medical setting (Levin, White, Bialer, Charlson, & Kissane, 2014). In recent years, concerted attempts have been made to introduce CBT as an effective part of enhancing the psychological care of patients with cancer (Horne & Watson, 2011). Normalizing stress reactions, challenging negative thinking, and promoting problem solving can enhance care of the patient with cancer (Moorey & Watson, 2015). It has been helpful in treating adjustment reactions in patients with cancer (Adler & Page, 2008).

## Supportive Psychotherapy

Supportive psychotherapy is a therapeutic approach that uses interventions to help patients deal with distressing emotions, reinforce preexisting strengths, and promote adaptive coping with the illness. It explores patients' self, body image, and role changes within a relationship of mutual respect and trust (Lederberg & Holland, 2011). This therapy is the most extensively practiced form of individual psychotherapy (Winston, 2014). Its approach involves providing emotional support and encouragement, focusing on emotional responses, and encouraging adaptive coping. Goals of supportive psychotherapy often include enhancement of self-esteem and coping as well as prevention of relapse of emotional problems rather than changing the personality (Winston, 2014). Supportive psychotherapy emphasizes an ongoing relationship with the patient to address distress and coping. By working through the problems in an ongoing relationship with the therapist, the patient gains confidence and skills to face the challenges ahead. Lederberg, Greenstein, and Holland (2015) reported that this form of therapy has been used to effectively manage depression, anxiety, and distress across all stages of cancer. Supportive psychotherapy may be the home base for patients through difficult times, and referrals to other specific forms of therapy are made as needed.

## Group Therapy

Group therapy comprises clients meeting together regularly with a therapist for purposes of sharing, gaining personal insight, and improving interpersonal coping strategies (Townsend, 2015). Group therapy differs from support groups in that group therapy is led by someone with advanced degrees in the psychology field (e.g., psychologists, psychiatrists, social workers, advanced practice psychiatric nurses) to seek improvement of function on an interpersonal level. Generally, the group is based on a theoretical framework, such as psychodynamics and cognitive. Group therapy allows patients to work through interpersonal issues through relating to others in the group.

## Dignity Therapy

Dignity therapy is a patient-affirming psychotherapeutic intervention designed to address existential and psychosocial distress in people who have only a short time left to live. Dignity is promoted by physical comfort, interpersonal relationships, spiritual peace, belongingness, and hope (see Chapter 9). Dignity therapists help patients to recall events from their lives, along with important thoughts, feelings, values, and life accomplishments. The focus can be on addressing relationships, leaving a legacy, and sharing ways to express love. Patients are invited to share their hopes and dreams for loved ones, pass along advice or guidance to the important people in their lives, and how they wish to be remembered (Chocinov & McKeen, 2011). Using a structured interview format, dignity therapists encourage patient participation. It is unique in that it aims to improve the quality of life in terminally ill patients by encouraging them to reflect on important or memorable life events.

Sessions are transcribed and edited, with a returned final version that they can bequeath to loved ones (Chochinov et al., 2006). This therapeutic intervention has its roots in the right to die movement, when "death with dignity" became a commonly heard phrase. Defining what is dignity led to the development of this therapeutic approach. This therapy is appropriate for patients near the end who are struggling with existential issues. It has multiple benefits, including promotion of spiritual and psychological well-being, mitigation of suffering, and engendering meaning and purpose. In some instances, it helps people prepare for death or provides them comfort in the time they have remaining. For family survivors, dignity therapy can help ease bereavement by giving them a document that expresses the feelings and thoughts of their departed loved one (Chocinov & McKeen, 2011).

Dignity therapy is fairly new with limited research data. Randomized controlled trials are difficult to perform given the sensitive nature of the patient population. A recent review of the literature found dignity therapy led to high satisfaction and benefits for patients and their families, including increased sense of meaning and purpose. The effects on physical or emotional symptoms, however, were inconsistent (Fitchett, Emanuel, Handzo, Boyken, & Wilkie, 2015). Chochinov and colleagues developed a Patient Dignity Inventory tool to track dignity-related distress. Dignity therapy has grown to be used in many palliative care settings, both as individual and group formats (Chochinov & Kredentser, 2015).

## Meaning-Centered Psychotherapy

Clinicians often are at a loss with patients who are facing death and are struggling with a sense of loss of meaning and despair. Facing death can bring about fear, hopelessness, and a loss of purpose in living. These feelings can contribute to suffering. An increasingly important concern for clinicians who care for patients at the end of life is their spiritual well-being and sense of meaning and purpose in life. Meaning-centered therapy has been developed to provide short-term, structured interventions to address spiritual well-being.

The therapy format involves the use of didactic and experiential exercises for the patient and therapist to work together to understand the importance and relevance of sustaining, reconnecting with, and creating meaning in their lives through common and reliable sources of meaning. Patients learn ways to shift from one source of meaning to another as the disease progresses. Lichtenthal, Applebaum, and Breitbart (2015) suggested that therapists support their patients to move away from actively doing things to just being present so that meaning can be derived from more passive ways as the disease progresses. Patients are taught that these sources of meaning may serve as resources during difficult times to address despair. Both individual and group formats have been developed (Lichtenthal et al., 2015). This therapy has also been used with family caregivers. Breitbart et al. (2015) found, in a sample of 253 patients with advanced cancer, those receiving meaning-centered psychotherapy had improvement in depression and quality of life. Applebaum, Kulikowski, and Breitbart (2015) reported that the use of meaning-centered therapy helped a spouse of a patient with cancer address personal existential distress and sense of burden. This therapy has been studied in a randomized controlled trial to show improved spiritual well-being and meaning and decreased anxiety, hopelessness, and desire for death (Breitbart et al., 2010).

## Mind–Body Practices

Mind–body practices are sometimes known as integrative therapies or as behavioral therapies. These therapies can help patients to recognize the role of the interaction between the mind and body as an important component of cancer treatment. Behavioral therapies use a variety of techniques, including relaxation, guided imagery, hypnosis, and biofeedback (Fawzy & Fawzy, 2011).

Rosenbaum and Van de Velde (2016) found that integrative techniques of yoga and massage reduced patients' stress and anxiety, improved their moods, and had a positive effect on overall health and quality of life.

### Relaxation Therapy

Relaxation therapy comprises learning different ways to reduce the body's stress response to induce the "relaxation response." This response is characterized by feelings of both physical and psychological relaxation (Lewis & Sharp, 2011). Relaxation therapy often includes progressive muscle relaxation as well as the incorporation of breathing exercises to focus one's attention within and reduce the reaction to outside stimuli. The relaxation response is an integrated psychobiologic phenomenon associated with reduced heart rate, peripheral vasodilatation, diaphragmatic breathing, increased alpha activity in the brain, and reduced muscle tone (Lewis & Sharp, 2011). Some advantages of using relaxation techniques for patients with cancer include promotion of well-being, prevention and control of distress, and a sense of mastery over distress during cancer treatment (Lewis & Sharp, 2011).

## Mindfulness

Mindfulness is a component of meditation and is based on the experience of yoga and Buddhist philosophy. It is a contemplative practice of being fully aware of what is occurring in the present moment (Bishop et al., 2004). It has two components: the self-regulating attention of immediate experience, thereby allowing for greater awareness of mental events in the present moment; and adopting a curiosity, openness, and acceptance toward one's experiences in this moment (Bishop et al., 2004). According to Shapiro and Carlson (2009), mindfulness has three objectives: intention, attention, and attitude. Mindfulness is the idea of learning to be present in life as it is occurring. Mental energy spent on regret and worry about the future contribute to depression and anxiety (Carlson, 2015). Mindfulness counteracts the experience of automatically reacting to experience, ruminating about the past, and worrying about the future, which may be prominent in individuals facing a life-threatening diagnosis (Carlson & Speca, 2010).

Mindfulness is achieved by paying attention to types of thoughts and feelings and body sensations. Techniques usually include sitting meditation, body scan, yoga, and breathing to focus attention inward. The person is encouraged to incorporate this into daily life. Incorporating yoga can include focus on yoga positions, breathing techniques, and meditation training. Yoga postures are used to focus attention inward. Mindfulness-based stress reduction (MBSR) is an approach to teach the use of mindfulness techniques in a more formal group setting, where skills can be effectively taught (Bishop et al., 2004). This can include group reflection, relaxation skills, awareness of breath, healing imagery, and mindful yoga practice. This program can also include cognitive behavior strategies to better understand one's response to illness (Charlson et al., 2014). Fish, Ettridge, Sharplin, Hancock, and Knott (2014) found MBSR to be effective in reducing distress and improving quality of life in patients with cancer. Facilitating MBSR requires specialized training.

Learning fundamentals of mind–body connection and how one's interpretations of the world can cause both physical and mental suffering are components of mindfulness. By focusing on the present, patients receive help controlling cancer-related fears, such as disease progression. Mindfulness has been combined with other therapies, including psychotherapies, as well as music and art therapies. Mindfulness-based concepts and techniques can be successfully integrated into standard psychotherapy. This will be most effective when therapists have a personal appreciation and practice of these skills (Payne, 2011). Mindfulness is also part of relaxation techniques and guided imagery.

## Guided Imagery

This technique is aimed at enhancing and anchoring the relaxation response in patients to increase the potency and controllability of it (Lewis & Sharp, 2011). Once the patient has obtained the optimal level of relaxation, the next step is to image or imagine a "special place." This can be a place that the patient is familiar with or an imaginary one to help induce a sense of calm and peacefulness. The aim is to allow patients to develop an image in their minds that is associated with safety and represents an escape from present concerns. Producing an image associated with relaxation then becomes another cue to induce the relaxation response. Relaxation is generally thought to be necessary for imagery to be successful, as it allows the mind to be open and receptive to new information. This can enhance the ability to produce an image. However, little empirical evidence supports such assertions (Lewis & Sharp, 2011). Guided imagery has been found to be helpful to facilitate rest and sleep for hospitalized patients (Nooner, Dwyer, DeShea, & Yeo, 2016).

A variation of guided imagery is known as visualization. Visualization is a cognitive tool that accesses one's imagination to realize all aspects of an object, action, or outcome. This may include recreating a mental sensory experience of sound, sight, smell, taste, or touch. In psychological practice, visualization is often used to mentally rehearse an action or bring a patient to a state of relaxation. In cancer care, visualization is also a technique to visualize the body's natural defenses to fight the cancer (Lewis & Sharp, 2011).

## Hypnosis

Hypnosis is a psychophysiological state of attentive, receptive concentration with relative suspension of peripheral awareness (Maldonado, 2015). Hypnosis has been used to treat a variety of cancer-related anxieties, such as needle phobia, chemotherapy side effects, anticipatory anxiety, and pain. Some individuals can enter a trance state much easier than others. By including posthypnotic suggestions, patients can gain some control over fears or negative behaviors. Hypnosis can be incorporated into psychotherapy if the therapist has that training.

## Massage

Massage is one of the oldest healthcare practices (Kravits, 2015). Massage involves the manual techniques of rubbing, stroking, tapping, or kneading the body's soft tissues to influence the whole person and promote well-being and relaxation (Wilkinson, Barnes, & Storey, 2008). In a review article, Field (2016) found evidence that massage therapy provides more stimulation of pressure receptors. This, in turn, enhances vagal activity and reduces cortisol levels. Despite limited research in the United States, the massage therapy profession has grown significantly. Massage therapy is increasingly practiced in traditional medical settings, highlighting the need for more rigorous research. Benefits include relaxation, pain relief, reduction of anxiety and depression, increased energy, and improved circulation (Kravits, 2015). Massage therapists working with patients with cancer need to have special training to safely provide the therapy in the presence of the many complexities, such as bone metastasis and altered platelet activity (Kravits, 2015).

# Behavior Modification Techniques

Behavior modification techniques include positive and negative reinforcement to modify negative behaviors. The most commonly used technique in oncology is systematic desensitization, a treatment for phobias in which the individual is taught to relax and then imagine various components of the phobic stimulus on a graded hierarchy, moving from that which produces the least fear to the most (Townsend, 2015). It is systematic in that individuals are able to identify a hierarchy of anxiety-producing events through which they progress during therapy. It may be used to treat phobias like fear of elevators or spiders. Through relaxation techniques paired with thinking or exposure to the stressful item, the anxiety can be reduced. For example, for an individual's fear of elevators, the first step might be to look at a picture of an elevator, then a lobby of a building with an elevator. By pairing these exposures with relaxation, the cycle of anxiety can be reduced or broken (Townsend, 2015). This approach teaches techniques to identify the early signs of building tension and ways to reduce the stress response. Generally, the person does not progress to experiencing the stressor (e.g., elevator ride) until he or she has mastered the ability to control the anxiety at the earlier stages. Systematic desensitization has been used to address fears of patients with cancer. Some common fears include needles, getting in an elevator at the oncologist's office, lying in the magnetic resonance imaging machine, or entering the chemotherapy treatment area. It has been effective in treating anxiety and phobias (Greer, MacDonald, & Traeger, 2015).

# Other Therapies

## Pastoral Counseling

Pastoral counseling generally is provided by a religious leader who is trained in traditional mental health theories and modalities. This form of counseling can include aspects of traditional psychotherapy and address spiritual support. It also can be particularly helpful in challenging misinformed spiritual beliefs that are contributing to the patient's psychological distress.

## Pet Therapy

Pet therapy, or animal-assisted therapy, is a formal guided interaction between a trained animal, a handler, and the patient. Unconditional love from an animal can provide support, enhance self-esteem, reduce anxiety and depression, and develop social skills. Patients who might be sensitive about their appearance after cancer treatment have benefitted from the nonjudgmental response from animals (Fleishman et al., 2015). Generally incorporated as part of a volunteer program, animal handlers require extensive training to be sensitive to the needs of patients with cancer. Animal-assisted therapy can be confused with animal-assisted activities that generally include an animal and its handler interacting with one or more people for comfort or recreation. Extensive anecdotal evidence supports the benefits of pet therapy, but more research is needed to demonstrate the long-term benefits of this therapy for people with cancer (Barger, 2016).

## Music Therapy

Music therapy is purposeful use of music to address physical, emotional, cognitive, social, and spiritual needs of individuals. Music is an important part of life and has been found to enhance quality of life. It is recognized as a nonpharmacologic modality offering soothing and expressive benefits (Luzzatto & Magill, 2015). Music can enhance the expression of feelings and memories. Music therapy includes the self-expression of feelings through music and can include listening to music, singing, composing, and playing instruments. Board-certified music therapists have advanced education in music as well as psychology and counseling. They can address anxiety, grief, depression, and isolation among other forms of distress through music. The goal is to get in touch with feelings and emotions that the patient is unable to experience in other ways (Townsend, 2015). Limited research exists on the effects of music as an intervention to minimize cancer pain (Keenan & Keithley, 2015).

## Art Therapy

Art therapy is based on the idea that the imagination is an essential part of mental function. Individuals project their internal world into visual images. Art therapy has its roots in psychoanalysis, where art was used to express the unconscious and facilitate access to the patient's inner world (Luzzatto & Magill, 2015). Professional art therapists are trained both in expressive use of art materials and in the psychotherapeutic process. Some outcomes of art therapy have been a calming effect, self-confidence, learning new coping strategies, new insight into one's behavior, and an increased ability to deal with existential issues (Luzzatto & Magill, 2015). Examples of the use of art therapy with patients with cancer can include the self-expression of building a collage or a free drawing. Talking about one's artwork can be a distraction as well as a way to express feelings and discover new meanings in life.

## The Future of Therapeutic Modalities

The development of new modalities is constantly evolving. Interestingly, some new modalities are based on combining therapies in new ways to enhance the therapeutic effect. For example, psychoeducation may be part of relaxation therapy, as education provided on the physiology of anxiety is incorporated in the relaxation session. Mindfulness has been combined with music therapy to expand the effect of each therapy (Lesiuk, 2015). Many other combinations of approaches are currently being used or will be considered in the future.

## Conclusion

The variety of therapeutic modalities for patients with cancer continues to grow. Patients need to be informed and provided access to a variety of therapies that meet their specific needs. The oncology nurse needs to maintain current knowledge of the range of therapies available and how to get access to these for appropriate patients.

## References

Adler, N.E., & Page, A.E.K. (Eds.). (2008). *Cancer care for the whole patient: Meeting psychosocial health needs.* Washington, DC: National Academies Press.

American Psychological Association. (n.d.). Psychoanalysis in psychology. Retrieved from http://www.apa.org/ed/graduate/specialize/psychoanalytic.aspx

Applebaum, A.J., & Breitbart, W.S. (2013). Care for the cancer caregiver: A systematic review. *Palliative and Supportive Care, 11,* 231–252. doi:10.1017/S1478951512000594

Applebaum, A.J., Kulikowski, J.R., & Breitbart, W.S. (2015). Meaning-centered psychotherapy for cancer caregivers: Rationale and overview. *Palliative and Supportive Care, 13,* 1631–1641. doi:10.1017/S1478951515000450

Barger, T.S. (2016). Pet project: Trained therapy animals boost the moods of hospitalized patients with cancer. *Cure, 15,* 48–52.

Bäuml, J., Froböse, T., Kraemer, S., Rentrop, M., & Pitschel-Walz, G. (2006). Psychoeducation: A basic psychotherapeutic intervention for patients with schizophrenia and their families. *Schizophrenia Bulletin, 32*(Suppl. 1), S1–S9. doi:10.1093/schbul/sbl017

Bishop, S.R., Lau, M., Shapiro, S., Carlson, L., Anderson, N.D., Carmody, J., ... Devins, G. (2004). Mindfulness: A proposed operational definition. *Clinical Psychology: Science and Practice, 11,* 230–241. doi:10.1093/clipsy.bph077

Breitbart, W.S., Rosenfeld, B., Gibson, C., Pessin, H., Poppito, S., Nelson, C., ... Olden, M. (2010). Meaning-centered group psychotherapy for patients with advanced cancer: A pilot randomized controlled trial. *Psycho-Oncology, 19,* 21–28. doi:10.1002/pon.1556

Breitbart, W.S., Rosenfeld, B., Pessin, H., Applebaum, A., Kulikowski, J., & Lichtenthal, W.G. (2015). Meaning-centered group psychotherapy: An effective intervention for improving psychological well-being in patients with advanced cancer. *Journal of Clinical Oncology, 33,* 749–754. doi:10.1200/JCO.2014.57.2198

Carlson, L.E. (2015). Mindfulness meditation and yoga for cancer patients. In J.C. Holland, W.S. Breitbart, P.N. Butow, P.B. Jacobson, M.J. Loscalzo, & R. McCorkle (Eds.), *Psycho-oncology* (3rd ed., pp. 492–496). New York, NY: Oxford University Press.

Carlson, L.E., & Speca, M. (2010). *Mindfulness-based cancer recovery: A step-by-step MBSR approach to help you cope with treatment and reclaim your life.* Oakland, CA: New Harbinger Publications.

Charlson, M.E., Loizzo, J., Moadel, A., Neale, M., Newman, C., Olivo, E., … Peterson, J.C. (2014). Contemplative self-healing in women breast cancer survivors: A pilot study in underserved minority women shows improvement in quality of life and reduced stress. *BMC Complementary and Alternative Medicine, 14,* 349. doi:10.1186/1472-6882-14-349

Chochinov, H.M., Hack, T., Hassard, T., Kristjanson, L.J., McClement, S., & Harlos, M. (2006). Dignity therapy: A novel psychotherapeutic intervention for patients near the end of life. *Journal of Clinical Oncology, 23,* 5520–5525. doi:10.1200/JCO.2005.08.391

Chochinov, H.M., & Kredentser, M.S. (2015). Dignity in the terminally ill. In J.C. Holland, W.S. Breitbart, P.N. Butow, P.B. Jacobson, M.J. Loscalzo, & R. McCorkle (Eds.), *Psycho-oncology* (3rd ed., pp. 480–486). New York, NY: Oxford University Press.

Chochinov, H.M., & McKeen, N.A. (2011). Dignity therapy. In M. Watson & D.W. Kissane (Eds.), *Handbook of psychotherapy in cancer care* (pp. 79–88). West Sussex, United Kingdom: Wiley-Blackwell.

de Vries, M., & Stiefel, F. (2014). Psycho-oncological interventions and psychotherapy in the oncology setting. In U. Goerling (Ed.), *Psycho-oncology* (pp. 121–135). doi:10.1007/978-3-642-40187-9_9

Fawzy, F.I., & Fawzy, N.W. (2011). A short-term, structured, psychoeducational intervention for newly diagnosed cancer patients. In M. Watson & D.W. Kissane (Eds.), *Handbook of psychotherapy in cancer care* (pp. 119–135). West Sussex, United Kingdom: Wiley-Blackwell.

Field, T. (2016). Massage therapy research review. *Complementary Therapies in Clinical Practice, 24,* 19–31. doi:10.1016/j.ctcp.2016.04.005

Fish, J.A., Ettridge, K., Sharplin, G.R., Hancock, B., & Knott, V.E. (2014). Mindfulness-based cancer stress management: Impact of a mindfulness-based programme on psychological distress and quality of life. *European Journal of Cancer Care, 23,* 413–421. doi:10.1111/ecc.12136

Fitchett, G., Emanuel, L., Handzo, G., Boyken, L., & Wilkie, D.J. (2015). Care of the human spirit and the role of dignity therapy: A systematic review of dignity therapy research. *BMC Palliative Care, 14,* 8. doi:10.1186/s12904-015-0007-1

Fleishman, S.D., Jonel, P., Chen, M.R., Rosenwalk, V., Abolencia, V., Gerber, J., & Nadesan, S. (2015). Beneficial effects of animal-assisted visits on quality of life during multimodal radiation-chemotherapy regimens. *Journal of Community and Supportive Oncology, 13,* 22–26. doi:10.12788/jcso.0102

Garchinski, C.M., DiBiase, A.-M., Wong, R.K., & Sagar, S.M. (2014). Patient-centered care in cancer treatment programs: The future of integrative oncology through psychoeducation. *Future Oncology, 10,* 2603–2614. doi:10.2217/fon.14.186

Greer, J.A., MacDonald, J., & Traeger, L. (2015). Anxiety disorders. In J.C. Holland, W.S. Breitbart, P.N. Butow, P.B. Jacobson, M.J. Loscalzo, & R. McCorkle (Eds.), *Psycho-oncology* (3rd ed., pp. 296–303). New York, NY: Oxford University Press.

Horne, D., & Watson, M. (2011). Cognitive-behavioural therapies in cancer care. In M. Watson & D.W. Kissane (Eds.), *Handbook of psychotherapy in cancer care* (pp. 15–26). West Sussex, United Kingdom: Wiley-Blackwell.

Keenan, A., & Keithley, J.K. (2015). Integrative review: Effects of music on cancer pain in adults [Online exclusive]. *Oncology Nursing Forum, 42,* E368–E375. doi:10.1188/15.ONF.E368-E375

Kravits, K. (2015). Complementary and alternative therapies in palliative care. In B.R. Ferrell, N. Coyle, & J.A. Paice (Eds.), *Oxford textbook of palliative nursing* (pp. 449–462). New York, NY: Oxford University Press.

Lederberg, M.S., Greenstein, M., & Holland, J.C. (2015). Supportive psychotherapy and cancer. In J.C. Holland, W.S. Breitbart, P.N. Butow, P.B. Jacobson, M.J. Loscalzo, & R. McCorkle (Eds.), *Psycho-oncology* (3rd ed., pp. 443–448). New York, NY: Oxford University Press.

Lederberg, M.S., & Holland, J.C. (2011). Supportive psychotherapy in cancer care: An essential ingredient in all therapies. In M. Watson & D.W. Kissane (Eds.), *Handbook of psychotherapy in cancer care* (pp. 3–14). West Sussex, United Kingdom: Wiley-Blackwell.

Lesiuk, T. (2015). The effect of mindfulness-based music therapy on attention and mood in women receiving adjuvant chemotherapy for breast cancer: A pilot study. *Oncology Nursing Forum, 42,* 276–282. doi:10.1017/S1478951513000618

Levin, T.T., White, C.A., Bialer, P., Charlson, R.W., & Kissane, D.W. (2014). A review of cognitive therapy in acute medical settings. Part II: Strategies and complexities. *Palliative and Supportive Care, 11,* 253–266.

Lewis, E.J., & Sharp, D.M. (2011). Relaxation and image-based therapy. In M. Watson & D.W. Kissane (Eds.), *Handbook of psychotherapy in cancer care* (pp. 49–58). West Sussex, United Kingdom: Wiley-Blackwell.

Lichtenthal, W.G., Applebaum, A.J., & Breitbart, W.S. (2015). Meaning-centered therapy. In J.C. Holland, W.S. Breitbart, P.N. Butow, P.B. Jacobson, M.J. Loscalzo, & R. McCorkle (Eds.), *Psycho-oncology* (3rd ed., pp. 475–479). New York, NY: Oxford University Press.

Luzzatto, P.M., & Magill, L. (2015). Art and music therapy. In J.C. Holland, W.S. Breitbart, P.N. Butow, P.B. Jacobson, M.J. Loscalzo, & R. McCorkle (Eds.), *Psycho-oncology* (3rd ed., pp. 497–501). New York, NY: Oxford University Press.

Maldonado, J.R. (2015). Hypnosis in psychosomatic medicine. In B.S. Fogel & D.B. Greenberg (Eds.), *Psychiatric care of medical patients* (3rd ed., pp. 266–300). New York, NY: Oxford University Press.

Moorey, S., & Watson, M. (2015). Cognitive therapy. In J.C. Holland, W.S. Breitbart, P.N. Butow, P.B. Jacobson, M.J. Loscalzo, & R. McCorkle (Eds.), *Psycho-oncology* (3rd ed., pp. 458–463). New York, NY: Oxford University Press.

Nooner, A.K., Dwyer, K., DeShea, L., & Yeo, T.P. (2016). Using relaxation and guided imagery to address pain, fatigue, and sleep disturbances: A pilot study. *Clinical Journal of Oncology Nursing, 20,* 547–552. doi:10.1188/16.CJON.547-552

Norcross, J.C. (1990). An eclectic definition of psychotherapy. In J.K. Zeig & W.M. Munion (Eds.), *What is psychotherapy? Contemporary perspectives* (pp. 218–220). San Francisco, CA: Jossey-Bass.

Oncology Nursing Society. (n.d.). Psychoeducation/psychoeducational interventions. Retrieved from https://www.ons.org/intervention/psychoeducationpsychoeducational-interventions

Payne, D. (2011). Mindful interventions for cancer patients. In M. Watson & D.W. Kissane (Eds.), *Handbook of psychotherapy in cancer care* (pp. 39–47). West Sussex, United Kingdom: Wiley-Blackwell.

Rosenbaum, M.S., & Van de Velde, J. (2016). The effects of yoga, massage, and Reiki on patient well-being at a cancer resource center [Online exclusive]. *Clinical Journal of Oncology Nursing, 20,* E77–E81. doi:10.1188/16.CJON.E77-E81

Schou, B.I., Karesen, R., Smeby, N.A., Espe, R., Sorensen, E.M., Amundsen, M., ... Ekeberg, O. (2014). Effects of a psychoeducational versus a support group intervention in patients with early-stage breast cancer: Results of a randomized controlled trial. *Cancer Nursing, 37,* 198–207. doi:10.1097/NCC.0b013e31829879a3

Shapiro, S., & Carlson, L. (2009). *The art and science of mindfulness: Integrating mindfulness into psychology and the helping professions.* Washington, DC: American Psychological Association.

Strada, E.A., & Sourkes, B.M. (2015). Principles of psychotherapy. In J.C. Holland, W.S. Breitbart, P.N. Butow, P.B. Jacobson, M.J. Loscalzo, & R. McCorkle (Eds.), *Psycho-oncology* (3rd ed., pp. 431–436). New York, NY: Oxford University Press.

Townsend, M.C. (2015). *Psychiatric mental health nursing* (8th ed.). Philadelphia, PA: F.A. Davis.

Wilkinson, S., Barnes, K., & Storey, L. (2008). Massage for symptom relief in patients with cancer: Systematic review. *Journal of Advanced Nursing, 63,* 430–439. doi:10.1111/j.1365-2648.2008.04712.x

Winston, A. (2014). Psychotherapy. In R.E. Hales, S.C. Yudofsky, & R. Weiss (Eds.), *American Psychiatric Publishing textbook of psychiatry* (6th ed.). Washington, DC: American Psychiatric Association.

# SECTION V

# Dimensions of Caring

Chapter 26. The Close of Life
Chapter 27. Ethical Issues
Chapter 28. Caring for the Family

**CHAPTER 26**

# The Close of Life

*Linda M. Gorman, RN, MN, PMHCNS-BC, CHPN, FPCN*

> *Endings matter, not just for the person, but perhaps even more, for those left behind.*
>
> —Atul Gawande

When patients and their families face the news that the cancer cannot be cured and is, in fact, advancing, end-of-life care needs to move into the primary treatment mode. Despite a declining death rate from cancer in recent years, 23% of deaths in the United States are cancer related (Siegel, Miller, & Jemal, 2017). In recent years, much has been published about the importance of good end-of-life care; however, it continues to elude some patients (Institute of Medicine [IOM], 2015). As a society, we continue to struggle with bringing death into the mainstream. Despite the growth of hospice and palliative care programs in the last 20 years, many patients remain unprepared for facing the final chapter of their disease.

As advances in cancer treatment are constantly being made, delays often occur in discussing end-of-life wishes or planning for the last phase of the disease. Even with an uncertain impact on quality, the possible chance at some extension of life may become the focus. Talking about end-of-life wishes may be viewed as negative and needing to be avoided until a later date. The administration of chemotherapy within 30 days of death is now being tracked by some researchers (Pacetti et al., 2015). Patients may be motivated to pursue chemotherapy near the end of life, in part, because of a poor understanding of their disease, hope that chemotherapy will provide benefit, and unrealistic expectations (Kadakia, Moynihan, Smith, & Loprinzi, 2012). Weeks et al. (2012) found that unrealistic expectations of chemotherapy in the presence of metastatic lung and colorectal cancers were common. Patients often viewed their treatment as potentially curative. Oncology professionals sometimes use confusing terms that can be misinterpreted as being curative, such as *prolonging survival* or *tumor response* (Rabow, 2014). Mack et al. (2015) found that patients with advanced lung and colon cancers who wanted care directed at comfort were just as likely to receive chemotherapy near death as patients who preferred life-prolonging care. In this study, these patients were able to identify that the chemotherapy was not curative.

Wright, Zhang, Keating, Weeks, and Prigerson (2014) also reported that chemotherapy in the last month of life is associated with greater risk of more aggressive treatment at the end, including CPR and intensive care unit (ICU) admissions. In 2012, the American Society of Clinical Oncology identified that offering nonbeneficial cancer treatment at the end of life was one of the top five practice concerns (Schnipper et al., 2012). The recommendation is to not use cancer-directed therapy for patients with solid tumors who have the following characteristics: low performance status (3 or 4), no benefit from prior evidence-based interventions, not eligible for a clinical trial, and no strong evidence supporting the clinical value of further anticancer treatment. Prigerson et al. (2015) had caregivers rate patients' quality of life in the week prior to death. They found that patients with a variety of metastatic cancers receiving chemotherapy near the end of their lives had greater distress and poorer quality of life near death regardless of their performance status at the time of administration. In another study by Wright et al. (2016), among 1,146 family members of older patients with fee-for-service Medicare who died of lung or colorectal cancer, earlier hospice enrollment, avoidance of ICU admissions within 30 days of death, and death occurring outside the hospital were associated with perceptions of better end-of-life care. These findings are supportive of advance care planning consistent with the preferences of patients.

## Initiating Advance Care Planning Conversations

Advance care planning conversations are an essential part of good patient care for patients with cancer. These conversations often do not take place or are ineffective (IOM, 2015; Saiki, Ferrell, Longo-Schoeberlein, Chung, & Smith 2017). Oncology professionals can initiate discussions about goals on a regular basis rather than waiting for the right moment to have the frank serious talk that most want to avoid. Some recent studies supported that incorporating end-of-life discussions between the patient and oncologist has led to improvements in patients' preferences being followed, better quality of life at the end, and reduced use of the ICU as the place of death (Mack, Weeks, Wright, Block, & Prigerson, 2010; Wright et al., 2008). Of special note is that these discussions were not associated with increased depression or giving up, often cited as a fear (Wright et al., 2008). However, Gawande (2016) noted that physicians and other health professionals—even those with substantial experience caring for the seriously ill—commonly lack skills in eliciting the goals, preferences, and values of their patients.

Transitioning from a "cure" mode to a "care" mode often is frightening. Patients and their loved ones may feel abandoned, helpless, panicked, and/or frustrated. Oncology nurses have an important role in promoting communication in advancing disease. Regularly assessing the presence of an advance directive, reviewing the content of that directive, promoting open discussion about the patient's hopes and fears, seeking out the patient's understanding of the treatment and prognosis, as well as promoting interprofessional communication about the patient's treatment plan, are all roles for nurses. Taking a more active role in communicating with patients, their families, and physicians about goals of care and prognosis takes special skills, and nurses may need to seek out more education and practice to develop them.

Some barriers to nurses taking a more active role in preparing patients may include a long-held belief that these conversations take away hope, fear of depressing the patient, uncertainty of what the physician has discussed with the patient, perception that the patient/family does not want to talk about these issues, and lack of skills (Boyd, Merkh, Rutledge, & Randall, 2011). These barriers can be addressed with development of better communication between the interprofessional team and patient/family. See Figure 26-1 for guidelines on enhancing communication with patients and their families.

As the end of life approaches, it is a key time to provide extra support and resources to the patient and family. Once the patient is reassured of this support, conversations about handling possible scenarios and reestablishing understanding of the patient's goals will help the oncology professional provide the appropriate support. As improved efforts are under way to provide oncology professionals with training in palliative care, more inroads will continue to be made to improve access to high quality end-of-life care. Oncology professionals need skills to help patients and their families identify and prepare for the advancing disease.

Because many patients will be physically and/or cognitively impaired as the end of life nears, final decisions may need to be made by others. Family members need to be aware of the patient's wishes (IOM, 2015).

## Components of High-Quality End-of-Life Care

Singer, Martin, and Kelner (1999) reported on the wishes of 126 people with advanced illnesses. Their wishes included (a) management of pain and other distressing symptoms of the illness, (b) a sense of control, (c) not wanting to be a burden, (d) avoidance of inappropriate prolongation of dying, and (e) strengthened relationships with loved ones. Steinhauser et al. (2000) studied a group of patients who expressed additional wishes, including having the opportunity to gain a sense of completion in their lives, wanting support from healthcare professionals beyond disease management, and wishing to be mentally aware. These points provide a rallying call to all oncology professionals to examine how they can address these quality-of-life issues for their patients. Kuhl (2009) suggested that the wishes of the dying reflect their own life journey and what they have valued throughout their lives. Few of these wishes can be achieved if advancing illness is not acknowledged and the opportunity to plan is not provided (Gawande, 2014).

---

- When the aggressive treatment phase is completed, offer resources and a concrete treatment plan for this next phase.
- Encourage the patient to share their goals with each phase of the illness.
- Introduce palliative care support early in the treatment. For patients who are clearly declining, introduce hospice information early rather than waiting for the last days.
- Identify what patients understand about their illness.
- Listen for openings the patient is willing to discuss concerns. For example, if a patient says, "I do not know how I will manage at home being so weak," this presents the opportunity to ask more about what he or she is worried about.
- If an opening does not present itself, make an observation about the patient's condition, such as, "I know things have been rough lately. What has the doctor said?" This will give the nurse a sense of the readiness to hear information about end-of-life care. You can also ask the doctor what discussions he or she has had in the past with the patient to give you more information.
- Move to more specific questions once the door to the conversation has been opened. For example, "I see how weak you are. What are you hoping for now?" This question can give you a clearer picture of what the patient and family are thinking.

**Figure 26-1. Addressing End-of-Life Care Wishes With Patients and Their Families**

The National Consensus Project for Quality Palliative Care (NCP, 2013) has been a leader in defining consistent and high standards as well as promoting continuity of care across settings. The guidelines this initiative developed were identified by the National Quality Forum as the preferred practices for palliative and hospice care quality. IOM (2015) proposed components of good end-of-life care based on NCP's guidelines (see Table 26-1).

**Table 26-1. Institute of Medicine Committee's Proposed Core Components of Quality End-of-Life Care**

| Component | Rationale |
| --- | --- |
| Frequent assessment of the patient's physical, emotional, social, and spiritual well-being | Interventions and assistance must be based on accurately identified needs. |
| Management of emotional distress | All clinicians should be able to identify distress and direct its initial and basic management. This is part of the definition of palliative care, a basic component of hospice, and clearly of fundamental importance. |
| Offer referral to expert-level palliative care | People with palliative needs beyond those that can be provided by non-specialist-level clinicians deserve access to appropriate expert-level care. |
| Offer referral to hospice if the patient has a prognosis of 6 months or less | People who meet the hospice eligibility criteria deserve access to services designed to meet their end-of-life needs. |
| Management of care and direct contact with patient and family for complex situations by a specialist-level palliative care physician | Care of people with serious illness may require specialist-level palliative care physician management, and effective physician management requires direct examination, contact, and communication. |
| Round-the-clock access to coordinated care and services | Patients in advanced stages of serious illness often require assistance, such as with activities of daily living, medication management, wound care, physical comfort, and psychosocial needs. Round-the-clock access to a consistent point of contact that can coordinate care obviates the need to dial 911 and engage emergency medical services. |
| Management of pain and other symptoms | All clinicians should be able to identify and direct the initial and basic management of pain and other symptoms. This is part of the definition of palliative care, a basic component of hospice, and clearly of fundamental importance. |
| Counseling of patient and family | Even patients who are not emotionally distressed face problems in areas such as loss of functioning, prognosis, coping with diverse symptoms, finances, and family dynamics, and family members experience these problems as well, both directly and indirectly. |
| Family caregiver support | A focus on the family is part of the definition of palliative care; family members and caregivers both participate in the patient's care and require assistance themselves. |

*(Continued on next page)*

**Table 26-1. Institute of Medicine Committee's Proposed Core Components of Quality End-of-Life Care** *(Continued)*

| Component | Rationale |
|---|---|
| Attention to the patient's social and cultural context and social needs | Person-centered care requires awareness of patients' perspectives on their social environment and of their needs for social support, including at the time of death. Companionship at the bedside at time of death may be an important part of the psychological, social, and spiritual aspects of end-of-life care for some individuals. |
| Attention to the patient's spiritual and religious needs | The final phase of life often has a spiritual and religious component, and research shows that spiritual assistance is associated with quality of care. |
| Regular personalized revision of the care plan and access to services based on the changing needs of the patient and family | Care must be person-centered and fit current circumstances, which may mean that not all of the above components will be important or desirable in all cases. |

*Note.* From *Dying in America: Improving Quality and Honoring Individual Preferences Near the End of Life* (pp. 8–9), by Institute of Medicine, 2015, pp. 8–9, Washington, DC: National Academies Press. Copyright 2015 by National Academy of Sciences. Reprinted with permission.

# End-of-Life Programs

## Palliative Care

In recent years, the proliferation of palliative care programs has played a role in transitioning patients from cure-oriented treatment to supportive care. Though palliative care is available for patients who are still receiving curative treatment, it is an important part of end-of-life care. Palliative care programs can be instrumental in providing expert symptom management, advance care planning, and effective use of resources, as well as helping patients to achieve their goals. Palliative care support in the hospital, nursing home, outpatient clinic, or at home can provide the expertise to transition the patient to hospice care when appropriate (see Chapter 1 for in-depth discussion of palliative care).

## Hospice

Hospice is a philosophy of care for terminally ill patients and their families that focuses on palliating symptoms and enhancing the quality of life for patients at the end of life. Based on the Medicare model, hospice care generally is for patients with a life expectancy of six months or less if the disease takes its expected course. Hospice affirms life and neither hastens nor postpones death. Generally, all curative treatments are no longer provided.

The modern hospice movement began in London, England, in 1967 when Dame Cicely Saunders established St. Christopher's Hospice. The first U.S. hospice was started in 1974 in New Haven, Connecticut. Hospice care in the United States usually is a home-based program. "Home" can be a nursing home or an assisted living setting. The National Hospice and Palliative Care Organization (NHPCO, 2016) reported that more than 4,100 hospice programs exist in the United States.

Many of the early U.S. hospices were small agencies largely made up of volunteers who provided services in the home. Dedicated people who believed in the hospice concept were the backbone of this grassroots movement. In 1981, the National Hospice Study attempted to validate the impact of hospice care (Mor & Kidder, 1985). The study compared the care and costs involved in meeting the needs of the dying in traditional oncology units and hospices. The study revealed that hospice care, particularly home hospice care, was significantly less costly than conventional care in the final two months of life. It also revealed that improved symptom control and increased caregiver satisfaction existed in the hospice program. This study led to Congress passing the Medicare Hospice Benefit in 1983.

Medicare's coverage of hospice has played a major role in shaping hospice care as it exists today. The regulations and specifics can be found at the Centers for Medicare and Medicaid Services website (CMS, 2008). At least 80% of hospice patients are Medicare beneficiaries (NHPCO, 2016). Medicare beneficiaries who are certified by a physician to have less than six months to live and who are receiving no curative treatment for the illness can select the benefit. Hospice patients are able to receive noncurative medical and support services, many of which would not otherwise be covered in regular home care. Hospice care allows for ongoing visits by a hospice nurse without the need to identify a skilled need for care (as is required in home health care). Signing up for the hospice benefit means that the beneficiary waives all rights to Medicare payment for curative treatment of the terminal condition. The individual can revoke the benefit at any time to pursue aggressive treatment or because of a change in condition. The patient or surrogate usually signs a do-not-resuscitate form and is advised to call the hospice agency rather than emergency medical services in case of an emergency. If the patient or surrogate wishes to pursue aggressive treatment at any time, hospice can be discontinued, and the patient can pursue aggressive treatment.

Hospices are paid on a daily basis per patient rather than per visit, and Congress determines the amount that Medicare pays (CMS, 2016). The daily rate paid to hospices covers all services, including nursing, equipment, symptom management medications, home health aides, social work, and clergy visits.

Since the inception of the Medicare hospice benefit, many private insurers and state systems of Medicaid also have a hospice benefit. The Medicare benefit continues to pay for hospice care beyond the six-month life expectancy if patients continue to meet the qualifications.

The benefit provides for different levels of care depending on the variations in care intensity needed by the patient and family. *Routine home care* is the most common level of care provided by the interprofessional team in the patient's residence (place of residence can include assisted living or nursing home). *Inpatient respite care* covers patients who need a short stay in an inpatient facility to relieve their caregivers. Respite care can be provided for up to five days. *General inpatient care* is appropriate when patients need symptom management that requires an inpatient setting. The hospice can arrange admission to a contracted nursing home, hospice facility, or acute hospital. This is particularly useful if the patient's symptoms become too complex to manage in the home. *Continuous care* covers patients in brief periods of crisis by providing a minimum of eight hours per day of care in the home, at least 50% of which must be provided by a licensed nurse. Continuous care can be provided most often in the last days of life, when patients require symptom management and caregiver education and support, or if caregiver breakdown occurs, which may precipitate a period of crisis. Continuous care can be the key to supporting a person's wish to die at home surrounded by loved ones and supported by hospice (Newman, Thompson, & Chandler, 2013).

Hospice programs must provide care using an interprofessional team. This team provides a variety of services, including pain and symptom management, psychosocial and spiritual support, and bereavement services. All members of the team should participate in providing these services. These components contribute to meeting the goal of administering comfort care to patients and support to family members. Symptom management is key to providing good hospice care. Quality measures in hospice include rating patients' comfort at an acceptable level within 48 hours of admission (NHPCO, 2016). See Figure 26-2 for components of hospice care.

The picture of hospice care for patients with cancer has changed over the last few decades. In the early years of hospice, cancer was the most common diagnosis by far. This has declined over the past few years and is perhaps related to the many new treatment options available for end-stage patients and the clearer guidelines for hospice appropriateness for other diagnoses, such as dementia and heart disease. The most recent data available find about 28% of all hospice patients have a cancer diagnosis (NHPCO, 2016). In a large study of Medicare beneficiaries with cancer, those receiving hospice care had significantly lower rates of hospitalization, ICU admissions, and invasive procedures at the end of life, along with significantly lower total costs during the last year of life (Obermeyer et al., 2014).

The median length of stay on hospice was 23 days in 2015 (NHPCO, 2016). This is considerably less time on the program than the six-month benefit, which reflects that hospice often remains an underutilized benefit for many. Despite the benefits of the program, many barriers to accessing hospice care still exist (see Figure 26-3).

When to bring up hospice to a patient and family can be challenging for the oncology team because of the many barriers. Often, the referral is made when the patient is near death and the family is overwhelmed. Some approaches to bringing in hospice to the family discussion include the following:
- Introduce a discussion about the patient's goals for the future. Hospice can be included as one alternative for the future. If the patient is in the hospital, hospice can be presented as

---

- Patient and family as unit of care
- Focus on symptom management, addressing physical, psychosocial, and spiritual distress
- Interprofessional team including physician, nurses, social workers, pharmacist, chaplain, dietitian, physical therapists, and others
- Service available 24 hours a day, seven days a week
- Physician-directed, nurse-coordinated care
- Volunteers, family, and friends active in providing care and support
- Bereavement services for survivors
- Coordinated homecare services with inpatient care available

**Figure 26-2. Components of Hospice Care**

*Note.* Based on information from Centers for Medicare and Medicaid Services, 2008, 2016a, 2016b.

---

- Fear of giving up treatments
- Hospice is often viewed as program for the last few days of life despite being a six-month (or longer) program.
- May be viewed as hastening death
- People think it is a place rather than a program.
- Patients and families are unprepared for the concept of home death.
- Lack of funding for hired caregivers
- Irrational fears that use of analgesics will hasten death
- Unrealistic expectations
- Unwilling to give up certain treatments that may not be covered under hospice (e.g., total parenteral nutrition, chemotherapy)

**Figure 26-3. Barriers to Hospice Care**

a way to get home with more support. Many patients worry that being at home will add to the burden of their loved ones/caregivers. Emphasizing the support of hospice can be a relief. Even if the patient is unrealistic about the future, giving this information as an option can give him or her something to consider in the future.
- "Have you ever heard of hospice?" is an important follow-up question. This gives the nurse the opportunity to identify the barriers and correct any misinformation. Most people have heard of it, but some may have negative associations with the focus on death or presume that it is just for the last few days of life. Providing information about what hospice provides (rather than focus on what they do not do) and education that the services are provided for weeks or months at home can lead to obtaining a referral. Once some interest is expressed, the patient and family may be more open to meet with the hospice provider.
- Introduce hospice before the patient's condition is close to end stage. Arrange a visit by a hospice provider so the patient and family can put a face to the program and learn about it without being in a position of making a decision at that time. Including palliative care in the treatment plan when appropriate in the earlier stages of disease course can also be a way to make the introduction of hospice less frightening.

CMS (2017) has implemented a pilot program called Medicare Care Choices Model, which is available in some areas of the country and allows patients to receive some aggressive treatments along with hospice. This program is being examined and may be the model for the future. This alternative addresses the major fear of giving up aggressive treatment too soon.

## Where People Die

When surveyed, most Americans express a preference to die in their homes (George H. Gallup International Institute, 1997; Teno et al., 2013). However, most die in institutional settings, such as nursing homes, assisted living and hospitals (Gruneir et al., 2007).

A person's place of death is decided by a complex interplay of many factors, including cultural beliefs, individual preferences, social support, access to care, age at death, cause of death, health coverage, and the services being used around the time of death (National Center for Health Statistics, 2010). For those on hospice, 44% died in their own home and 32% died in assisted living and nursing facilities (NHPCO, 2016).

Historically, family members cared for the sick in their own homes throughout the dying process. After World War II, as advances in healthcare technology grew, the hospital became the most frequent location of death. Today, nearly all Medicare beneficiaries spend at least some time in a hospital during their last year of life (Teno et al., 2013). Being in the hospital increases access to technologic advances and therefore increases the likelihood that they will be used to treat problems when a patient is close to death.

A trend toward less acute hospital deaths has occurred for the past few years. This is perhaps related to increased education and access to palliative care and hospice. Teno et al. (2013) found that for Medicare fee-for-service beneficiaries, the percentage who died in acute care hospitals declined from 33% in 2000 to 25% in 2009. In 2009, 33% of Medicare deaths occurred in private residences, 28% in nursing homes, and approximately 14% elsewhere. Bekelman et al. (2016) found that the percentage of Americans dying in acute hospitals has decreased to 22% over the last decade.

Nursing homes have exhibited a steady increase as a location of death (National Center for Health Statistics, 2010). Reasons for this include shorter lengths of stay in the acute hospital setting and patients discharged from the acute hospital with care needs that are beyond the level of care available at home (e.g., IV antibiotics, high-flow oxygen). At times, insurance (e.g., Medicare) may cover nursing home costs if the patient meets certain criteria. This avoids the financial costs of home caregivers. For many, the delivery of end-of-life care in the nursing home setting will be increasingly more common. The hospice benefit can be provided in a nursing home under some circumstances, but it often is underutilized. Underutilization, in part, may be caused by reimbursement policies that encourage nursing homes to focus on restorative care (Unroe, Ersek, & Cagle, 2015). The nursing home environment presents many challenges, including staff with many different knowledge and education levels and a high turnover rate. Regulations and reimbursement can impede quality end-of-life care in nursing homes (IOM, 2015; Unroe et al., 2015). For example, giving sedatives or analgesics may require additional documentation to justify their administration in the skilled nursing setting. In addition, infrequent physician visits also may contribute to poor symptom management. The environment may not be set up for family involvement or unrestricted visitors, which can contribute to family anxiety.

Another recent trend is an increase in the number of transitions in the last three days of life (Teno et al., 2013). Examples of transitions may include transfer from home to hospital, to nursing home, back to the emergency department, and then home all in the last few days of life. These transitions may be indicative of an unclear end-of-life plan; inadequate resources, including caregiving; uncertain life expectancy; and more treatment options being offered.

## Coping With a Death at Home

Identifying the patient's preference for location of death is an important component of good end-of-life care. Because many people express the wish for a home death, achieving it can support a patient's desire for autonomy. Anticipating a home death can provide the patient and family with an intimate, personal experience that brings them closer together during a time of tremendous stress. The close presence of the family may allow time for working through conflicts and obtaining forgiveness for past hurts. Being in one's home surrounded by family, friends, pets, and cherished possessions can provide a sense of peace and control for the patient. The family can gain a sense of accomplishment by knowing that they helped to meet the patient's wish to die at home. Wright et al. (2014) found improved quality of life for those dying at home rather than in the hospital setting.

A romanticized image of being surrounded by loved ones at the end can lead to this preference, but many factors need to be considered before embarking on this plan. A major concern is the need for adequate caregivers, which may include family, friends, and/or hired individuals. In fact, caregiver preference may be a stronger predictor of home death than patient preference (Funk et al., 2010). A 2015 study found the following caregiver needs: what to expect, how to provide care, and how to access help (Funk, Stajduhar, & Outcalt, 2015). These caregivers can become overwhelmed by the patient's care needs and presence of uncertainty, even with the presence of hospice support. However, the satisfaction of providing this care may compensate for the stress. Wright et al. (2014) identified that less psychiatric illness was evident in bereaved family members after a home death rather than a hospital death.

Gott, Seymour, Bellamy, Clark, and Ahmedzai (2004) interviewed older adults in the United Kingdom and found that being viewed as a burden was a great concern. Patients need to feel safe and nurtured. Patients' symptoms and physical needs must be met, and caregivers must feel supported and competent in meeting patients' needs (Lysaght & Ersek, 2013). Patients can receive comfort from seeing that their caregivers are prepared.

Nurses can help patients and their families identify the site of death in advance that best meets the realistic support available. Incorporating this into goal discussions is important and should be done regularly when the patient and/or family are ready to consider it. Families need reassurance that the inability to support a home death is not a failure. Some family caregivers do experience distress if hospitalization becomes necessary (Topf, Robinson, & Bottoroff, 2013). Gott et al. (2004) suggested that the hospital not be demonized as a bad place to die if the home is not ideal.

## Pediatric End-of-Life Care

Much has been written about the end-of-life care for adults, but the needs of dying infants and children have long been underemphasized and understudied. In 2003, IOM released *When Children Die: Improving Palliative and End-of-Life Care for Children and Their Families*, which provided empirical evidence that the U.S. healthcare system was failing to meet the physical, emotional, cultural, spiritual, and psychosocial needs of children with life-threatening illness and their families. Although pediatric palliative care has grown in the last few years to address these issues, many gaps still exist (Feudtner et al., 2013). Advancing pediatric palliative care is needed to support the children and families who live with life-threatening illnesses (O'Shea & Kanarek, 2013). Pediatric palliative care should include the following: providing pain and symptom management in the broad pediatric range from neonate to adolescent, caring for and interacting with developmentally distinct groups, engaging in shared decision making with parents and adolescents, providing accommodations for prognoses that are often more uncertain than in adult patients, and delivering concurrent disease-directed therapy with palliative care (Levine et al., 2013).

Cancer is the leading cause of nonaccidental/nontraumatic death in childhood (Levine et al., 2013; Siegel et al., 2017). Facing the loss of a child may be the most traumatic event in a person's life (Ashton & Ashton, 2000). Parents face multiple losses; not only do they lose the relationship with the child, they also lose what the child represented for the family's hopes and dreams. Pediatric oncology professionals must develop special skills to address the needs of the children, parents, and siblings. Traditionally, children receive aggressive treatment until the very end. Accepting when it is time to stop aggressive treatment may be unthinkable for parents (Wolfe et al., 2000). Parents may resist facing the reality of the poor prognosis. At times, communication within a family can be difficult if the child wants to address their fears and concerns and the parents are unable to bear this. Other families may feel abandoned by their healthcare team if the team is unable to address the needs of the patient and family when the end is near.

Because most pediatric deaths occur in the home, access to hospice care is essential (Levine et al., 2013). Hospice care for children has been underutilized by parents and healthcare professionals, Many hospices do not have the capacity or experience to care for infants, children, and adolescents. Pediatric treatment plans are also sometimes too unfamiliar, complex, and costly for traditional hospice programs (American Academy of Pediatrics, 2013). In addition, life expectancy often is more difficult to estimate in children; aggressive treatment is more likely to be continued because of the patient's age or denial of the prognosis; parents often do not have experience with death, resulting in fear of hospice care; and insurance coverage is often restricted. In some communities, the hospice care may be provided by staff who are not specifically trained in pediatrics (Levine et al., 2013).

## End-of-Life Nursing

Along with the increase in research and education on the close-of-life phase of illness, the specialty of palliative and hospice nursing has grown and developed. The specialty of palliative nursing is newer than other specialties and includes nurses in a variety of settings: hospitals, radiation therapy, clinics, nursing homes, hospices, and home health. In reality, many nurses who work in palliative care are not in an identified palliative care program. In particular, critical care nurses and oncology nurses may consider themselves to be palliative care specialists as they address patient comfort and goals in the face of advanced illness. Palliative care nurses are generally members of an interprofessional team. The role of advanced practice nurses in palliative care has grown in the past decade to lead teams, work as a clinical leader in hospices, and conduct research. Many palliative care nurses work in hospices, often in the role of a case manager. These nurses generally function as coordinators of the interprofessional treatment plan with the goal of maintaining comfort for hospice patients. Because they are often asked to make treatment decisions, hospice nurses need a wide range of skills in areas such as home health, oncology, pain management, and skin care, in addition to having excellent psychosocial skills. Skills that palliative and hospice nurses need include assessment and management of symptoms of advanced illness, communication (often around death and dying), application of ethical principles, and the ability to work effectively in the organization (Hospice and Palliative Nurses Association [HPNA], 2015; IOM, 2014).

In 2014, HPNA developed *Palliative Nursing: Scope and Standards of Practice*. These standards helped to define the specialty of palliative nursing. Certification examinations exist for advanced practice nurses, RNs, and nurses' aides through the Hospice and Palliative Credentialing Center.

Many specialties in nursing provide care for patients at the end of life. The specialty of palliative nursing is leading the way to develop important tools to assist nurses to meet the needs of patients in a variety of settings and specialties.

## Conclusion

The importance of addressing the care needs of patients at the end of life is beginning to attain more attention and research. Palliative care and hospice nursing can provide care and services to patients and their families to help them to achieve their goals of comfort and enhanced quality of life throughout the disease progression. Oncology professionals are in key positions to promote improved end-of-life care. In cancer centers, clinics, hospitals, nursing facilities, and homes, patients with cancer can receive high-quality care throughout the progression of their disease.

# References

American Academy of Pediatrics. (2013). Pediatric palliative care and hospice care commitments, guidelines, and recommendations. *Pediatrics, 132,* 966–972. doi:10.1542/peds.2013-2731

Ashton, J., & Ashton, D. (2000). Dealing with chronic/terminal illness or disability of a child: Anticipatory mourning. In T.A. Rando (Ed.), *Clinical dimensions of anticipatory mourning: Theory and practice in working with the dying, their loved ones, and their caregivers* (pp. 415–454). Champaign, IL: Research Press.

Bekelman, J.E., Halpern, S.D., Blankart, C.R., Bynum, J.P., Cohen, J., Fowler, R., … Emanuel, E.J. (2016). Comparison of site of death, health care utilization, and hospital expenditures for patients dying with cancer in 7 developed countries. *JAMA, 315,* 272–283. doi:10.1001/jama.2015.18603

Boyd, D., Merkh, K., Rutledge, D.N., & Randall, V. (2011). Nurses' perceptions and experiences with end-of-life communication and care [Online exclusive]. *Oncology Nursing Forum, 38,* E229–E239. doi:10.1188/11.ONF.E229-E239

Centers for Medicare and Medicaid Services. (2008). Hospice condition of participation and interpretive guidelines. Retrieved from https://www.gpo.gov/fdsys/pkg/FR-2008-06-05/pdf/08-1305.pdf

Centers for Medicare and Medicaid Services. (2016a). Hospice payment system. Retrieved from https://www.cms.gov/Outreach-and-Education/Medicare-Learning-Network-MLN/MLNProducts/Downloads/hospice_pay_sys_fs.pdf

Centers for Medicare and Medicaid Services. (2016b). Medicare hospice benefits. Retrieved from https://www.medicare.gov/Pubs/pdf/02154.pdf

Centers for Medicare and Medicaid Services. (2017). Medicare Care Choices Model. Retrieved from https://innovation.cms.gov/initiatives/Medicare-Care-Choices

Feudtner, C., Womer, J., Augustin, R., Remke, S., Wolfe, J., Friebert, S., & Weissman, D. (2013). Pediatric palliative care programs in children's hospitals: A cross-sectional national survey. *Pediatrics, 132,* 1063–1070. doi:10.1542/peds.2013-1286

Funk, L., Stajduhar, K., & Outcalt, L. (2015). What family caregivers learn when providing care at the end of life: A qualitative secondary analysis of multiple datasets. *Palliative and Supportive Care, 13,* 425–433. doi:10.1017/S1478951513001168

Funk, L., Stajduhar, K., Toye, C., Aoun, S., Grande, G., & Todd, C. (2010). Part 2: Home-based family caregiving at the end of life: A comprehensive review of published qualitative research (1998–2008). *Palliative Medicine, 24,* 594–607. doi:10.1177/0269216310371411

Gawande, A. (2014). *Being mortal: Medicine and what matters in the end.* New York, NY: Metropolitan Books.

Gawande, A. (2016). Quantity and quality of life: Duties of care in life-limiting illness. *JAMA, 315,* 267–269. doi:10.1001/jama.2015.19206

George H. Gallup International Institute. (1997). *Spiritual beliefs and the dying process: A report on a national survey.* Princeton, NJ: Princeton Research Center.

Gott, M., Seymour, J., Bellamy, G., Clark, D., & Ahmedzai, S. (2004). Older people's views about home as a place of care at the end of life. *Palliative Medicine, 18,* 460–467. doi:10.1191/0269216304pm889oa

Gruneir, A., Mor, V., Weitzen, S., Truchil, R., Teno, J., & Roy, J. (2007). Where people die: A multilevel approach to understanding influences on site of death in America. *Medical Care and Research Review, 64,* 351–378. doi:10.1177/1077558707301810

Hospice and Palliative Nurses Association. (2015). *Value of the advanced registered nurse in palliative care* [Position statement]. Retrieved from http://hpna.advancingexpertcare.org/wp-content/uploads/2015/08/Value-of-the-Advanced-Practice-Registered-Nurse-in-Palliative-Care.pdf

Institute of Medicine. (2015). *Dying in America: Improving quality and honoring individual preferences near the end of life.* Washington, DC: National Academies Press.

Kadakia, K.C., Moynihan, T.J., Smith, T.J., & Loprinzi, C.L. (2012). Palliative communications: Addressing chemotherapy in patients with advanced cancer. *Annals of Oncology, 23*(Suppl. 3), 29–32. doi:10.1093/annonc/mds085

Kuhl, D. (2009). What dying people want. In H.M. Chocinov & W. Breitbart (Eds.), *Handbook of psychiatry in palliative medicine* (2nd ed., pp. 141–156). New York, NY: Oxford University Press.

Levine, D., Lam, C.G., Cunningham, M.J., Remke, S., Chrastek, J., Klick, J., … Backer, J.N. (2013). Best practices for pediatric palliative cancer care: A primer for clinical providers. *Journal of Community and Supportive Oncology, 11,* 114–125. doi:10.12788/j.suponc.0012

Lysaght, S., & Ersek, M. (2013). Settings of care within hospice: New options and questions about dying "at home." *Journal of Hospice and Palliative Nursing, 15,* 171–176. doi:10.1097/NJH.0b013e3182765a17

Mack, J.W., Walling, A., Dy, S., Antonio, A.L.M., Adams, J., Keating, N.L., & Tisnado, D. (2015). Patient beliefs that chemotherapy may be curative and care received at the end of life among patients with metastatic lung and colorectal cancer. *Cancer, 121,* 1891–1897. doi:10.1002/cncr.29250

Mack, J.W., Weeks, J.C., Wright, A.A., Block, S.D., & Prigerson, H.G. (2010). End-of-life discussions, goal attainment, and distress at the end of life: Predictors and outcomes of receipt of care consistent with preferences. *Journal of Clinical Oncology, 28,* 1203–1208. doi:10.1200/JCO.2009.25.4672

Mor, V., & Kidder, D. (1985). Cost savings in hospice: Final results of the National Hospice Study. *Health Services Research, 20,* 407–422.

National Center for Health Statistics. (2010). *Health, United States, 2010: With special feature on death and dying.* Retrieved from https://www.cdc.gov/nchs/data/hus/hus10.pdf

National Consensus Project for Quality Palliative Care. (2013). *Clinical practice guidelines for quality palliative care* (3rd ed.). Pittsburgh, PA: Author.

National Hospice and Palliative Care Organization. (2016). *NHPCO facts and figures, 2016.* Retrieved from http://www.nhpco.org/sites/default/files/public/Statistics_Research/2016_Facts_Figures.pdf

Newman, A., Thompson, J., & Chandler, E.M. (2013). Continuous care: A home hospice benefit. *Clinical Journal of Oncology Nursing, 17,* 19–20. doi:10.1188/13.CJON.19-20

Obermeyer, Z., Makar, M., Abujaber, S., Dominici, F., Block, S., & Cutler, D.M. (2014). Association between the Medicare hospice benefit and health care utilization and costs for patients with poor-prognosis cancer. *JAMA, 312,* 1888–1896. doi:10.1001/jama.2014.14950

O'Shea, E.R., & Kanarek, R.B. (2013). Understanding pediatric palliative care. *Journal of Pediatric Oncology Nursing, 30,* 34–40. doi:10.1177/1043454212471725

Pacetti, P., Paganini, G., Orlandi, M., Mambrini, A., Pennucci, M.C., Del Freo, A., & Cantore, M. (2015). Chemotherapy in the last 30 days of life of advanced cancer patients. *Supportive Care in Cancer, 23,* 3277–3280. doi:10.1007/s00520-015-2733-6

Prigerson, H.G., Bao, Y., Shah, M.A., Paulk, E., LeBlanc, R.W., Schneider, B.J., ... Maciejewski, P.K. (2015). Chemotherapy use, performance status, and quality of life at the end of life. *JAMA Oncology, 1,* 778–784. doi:10.1001/jamaoncol.2015.2378

Rabow, M. (2014). Chemotherapy at the end of life. *BMJ, 348,* 1529. doi:10.1136/bmj.g1529

Saiki, C., Ferrell, B., Longo-Schoeberlein, D., Chung, V., & Smith, T.J. (2017). Goals-of-care discussions. *Journal of Community and Supportive Oncology, 15,* e190–e194. doi:10.12788/jcso.0355

Schnipper, L.E., Smith, T.H., Raghavan, D., Blayney, D.W., Ganz, P.A., Mulvey, T.M., & Wollins, D.S. (2012). American Society of Clinical Oncology identifies five key opportunities to improve care and reduce costs: The top five list for oncology. *Journal of Clinical Oncology, 30,* 1715–1724. doi:10.1200/JCO.2012.42.8375

Siegel, R.L., Miller, K.D., & Jemal, A. (2017). Cancer statistics, 2017. *CA: A Cancer Journal for Clinicians, 65,* 7–30. doi:10.3322/caac.21387

Singer, P.A., Martin, D.K., & Kelner, M. (1999). Quality end-of-life care: Patients' perspectives. *JAMA, 281,* 163–168. doi:10.1001/jama.281.2.163

Steinhauser, K.E., Christakis, N.A., Clipp, E.C., McNeilly, M., McIntyre, L., & Tulsky, J.A. (2000). Factors considered important at the end of life by patients, family, physicians, and other care providers. *JAMA, 284,* 2476–2482. doi:10.1001/jama.284.19.2476

Teno, J.M., Gozalo, P.L., Bynum, J.P., Leland, N.E., Miller, S.C., Morden, N.E., ... Mor, V. (2013). Change in end-of-life care for Medicare beneficiaries: Site of death, place of care, and health care transitions in 2000, 2005, and 2009. *JAMA, 309,* 470–477. doi:10.1001/jama.2012.207624

Topf, L., Robinson, C.A., & Bottorff, J.L. (2013). When a desired home death does not occur: The consequences of broken promises. *Journal of Palliative Medicine, 16,* 875–880. doi:10.1089/jpm.2012.0541

Unroe, K.T., Ersek, M., & Cagle, J. (2015). The IOM report on dying in America: A call to action for nursing homes. *Journal of the American Medical Directors Association, 16,* 90–92. doi:10.1016/j.jamda.2014.11.010

Weeks, J.C., Catalano, P.J., Cronin, A., Finkelman, M.D., Mack, J.W., Keating, N.L., & Schrag, D. (2012). Patients' expectations about effects of chemotherapy for advanced cancer. *New England Journal of Medicine, 367,* 1616–1625. doi:10.1056/NEJMoa1204410

Wolfe, J., Klar, N., Grier, H.E., Duncan, J., Salem-Schatz, S., Emanuel, E.J., & Weeks, J.C. (2000). Understanding of prognosis among parents of children who died of cancer. *JAMA, 284,* 2469–2475. doi:10.1001/jama.284.19.2469

Wright, A.A., Keating, N.L., Ayanian, J.Z., Chrischilles, E.A., Kahn, K.L., Ritchie, C.S., ... Landrum, M.B. (2016). Family perspective of aggressive cancer care at the end of life. *JAMA, 315,* 284–292. doi:10.1001/jama.2015.18604

Wright, A.A., Zhang, B., Keating, N.L., Weeks, J.C., & Prigerson, H.G. (2014). Associations between palliative chemotherapy and adult cancer patients' end of life care and place of death: Prospective cohort study. *BMJ, 348,* 1219. doi:10.1136/bmj.g1219

Wright, A.A., Zhang, B., Ray, A., Mack, J.W., Trice, E., Balboni, T.A., ... Prigerson, H.G. (2008). Associations between end-of-life discussions, patient mental health, medical care near death, and caregiver bereavement adjustment. *JAMA, 300,* 1165–1173. doi:10.1001/jama.300.14.1665

# CHAPTER 27

# Ethical Issues

Rita Hand, RN, MSN, GNP-BC

> *We do not act rightly because we have virtue or excellence, but we rather have those because we have acted rightly.*
>
> —Aristotle

Nurses assume a prominent role in care of persons throughout the cancer trajectory and, as such, possess a responsibility to model, guide, and provide ethically sound care. Attention to the ethical dimensions of cancer care is central to the well-being of patients, families, and the provision of high-quality nursing care (Pavlish, Brown-Saltzman, Jakel, & Fine, 2014). By virtue of their distinct advocacy relationship with patients and their families and the centrality in their provision of care, nurses bring a unique perspective to understanding and evaluating the ethical dimensions of cancer care (McSteen & Peden-McAlpine, 2006).

Unprecedented advances in medical science have created great promise for prolonging individual health but also rivet oncology care with new and complex ethical quandaries. Among some of the most perplexing ethical challenges confronting the cancer care continuum are the distinction between medical paternalism and patient autonomy, what is an ordinary versus extraordinary means of preserving life, defining when to withhold and withdraw treatment, hastening death, equal distribution of healthcare resources versus rationing of care and services, and the increased moral distress and resulting burden placed on caregivers (Chow, 2014; Pavlish, Brown-Saltzman, Fine, & Jakel, 2015; Shepard, 2010).

The focus of this chapter is on the ethical dilemmas that challenge nurses, patients, and the greater healthcare community related to prevention, detection, education, treatment options and outcomes, and palliation in cancer care.

## Defining Ethics

*Ethics* is concerned with systematically evaluating varying viewpoints as it relates to what is morally "right or wrong" or "good or bad" in the context of fairness, rights, obligations, benefits to society, or specific virtues that enjoin honesty, compassion, and loyalty. The study of ethics as it intersects with health care is termed *bioethics*. The evolution of bioethics was a natural extension of the move away from a mechanistic model to a holistic approach toward caring for ill people. Over time, a myriad of ethical theories and methodologies have arisen, shaped by the gender, socioeconomic strata, and culture of philosophers. However, common to many of the ethical theories are frameworks constructed by foundational ethical principles.

Ethical decision making and consequential actions are traditionally defined by four primary principles: autonomy (respect for the decisions made by an autonomous person), beneficence (actions performed that contribute to the welfare of others), nonmaleficence (an obligation not to inflict harm intentionally), and justice (the fair, equitable, and appropriate treatment in light of what is due or owed to a person) (Beauchamp & Childress, 2013).

Ethical dilemmas emerge across the specialties as nurses work to provide the best possible care while responding to threats to their own personal, professional, or community value structures. Personal beliefs about what is "right or wrong" or "good or bad" are largely embedded in personal values, beliefs, societal norms, and past experiences. Daily healthcare encounters require the application of ethical principles and choices that embrace complex decision making and different personally held values. Differences of opinions within the healthcare team regarding continued treatment or types of care as well as differences in value systems with those of the employing organization are sources of daily ethical challenges facing the nursing profession (Chow, 2014). Determining a course of action when principles conflict contributes to the actions and omissions that generate the greatest controversies in ethics at the bedside (Cohen & Erickson, 2006). In the clinical setting, a bioethics consultation is typically requested when a clinical situation presents competing values and/or principles. The sources can exist within the healthcare team, with the patient/family and the healthcare team, when a patient's decisional capacity or surrogate is in question, and/or if clarification is needed regarding patient preferences or achievement of realistic outcomes using the appropriate direction or options of treatment (Dalinis, 2004).

Continued exposure by the nurse to ethical challenges can lead to moral distress and conflict when the situation (or institution) dictates one act contrary to an individual's core values. Examples of situations contributing to moral distress include involvement in complex end-of-life scenarios, medically inappropriate treatment, delayed prognostic discussions, and lack of staff education related to available resources or options (Pavlish et al., 2014).

## Ethical Nursing Practice

The many ethical challenges that confront nurses have propelled the formation of several professional statements that articulate the shared values upheld by the nursing profession. The American Nurses Association's (ANA, 2015) *Code of Ethics for Nurses With Interpretive Statements* provides a framework of ethical standards for the nursing profession. It outlines the ethical obligations and duties of every individual who enters the nursing profession, identifies the profession's non-negotiable ethical standards, and describes the profession's commitment to society.

Similarly, the Oncology Nursing Society's (ONS's) *Statement on the Scope and Standards of Oncology Nursing Practice* (Brant & Wickham, 2013) states that oncology nurses' decisions and actions are portrayed in an ethical manner. Oncology nurses need to examine personal philosophy; discuss ethical issues with colleagues; address advance directives with patients and families; serve as a patient advocate; maintain sensitivity to patients' cultural differences;

preserve patient autonomy, dignity, and rights; find resources to examine issues; and engage in ethical decision making.

These organizational statements provide a starting point for ethical insight; however, they do not provide explicit answers to the troubling ethical realities that confront nurses in practices. In 2014, a group of nursing ethics leaders, along with ANA, convened at the National Nursing Ethics Summit. These participants produced a blueprint for 21st century nursing ethics (Johns Hopkins Berman Institute of Bioethics, 2014) to develop ideas and move nursing ethics issues forward in the following four key domains: clinical practice, nursing education, nursing ethics research, and nursing policy. The goal was to help strengthen the ethical foundation of nursing and create healthy, sustainable, ethically principled environments for the populations served.

# Autonomy, Informed Consent, Truth Telling, and Advance Directives

In recent decades, autonomous decision making has challenged the long-held model of paternalism in which one person determines what is good for another instead of facilitating the other person's involvement. At times, paternalistic decisions may be justified in public health issues, such as in the case of school age vaccinations (Buchanan, 2008). However, research has indicated that patients want to be informed of their diagnosis and prognosis as well as be active participants in care-related decision making (Hoerger et al., 2013; Mack et al., 2012; Parker et al., 2007; Walczak et al., 2014). Autonomy, the ability to govern oneself, is a central paradigm for individual rights. The demand for more autonomy has resulted in an increase in shared healthcare information and decision making. Shared decision making is producing increased understanding of treatment options, realistic expectations of disease trajectory, improved adherence, and enhanced patient satisfaction (Allen et al., 2012; Politi, Studts, & Haylip, 2012; Zalonis & Slota, 2014).

The doctrine of informed consent, the right to accept or reject treatment, is a cornerstone in clinical care of the ethical and legal rights of the individual to make autonomous healthcare decisions (Hall, Prochazka, & Fink, 2012). The philosophical, sociological, and legal doctrine of informed consent prevents forced, coerced, or manipulated decision making. However, there may be times when healthcare interventions occur without the patient's informed consent. This results when the individual's capacity for decision making is lost during emergencies when there is no time for complete disclosure, or when patients waive their right to give informed consent (Wiegand & Grant, 2014).

Disease-related or treatment-induced alterations in one's capacity for autonomous decision making may occur along the cancer continuum. Nurses, because of their enduring relationship with patients over time, play a vital role in clarifying patients' decisional capacity and are in an ideal position to assist the medical team in this process (Walczak et al., 2014).

Written or oral advance directives are foundational to the preservation of self-determination when decisional capacity is impaired. Advance directives afford patients the opportunity to provide treatment instructions and/or appoint a decision maker, called a *healthcare power of attorney* or *surrogate*. In 1991, the Patient Self-Determination Act was enacted into federal legislation, mandating that all patients be informed of their prerogative to accept or refuse treatment and to execute advance directives. This act led to improved education, communication, and legislation, which contributed to an increase in documentation and prevention of resuscitation at the end of life. However, overall completion of advance directives remains low (Garrido, Balboni, Maciejewski, Bao, & Prigerson, 2014). To date, studies have not confirmed that advance directives facilitate decision making or truly direct care (Castillo et al., 2011; Evangelista et al., 2012; Kossman, 2014; Silveira, Wiitala, & Piette, 2014; Yung, Walling, Min, Wenger, & Ganz, 2010). In situations where an individual has lost the capacity for self-determination and communication of treatment preferences with no advance directive, the responsibility for healthcare decision making generally is assigned to family members, particularly the next of kin. The surrogate decision maker attempts to use substituted judgment (i.e., making the decision the patient would have made if he/she were capable). The role of the surrogate decision maker is legally recognized in the United States (Wiegand & Grant, 2014).

Despite the transition from medical paternalism to shared decision making, ethical challenges surround the promotion of patient autonomy. As the paradigm of shared decision making becomes a more accepted model, the issue remains of how much information should be given to patients. An imbalance of power exists between patients and the healthcare team. The ability of patients to enact autonomous decision making is wholly dependent on the range of choices presented by the healthcare team. These choices revolve around the divulgence of information by the team members and the healthcare system (Russell & Ward, 2011).

Disparities persist in the cancer care arena between the type and amount of information patients wish to receive to assist their decision making and the amount of information shared by the healthcare team (Koedoot et al., 2004; Russell & Ward, 2011; Wilson, Gott, & Ingleton, 2013; Zamichow, 2015). Some studies support that patients with cancer initially prefer to receive honest, specific information about their condition, regardless of whether the information is good or bad (Harrington & Smith, 2008). However, some oncology care providers continue to avoid communicating negative prognostic information because of cultural considerations and the potential to threaten patients' hope (Robinson et al., 2008; Taddonio, 2014; Zahedi, 2011).

A systematic review performed by Clayton et al. (2008) found that the skill of balancing honesty with hope was beneficial. Although patients with advanced cancers may hope for a cure, they often are fully aware of the terminal aspect of their illness. Hope may change and adopt different meanings as the illness progresses. Physicians' lack of clarity and truth telling is associated with a majority of ethical dilemmas and increased burdens for the entire healthcare team (Cheon, Coyle, Wiegand, & Welsh, 2015; Pavlish et al., 2015). Conversely, research has indicated that healthcare providers frequently remain unaware of patients' wishes (Barakat et al., 2013; Mack et al., 2012; Snyder, Hazelett, Allen, & Radwany, 2013). Improving the cornerstone of communication around difficult issues in cancer care through early, open, honest, sensitive, and direct dialogue reduces patient anxiety and facilitates autonomy and maintenance of a therapeutic relationship between the healthcare provider and the patient (Nakajima, Hata, Onishi, & Ishida, 2013; Parker et al., 2007).

## Medically Inappropriate Treatment: Determining Life and Death

Remarkable advances in medical technology are responsible for prolongation of life. These scientific advances, along with increased access to medical information by patients, have fostered an expectation that limitless treatment options and cures are available. At times, the extension of life may lead to the meaningful attainment of goals and the return of functional capacity. However, patients may sometimes never achieve the return of functional capabilities or potential for life that is independent of applied life-sustaining interventions and merely prolong terminal illness and the dying process. Therapies that prolong life simply for the sake of prolongation in which the patient does not have the capacity to ever appreciate life lead to outcomes that are ethically and medically unacceptable, inappropriate, and often described as *futile* (Schneiderman, 2011). Serious ethical, medical, and societal dilemmas result from the application of medically inappropriate treatment (also referred to as *nonbeneficial medical treatment*) (Schneiderman, 2011).

Patients with advanced cancer and their families are confronted with many difficult emotions in the face of an often-bleak prognosis. The conflict between hope and reality can multiply the stress that patients and families are experiencing. Cultural and religious faith, perceived racial or socioeconomic status prejudices, or health providers' financial incentive factors may contribute to patients' confusion and inability to make informed and calculated decisions about treatment (Burkle & Benson, 2012). The dilemma of autonomy versus medical paternalism is sometimes at the core of nonbeneficial medical treatment. How far does patient autonomy extend? Do patients and family members have the right to sway the hand of the healthcare professionals with demands for certain interventions or treatments? Or should the medical professionals with specialty expertise have the final say in what treatment is appropriate?

Another issue is whether healthcare professionals have an obligation to provide every available intervention simply because they exist, even when they may be medically unreasonable, might incur greater harm, and/or have little chance of achieving the desired outcome. Is it within the domain of health care to withhold or even withdraw therapies deemed to be inappropriate without subjecting such a decision to the patient's approval? Ethically, what is the deciding principle when conflicts arise between a healthcare professional's duty to do good and prevent harm and a patient's or family's right to self-determination? Additionally, consideration must be given to society's concern with justice, equal distribution of limited resources, and the denial of treatment based on economic interests.

The concept of futility in medicine does not have a universally recognizable and clinically applicable meaning. The American Thoracic Society (1991) described a situation as "medically futile" if reasoning and experience indicate that the intervention would be highly unlikely to result in a meaningful survival for the patient. In 1997, the Society of Critical Care Medicine stated that treatments should be defined as futile only when their intended goals cannot be accomplished. Schneiderman (2011) has researched medical futility extensively and has maintained that treatment is a failure and futile "if the best outcome physicians achieve is to maintain survival, which requires keeping the patient perpetually confined to the intensive care unit or the acute care setting" (p. 126).

Futility is a concept that does not stand well alone and is situation dependent. When conflicts arise, as they inevitably do, futility remains the most common justification for the withholding or withdrawal of therapies (Bloomer, Tiruvoipati, Tsiripillis, & Botha, 2010). The conundrum lies in the meaning of acceptable outcomes or meeting goals. Whose goals are we addressing? The physician's treatment plan goals are based on empirical science and experience with the hope of healing. The patient's goal may be to prolong life at all costs to wait for a cure.

The definition that has gained momentum with the patient autonomy movement in reaction to medical paternalism is that futility should depend on the likelihood of achieving the patient's goals, which may simply be to prolong life and await a miracle, with little likelihood of achieving the goal of the treatment plan (Schneiderman, 2011).

The notion of not declaring treatment futile so long as it can prolong life, even a permanently unconscious life, is not supported by the Hippocratic Oath nor the classical tradition of medicine (Schneiderman, 2011). The claim that the goal of medicine is to preserve life has ambiguous meaning and dubious roots in religious historical tradition. Physicians and healthcare providers have struggled to maintain patient autonomy while practicing under the guidance of treatments based on beneficial care. However, almost all futility policies agree that physicians are not obligated to continue life-sustaining treatment of patients who have reliably been determined to be permanently unconscious (Schneiderman, 2011).

Collaborative practice involves the entire healthcare team. The presence of medically inappropriate treatment can negatively affect the entire team and interfere with collaboration. Bedside nurses are particularly vulnerable to moral distress created by futility (Sirilla, 2014). Forced treatment is unhealthy for the patient and the healthcare team, whether the coercion is directed against the patient by overriding his or her wishes or against the healthcare team by commanding them to act against instinct and conscience. Institutional policies regarding futile treatment, ethics committees, and palliative care teams are helpful navigational resources. Maintaining early, timely, open communication with the family and patient regarding patient wishes, achievable medical treatment goals, and frequently reinforced realistic expectations reduces stress, post-traumatic anxiety, depression, and bereavement (Adolph, Frier, Stawicki, Gerlach, & Papadimos, 2011).

Oncology nurses are often a principal liaison between the patient and family and the medical team. As such, they play a key role in family support, patient advocacy, and the communication of nonabandonment. They are the primary source for supplying education, clarifying information, and providing compassionate, supportive care throughout the illness continuum.

## Hastened Death: Assisted Suicide and Euthanasia

The ability to exercise autonomy in healthcare decision making has extended into the arena of self-determination over the events that will lead to one's death. Few issues in health care remain as controversial as efforts to hasten death through assisted suicide and euthanasia (see Table 27-1). The focus of ethical scrutiny related to assisted suicide and euthanasia is on the patient–healthcare provider relationship because of the conflicting ethical principles of autonomy, beneficence, and nonmaleficence.

The experience of facing a potentially life-limiting illness such as cancer is a common catalyst for the contemplation of one's mortality. Fears of living or dying with distressing symptoms, being stripped of dignity, losing self-control, or becoming a burden to family and friends may provoke an individual with cancer to consider suicide (see Chapter 17 for more information on depression and suicide). It is not uncommon for the healthcare team, as a result of their enduring relationships with patients, to receive requests to actively aid a patient in hastening death (Lachman, 2010).

Overwhelming emotional distress manifested through hopelessness and depression are key factors at the center of one's desire to hasten death (Rodin et al., 2007), often with the hope of avoiding suffering, maintaining control over potentially frightening and unknown circumstances, or forgoing the family's burden of care (Monforte-Royo, Villavicencio-Chavez, Tomas-Sabado, Mahtani-Chugani, & Balaguer, 2012). Autonomy supports a patient's right to discontinue life-sustaining treatments, request high-dose opioids to treat intractable pain, or select palliative sedation to treat suffering (Hospice and Palliative Nurses Association [HPNA], 2017a). Patients may choose to stop eating and drinking to hasten death. Actively assisting a patient to die is different than passive participation.

Assisted suicide is also referred to as aid in dying, assisted dying (AD), or physician-assisted suicide (PAS). Proponents for AD argue that the ability to choose death is a moral extension

## Table 27-1. Definitions of Ethical Issues

| Term | Definition |
| --- | --- |
| Assisted suicide | Someone provides the means by which one takes his or her life (e.g., a physician prescribes a lethal dose of medication with the understanding that the patient intends to use it to commit suicide). |
| Conscientious objection | Rejection of an action because the action would violate a deeply held moral, religious, or ethical value about what is right or wrong (i.e., the refusal to perform abortions based on the belief that life begins at conception). |
| Ethical dilemma | A conflict of two or more ethical principles. |
| Euthanasia | A person commits to an action with the intent of ending the patient's life (e.g., a physician injects a patient with a lethal dose of medication). |
| Involuntary euthanasia | The healthcare provider, without the consent of the terminally ill patient, intentionally causes the patient's death (mercy killing). |
| Moral distress | One understands the right thing or course of action but is unable to act in accordance with core values and obligation because of institutional constraints. Frequent recurrences may threaten self-worth. |
| Palliative care | A board-certified branch of medicine and nursing whose goal is to improve the quality of life for patients and families facing a life-threatening illness through prevention (advance directives, counseling), assessment, and treatment of physical (pain), psychological (depression), and spiritual problems (fear of dying). |
| Palliative sedation | The controlled and monitored use of medications (nonopioid) intended to lower a patient's consciousness for relief of refractory and unendurable symptoms. To palliate the symptoms to sedation. A legal remedy for intractable symptoms (terminal sedation). |
| Principle of double effect | The permission to commit an action that may cause serious harm as a side effect of promoting some good end. According to the principle of double effect, it is sometimes permissible to cause a harm as a side effect of bringing about a good result as long as the intention and the proportion of the good effect outweighs the bad (i.e., saving a mother's life at the cost of fetal death or increasing a pain medication at risk of hastened death with the intent of comfort in a terminal patient). |
| Shared decision making | A model of collaboration between healthcare providers and patients to reach agreement regarding multiple medically appropriate treatment options. |
| Suicide | The taking of one's own life. |
| Voluntary euthanasia | The healthcare provider, with the consent of the terminally ill patient, intentionally causes the patient's death. |

of autonomy, and violation of one's autonomy infringes upon patients' rights (Bergh, Dierckx de Casterlé, & Gastmans, 2005). Additionally, AD is a compassionate and merciful response to one's suffering at the end of life (Zenz, Tryba, & Zenz, 2014). Other advocates for AD propose that it is consistent with the legitimate medical desire to prevent suffering and exercise beneficence in aiding in the achievement of a "good death" (Lickerman, 2015). Patients may consider the option of their own death as a type of control, all that remains of their autonomy, or "the last ace up their sleeve" (Monforte-Royo et al., 2012). Giving patients the choice to decide their fate returns a little of the control that has been lost, which in turn allows for the hope that they can lead the best life that they have left.

Those opposing the argument of AD do not find this practice to be a normal, beneficent part of their healthcare practices and vehemently proclaim that it violates the Hippocratic Oath. Opponents cite evidence that aid in dying opposes "normal" healthcare practices, ethical concepts of nonmaleficence, and respect of the sanctity of life. Patient autonomy, self-determination, and the right to choose freely are refuted with the argument that solely because an individual has a right to choose something does not mean that what one chooses is morally justified (Pritchard, 2012). It does not oblige someone to assist another person to die (Putnam, 2009). Others insist that it is illogical to consider the role of a physician healer, who is educated to preserve life, with the task of hastening death (Randall & Downie, 2010). In addition, some foes to AD fear it will lead to the "slippery slope" argument, where it will become easier to hasten death in marginalized individuals in society (Randall & Downie, 2010).

Of additional concern are studies that indicate some requests for hastened death are a response to overwhelming emotional distress with different meanings that do not necessarily imply a true wish to hasten one's death. Rather, considering the possibility of death allows for the individual's immediate need to draw attention for more control over their life (Monforte-Royo et al., 2012; Ohnsorge, Gudat, & Rehmann-Sutter, 2014; Ternestedt, 2005). Careful exploration and attention to the reasons surrounding the request, providing information regarding options, prognosis, and the ability to control these decisions, should be considered in the design and formation of any comprehensive care plan (Monforte-Royo et al., 2012).

The increasing presence of palliative care teams and hospice support to offer expertise to address physical, psychosocial, and spiritual suffering needs to be available to all patients (Zenz et al., 2014). For intractable symptoms, palliative care professionals may use palliative sedation to induce somnolence and reduce suffering while awaiting an inevitable death. Based on the doctrine of double effect, that it is morally permissible to perform an action in pursuit of a good end with full knowledge that the action will also bring about bad results, palliative sedation is viewed as ethically and legally acceptable in appropriate situations (HPNA, 2016).

## Hastened Death: Legal Matters

Although the practice of hastening death is a widely debated topic, the actual incidence of occurrence is unknown. Public debate regarding the issues of euthanasia and assisted suicide continues to evolve. Euthanasia, or *mercy killing*, to date remains illegal in the United States. Currently, the Netherlands, Belgium, and Luxembourg allow euthanasia in specific conditions in patients with a terminal diagnosis. Switzerland, Germany, Albania, Colombia, Japan, and, most recently, Canada are on the growing list of countries that allow assisted suicide. In the United States, Oregon was the first state to legalize PAS, allowing a physician or nurse practitioner to prescribe a lethal dose of medication for a patient with a terminal illness with less than six months to live. Several years later, other states, including Washington, Montana, Vermont, and New Mexico, joined the list of states to permit PAS (MacLeod, Wilson, & Malpas, 2012). California passed AD legislation in 2015 and Colorado in 2016 (Strouse, 2017). Other states are in the process of trying to expand this further. Patients must meet a number of strict requirements before the practitioner can prescribe a lethal dose of medication (Oregon Public Health Division, 2016).

AD is responsible for less than 1% of deaths in Oregon (Oregon Public Health Division, 2016). Of those who do obtain the lethal prescription, some never actually take the medication to end their life (Gawande, 2014; Oregon Public Health Division, 2016). In the Netherlands, where euthanasia and PAS have been in practice for a number of years, no significant increase has been noted in either practice over time. Statistically, it remains at 2%–3% of total mortality (Abrahm, 2008; Steck, Egger, Maessen, Reisch, & Zwahlen, 2013). In 2002, the Netherlands legalized advance directives for euthanasia for patients with dementia. Despite legalization and support to limit life-sustaining interventions, both physicians and relatives are reluctant to adhere to advance directives for euthanasia in dementia patients. The primary reason that is given is patients' inability to engage in meaningful communication (de Boer, Dröes, Jonker, Eefsting, & Hertogh, 2011). In a comparison study of vulnerable populations in Oregon and the Netherlands, no evidence exists that vulnerable populations are more likely to be affected mitigating the "slippery slope" argument (Battin, van der Heide, Ganzini, van der Wal, & Onwuteaka-Philipsen, 2007).

Nurses may experience moral distress in caring for patients requesting PAS, especially if the action is incongruent with the nurse's religious values (Abrahm, 2008; Lachman, 2014). In states that allow PAS, nurses retain the prerogative to conscientiously object to remain involved in that patient's care (ANA, 2013; ONS, 2010). Conscientious objection in health care is based on the rejection of some action by the healthcare provider because the action would violate a deeply held ethical or moral value (Lachman, 2014).

However, refusal to provide care based on self-interest, discrimination, or prejudice is never grounds for conscientious objection. Current research of nurses in Washington, where the Death With Dignity Act is legal, indicates that nurses lack information and formal education regarding the laws surrounding it. Unclear professional guidelines create ethical conflicts, which result in most nurses referring the patient to another source if asked about Death With Dignity (Jablonski, Clymin, Jacobson, & Feldt, 2012). Professional guidelines explicitly forbid nurse participation in AD. However, nurses must maintain the role of patient advocate. It is the nurse's obligation to be knowledgeable about the consequences of healthcare decisions and the legal and moral rights associated with patient's self-determination (ANA, 2013). Therefore, nurses must remain fully informed and able to impart comprehendible, accurate, and complete information to patients to facilitate decision making.

## Response of Professional Organizations to Hastened Death

Many professional organizations have developed responses to the ethical, legal, and social debates arising in response to assisted suicide. As the largest professional body representing nursing, ANA prohibits nurses' participation in assisted suicide and euthanasia (ANA, 2013). HPNA's position statement (2017b) does not support the legalization of hastened death. Rather, it focuses on the provision of aggressive palliative care, nonjudgmental respect for patient choices, and continually meeting health needs with timely transfer of care in the event of conscientious moral objection. ONS's position statement on nurses' responsibility to patients requesting assistance in hastening death (2010) adopts a strong position of support, nonabandonment, and advocacy. Although professional societies formalize their responses for those they represent, it remains imperative that individuals examine their own beliefs and formulate a response that will personally guide their delivery of health care. However, guidelines are unclear as to the specific nursing role related to what is participation and patient education as AD becomes more accepted. This creates a confusing situation and a potential barrier regarding nurses' ability to provide patients with accurate information about the law (Jablonski et al., 2012). How to balance the patient's view of quality versus quantity of life against the historical and culturally developed roles and responsibilities of the healthcare profession to support life and prevent suffering remains the dilemma (MacLeod et al., 2012).

# The Injustice of Health Disparities

Despite the fact that cancer rates continue to decline (Kohler et al., 2011) and medical science progress has resulted in increased longevity and improved quality of life, vast healthcare disparities continue to be present throughout the entire cancer continuum, from prevention to palliation (Edwards et al., 2014; Kagawa-Singer, Valdez-Dadia, Yu, & Surbone, 2010). A heavier burden of illness is borne by some groups, particularly the poor, older adults, and ethnic minorities (e.g., African American, Latino/Hispanic, American Indian/Alaskan Native, Asian American, Pacific Islander). Ethnic minorities are an increasing percentage of the U.S. population (Kaiser Family Foundation, 2010). The unequal burden of disease in our society is a challenge to medicine. Multiple factors such as poverty, lack of resources, inadequate education, social class, lack of health insurance, age, lifestyle, diet, environment, and physician bias all contribute to this phenomenon. Smedley, Stith, and Nelson (2003) identified that cultural, economic and social factors interplay in healthcare disparities and increase cancer risk. Although no definite answer exists as to why some populations have higher morbidity and mortality, it is known that serious research is lacking on ethnic minorities, women, and older adults. Throughout time, the exploitation of racial and ethnic minority groups, children, prisoners, and the poor has occurred without consent or knowledge for unethical medical research. Currently, American pharmaceutical companies outsource more than half of their clinical trials to third world countries with large populations that lack the access to basic health services and cancer resources and where clinical trials may be their only access to health care (Adashi, 2011). These foreign trials cost 40% less than American drug trials, lack oversight, and beg the same ethical questions that have contributed to lack of current U.S. trial participation (Virk, 2010). The older African American population witnessed the same unethical treatment epitomized by the Tuskegee Syphilis Experiment, which contributes to current mistrust of the healthcare establishment (Owens, Jackson, Thomas, Friedman, & Hebert, 2013).

Although 66% of patients with cancer are over the age of 65, this group is represented by only 25% of cancer clinical trial enrollees (Herrara et al., 2010). Physical health impairments, comorbidities, and low health literacy are major barriers to trial participation exhibited by older, racial, or ethnic populations that have less healthcare access, know less about their diseases, exhibit poorer self-management or knowledge of availability of credible treatments, and have a greater reliance on physician care.

Of all racial or ethnic minorities, African American men have the highest overall cancer incidence rate. In prostate cancer alone, incidence is 60% higher and mortality is 150% higher when compared to Caucasians (Owens et al., 2013). Younger African American patients experienced more aggressive tumors with higher recurrence rates, which contributed to the greater mortality (Wagner et al., 2012). When factors were adjusted to provide easy access and equal treatment at the Veterans Administration (Andaya et al., 2013), African American patients still had a statistically significant worse overall survival rate. Although these studies were primarily male dominated, similar results were seen in female breast cancer studies (Blackman & Masi, 2006). Disparities exist in other groups as well, and reporting incidence and mortality remains geographically diverse (see Chapter 5 for more informaton on cultural issues).

Health disparities are challenges that federal, state, and private organizations are working to eliminate. The Centers for Disease Control and Prevention Healthy People 2020 initiative serves to guide national health promotion and disease prevention efforts to improve the health of all people in the United States (see Figure 27-1).

On a global scale, developing countries produce a 60% higher rate of cancer (Jones, Chilton, Hajek, Iammarino, & Laufman, 2006) and are quantitative leaders because of dense

## Economic Stability
- Poverty
- Employment
- Food security
- Housing security

## Education
- High school graduation
- Enrollment in higher education
- Language and literacy
- Early childhood education

## Health Care
- Access to health care
- Access to primary care
- Health literacy

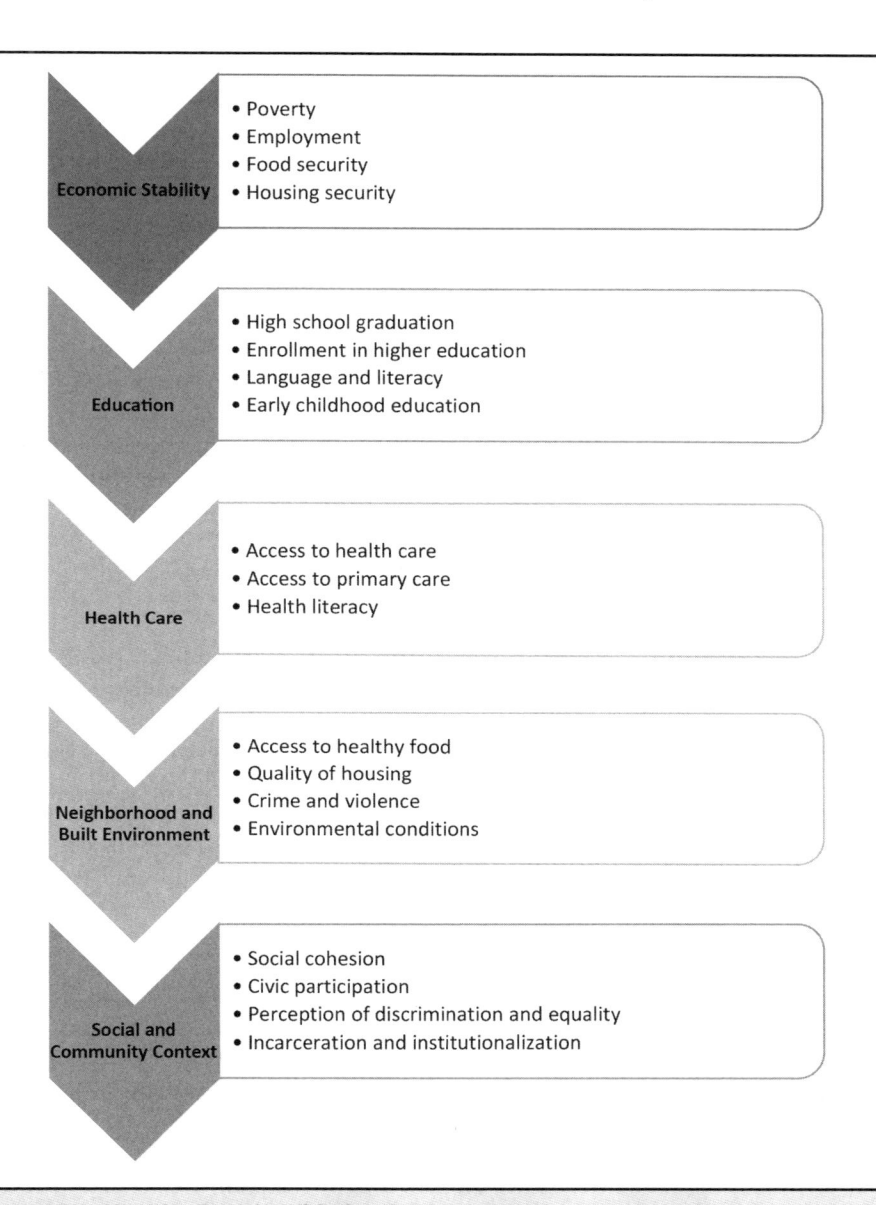

## Neighborhood and Built Environment
- Access to healthy food
- Quality of housing
- Crime and violence
- Environmental conditions

## Social and Community Context
- Social cohesion
- Civic participation
- Perception of discrimination and equality
- Incarceration and institutionalization

**Figure 27-1. Healthy People Initiative Social Determinants of Health**

*Note.* Based on information from Centers for Disease Control and Prevention, 2017.

populations, environmental factors, and lack of adequate sanitation. However, similar qualitative etiologies can be identified in both developing nations and developed western countries, such as environmental pollution, the need for social justice, the lack of resources, economic inequalities, the industrialization and urbanization contributing to cancer exposure, and increased mortality rates (Jones et al., 2006). Although no one model can serve all societies, allocating resources appropriately and focusing on improvement of similar factors on a local level can provide for generalizable information and formats that can be adapted to various cultures and environments (Jones et al., 2006).

## Justice and the Allocation of Health Resources

The 21st century has been fraught with healthcare costs that are escalating beyond control. Expensive, state-of-the-art medical facilities, rising costs of medical education, advancement of novel technologies, new and expensive medications, and increasing morbidity among an aging population are factors that have directly increased healthcare costs. The traditional fee-for-service system of healthcare reimbursement offers no incentive for reducing healthcare expenditures and conspires to escalate the price tag for health services; therefore, reform has long been needed.

On March 2010, the Obama administration signed the Patient Protection and Affordable Care Act into law to expand access to care and to provide health care to all Americans. Specific provisions mandated employer provision of health care, expanded Medicaid, and increased subsidies to individuals to help pay premiums (U.S. Department of Health and Human Services, 2017). The law prohibited denying insurance based on preexisting conditions, and lifetime caps were eliminated, which was of major importance to patients with cancer. As society wrestles with how to provide adequate healthcare coverage for the uninsured, challenges remain. Many Americans are uninsured for a variety of reasons, and the continued high costs of co-pays and pharmacy costs for cancer therapies remain barriers to improved access.

The Affordable Care Act created an ethical dilemma between individual autonomy versus federal paternalism regarding the requirement that all persons purchase health insurance and the states' rights on funding to deny or create state marketplaces. There continues to be disagreement in the United States as to how to address this issue. How health care is provided continues to be a major area of controversy.

Managed care is the primary response to the dilemma of rising healthcare costs; one of its chief aims is to manage costs. The creation of shared risk by both the managed care organization and the healthcare professional invokes dual responsibility for cost containment and the allocation of healthcare resources. Healthcare providers share a dual and seemingly incompatible role of honoring the principles of beneficence and nonmaleficence in caring for patients while pleasing their boss (managed care organization) in carrying out its cost-controlling agenda. In reality, the ethical principle of justice may be violated, as healthcare providers are asked to serve two potentially differing interests (DeCamp & Soleymani-Lehmann, 2015).

Managed care is not inherently unethical, but it does introduce some ethical conundrums. Healthcare professionals, who share responsibility for husbanding resources, may succumb to financial pressures from the managed care organization regarding referral practices and rationing or restricting treatment options not covered by the plan (DeCamp & Soleymani-Lehmann, 2015). Trust between healthcare professionals and their patients may diminish as patients learn that their care providers are interested in potentially withholding care to reduce costs. Treatment protocols may not cover or permit the use of expensive or novel therapies; this is particularly troublesome for cancer care (DeCamp & Soleymani-Lehmann, 2015). Finally, managed care has a tendency to find it more cost effective to prescribe a medication rather than offer more time-consuming counseling for mental or emotional anguish (Rosenberg & DeMaso, 2008; Syrjala et al., 2014). The evolution of managed care has resulted in a shift away from the primacy of the patient–provider relationship and created new ethical challenges. The managed care marketplace is changing the delivery of cancer care. Treatment for cancer is undergoing much scrutiny, as managed care reviewers require detailed reviews of treatment plans to provide initial verification and recertification for a provider's recommended course of therapy. Therapies that are expensive, new on the market, or investigational undergo particular inquiry. The evolution of managed care has created shorter hospital stays that result in sicker patients being returned into the community where families have an increasing responsibility to provide care. Oncology nurses must remain aware of the impact that managed care has on patients and families clinically, fiscally, and practically.

## Conclusion

The "good and bad" and "right and wrong" are increasingly blurred by the ethical complexity of care in today's healthcare delivery system. Oncology nurses are faced with a variety of new ethical challenges propagated by scientific advancement, new legislation, societal changes, and fewer resources to accomplish the privilege of caring well for those living with cancer. The ethical principles of autonomy, beneficence, nonmaleficence, and justice are the foundation of knowledge that propose examination of a variety of dilemmas. These principles provide catalysts, which proliferate dissent in the ethics of health care on topics such as paternalism and self-determination, ordinary versus extraordinary means of preserving life, delaying or hastening death, and rationing versus good stewardship. Oncology nurses have an invaluable role in the discussion of ethical issues in the arena of cancer care. They serve as patient advocates, a liaison between the provider and the patient, and representatives of community and the healthcare system; as such, oncology nurses have a voice in any ethical deliberation and a duty to speak up.

*The author would like to acknowledge Libby Bowers, RN, MSN, CHPN, CCRN, for her contribution to this chapter from the previous edition of this book.*

## References

Abrahm, J.L. (2008). Patient and family requests for hastened death. *Hematology, 1,* 475–480. doi:10.1182/ash education-2008.1.475

Adashi, E.Y. (2011). International human subject research. Taking stock in the wake of the Guatemala affair. *Contemporary Clinical Trials, 32,* 605–607. doi:10.1016/j.cct.2011.05.001

Adolph, M.D., Frier, K.A., Stawicki, S.P.A., Gerlach, A.T., & Papadimos, T.J. (2011). Palliative critical care in the intensive care unit: A 2011 perspective. *International Journal of Critical Illness and Injury Science, 1,* 147–153. doi:10.4103/2229-5151.84803

Allen, L.A., Stevenson, L.W., Grady, K.L., Goldstein, N.E., Matlock, D.D., Arnold, R.M., … Spertus, J.A. (2012). Decision making in advanced heart failure: A scientific statement from the American Heart Association. Endorsed by Heart Failure Society of America and American Association of Heart Failure. *Nurses, 125,* 1928–1952. doi:10.1161/cir.0b013e31824f2173

American Nurses Association. (2013). *Euthanasia, assisted suicide, and aid in dying* [Position statement]. Retrieved from http://www.nursingworld.org/euthanasiaanddying

American Nurses Association. (2015). *Code of ethics for nurses with interpretive statements.* Retrieved from http://www.nursingworld.org/MainMenuCategories/EthicsStandards/CodeofEthicsforNurses/Code-of-Ethics-For-Nurses.html

American Thoracic Society. (1991). Withholding and withdrawing life sustaining therapy. *Annals of Internal Medicine, 115,* 478–485. doi:10.7326/0003-4819-115-6-478

Andaya, A.A., Enewold, L., Zahm, S.H., Shriver, C.D., Stojadinovic, A., McGlynn, K.A., & Zhu, K. (2013). Race and colon cancer survival in an equal-access health care system. *Cancer Epidemiology, Biomarkers and Prevention, 22,* 1030–1036. doi:10.1158/1055-9965.EPI-13-0143

Barakat, A., Barnes, S.A., Cassanova, M.A., Stone, M.J., Shuey, K.M., & Miller, A.M. (2013). Advance care planning knowledge and documentation in a hospitalized cancer population. *Proceedings, 26,* 368–372.

Battin, M.P., van der Heide, A., Ganzini, L., van der Wal, G., & Onwuteaka-Philipsen, B.D. (2007). Legal physician-assisted dying in Oregon and the Netherlands: Evidence concerning the impact on patients in "vulnerable" groups. *Journal of Medical Ethics, 33,* 591–597. doi:10.1136/jme.2007.022335

Beauchamp, T.L., & Childress, J.F. (2013). *Principles of biomedical ethics* (7th ed.). New York, NY: Oxford University Press.

Bergh, M., Dierckx de Casterlé, D., & Gastmans, C. (2005). The complexity of nurses' attitudes toward euthanasia: A review of literature. *Journal of Medical Ethics, 31,* 441–446. doi:10.1136/jme.2004.009092

Blackman, D.J., & Masi, C.M. (2006). Racial and ethnic disparities in breast cancer mortality. Are we doing enough to address the root causes? *Journal of Clinical Oncology, 24,* 2170–2178. doi:10.1200/JCO.2005.05.4734

Bloomer, M.J., Tiruvoipati, R., Tsiripillis, M., & Botha, J.A. (2010). End of life management of adult patients in an Australian metropolitan intensive care unit: A retrospective observational study. *Australian Critical Care, 23,* 13–19. doi:10.1016/j.aucc.2009.10.002

Brant, J.M., & Wickham, R. (Eds.). (2013). *Statement on the scope and standards of oncology nursing practice: Generalist and advanced practice.* Pittsburgh, PA: Oncology Nursing Society.

Buchanan, D.R. (2008). Autonomy, paternalism and justice: Ethical priorities in public health. *American Journal of Public Health, 98,* 15–21. doi:10.2105/AJPH.2007.110361

Burkle, C.M., & Benson, J.J. (2012). End-of-life care decisions: Importance of reviewing systems and limitation of 2 recent North American cases. *Mayo Clinic Proceedings, 87,* 1098–1105. doi:10.1016/j.mayocp.2012.04.019

Castillo, L.S., Williams, B.A., Hooper, S.M., Sabatino, C.P., Weithorn, L.A., & Sudore, R.L. (2011). Lost in translation: The unintended consequences of advance directive law on clinical care. *Annals of Internal Medicine, 154,* 121–128. doi:10.7326/0003-4819-154-2-201101180-00012

Centers for Disease Control and Prevention. (2017). Healthy people. Retrieved from https://www.cdc.gov/nchs/healthy_people

Cheon, J., Coyle, N., Wiegand, D.L., & Welsh, S. (2015). Ethical issues experienced by hospice and palliative nurses. *Journal of Hospice and Palliative Nursing, 17,* 7–13. doi:10.1097/NJH.0000000000000129

Chow, K. (2014). Ethical dilemmas in the intensive care unit: Treating pain and symptoms in the noncommunicative patient at end of life. *Journal of Hospice and Palliative Nursing, 5,* 256–260. doi:10.1097/NJH.0000000000000069

Clayton, J.M., Hancock, K., Parker, S., Butow, P.N., Walder, S., Carrick, S., ... Tattersall, M.H. (2008). Sustaining hope when communicating with terminally ill patients and their families: A systematic review. *Psycho-Oncology, 17,* 641–659. doi:10.1002/pon.1288

Cohen, J.S., & Erickson, J.M. (2006). Ethical dilemmas and moral distress in oncology nursing practice. *Clinical Journal of Oncology Nursing, 10,* 775–780. doi:10.1188/06.CJON.775-780

Dalinis, P.M. (2004). Bioethics consultation: Appropriate uses in end-of-life care. *Journal of Hospice and Palliative Nursing, 6,* 117–122.

de Boer, M.E., Dröes, R.M., Jonker, C., Eefsting, J.A., & Hertogh, C.M. (2011). Advance directives for euthanasia in dementia: How do they affect resident care in Dutch nursing homes? Experiences of physicians and relatives. *Journal of the American Geriatrics Society, 59,* 989–996. doi:10.1111/j.1532-5415.2011.03414.x

DeCamp, M., & Soleyman-Lehmanni, L. (2015). Guiding choice—Ethical influencing referrals in ACOs. *New England Journal of Medicine, 372,* 205–207. doi:10.1056/NEJMp1412083

Edwards, B.K., Noone, A.M., Mariotto, A.B., Simard, E.P., Boscoe, F.R., Henley, S.J., ... Ward, E.M. (2014). Annual report to the nation on the status of cancer, 1975–2010: Featuring prevalence of comorbiditiy and impact on survival among persons with lung, colorectal, breast, or prostate cancer. *Cancer, 120,* 1290–1314. doi:10.1002/cncr.28509

Evangelista, L.S., Motie, M., Lombardo, D., Ballard-Hernandez, J., Malick, S., & Liao, S. (2012). Does preparedness planning improve attitudes and completion of advance directives in patients with symptomatic heart failure? *Journal of Palliative Medicine, 15,* 1316–1320. doi:10.1089/jpm.2012.0228

Garrido, M.M., Balboni, T.A., Maciejewski, P.K., Bao, Y., & Prigerson, H.G. (2014). Quality of life and cost of care at end of life: The role of advance directives. *Journal of Pain and Symptom Management, 49,* 828–835. doi:10.1016/j.jpainsymman.2014.09.015

Gawande, A. (2014). *Being mortal: Medicine and what matters in the end.* New York, NY: Metropolitan Books.

Hall, D.E., Prochazka, A., & Fink, A.S. (2012). Informed consent for clinical treatment. *Canadian Medical Association Journal, 184,* 533–540. doi:10.1503/cmaj.112120

Harrington, S.E., & Smith, T.J. (2008). The role of chemotherapy at the end of life. "When is enough, enough?" *JAMA, 299,* 2667–2668. doi:10.1001/jama.299.22.2667

Herrara, A.P., Snipes, S.A., King, D.W., Torres-Vigil, I., Goldberg, D.S., & Weinberg, A.D. (2010). Disparate inclusion of older adults in clinical trials: Priorities and opportunities for policy and practice change. *American Journal of Public Health, 100,* 105–112. doi:10.2105/AJPH.2009.162982

Hoerger, M., Epstein, R.M., Winters, P.C., Fiscella, K., Duberstein, P.R., Gramlin, R., ... Kravitz, R.L. (2013). Value and options in cancer care (VOICE): Study design and rationale for a patient-centered communication and decision-making intervention for physicians, patients with advanced cancer, and their caregivers. *BMC Cancer, 13,* 188. doi:10.1186/1471-2407-13-188

Hospice and Palliative Nurses Association. (2016). *Palliative sedation* [Position statement]. Retrieved from http://advancingexpertcare.org/wp-content/uploads/2016/01/Palliative-Sedation.pdf

Hospice and Palliative Nurses Association. (2017a). *Guidelines for the role of the registered nurse and advanced practice registered nurse when hastened death is requested* [Position statement]. Retrieved from http://advancingexpertcare.org/wp-content/uploads/2017/07/Guidelines-for-RN-and-APRN-When-Hastened-Death-Requested.pdf

Hospice and Palliative Nurses Association. (2017b). *Physician assisted death/physician assisted suicide* [Position statement]. Retrieved from http://advancingexpertcare.org/wp-content/uploads/2017/07/Physician-Assisted-Death-Physician-Assisted-Suicide.pdf

Jablonski, A., Clymin, J., Jacobson, D., & Feldt, K. (2012). The Washington State Death With Dignity Act: A survey of nurses knowledge and implications for practice part 1. *Journal of Hospice and Palliative Nursing, 14,* 45–52. doi:10.1097/NJH.0b013e3182350f32

Johns Hopkins Berman Institute of Bioethics. (2014). A blueprint for 21st century nursing ethics: Report of the National Nursing Summit. Retrieved from http://www.bioethicsinstitute.org/nursing-ethics-summit-report

Jones, L.A., Chilton, J.A., Hajek, R.A., Iammarino, N.K., & Laufman, L. (2006). Between and within: International perspective on cancer and health disparities. *Journal of Clinical Oncology, 24,* 2204–2208. doi:10.1200/JCO.2005.05.1813

Kagawa-Singer, M., Valdez-Dadia, A., Yu, M.C., & Surbone, A. (2010). Cancer, culture, and health disparities: Time to chart a new course. *CA: A Cancer Journal for Clinicians, 60,* 12–39. doi:10.3322/caac.20051

Kaiser Family Foundation. (2010). Health reform and communities of color: Implication for racial and ethnic health disparities. Facts on health reform. Retrieved from http://kff.org/disparities-policy/issue-brief/health-reform-and-communities-of-color-implications

Koedoot, C.G., Oort, F.J., de Haan, R.J., Bakker, P.J., de Graeff, A., & de Haes, J.C. (2004). The content and amount of information given by medical oncologists when telling a patient with advanced cancer what their treatment options are. *European Journal of Cancer, 40,* 225–235. doi:10.1016/j.ejca.2003.10.008

Kohler, B.A., Ward, E., McCarthy, B.J., Schymura, M.J., Ries, L.A., Eheman, C., ... Edwards, B.K. (2011). Annual report to the nation on the status of cancer, 1975–2007. *Journal of the National Cancer Institute, 103,* 714–736. doi:10.1093/jnci/djr077

Kossman, D.A. (2014). Prevalence, view, and impact of advance directives among older adults. *Journal of Gerontology Nursing, 40,* 44–50. doi:10.3928/00989134-20140310-01

Lachman, V.D. (2010). Physician-assisted suicide: Compassionate liberation or murder? *MEDSURG Nursing, 19,* 121–125.

Lachman, V.D. (2014). Conscientious objection in nursing: Definition and criteria for acceptance. *MEDSURG Nursing, 23,* 196–198.

Lickerman, A. (2015). Achieving a good death. Retrieved from http://www.slate.com/articles/health_and_science/medical_examiner/2015/02/end_of_life_decisions_achieving_a_good_death_with_the_help_of_a_doctor_and.html

Mack, J.W., Cronin, A., Taback, N., Huskamp, H.A., Keating, N.L., Malin, J.L., ... Weeks, J.C. (2012). End-of-life discussions among patients with advanced cancer: A cohort study. *Annals of Internal Medicine, 156,* 204–210. doi:10.7326/0003-4819-156-3-201202070-00008

MacLeod, R.D., Wilson, D.M., & Malpas, P. (2012). Assisted or hastened death: The healthcare practitioner's dilemma. *Global Journal of Health Science, 4,* 87–98. doi:10.5539/gjhs.v4n6p87

McSteen, K., & Peden-McAlpine, C. (2006). The role of the nurse as advocate in ethically difficult care situations with dying patients. *Journal of Hospice and Palliative Nursing, 8,* 259–269. doi:10.1097/00129191-200609000-00011

Monforte-Royo, C., Villavicencio-Chavez, C., Tomas-Sabado, J., Mahtani-Chugani, V., & Balaguer, A. (2012). What lies behind the wish to hasten death? A systematic review and meta-ethnography from the perspective of patients. *PLOS ONE, 7,* e37117. doi:10.1371/journal.pone.0037117

Nakajima, N., Hata, Y., Onishi, H., & Ishida, M. (2013). The evaluation of the relationship between the level of disclosure of cancer in terminally ill patients with cancer and the quality of terminal care in these patients and their families using the support team assessment schedule. *American Journal of Hospice and Palliative Care, 30,* 370–376. doi:10.1177/1049909112452466

Ohnsorge, K., Gudat, H., & Rehmann-Sutter, C. (2014). Intentions in wishes to die: Analysis and a typology—A report of 30 qualitative case studies of terminally ill cancer patients in palliative care. *Psycho-Oncology, 23,* 1021–1026. doi:10.1002/pon.3524

Oncology Nursing Society. (2010). Nurses' responsibility to patients requesting assistance in hastening death. *Oncology Nursing Forum, 37,* 249–250.

Oregon Public Health Division. (2016). Death with Dignity Act. Retrieved from https://www.oregon.gov/oha/PH/ProviderPartnerResources/EvaluationResearch/DeathwithDignityAct/Documents/year17.pdf

Owens, O.L., Jackson, D.D., Thomas, T.L., Friedman, D.B., & Hebert, J.R. (2013). African American men's and women's perceptions of clinical trials research: Focusing on prostate cancer among a high-risk population in the south. *Journal of Health Care for the Poor and Underserved, 24,* 1784–1800. doi:10.1353/hpu.2013.0187

Parker, S.M., Clayton, J.M., Hancock, K., Walder, S., Butow, P.N., Carrick, D., ... Tattersall, M.H. (2007). A systematic review of prognostic/end-of-life communication with adults in the advanced stages of a life-limiting illness: Patient/caregiver preferences for the content, style, and timing of information. *Journal of Pain and Symptom Management, 34,* 81–93. doi:10.1016/j.jpainsymman.2006.09.035

Pavlish, C., Brown-Saltzman, K., Fine, A., & Jakel, P. (2015). A culture of avoidance: Voices from inside ethically difficult clinical situations. *Clinical Journal of Oncology Nursing, 19,* 1–7. doi:10.1188/15.CJON.19-02AP

Pavlish, C., Brown-Saltzman, K., Jakel, P., & Fine, A. (2014). The nature of ethical conflicts and the meaning of moral community in oncology practice. *Oncology Nursing Forum, 41,* 130–138. doi:10.1188/14.ONF.130-140

Politi, M.C., Studts, J.L., & Hayslip, J.W. (2012). Shared decision making in oncology practice: What do oncologists need to know? *Oncologist, 17,* 91–100. doi:10.1634/theoncologist.2011-0261

Pritchard, J. (2012). Euthanasia: A reply to Bartel and Otlowski. *Journal of Law and Medicine, 19,* 610–621.

Putnam, C. (2009). What kind of a right is the "right to die?" *European Journal of Mental Health, 4,* 165. doi:10.1556/EJMH.4.2009.2.1

Randall, F., & Downie, R. (2010). Assisted suicide and voluntary euthanasia: Role contradictions for physicians. *Clinical Medicine, 10,* 323–325. doi:10.7861/clinmedicine.10-4-323

Robinson, T.M., Alexander, S.C., Hays, M., Jeffreys, A.S., Olsen, M.K., Rodriguez, K.L., ... Tulsky, J.A. (2008). Patient–oncologist communication in advanced cancer: Predictors of patient perception of prognosis. *Supportive Care in Cancer, 16,* 1049–1057. doi:10.1007/s00520-007-0372-2

Rodin, G., Zimmerman, C., Rydall, A., Jones, J., Shepard, F.A., Moore, M., ... Gagliese, L. (2007). The desire for hastened death in patients with metastatic cancer. *Journal of Pain and Symptom Management, 33,* 661–675. doi:10.1016/j.jpainsymman.2006.09.034

Rosenberg, E., & DeMaso, D.R. (2008). A doubtful guest: Managed care and mental health. *Child and Adolescent Psychiatry Clinics of North America, 17,* 53–66. doi:10.1016/j.chc.2007.07.005

Russell, B.J., & Ward, A.M. (2011). Deciding what information is necessary: Do patients with advanced cancer want to know all the details? *Cancer Management and Research, 3,* 191–199. doi:10.2147/CMAR.S12998

Schneiderman, L.J. (2011). Defining medical futility and improving medical care. *Journal of Bioethical Inquiry, 8,* 123–131. doi:10.1007/s11673-011-9293-3

Shepard, A. (2010). Moral distress: A consequence of caring. *Clinical Journal of Oncology Nursing, 14,* 25–27. doi:10.1188/10.CJON.25-27

Silveira, M.J., Wiitala, W., & Piette, J. (2014). Advance directive completion by elderly Americans: A decade of change. *Journal of the American Geriatrics Society, 62,* 706–710. doi:10.1111/jgs.12736

Sirilla, J. (2014). Moral distress in nurses providing direct care in inpatient oncology units. *Clinical Journal of Oncology Nursing, 18,* 536–541. doi:10.1188/14.CJON.536-541

Smedley, B.D., Stith, A.Y., & Nelson, A.R. (Eds.). (2003). *Unequal treatment: Confronting racial and ethnic disparities in health care.* Washington, DC: National Academies Press.

Snyder, S., Hazelett, S., Allen, K., & Radwany, S. (2013). Physician knowledge, attitude, and experience with advance care planning, palliative care, and hospice: Results of a primary care study. *American Journal of Hospice and Palliative Care, 30,* 419–424. doi:10.1177/1049909112452467

Society of Critical Care Medicine. (1997). Consensus statement of the Society of Critical Care Medicine's Ethics Committee regarding futile and other possible inadvisable treatments. *Critical Care Medicine, 24,* 887–891.

Sryjala, K.L., Jensen, M.P., Mendoza, M.E., Yi, J.C., Fisher, H.M., & Keefe, F.J. (2014). Psychological and behavioral approaches to cancer pain management. *Journal of Clinical Oncology, 32,* 1703–1711. doi:10.1200/JCO.2013.54.4825

Steck, N., Egger, M.M., Maessen, M., Reisch, T., & Zwahlen, M. (2013). Euthanasia and assisted suicide in selected European countries and US states: Systematic literature review. *Medical Care, 51,* 938–944. doi:10.1097/mlr.0b013e3182a0f427

Strouse, T. (2017). End-of-life options and the legal pathways to physician aid in dying. *Journal of Community and Supportive Oncology, 15,* 1–3.

Taddonio, P. (2014). How should doctors help terminally ill patients prepare for death? Retrieved from http://www.pbs.org/wgbh/frontline/article/how-should-doctors-help-terminally-ill-patients-prepare-for-death

Ternestedt, B.M. (2005). Expressed desire for hastened death by patients with advanced cancer had several meanings and uses. *Evidence-Based Nursing, 8,* 96. doi:10.1136/ebn.8.3.96

U.S. Department of Health and Human Services. (2017, July 3). About the Affordable Care Act. Retrieved from http://www.hhs.gov/healthcare/facts/timeline/index.html

Virk, K.P. (2010). Addressing issues affecting clinical trials in Brazil. *Clinical Research and Regulatory Affairs, 27,* 52–59. doi:10.3109/10601333.2010.480974

Wagner, S.E., Hurley, D.M., Hebert, J.R., McNamara, C., Bayakly, A.R., & Vena, J.E. (2012). Cancer mortality-to-incidence ratios in Georgia: Describing racial cancer disparities and potential geographic determinants. *Cancer, 118,* 4032–4045. doi:10.1002/cncr.26728

Walczak, A., Butow, P.N., Clayton, J.M., Tattersall, M.H.N., Davidson, P.M., Young, J., & Epstein, R.M. (2014). Discussing prognosis and end-of-life care in the final year of life: A randomized controlled trial of a nurse-led communication support program for patients and caregivers. *BMJ Open, 4,* e005745. doi:10.1136/bmjopen-2014-005745

Wiegand, D.L., & Grant, M.S. (2014). Bioethical issues related to limiting life-sustaining therapies in the intensive care unit. *Journal of Hospice and Palliative Nursing, 16,* 60–64. doi:10.1097/NJH.0000000000000049

Wilson, F., Gott, M., & Ingleton, C. (2013). Perceived risks around choice and decision making at end of life: A literature review. *Palliative Medicine, 27,* 38–53. doi:10.1177/0269216311424632

Yung, V.Y., Walling, A.M., Min, L., Wenger, N.S., & Ganz, D.A. (2010). Documentation of advance care planning for community-dwelling elders. *Journal of Palliative Medicine, 13,* 861–867. doi:10.1089/jpm.2009.0341

Zahedi, F. (2011). The challenge of truth telling across cultures: A case study. *Journal of Ethics and History of Medicine, 4,* 11.

Zalonis, R., & Slota, M. (2014). The use of palliative care to promote autonomy in decision making. *Clinical Journal of Oncology Nursing, 18,* 707–711. doi:10.1188/14.CJON.707-711

Zamichow, N. (2015, February 15). Saying the D-word. Op-ed for Sunday. *Los Angeles Times,* p. A27.

Zenz, J., Tryba, M., & Zenz, M. (2014). Physician-assisted dying: Acceptance by physicians only for patients close to death. *Pain and Therapy, 3,* 103–112. doi:10.1009/s40122-014-0029-z

CHAPTER 28

# Caring for the Family

*Sheila M. Ferrall, MS, RN, AOCN®*

> *Behold, I am going to send an angel before you to guard you along the way.*
>
> —Exodus 23:20

Cancer is widely considered to be a disease of both individuals and their families. Approximately 1.68 million in the United States will be diagnosed with cancer in 2017 (American Cancer Society, 2017); spouses, children, parents, and partners are among those who will be profoundly affected by the diagnosis. Family members have always played a role in the care of patients with cancer. However, changes in health care have served to significantly increase demands on these caregivers. Technologic advances allow for the management of cancers that were previously considered untreatable. With an eye toward cost savings, patients are being discharged earlier from inpatient settings. Treatments once provided only during an inpatient hospitalization now are given on an outpatient basis and often at home. The increasing availability of oral chemotherapy further contributes to the shift from managing care in a medical setting to the home. In light of these changes, family caregivers are assuming growing responsibility for the care of loved ones, often with little preparation.

The range of potential caregivers for patients with cancer is wide. Spouses, parents, children, and siblings are all possible caregivers. The Institute for Patient- and Family-Centered Care defines family as two or more persons who are related in any way—biologically, legally, or emotionally (Clay & Parsh, 2016). This definition includes those not related to the individual in the traditional sense but designated by the patient as family. With that in mind, friends, neighbors, lovers, or partners may play significant roles as family caregivers for patients with cancer.

According to statistics published by the Family Caregiver Alliance (2015), approximately 43.5 million Americans provide unpaid care each year to ill, disabled, or aged family members or friends. The value of these services provided by family caregivers is estimated to be $450 billion per year, which is more than double what it was in 1996 (Feinberg, Reinhard, Houser, & Choula, 2011). Individuals assuming the caregiver role experience unique challenges. Accurate and thorough assessment of these challenges will allow oncology nurses to structure interventions to support this diverse and vital group.

## Assessment of Caregiver Challenges

Regardless of the type of cancer or stage at diagnosis, caregivers must cope with inevitable challenges. A roller coaster analogy aptly depicts both patients' and caregivers' feelings during this time, with highs and lows throughout the illness. Patients' and caregivers' quality of life can be affected by their responses to the situation. A caregiver assessment should be routinely included for every patient with cancer to evaluate if the caregiver is willing and capable of providing care (Given, Given, & Sherwood, 2012). Further, caregiver assessment should occur at regular intervals to evaluate and respond to the changing needs of the family caregiver (Glajchen, 2012; Grant et al., 2013; Northouse, Katapodi, Schafenacker, & Weiss, 2012).

A number of instruments are available that specifically assess the needs of family caregivers. Prue, Santin, and Porter (2015) identified seven caregiver self-report needs assessment tools. Of the seven tools identified, the authors recommended the Needs Assessment of Family Caregivers–Cancer (NAFC-C) as having the greatest potential for both clinical and research use. NAFC-C is a 27-item scale that measures needs in terms of both the importance of the need and to what extent the need has been met. Although it requires further psychometric testing, the tool is short and relevant across the cancer caregiving trajectory, which makes it ideally suited for clinical use.

### Diagnosis

In a seminal article, Sales (1991) reviewed literature on the psychosocial impact of cancer on the family and presented the information within a framework of six phases of cancer. During the initial or diagnosis phase of illness, caregivers face many of the same feelings of anxiety, anger, and helplessness as patients. Caregivers may feel ignored or excluded by medical personnel who attend to the patient and may have difficulty communicating their questions and information needs. Caregivers of hospitalized patients find themselves in the position of helping patients to cope with the physical and emotional impact of surgery, radiation, and chemotherapy. In addition to visiting and providing emotional support, caregivers often must assume multiple roles vacated by the patient during hospitalization, resulting in feelings of overload and exhaustion. As the patient leaves the hospital, caregivers face a new problem: how to deal with the patient's day-to-day challenges of living with cancer. If the patient has physical limitations, the caregiver has the task of adapting their preexisting lifestyle to the patient's needs. Direct caregiving tasks may take priority over the caregiver's usual activities. The economic realities of treatment become clear and may involve significant financial burden. Family disagreement over treatment decisions may further complicate this difficult period (Shin et al., 2013, 2015; Zhang & Siminoff, 2003).

### Treatment

During the active treatment phase, patients and caregivers find themselves interacting repeatedly with healthcare providers. Frequent visits for treatments may pose scheduling and transportation problems. Caregivers must coordinate treatment visits for the patient while maintaining some connection to their own work or personal commitments. Both caregivers and patients may feel unprepared to manage treatment effects (Harden et al., 2002; Hendrix et al., 2016).

In 2011, van Ryan et al. studied the cancer care delivered by informal caregivers to newly diagnosed patients with lung and colorectal cancer. In addition to assisting with the activities of daily living, the caregivers reported participating in a variety of tasks, including watching for treatment side effects (68%), administering medications (34%), and determining whether to call a healthcare provider (30%). Nearly half of the caregivers surveyed reported that they did not receive training for the care they provided. In a study of 194 caregivers of patients receiving outpatient treatment for leukemia (Tamayo, Broxson, Munsell, & Cohen, 2010), caregivers rated the following as "very important": learning how to manage side effects of medications (84%), administering medications (72%), and learning how to manage symptoms such as fatigue (82%) among others. Studies of caregivers of other patient populations echo the need for education and preparation for the caregiving role (Coolbrandt et al., 2014; Von Ah, Spath, Nielsen, & Fife, 2016).

## Recurrence and Advanced Cancer

Cancer recurrence creates emotional distress that rivals the stress that occurs during the initial diagnosis. Options for treatment may be restricted to more aggressive, higher risk modalities that require closer monitoring and more caregiver involvement. Progressive deterioration and physical decline are hallmarks of advanced cancer. As the disease interferes with normal functioning, caregivers, by necessity, assume added responsibilities.

As cancer progresses, the caregiving burden increases. Bowman, Rose, Radziewicz, O'Toole, and Berila (2009) examined family caregiver engagement in an intervention tailored to patients with advanced cancer and their families. Caregivers in this study identified caregiving tasks as their most significant problem (84%), followed by practical problems (36%), communication with healthcare providers (39%), and psychological issues (32%). Home care of patients with advanced cancer can have a negative impact on caregivers' health, schedule, anxiety, and energy (Aranda & Hayman-White, 2001). Weitzner, McMillan, and Jacobsen (1999) compared the impact of cancer caregiving in curative and palliative settings on caregiver quality of life. Not surprisingly, caregivers of patients receiving palliative care had significantly lower quality-of-life and physical health scores. These seminal works provide evidence that, beyond some social work availability, the provision of supportive services in hospice and palliative home care remain limited (Connor, 2015).

Likewise, a significant relationship exists between caregiver stressors and caregiver outcomes. In a study of coping and its effect on cancer caregiving (Gaugler, Eppinger, King, Sandberg, & Regine, 2013), the researchers sought to determine how different coping strategies were associated with caregiver stress and health outcomes. Caregivers who used negative expectation coping (e.g., worrying, expecting the worst) were more likely to feel entrapped by their caregiving role and suffer feelings of anxiety, depressive symptoms, and guilt. Redinbaugh, Baum, Tarbell, and Arnold (2003) examined caregiver stressors, coping, and caregiver strain in a sample of 31 family caregivers and their terminally ill loved ones enrolled in home hospice programs. Higher levels of caregiver strain were noted when patients had greater physical needs, greater psychological distress, and poorer existential quality of life. Caregivers were better able to define problems related to their patients' illness when they believed that families accepted the illness. They also felt more capable of managing and resolving illness-related stressors and reported lower levels of strain. In the settings of palliative and hospice care, Connor (2015) stressed that the focus of care must be on immediate family needs that are helpful for patient support and on achieving closure while promoting adaptive coping mechanisms for the family.

## Spiritual Assessment

Caregivers have been observed to have spiritual needs similar to those of their patients (Taylor, 2003), yet this is an area that oncology nurses may overlook. Kuuppelomäki (2002) studied 166 nurses from five hospitals in Finland. Although the majority of the participating nurses agreed that the patient's family should be given spiritual support, half of the nurses were not willing to offer that support. The nurses identified many obstacles to providing spiritual support, including family members turning to other experts with their spiritual needs, lack of time, and family members being unable to express their spiritual needs. Connor (2015) discussed the limited spiritual care services in the patient's home, especially at the end of life. The author cited that in 2012, only 4.3% of hospice workers were identified as spiritual-care providers. Therefore, it is imperative that nursing care provide assessment of the spiritual needs of patients and caregivers. Ferrell and Baird (2012) asserted that oncology nurses are positioned to screen caregivers for spiritual needs and respond with the foundations of spiritual care: being fully present, listening for what is said and what is intended, and bearing witness to suffering and compassion in action (see Chapter 9 for information on spiritual and religious support).

## Cultural Assessment

Healthcare providers must consider cross-cultural issues when assessing caregiver needs and structuring interventions. Patterns of resource utilization, lack of trust in social services providers, and varying interpretations of pain and social support are just a few areas where culture may influence the role of the caregiver (Glajchen, 2004; Leow, Chan, & Chan, 2014) (see Chapter 5 on cultural influences).

# Caregiver Quality of Life

The intense nature of cancer caregiving puts caregivers at risk for poor quality of life (Lapid et al., 2015). Psychological distress for caregivers may rival and, in some cases, exceed that of patients. Kim, Carver, Spillers, Love-Ghaffari, and Kaw (2012) examined the fear of cancer recurrence among 455 cancer survivor and caregiver pairs. Patients two years after diagnosis were targeted for the study. Although survivors and caregivers both experienced fear of recurrence, the relationship between fear of recurrence and cancer severity was greater for caregivers than for cancer survivors. In an important study by Matthews (2003), role (caregiver or survivor), gender, and psychological distress were evaluated in 135 caregiver–patient dyads. Matthews found significantly higher overall distress levels for caregivers than cancer survivors. Caregiver scores were significantly higher than survivors' on distress for diagnosis and fear of cancer recurrence. Additionally, Matthews reported that female caregivers scored higher than their male counterparts on cancer-related anxiety, future uncertainties, fear of recurrence, and future diagnostic tests. In a study of caregivers of patients undergoing hematopoietic stem cell transplantation, Sabo, McLeod, and Couban (2013) described the uncertainty and stress related to the unknown as a significant source of distress for caregivers.

The following studies demonstrated the need to carry out assessment to identify perceptions of the caregiving role and preparedness. In a review of the psychological impact of cancer on patients' partners and other key relatives, Pitceathly and Maguire (2003) suggested that certain caregivers are particularly vulnerable to stresses associated with the caregiver role. Specifically, those in conflicted relationships and those who have a negative view of illness-related events or of the impact of the caring role on their life are more likely to experience problems. In a study of 87 caregivers of adult patients receiving treatment for lymphoma or solid tumors, Schumacher et al. (2008) studied the effects of demand, mutuality, and preparedness on caregiver outcomes. Not surprisingly demand, or the time dedicated to the tasks of caregiving, was a significant predictor of the outcomes of perceived difficulty, global strain, and, to a lesser extent, depression, fatigue, and mood disturbance. Mutuality, or the quality of the relationship between the caregiver and patient, was strongly associated with anger. This suggests that poor relationship quality could create a particularly difficult caregiver experience. Mutuality and preparedness, or the perceived readiness to take on the caregiver role, were both associated with global strain, confusion, and mood disturbance. Further, mutuality was linked to tension, depression, and anger, while preparedness was linked to vigor and fatigue. Both studies underscored the need to include caregiver assessment as an essential aspect of care and to structure interventions based on assessment findings.

In a comprehensive review of the literature focused on the effects of caring on the family caregiver, Stenberg, Ruland, and Miaskowski (2010) identified more than 200 problems associated with caregiving responsibilities. The problems or burdens identified from the 192 articles that met the inclusion criteria fell into the following broad categories: physical caregiver health problems, social problems and need for information, emotional issues, and burden related to the caregiving responsibilities. Social and emotional issues related to caregiving were studied most frequently. Examples of social problems related to financial difficulties, problems with work and/or education, challenges related to role, feelings of isolation, and the need for information about a number of topics. Kim and Given (2008) also reviewed literature on caregiver quality of life and reported that psychological distress is the most studied dimension. Zaider and Kissane (2015) advocated for routine assessment of the "family environment" to determine the risk of morbidity within each family. They suggested the use of screening in the clinical setting with a tool such as the Family Relationship Index, which has proven to be valid and reliable in detecting family cohesiveness, communication, and conflict resolution.

Caregivers often report significant issues related to depression and sleep (Kotronoulas, Wengstrom, & Kearney, 2013; Stenberg et al., 2010). Sleep disorders in caregivers has received little attention in the past but is most important because of the negative impact that sleep deprivation can have on caregiver functioning (Lowery, 2015). Carter and Chang (2000) administered the Center for Epidemiological Studies Depression Scale and the Pittsburgh Sleep Quality Index to 51 caregivers of patients with cancer. Their purpose was to describe sleep problems and depression levels of caregivers and explore the relationship between those two variables. Caregivers in this descriptive study primarily were white female spouses. More than half of the caregivers experienced depressive symptoms at a level that suggested a risk for clinical depression, and 95% reported severe sleep problems. Caregivers who reported higher levels of sleep problems reported higher levels of depression. Carter (2002) sought to describe caregiver sleep problems and depression levels using narratives. Forty-seven caregivers of patients with advanced cancer were interviewed in person or via telephone. Carter (2002) reported that caregivers described significant fluctuations in sleep patterns over time.

Caregivers also described how chronic sleep loss set into motion the downward movement toward depressive symptoms. Emanuel, Fairclough, Slutsman, and Emanuel (2000) conducted a national study looking at a number of factors impacting patients (50% who had cancer). They found that caregivers of patients with advanced and terminal illnesses were significantly more depressed. Of terminally ill patients with high care needs, 15% gave serious thought to euthanasia/physician-assisted suicide because of the perceived burden created by their illness. Financial burden also was significant for patients with terminal illness. More recent research points to a majority of caregivers reporting moderate to severe sleep deprivation associated with depression, ineffective coping, lower optimism, less mastery, and higher neuroticism (Kotronoulas et al., 2013; Lowery, 2015; Northouse, Williams, Given, & McCorkle, 2012).

Given the significant impact of a cancer diagnosis of a loved one, assessment of caregiver quality of life is essential. Deeken, Taylor, Mangan, Yabroff, and Ingham (2003) conducted a comprehensive review of self-report instruments developed to measure the burden, needs, and quality of life of informal caregivers. After extensive literature review, the researchers identified 28 instruments, which they evaluated in terms of development, content, and psychometric properties. The researchers concluded that several instruments are available to both clinicians and researchers to evaluate caregiver burden, quality of life, and, to a lesser extent, needs. Waller, Boyes, Carey, and Sanson-Fisher (2015) provided a comprehensive list and psychometric properties of available tools to screen unmet needs of caregivers, family, and patient supports. One screening tool specifically cited by these researchers for having the best performance for caregiver screening was the Support Person's Unmet Needs Survey (Waller et al., 2015).

Zwahlen, Hagenbuch, Carley, Recklitis, and Buchi (2008) validated the use of the Distress Thermometer as a screening instrument for depression and anxiety in family caregivers. The Distress Thermometer a self-report measure of distress, has been widely used in patients. Approximately 321 family members of patients with cancer completed the Distress Thermometer and the Hospital Anxiety and Depression Scale (HADS) via mail. HADS has been used to validate the Distress Thermometer in the oncology setting. Based on their results, the authors suggested the Distress Thermometer as an efficient and valid tool to assess depression and anxiety in family members.

# Strategies to Facilitate Caregiver Coping

Oncology nurses hold key positions in terms of assessing caregiver coping and developing interventions to support them in their roles. Interventions vary according to the specific issues for each caregiver, but they generally fall into one of four categories: providing information, providing psychological support, providing physical support, and mobilizing resources.

## Providing Information

Studies have repeatedly identified information or cognitive needs as a primary area of concern for caregivers (Friesen, Pepler, & Hunter, 2002; Fukui, 2002; Harrington, Lackey, & Gates, 1996; Rees & Bath, 2000; Steele & Fitch, 1996; Stenberg et al., 2010; Stetz, McDonald, & Compton, 1996; Tamayo et al., 2010). During the initial phase of illness, obtaining information about the disease and its treatment can serve as a useful coping strategy for caregivers and patients. However, some patients and families may prefer limited information initially, delaying negative information that they have not asked for and are not prepared to hear (Wideheim, Edvardsson, Pahlson, & Ahlstrom, 2002).

Wittenberg-Lyles, Goldsmith, Oliver, Demiris, and Rankin (2012) reviewed case studies to better understand the types of communication of cancer caregivers. They examined caregiver communication in terms of the degree of family conversation and family conformity. The dimension of conversation refers to the degree to which families talk openly about illness and engage in free, spontaneous conversation versus avoiding or limiting conversation about illness. Hierarchy within the family establishes family conformity. High family conformity translates to uniform beliefs and harmony, while families with low conformity do not emphasize obedience to elders. Four patterns of communication were identified: manager, carrier, partner, and loaner. The authors applied case studies to illustrate the four communication patterns and provided strategies to enhance communication within each pattern. Although the authors acknowledged more research around communication patterns of cancer caregivers is needed, they highlighted the importance of recognizing that communication styles and needs differ, and these differences should be considered when using communication interventions to reduce caregiver burden.

Evidence suggests that a structured psychoeducational caregiver intervention can improve caregiver quality of life and positively impact caregiver outcomes (Leow, Chan, & Chan, 2015). In a pilot randomized, controlled trial of the effectiveness of a psychoeducational intervention used with hospice patients in Singapore, the researchers found that the intervention group reported significantly higher quality of life, self-efficacy in self-care, social support, and closeness with the patient, as well as lower stress and depression (Leow et al., 2015). The psychoeducational intervention included a one-hour face-to-face session in which a video clip was reviewed and a care plan developed. After the initial session, two follow-up phone calls were made that ranged from 15 to 30 minutes depending on the needs of the caregiver. Caregivers were also invited to participate in a caregiver forum as part of the intervention. Data were collected over the course of eight weeks (baseline, week 4, and week 8). Those caregivers who received the intervention showed improvement in all areas measured. The researchers suggested further study of the psychoeducational intervention, but acknowledged that it showed promise and could be used as part of standard care for hospice caregivers.

Given, Given, and Kozachik (2001) suggested that interventions such as family conferences, skills training, problem-solving strategies, caregiver training, help sheets, books, videos, CDs, and websites can address the information needs of family caregivers. In this era of increasing outpatient treatments and fewer hospital admissions, caregiver interactions with the healthcare team often are limited. However, allowing time for specific questions is critical. Asking caregivers to identify specific information needs will help ensure that the areas of greatest concern are addressed. Encouraging appropriate decision making, providing advance care planning, and supporting home care are ways in which healthcare providers can be of service to caregivers as patients approach the end of life (Rabow, Hauser, & Adams, 2004).

The Oncology Nursing Society has published evidence-based practice guidelines that outline interventions designed to reduce caregiver strain and burden (Honea et al., 2008). Research supports offering structured programs of information for caregivers as effective interventions. Topical areas might include managing symptoms, discussing psychosocial issues, identifying resources, discussing coordination of service, and teaching caregiver self-care strategies.

## Providing Psychological Support

As professional caregivers become more involved in the high-tech aspect of cancer care, the potential to neglect psychological needs of family caregivers exists. Historically, caregivers have indicated that they have considerable psychological needs (Blanchard,

Albrecht, & Ruckdeschel, 1997). In a systematic review of the literature, Honea et al. (2008) identified that supportive interventions that allow caregivers to discuss issues and feelings about the experience of caregiving may be effective in reducing caregiver burden. Caregivers may benefit from psychotherapy in which a therapeutic relationship with a professional therapist develops and caregivers are assisted in identifying strategies to manage distress. Cognitive behavioral interventions involve teaching caregivers self-monitoring skills and facilitate problem solving by focusing on time, overload, and emotional reactivity management. This approach helps caregivers to reengage in positive experiences and pleasant activities. Telephoning patient caregivers rather than waiting for them to initiate contact is one way to convey support (Applebaum & Breitbart, 2013; Badger, Segrin, Dorros, Meek, & Lopez, 2007; Lapid et al., 2015; Shaw et al., 2016). Scheduled contact via telephone allows caregivers to ventilate and discuss problems as they arise. Offering caregivers the opportunity for individual, group, or peer counseling may help them to identify and resolve issues. Oncology nurses can provide caregivers with ongoing information about stress management and coping with role changes, anxiety, and depression. Community resources such as the Cancer Support Community provide family support groups (see Appendix).

Targeted interventions for caregivers of patients with cancer have shown to positively impact caregiver outcomes (Northouse, Katapodi, Song, Lingling, & Mood, 2010) according to a meta-analysis of data from 29 randomized clinical trials of cancer caregiver interventions. Caregiver self-care was addressed in 27 of the 29 trials and was aimed at the support needed by caregivers to manage their own physical and emotional health needs. Among the positive outcomes noted, caregivers reported less caregiver burden, use of more effective coping strategies, and less distress and anxiety.

As with identifying information needs, asking caregivers to talk about their stressors allows specific concerns to be addressed. Isolating some time alone with the caregiver during an outpatient visit or over the phone may provide an opportunity for catharsis. Asking questions such as "How are you coping with this situation?"; "What do you find most difficult to deal with?"; and "How are you taking care of yourself?" gives caregivers permission to discuss issues that they might otherwise feel guilty mentioning. Finally, recognizing depressive symptoms that require further intervention and making appropriate referrals will further support caregivers.

## Providing Physical Support

Caregivers may need assistance with the physical demands of caring for a patient with cancer at home. When asked, caregivers identified time away from the house, time for personal needs, time for rest, and adequate sleep as significant needs (Steele & Fitch, 1996; Stenberg et al., 2010). Caregivers of patients in the terminal phase may demonstrate a need for overnight respite to prevent exhaustion. Patients receiving the Medicare hospice benefit may have access to short-term respite care in a skilled nursing facility so that caregivers can have some time away from caring for the patient. Nurses should work with caregivers and team members to determine whether hired caregivers are needed. Although often not covered by insurance, this may be necessary to keep the patient out of the hospital at any stage of the illness.

In addition to evaluating the physical demands of caregiving, oncology nurses should assess the availability of appropriate equipment in the home. Harrington et al. (1996) studied the needs of 55 caregivers of clinic and hospice patients. The caregivers of hospice patients ranked equipment to help with patient care as a top need. Routine assessment of the home environment will ensure that required equipment is available to meet the patient's changing needs.

## Mobilizing Resources

Exploring avenues of support for caregivers is an important intervention for oncology nurses. Caregivers today are more sophisticated than ever in terms of seeking information via the Internet and other sources. Despite this level of sophistication, caregivers may be unaware of resources available in their own communities. Maintaining a current list of community aids and distributing it to caregivers will make them aware of resources. Likewise, keeping track of local support group meetings for caregivers may be helpful.

In addition to seeking community resources, caregivers should explore their personal resources for support. Extended family, friends, and church members are a few examples of people who can offer support after a cancer diagnosis. Encourage caregivers to identify specific ways in which these people can help, such as providing transportation one or two days a week for radiation treatments, light housekeeping duties, preparing meals, shopping, and spending time with the patient. Oncology nurses should seize the opportunity to have frank discussions about personal resources with caregivers and encourage them to ask for help.

## Conclusion

An increasing number of family caregivers are being called upon to care for patients with cancer throughout their illness. Assuming this role as caregiver entails many challenges. Yet, caregivers take on this burden without question and often with little help or preparation. Adequate assessment of caregiver needs is central to identifying appropriate interventions. Although further research is required to help define which interventions would be most effective for this important group, existing evidence supports that providing structured education to caregivers, offering supportive interventions, and identifying strategies for respite may reduce the burden associated with caregiving. Oncology nurses play a vital role in supporting caregivers so they are equipped to make this difficult journey with their loved ones.

## References

American Cancer Society. (2017). *Cancer facts and figures 2017.* Retrieved from https://www.cancer.org/content/dam/cancer-org/research/cancer-facts-and-statistics/annual-cancer-facts-and-figures/2017/cancer-facts-and-figures-2017.pdf

Applebaum, A.J., & Breitbart, W. (2013). Care for the cancer caregiver: A systematic review. *Palliative and Supportive Care, 11,* 231–252. doi:10.1017/S1478951512000594

Aranda, S.K., & Hayman-White, K. (2001). Home caregivers of the person with advanced cancer: An Australian perspective. *Cancer Nursing, 24,* 300–307. doi:10.1097/00002820-200108000-00011

Badger, T., Segrin, C., Dorros, S.M., Meek, P., & Lopez, A.M. (2007). Depression and anxiety in women with breast cancer and their partners. *Nursing Research, 56,* 44–53. doi:10.1097/00006199-200701000-00006

Blanchard, C.G., Albrecht, T.L., & Ruckdeschel, J.C. (1997). The crisis of cancer: Psychological impact on family caregivers. *Oncology, 11,* 189–194.

Bowman, K.F., Rose, J.H., Radziewicz, R.M., O'Toole, E.E., & Berila, R.A. (2009). Family caregiver engagement in a coping and communication support intervention tailored to advanced cancer patients and families. *Cancer Nursing, 32,* 73–81. doi:10.1097/01.NCC.0000343367.98623.83

Carter, P.A. (2002). Caregivers' descriptions of sleep changes and depressive symptoms. *Oncology Nursing Forum, 29,* 1277–1283. doi:10.1188/02.ONF.1277-1283

Carter, P.A., & Chang, B.L. (2000). Sleep and depression in cancer caregivers. *Cancer Nursing, 23,* 410–415. doi:10.1097/00002820-200012000-00002

Clay, A.M., & Parsh, B. (2016). Patient- and family-centered care: It's not just for pediatrics anymore. *AMA Journal of Ethics, 18,* 40–44. doi:10.1001/journalofethics.2016.18.1.medu3-1601

Connor, S.R. (2015). Hospice and home care. In J.C. Holland, W.S. Breitbart, P.N. Butow, P.B. Jacobsen, M.J. Loscalzo, & R. McCorkle (Eds.), *Psycho-oncology* (3rd ed., pp. 249–258). New York, NY: Oxford University Press.

Coolbrandt, A., Sterckx, W., Clement, P., Borgenon, S., Decruyenaere, M., de Vleeschouwer, S., ... de Casterlé, B.D. (2014). Family caregivers of patients with a high-grade glioma: A qualitative study of their lived experience and needs related to professional care. *Cancer Nursing, 38,* 406–413. doi:10.1097/NCC.0000000000000216

Deeken, J.F., Taylor, K.L., Mangan, P., Yabroff, R., & Ingham, J.M. (2003). Care for the caregivers: A review of self-report instruments developed to measure the burden, needs, and quality of life of informal caregivers. *Journal of Pain and Symptom Management, 26,* 922–953. doi:10.1016/S0885-3924(03)00327-0

Emanuel, E.J., Fairclough, D.L., Slutsman, J., & Emanuel, L.L. (2000). Understanding economic and other burdens of terminal illness: The experience of patients and their caregivers. *Annals of Internal Medicine, 132,* 451–459. doi:10.7326/0003-4819-132-6-200003210-00005

Family Caregiver Alliance. (2015). Caregiver statistics: Demographics. Retrieved from https://www.caregiver.org/caregiver-statistics-demographics

Feinberg, L., Reinhard, S.C., Houser, A., & Choula, R. (2011). *Valuing the invaluable: 2011 update, the growing contributions and costs of family caregiving.* Retrieved from http://assets.aarp.org/rgcenter/ppi/ltc/i51-caregiving.pdf

Ferrell, B., & Baird, P. (2012). Deriving meaning and faith in caregiving. *Seminars in Oncology Nursing, 28,* 256–261. doi:10.1016/j.soncn.2012.09.008

Friesen, P., Pepler, C., & Hunter, P. (2002). Interactive family learning following a cancer diagnosis. *Oncology Nursing Forum, 29,* 981–987. doi:10.1188/02.ONF.981-987

Fukui, S. (2002). Information needs and the related characteristics of Japanese family caregivers of newly diagnosed patients with cancer. *Cancer Nursing, 25,* 181–186. doi:10.1097/00002820-200206000-00002

Gaugler, J.E., Eppinger, A., King, J., Sandberg, T., & Regine, W.F. (2013). Coping and its effects on cancer caregiving. *Supportive Care in Cancer, 21,* 385–395. doi:10.1007/s00520-012-1525-5

Given, B.A., Given, C.W., & Kozachik, S. (2001). Family support in advanced cancer. *CA: A Cancer Journal for Clinicians, 51,* 213–231. doi:10.3322/canjclin.51.4.213

Given, B.A., Given, C.W., & Sherwood, P. (2012). The challenge of quality cancer care for family caregivers. *Seminars in Oncology Nursing, 28,* 205–212. doi:10.3322/canjclin.51.4.213

Glajchen, M. (2004). The emerging role and needs of family caregivers in cancer care. *Journal of Supportive Oncology, 2,* 145–155.

Glajchen, M. (2012). Physical well-being of oncology caregivers: An important quality-of-life domain. *Seminars in Oncology Nursing, 28,* 226–235. doi:10.1016/j.soncn.2012.09.005

Grant, M., Sun, V., Fujinami, R., Sidhu, R., Otis-Green, S., Juarez, G., ... Ferrell, B. (2013). Family caregiver burden, skills preparedness, and quality of life in non-small cell lung cancer. *Oncology Nursing Forum, 40,* 337–346. doi:10.1188/13.ONF.337-346

Harden, J., Schafenacker, A., Northouse, L., Mood, D., Smith, D., Pienta, K., ... Baranowski, K. (2002). Couples' experience with prostate cancer: Focus group research. *Oncology Nursing Forum, 29,* 701–709. doi:10.1188/02.ONF.701-709

Harrington, V., Lackey, N.R., & Gates, M.F. (1996). Needs of caregivers of clinic and hospice cancer patients. *Cancer Nursing, 19,* 118–125. doi:10.1097/00002820-199604000-00006

Hendrix, C.C., Bailey, D.E., Jr., Steinhauser, K.E., Olsen, M.K., Stechuchak, K.M., Lowman, S.G., ... Tulsky, J.A. (2016). Effects of enhanced caregiver training program on cancer caregiver's self-efficacy, preparedness, and psychological well-being. *Supportive Care in Cancer, 24,* 327–336. doi:10.1007/s00520-015-2797-3

Honea, N.J., Brintnall, R., Given, B., Sherwood, P., Colao, D.B., Somers, S.C., & Northouse, L.L. (2008). Putting evidence into practice: Nursing assessment and interventions to reduce family caregiver strain and burden. *Clinical Journal of Oncology Nursing, 12,* 507–516. doi:10.1188/08.CJON.507-516

Kim, Y., Carver, C.S., Spillers, R.L., Love-Ghaffari, M., & Kaw, C. (2012). Dyadic effects of fear of recurrence on the quality of life of cancer survivors and their caregivers. *Quality of Life Research, 21,* 517–525. doi:10.1007/s11136-011-9953-0

Kim, Y., & Given, B. (2008). Quality of life of family caregivers of cancer survivors: Across the trajectory of illness. *Cancer, 112,* 2556–2568. doi:10.1002/cncr.23449

Kotronoulas, G., Wengstrom, Y., & Kearney, N. (2013). Sleep patterns and sleep-impairing factors of persons providing informal care for people with cancer. *Cancer Nursing, 36,* E1–E15. doi:10.1097/NCC.0b013e3182456c38

Kuuppelomäki, M. (2002). Spiritual support for families of patients with cancer: A pilot study of nursing staff assessments. *Cancer Nursing, 26,* 209–218. doi:10.1097/00002820-200206000-00007

Lapid, M.I., Atherton, P.J., Kung, S., Sloan, J.A., Shahi, V., Clark, M.M., & Rummans, T.A. (2015). Cancer caregiver quality of life: Need for targeted intervention. *Psycho-Oncology, 25,* 1400–1407. doi:10.1002/pon.3960

Leow, M., Chan, M., & Chan, S. (2014). Predictors of change in quality of life and family caregivers of patients near the end of life with advanced cancer. *Cancer Nursing, 37,* 391–400. doi:10.1097/NCC.0000000000000101

Leow, M., Chan, S., & Chan, M. (2015). A pilot randomized, controlled trial of the effectiveness of psychoeducational intervention on family caregivers of patients with advanced cancer [Online exclusive]. *Oncology Nursing Forum, 42,* E63–E72. doi:10.1188/15.ONF.E63-E72

Lowery, A.E. (2015). Sleep and cancer. In J.C. Holland, W.S. Breitbart, P.N. Butow, P.B. Jacobsen, M.J. Loscalzo, & R. McCorkle (Eds.), *Psycho-oncology* (3rd ed., pp. 225–238). New York, NY: Oxford University Press.

Matthews, B.A. (2003). Role and gender differences in cancer-related distress: A comparison of survivor and caregiver self-reports. *Oncology Nursing Forum, 30,* 493–499. doi:10.1188/03.ONF.493-499

Northouse, L.L., Katapodi, M.C., Schafenacker, A.M., & Weiss, D. (2012). The impact of caregiving on the psychological well-being of family caregivers and cancer patients. *Seminars in Oncology Nursing, 28,* 236–245. doi:10.1016/j.soncn.2012.09.006

Northouse, L.L., Katapodi, M.C., Song, L., Lingling, Z., & Mood, D.W. (2010). Interventions with family caregivers of cancer patients. *CA: A Cancer Journal for Clinicians, 60,* 317–339. doi:10.3322/caac.20081

Northouse, L.L., Williams, A.L., Given, B., & McCorkle, R. (2012). Psychosocial care for family caregivers of patients with cancer. *Journal of Clinical Oncology, 30,* 1227–1234. doi:10.1200/JCO.2011.39.5798

Pitceathly, C., & Maguire, P. (2003). The psychological impact of cancer on patients' partners and other key relatives: A review. *European Journal of Cancer, 39,* 1517–1524. doi:10.1016/S0959-8049(03)00309-5

Prue, G., Santin, O., & Porter, S. (2015). Assessing the needs of informal caregivers to cancer survivors: A review of the instruments. *Psycho-Oncology, 24,* 121–129. doi:10.1002/pon.3609

Rabow, M.W., Hauser, J.M., & Adams, J. (2004). Supporting family caregivers at the end of life. *JAMA, 291,* 483–491. doi:10.1001/jama.291.4.483

Redinbaugh, E.M., Baum, A., Tarbell, S., & Arnold, R. (2003). End-of-life caregiving: What helps family caregivers cope? *Journal of Palliative Medicine, 6,* 901–909. doi:10.1089/109662103322654785

Rees, C.E., & Bath, P.A. (2000). Exploring the information flow: Partners of women with breast cancer, patients, and healthcare professionals. *Oncology Nursing Forum, 27,* 1267–1275.

Sabo, B., McLeod, D., & Couban, S. (2013). The experience of caring for a spouse undergoing hematopoietic stem cell transplantation. *Cancer Nursing, 36,* 29–40. doi:10.1097/NCC.0b013e31824fe223

Sales, E. (1991). Psychosocial impact of the phase of cancer on the family: An updated review. *Journal of Psychosocial Oncology, 9,* 1–18. doi:10.1300/J077v09n04_01

Schumacher, K.L., Stewart, B.J., Archbold, P.G., Caparro, M., Mutale, F., & Agrawal, S. (2008). Effects of caregiving demand, mutuality, and preparedness on family caregiver outcomes during cancer treatment. *Oncology Nursing Forum, 35,* 49–56. doi:10.1188/08.ONF.49-56

Shaw, J.M., Young, J.M., Butow, P.N., Badgery-Parker, T., Durcinoska, I., Harrison, J.D., … Solomon, M.J. (2016). Improving psychosocial outcomes for caregivers of people with poor prognosis gastrointestinal cancers: A randomized controlled trial (Family Connect). *Supportive Care in Cancer, 24,* 585–595. doi:10.1007/s00520-015-2817-3

Shin, D.W., Cho, J., Kim, S.Y., Chung, I.J., Kim, S.S., Yang, H.K., … Park, J. (2015). Discordance among patient preferences regarding disclosure of terminal status and end-of-life choices. *Psycho-Oncology, 24,* 212–219. doi:10.1002/pon.3631

Shin, D.W., Cho, J., Roter, D.L., Kim, S., Sohn, S.K., Yoon, M.-S., … Park, J.-H. (2013). Preferences for and experiences of family involvement in cancer treatment decision-making: Patient–caregiver dyads study. *Psycho-Oncology, 22,* 2624–2631. doi:10.1002/pon.3339

Steele, R.G., & Fitch, M.I. (1996). Needs of family caregivers of patients receiving home hospice care for cancer. *Oncology Nursing Forum, 23,* 823–828.

Stenberg, U., Ruland, C.M., & Miaskowski, C. (2010). Review of literature on the effects of caring for a patient with cancer. *Psycho-Oncology, 19,* 1013–1025. doi:10.1002/pon.1670

Stetz, K.M., McDonald, J.C., & Compton, K. (1996). Family caregivers and the marrow transplant experience. *Oncology Nursing Forum, 23,* 1421–1427.

Tamayo, G., Broxson, A., Munsell, M., & Cohen, M. (2010). Caring for the caregiver [Online exclusive]. *Oncology Nursing Forum, 37,* E50–E57. doi:10.1188/10.ONF.E50-E57

Taylor, E.J. (2003). Nurses caring for the spirit: Patients with cancer and family caregiver expectations. *Oncology Nursing Forum, 30,* 585–590. doi:10.1188/03.ONF.585-590

van Ryan, M., Sanders, S., Kahn, K., van Houtven, C., Griffin, J., Martin, M., ... Rowland, J. (2011). Objective burden, resources, and other stressors among informal cancer caregivers: A hidden quality issue? *Psycho-Oncology, 20,* 44–52. doi:10.1002/pon.1703

Von Ah, D., Spath, M., Nielsen, A., & Fife, B. (2016). The caregiver's role across the bone marrow transplantation trajectory. *Cancer Nursing, 39,* E12–E19. doi:10.1097/NCC.0000000000000242

Waller, A., Boyes, A., Carey, M., & Sanson-Fisher, R. (2015). Screening and assessment for unmet needs. In J.C. Holland, W.S. Breitbart, P.N. Butow, P.B. Jacobsen, M.J. Loscalzo, & R. McCorkle (Eds.), *Psycho-oncology* (3rd ed., pp. 369–383). New York, NY: Oxford University Press.

Weitzner, M.A., McMillan, S.C., & Jacobsen, P.B. (1999). Family caregiver quality of life: Differences between curative and palliative cancer treatment settings. *Journal of Pain and Symptom Management, 17,* 418–428. doi:10.1016/S0885-3924(99)00014-7

Wideheim, A., Edvardsson, T., Pahlson, A., & Ahlstrom, G. (2002). A family's perspective on living with a highly malignant brain tumor. *Cancer Nursing, 25,* 236–244. doi:10.1097/00002820-200206000-00012

Wittenberg-Lyles, E., Goldsmith, J., Oliver, D., Demiris, G., & Rankin, A. (2012). Targeting communication interventions to decrease caregiver burden. *Seminars in Oncology Nursing, 28,* 262–270. doi:10.1016/j.soncn.2012.09.009

Zaider, T.I., & Kissane, D.W. (2015). Psychosocial interventions for couples and families coping with cancer. In J.C. Holland, W.S. Breitbart, P.N. Butow, P.B. Jacobsen, M.J. Loscalzo, & R. McCorkle (Eds.), *Psycho-oncology* (3rd ed., pp. 526–538). New York, NY: Oxford University Press.

Zhang, A.Y., & Siminoff, L.A. (2003). The role of the family in treatment decision making by patients with cancer. *Oncology Nursing Forum, 30,* 1022–1028. doi:10.1188/03.ONF.1022-1028

Zwahlen, D., Hagenbuch, N., Carley, M.I., Recklitis, C.J., & Buchi, S. (2008). Screening cancer patients' families with the distress thermometer (DT): A validation study. *Psycho-Oncology, 17,* 959–966. doi:10.1002/pon.1320

# SECTION VI

# Patient Support Systems

Chapter 29. Programmatic Approaches to Psychosocial Support
Appendix. Psychosocial Support Programs and Resources for People With Cancer and Their Families

CHAPTER 29

# Programmatic Approaches to Psychosocial Support

*Margaret I. Fitch, RN, MScN, PhD*

> *Separate reeds are weak and easily broken; but bound together they are strong and hard to tear apart.*
>
> —The Midrash

When cancer strikes, it has more than a physical impact. Cancer and its treatment also have emotional, psychological, social, and spiritual consequences that create myriad changes for an individual. For most, life is altered irrevocably when a definitive diagnosis of cancer is made. Dealing with the various changes can present many challenges and difficult issues for the person diagnosed with the disease and family members (Dunn et al., 2012; Grunfeld et al., 2004; Harrison, Young, Price, Butow, & Solomon, 2009; Pusa, Persson, & Sundin, 2012). Whether an individual has timely access to appropriate assistance will influence their ability to cope effectively and their quality of life (MacDonald, 2001).

Supportive care is the provision of the necessary services as defined by those living with or affected by cancer to meet their physical, informational, emotional, psychological, social, spiritual, and practical needs throughout the full spectrum of their experiences with cancer (Fitch, Gray, Godel, & Labreque, 2008). *Supportive care* is an overarching or umbrella term that encompasses a range of services and areas of expertise required for comprehensive, high-quality care of patients with cancer, including psychosocial oncology, rehabilitation oncology, and palliative care. Ultimately, supportive care services are designed to assist patients in meeting their needs, maintaining or improving quality of life, and optimizing their sense of well-being.

The specific focus of this chapter is on the psychosocial needs of patients with cancer and the programs designed to help meet those needs, as well as the background context for psychosocial support. The term *psychosocial* refers to the relationship between social conditions and mental health. It relates to how a person feels about the way the disease or its treatment has affected social functioning at work and home; relationships with partner/spouse, children, extended family, and friends; and one's self and body (Adler & Page, 2008; Nicholas & Veach, 2000). Disturbances and changes in these areas can evoke intense feelings of emotional distress.

In the past decade, the notion of person-centered care has gained considerable attention in health care and is seen as a hallmark of quality (Institute of Medicine, 2001; Picker Institute, 2014). Achieving person-centered care implies that healthcare providers adopt a "whole person" approach in their interactions with individuals (Balik, 2012; Epstein & Street, 2011). This trend has helped bring forth an increased concern about the psychosocial needs of patients with cancer. In addition, healthcare providers have gained an understanding of the impact of psychosocial distress, finding concrete strategies to provide effective psychosocial interventions. Patients and survivors have shown a keen interest in finding ways to enhance coping and to reduce the psychosocial distress they experience throughout the cancer journey and are speaking out about their concerns. The idea of embedding person-centered perspectives in cancer care planning and program development is gaining traction across the cancer system (Coulter, 2007). Unfortunately, rigorous systematic literature reviews or empirical research studies validating the use of specific interventions to reduce psychosocial distress have not kept pace with the popular enthusiasm for them.

## Background Context

Some individuals experience cancer as a single event with a defined beginning and ending. For others, the cancer experience takes on a chronic nature. Everyone undergoes a spectrum of experiences with a cancer care system that includes a peridiagnostic interval, diagnosis, treatment, and follow-up care. Depending on the situation, follow-up care may encompass long-term survivorship with no further clinical evidence of disease or recurrent disease, metastatic spread, and death. Throughout this spectrum of experiences, patients diagnosed with cancer and their family members are likely to confront social, psychological, and spiritual issues and require access to supportive care services (see Figure 29-1).

Individuals may enter the cancer care delivery system at different points and move through the system along various pathways. Some will enter at the point of screening and may never proceed further. Others will enter at the point of diagnosis and move through phases of treatment, rehabilitation, and follow-up. Some of those in follow-up will live without further evidence of disease, whereas others will face the cycle of recurrence and treatment several times, depending on the type of cancer. Some may require palliative care services at diagnosis. Death as a result of cancer remains the final outcome for approximately half of those diagnosed with the disease (Canadian Cancer Society, 2015), although the time between diagnosis and death can widely vary. Each person travels a unique and personal journey in living with cancer.

Regardless of the journey's pathway for any individual, that person carries physical, social, emotional, psychological, spiritual, informational, and practical needs. These needs will vary from person to person, as well as within the same person, as the course of the disease and treatment unfolds. No two individuals respond exactly the same way to the diagnosis of cancer and its impact on their lives or desire exactly the same assistance in dealing with their situation (see Figure 29-2).

The onset of an illness can influence a person's ability to meet their own needs. Physical discomfort, disability, emotional distress, and a sense of personal crisis may interfere with an individual's capacity to act, and the usual ways of meeting one's needs may be compromised. The patient may require new knowledge, new skills, or a different network of supports to manage the new demands of the illness situation, whether it is acute, chronic, or palliative. Having to learn new information and seek out resources in times of emotional vulnerabil-

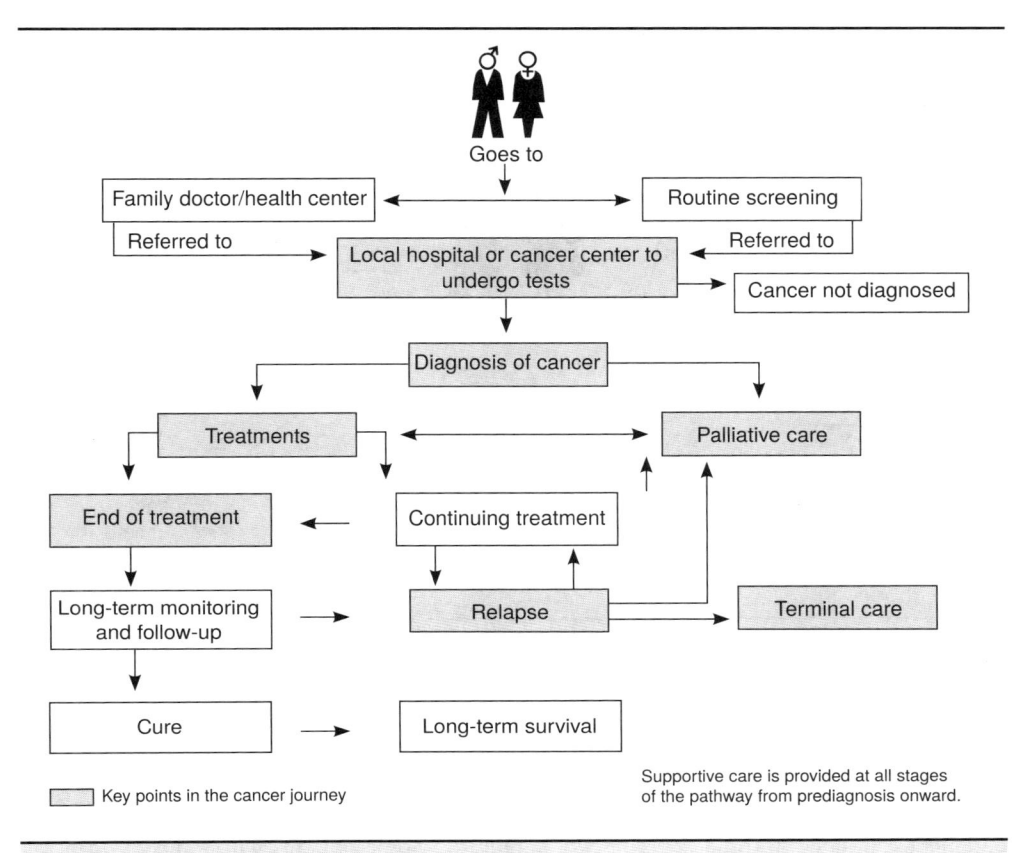

**Figure 29-1. Map of the Patient Pathway**

ity, especially when faced with a heightened sense of life threat, adds to the burden of suffering that patients feel (Coulter & Ellins, 2007; Sutherland, Hoey, White, Jefford, & Hegarty, 2008). Services to assist individuals in meeting this broad range of needs must be clearly visible and easily accessible to patients and their family members. Individuals may want to access these services at various points during their cancer journey.

One of the challenges in providing services to assist patients in meeting a broad range of needs is that needs are met in different ways from person to person. The intervention(s) that may be helpful to one person will not necessarily be useful to another person. People have different styles of learning and ways of dealing with what happens to them. Ideally, they ought to be able to choose specific interventional approaches from a menu of options.

A person's perception of the situation will influence how he or she copes with life-threatening illness and adapts to its aftermath (Lazarus & Folkman, 1984), as well as a number of factors, such as socioeconomic status, educational background, social support, culture, religion, and geographic location (Muzzin, Anderson, Figueredo, & Gudelis, 1994). The success of an intervention for an individual must be judged on the basis of whether it has been tailored sufficiently to attend to the person's unique situational factors. In the practice environment, this means the assessment process must identify the expectations and goals of the individual across all need areas within an existing situation and then tailor the intervention plan to those parameters in collaboration with the person. This process of assess-

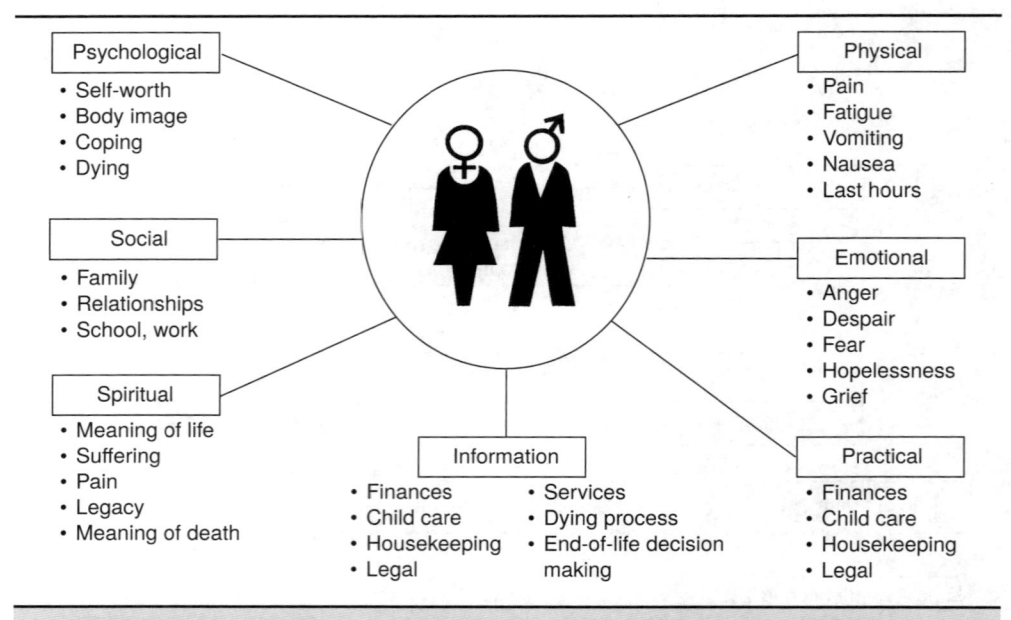

**Figure 29-2. Needs and Examples of Patients With Life-Threatening Illness**

**Psychological**
- Self-worth
- Body image
- Coping
- Dying

**Social**
- Family
- Relationships
- School, work

**Spiritual**
- Meaning of life
- Suffering
- Pain
- Legacy
- Meaning of death

**Information**
- Finances
- Child care
- Housekeeping
- Legal
- Services
- Dying process
- End-of-life decision making

**Physical**
- Pain
- Fatigue
- Vomiting
- Nausea
- Last hours

**Emotional**
- Anger
- Despair
- Fear
- Hopelessness
- Grief

**Practical**
- Finances
- Child care
- Housekeeping
- Legal

ment, mutual goal setting, and tailoring interventions is necessary throughout the course of a patient's cancer journey (Fitch, Porter, & Page, 2009).

Emotional or psychosocial distress is a natural response to life-threatening illness that all patients experience to some degree (see Chapter 18). Some patients with cancer, given relevant information, good symptom management, and good communication with their care providers, will mobilize their own supports or resources and cope effectively with their cancer situation (Bakker, Fitch, Gray, Reed, & Bennett, 2001). Others will require additional help to manage. If needs remain unmet, some will continue to experience ongoing distress and upheaval. This distress can escalate to significant levels, thus compromising compliance with tumor therapy, increasing use of other healthcare services, and elevating costs for care (Carlson et al., 2004; DiMatteo & Haskard-Zolnierek, 2011; Holland & Bultz, 2007; Zabora, BrintzenhofeSzoc, Curbow, Hooker, & Piantadosi, 2001).

For outpatients with various types of cancer, the prevalence of significant psychosocial distress (i.e., where intervention by professionals would be beneficial) has been reported as 20%–43% (Adler & Page, 2008; Armes et al., 2009; Zabora et al., 2001). Feelings of distress vary over the course of the cancer journey, with heightened levels occurring at certain points: at diagnosis, at the beginning and ending of treatment, at the time of recurrence, living with advanced disease, and when end of life becomes evident (Butow et al., 2012; Harrison et al., 2009; Howell et al., 2015). However, the presence of psychosocial distress in itself does not reveal the reason for that distress or point to a specific course of intervention. Nurses must talk with patients to uncover the reason for their distress and their desire for assistance.

Individuals who receive appropriate emotional or psychosocial care experience less anxiety and depression and generally are able to return to a productive life. Both patients and families experience significant improvement in quality of life (Galway et al., 2012; Goerling, Foerg, Sander, Schramm, & Schlag, 2011; Zimmerman, Heinrichs, & Baucom, 2007). Evidence also exists regarding the efficacy of interventions designed to augment coping skills, problem solving using behavioral training, stress management, cognitive therapy, and support of patients with cancer. Better outcomes have been reported in areas such as psychological state, coping response, quality of life, and compliance with therapy (Eaton & Tipton, 2009; Fawzy, 1999; Howell et al., 2015; Khan, Amatya, Pallant, Rajapaksa, & Brand, 2012; Richardson & Johnson, 1999; Stacey & Legare, 2015). Evidence has shown that heightened psychosocial distress, if left unchecked, is associated with poor prognosis (Kaasa, Mastekaasa, & Lund, 1989; Satin, Linden, & Phillips, 2009) and that psychosocial intervention potentially may extend survival (Carlson & Bultz, 2002; Cunningham et al., 2000).

## Helping Patients to Meet Their Psychosocial Needs

Patients and their families require comprehensive, quality cancer care or an integrated approach that ensures person-centered care is incorporated with tumor-centered disease care. Cancer programs must focus on biopsychosocial care and ensure that structures and processes are in place to allow (a) ongoing identification of needs in all domains, (b) a dialogue with patients and families about their desire for assistance, (c) provision of information about available resources, and (d) referral (if required). Cancer programs need to ensure psychosocial interventions/programs are available in addition to systemic, radiation, surgical, and symptom management interventions. This approach requires collaborative partnerships among a range of institution-based and community-based providers, as well as among professional and volunteer initiatives. Currently, there remains wide variation among cancer programs in the availability of psychosocial programming by professionals and uneven access for patients who live in different regions. Additionally, volunteer-based community support agencies offer different programs from region to region. Patients and families often feel that they do not know where to turn for help with psychosocial concerns.

Helping patients to meet their psychosocial needs must begin with their entry into the cancer care system (Stanton, 2006). Aspects of psychosocial care must be integral to the practice of all healthcare professionals and demonstrated in actions such as offering patients and family members emotional support and information during the course of their interactions, communicating in a person-centered and sensitive manner, and referring patients to psychosocial programs or experts as required. How sensitively that communication is handled is of importance to patients and can have a significant impact on their coping (Butow et al., 1996; Street, Makoul, Arora, & Epstein, 2009; Tattersall, Butow, & Clayton, 2002). In addition to the basic psychosocial interventions provided by nurses, oncologists, pharmacists, and radiation therapists, more focused and specialized therapeutic psychosocial interventions may be provided by social workers, psychologists, chaplains, advanced practice nurses, psychiatrists, and therapists in the fields of art, music, and touch. Peer support and volunteer-led initiatives also have an important role in helping patients to meet their psychosocial needs but should not be offered in place of professional services. Peers and volunteers provide a different type of support to patients.

Linking all of these providers in a way that allows patients with cancer and families easy access to the full range of services remains a challenge in many jurisdictions. Yet, this linkage is imperative if patients are to experience continuity and comprehensiveness in their care experience. Patients can find the array of service providers somewhat overwhelming and may not completely understand what each professional or service can do to help them. Providing information about available services, both within the healthcare institution and within the wider community, is an important strategy to assist patients and their family members. Patient navigation services (Campbell, Craig, Eggert, & Bailey-Dorton, 2010; Fillion et al., 2012; Korber, Padula, Gray, & Powell, 2011) and survivorship care plan initiatives (Clausen et al., 2012; Curcio, Lambe, Schneider, & Khan, 2012; Earle, 2006; Hill-Kaycer et al., 2013; Miller, 2008) have been designed with success to meet this type of need.

## Programmatic Approaches to Psychosocial Care

Successful cancer programs have created programmatic mechanisms to (a) provide basic information and support to all patients with cancer and their families, (b) identify those who need additional assistance, and (c) link those who need additional assistance with appropriate services in a timely fashion. Figure 29-3 provides an illustration of various psychosocial services that may be involved in meeting the psychosocial needs of patients with cancer and their families at some point in the illness experience. At the very least, healthcare providers need to know about the services available in their local areas and be able to talk with patients about the benefits of the services (i.e., how that service might be able to help).

The following descriptions present information about programmatic approaches designed to help patients and their families to meet psychosocial needs during the cancer experience. These can be brought together in one facility or coordinated within a geographic area (see Table 29-1 and Appendix).

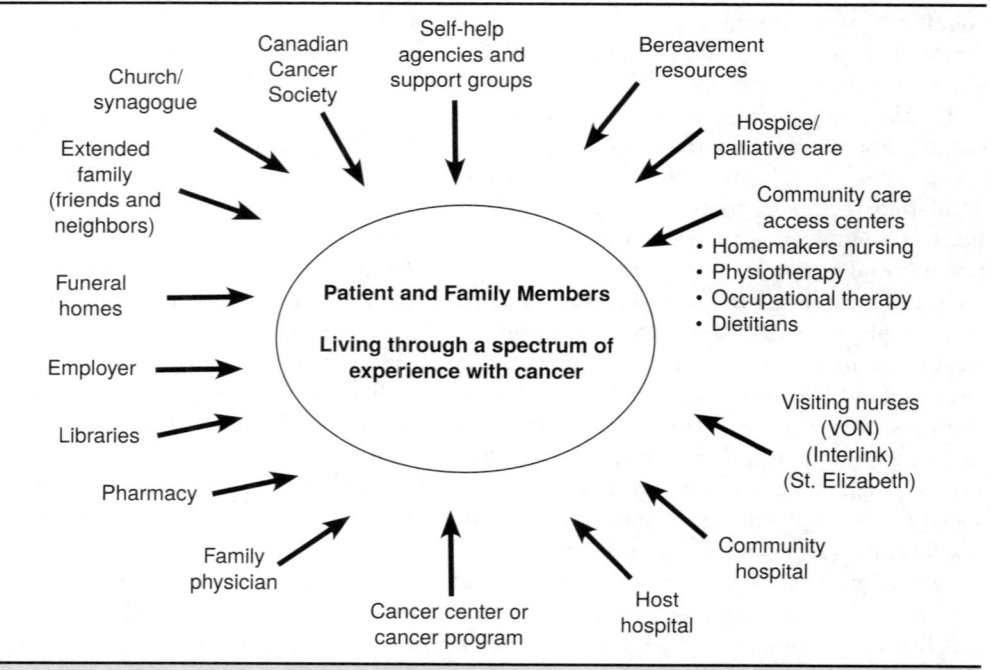

**Figure 29-3. Providers of Supportive Care**

*Note.* Based on information from Fitch et al., 2008.

## Table 29-1. Supportive Care Program Model

| Service or Activity | Target Group | Purpose | Leadership |
|---|---|---|---|
| Orientation | All new patients and family members | Introduces the cancer center and the cancer care system, offers information about resources, provides links to contacts to follow-up | Staff/patients and volunteers |
| Emotional support and peer information (e.g., Reach to Recovery, CanSurmount, self-help groups) | Individuals who wish to talk with another patient either in a group setting or on a one-to-one-basis | Provides an opportunity to talk with other patients with cancer about their experiences, feelings, concerns; allows sharing of experiences and information on a peer basis | Staff/patients and volunteers |
| Psychoeducational (group or one-to-one) | Individuals who want to learn new coping skills and express difficulty coping with the cancer experience | Provides an opportunity to learn coping skills and problem-solving skills regarding issues confronting them | Professionally trained group leaders |
| Adjustment/supportive counseling (group or one-to-one) | Individuals who require help to adjust to their diagnosis and treatment | Provides regular assistance/support for individuals during their treatment | Professional |
| Crisis intervention (one-to-one) | Individuals requiring immediate intervention regarding emotional, spiritual, or psychosocial distress | Provides immediate intervention focused on managing or resolving emotional/psychosocial distress crises | Professional |
| Psychotherapy (group or one-to-one)<br>• Short-term<br>• Long-term | Individuals requiring ongoing intervention regarding emotional, spiritual, or psychosocial distress | Provides ongoing intervention focused on managing or resolving significant emotional/psychosocial distress | Professional |
| Nutritional intervention | Individuals who want advice regarding nutrition and who are experiencing difficulties regarding eating | Provides advice regarding nutrition/intervention for those with eating difficulties | Nutritionist |
| Pain and symptom management | Individuals experiencing difficulties with management of pain or other symptoms (e.g., lymphedema, fatigue) | Reduces or eliminates distress caused by symptoms | Healthcare professional |
| Practical assistance | Individuals who require help with activities of daily living, child care, financial assistance, or transportation | Provides services designed to assist with practical matters | Staff/patients and volunteers |

*Note.* Based on information from Fitch et al., 2009.

## Patient Orientation, Information, and Education Approaches

Over the past two decades, reports from patients have consistently cited how timely access to relevant, understandable information has been a key element in their capacity to cope with their cancer and gain a sense of control over what is happening to them (Balmer, 2005; Brashers, Goldsmith, & Hsieh, 2002; Fitch, McAndrew, & Harth, 2013; Gray et al., 1998). However, the importance of providing information extends beyond this perceived need. Patients with cancer who receive information experience significant benefits, including increased participation in treatment decision making (Coulter & Ellins, 2007; Stacey & Legare, 2015); increased satisfaction with treatment choices and interactions with healthcare professionals (Hibbard & Greene, 2013; Mills & Davidson, 2002; Sutherland et al., 2008); increased control and coping with the stress of the diagnosis and treatment (Cappiello, Cunningham, Knobft, & Erdos, 2007; Rutten, Arora, Bakes, Aziz, & Rowlad, 2005; van de Molen, 2000); decreased levels of anxiety, mood disturbance, and affective distress (Chan, Richardson, & Richardson., 2011); and assistance in communicating illness-related information to their families (Skalla, Bakitas, Furstenberg, Ahles, & Henderson, 2004; Smith, Dickens, & Edwards, 2005).

Patients have identified the importance of receiving information about cancer, treatment options, side effects, and available resources from their healthcare providers, especially at the time of diagnosis (Ankem, 2006; Gray, Fitch, Phillips, Labrecque, & Fergus, 2000; Fitch, Gray, & Franssen, 2000; Vlossak & Fitch, 2008). Typically, satisfaction with the information provided about these topics is higher than for topics such as emotional issues, impact on personal and social relations, lifestyle and body-image changes, and emotional needs of family members (Faller et al., 2016; Fitch & McAndrew, 2011; Fitch et al., 2000). These latter topics tend to emerge with more intensity later in the course of the cancer experience (i.e., during or after treatment) (Fitch et al., 2008; Fitch, Nicoll, & Keller-Olman, 2007). Much of the work in reporting patient information needs focuses on newly diagnosed individuals, but the recognition is growing that information and education needs and topics of importance will change throughout the course of the cancer experience (Fitch & McAndrew, 2011). In particular, growth in the number of cancer survivors has sparked the need for educational approaches to meet their specific needs for information (Curtiss & Haylock, 2006; Feuerstein, 2007; Galbraith, Hays, & Tanner, 2012). Recommendations for program development emphasize the importance of targeting the information program to the stage of disease for maximum benefit (Ashbury, 1999; Kiesler & Auerbach, 2006). Recommendations are also emerging about the need to tailor education programs and delivery to the gender and age of the individuals (Fitch & Allard, 2007; Fitch, Gray, & Franssen, 2001; Gould, Grassau, Manthorne, Gray, & Fitch, 2006; Gray, Fergus, & Fitch, 2005).

Providing patient information and education programs has been identified as an important function of cancer programs for a number of years. As a result, healthcare professionals have organized initiatives in many forms, including written pamphlets, brochures, and books; patient/family libraries and resource centers; videos; teleconferences; audiotapes; web-based programs; CD-ROMs; education lectures/discussion groups; orientation programs; posters/bulletin boards; newsletters; and teaching cards and demonstration models (Agre, Dougherty, & Pirone, 2002; Davison, Szafron, Gutwin, & Visvanathan, 2014; Edgar, Greenberg, & Remmer, 2002; Hack et al., 1999; Jones et al., 2006; Shaw, McTavish, Hawkins, Gustafson, & Pingree, 2000; Till, 2003).

Recently, the stunning growth in the use of Internet and social media has opened the way for innovative programs in providing information and support. The vast majority of citizens in the United States are Internet users, have a smartphone, or use social media to access and share information. These vehicles have become a standard form of communication, especially for younger generations (Duggan, Ellison, Lampe, Lenhart, & Madden, 2015). This largely consumer-driven phenomenon has changed the demand for information and access to health information in particular (Gagnon & Sabus, 2015). The emergence of the Internet and social media has shifted information-seeking behaviors in society, influencing health behaviors, decision making, and access to supports.

The growth in digital avenues of communication has led to creation of a range of program approaches for supporting patients with cancer and their families. The use of the telephone or online approaches has grown significantly in recent years. Some programs offer the opportunity for patients to access their own health records and information about their test results (Kim et al., 2016). Others provide opportunity to access information (Foley et al., 2016), education programming (Beaunoyer, Arsenault, Lomanowska, & Guitton, 2016), virtual navigation (Loiselle et al., 2013), or support and counseling, either peer or professionally led (Melton, Brewer, Kolva, Joshi, & Bunch, 2016; Zhang, O'Carroll Bantum, Owen, Bakken, & Elhadad, 2016). These approaches have been met with success, especially for patients and caregivers who live in rural or remote settings, are unable to travel to cancer or support centers, or who may have a rare type of cancer and find it difficult to connect with peers (Collett, Kent, & Swain, 2006; Høybye, Johansen, & Tjørnhøj-Thomsen, 2005; Loiselle et al., 2013; Stephens et al., 2013).

Although not always specified in the literature, providing information and offering education have different goals or intended outcomes. Goals for providing patient information include the communication of facts and practical guidance. Most frequently, information programs are designed with the intent of helping patients to navigate the cancer system, reducing anxiety, and encouraging patients' active participation in decision making about their treatment and rehabilitation. Educational programs aim to influence attitudes and behavior and maintain or improve health. It is an active process that assists people in changing behavior and improving decision-making and coping skills (Friedman, Cosby, Boyko, Hatten-Bauer, & Turnball, 2011; Padilla & Bulcavage, 1991). Education programs can assist patients psychosocially by helping them to recognize their anxieties and develop strategies for dealing with them. Studies have demonstrated that anxiety decreases significantly when patients are informed and prepared emotionally for their treatment (Chan, Webster, & Marquart, 2012; Chien, Liu, Chien, & Liu, 2014). At the same time, benefit can be found in helping patients learn to determine how the information applies to their situation. Patients then can be discerning about what they are accessing and reading (Fitch et al., 2007).

The challenge for healthcare professionals is to be clear about the intended outcomes of the program of information provision or patient and family education. Each type of program requires appropriate methods of content delivery and outcome evaluation. These methods must be adjusted for the specific target audience. The notion of "one size fits all" is not useful. Programs need to be tailored to the specific patient population. Unfortunately, comparatively few rigorous evaluation studies have been undertaken to determine the most effective methods of designing and implementing patient education materials and the extent to which the materials influence patient outcomes, but the evidence is growing with regard to effective approaches and best practices for patient teaching (Friedman et al., 2011). Consensus exists regarding the principles of successful program development and delivery (see Figure 29-4).

This area of health care, providing information and education, remains challenging. The pace of knowledge development and availability of information is escalating exponentially. Healthcare professionals are no longer the sole provider of healthcare information and may have difficulty remaining current with all available information. They are struggling with ever-increasing caseloads. Patients are becoming educated consumers (Gagnon & Sabus, 2015; Tyson, 2000), and many individuals use the Internet for medical advice (Beaunoyer et

- Program development must include audience participation.
- Materials must be audience specific.
- Messages must be personalized.
- Materials must present information in plain language.
- Materials must be culturally sensitive.
- Active strategies to provide materials directly to patients are more successful.
- Materials should be introduced at key moments in the cancer trajectory.
- Materials should be relevant and comprehensive, present options, and facilitate communications with providers.
- Vehicles other than print can be beneficial.
- Dissemination of patient education materials must correspond to the needs of the patient audience.
- Multiple strategies are more effective than single strategies.

**Figure 29-4. Principles Associated With Successful Information and Education Program Development and Implementation**

*Note.* Based on information from Ashbury, 1999.

al., 2016; Fox & Rainie, 2002). This makes the Internet a critically important tool for information dissemination. However, patients can be overwhelmed with detailed information and experience difficulty knowing what truly applies to them; often, they desire help to sort through the information they have found and understand its relevance for their situation (Fitch et al., 2007). Given that the provision of relevant, understandable information is a critical influence on coping with cancer, finding local solutions to these challenges is important.

## Peer Information and Support Approaches

Although many patients with cancer want information from their healthcare providers, some also want information and support from fellow patients or peers. Many patients claim that the information and support gathered from peers is different from that provided by their healthcare professionals and find it tremendously helpful in coping and navigating the cancer system. This latter observation has been influential in the development and growth of self-help cancer organizations and the use of social media vehicles to seek peer support (Chou, Liu, Post, & Hesse, 2011; Duggan et al., 2015; Dunn, Steginga, Roseman, & Millichap, 2003).

Self-help groups often have objectives related to providing emotional support as well as nonmedical information. In addition to face-to-face group meetings, many groups have initiated other activities aimed at helping patients with cancer and their families. Examples of these include writing booklets, distributing newsletters, creating websites, providing one-on-one peer support, delivering telephone-based peer support, activating blogs, and publishing online journals (Collett et al., 2006; Hawkes, Hughes, Hutchison, & Chambers, 2010).

One-on-one peer support programs facilitate a patient's ability to interact with another patient who has undergone a similar experience. The matching of the patient and the peer may be made on the basis of cancer type (e.g., breast cancer), age, or life circumstance (e.g., rural dwelling, mother with children). Peer volunteers are trained for this role and, in most instances, focus on providing emotional support and practical information. Care is taken to not provide medical information. Evaluations of face-to-face peer support programs (Ashbury, 1999; Gottlieb & Wachala, 2007) and telephone peer support (Canadian Cancer Society, 2002) have cited benefits similar to those of self-help groups. The one-on-one approach works well for those who do not care for the group setting or who are unable to attend the group meetings. Internet-based peer support is now readily available (Lieberman et al., 2003; Stephens et al., 2013; Winzelberg et al., 2003).

A solid body of evidence has accumulated regarding the positive relationship between social support and health (Cohen, 2004) as well as the effect that social support has on helping individuals to adjust to and cope with cancer (Hasson-Ohayson, Goldzweig, Braun, & Galinsky, 2010; Kim, Sherman, & Taylor, 2008; Kroenke, Kubzansky, Schernhammer, Holmes, & Kawachi, 2006; Wenzel et al., 2012). Various definitions of social support exist but all share the common theme of being cared for by others and feeling emotionally connected. A social network can provide both tangible and intangible support. When coping with new situations, human beings often search out others who have similar experiences as an avenue to finding meaningful support. Individuals can feel an intense sense of isolation and loneliness, especially with diseases that carry an element of stigma.

Self-help groups are defined as "member-governed voluntary associations of persons who share a common problem, and who rely on experiential knowledge at least partly to mutually solve or cope with their common concerns" (Borkman, 1990, p. 321). Specifically excluded are support or psychoeducational groups led by healthcare professionals or cofacilitated by healthcare professionals and a volunteer peer. From the self-help perspective, these are quite different models, with distinct philosophies, goals, and approaches (Dunn et al., 2003).

Self-help peer groups exist because of a belief in the value of peer information and support, as well as perceived gaps in the cancer system. In many instances, the groups are organized for individuals with a particular cancer (e.g., breast, prostate, colon). The groups range from those that are highly structured in terms of time and membership to drop-in groups that are rather loosely structured. Usually, leaders have had some preparation for or orientation to leading a group and are survivors themselves. Several studies have described the benefits that patients and survivors feel from attending self-help groups in person (Ashbury, Cameron, Mercer, Fitch, & Nielsen, 1998; Cyr, McKee, O'Hagan, & Priest, 2016; Gray, Fitch, Davis, & Phillips, 1996, 1997a, 1997b) or online (Eysenbach, Powell, Englesakis, Rizo, & Stern, 2004). These benefits include sharing common experiences/talking about difficulties, being accepted and affirmed, feeling supported, sharing information, reconstructing a positive identity, gaining a sense of affiliation and community, experiencing personal transformation, and finding opportunities for advocacy and empowerment. Attendees also have cited some drawbacks in attending a self-help group: dominance by some members, inability to help with complex or intimate issues, and lack of training and poor facilitation by group leaders.

Many of the established self-help groups have an interest in linking with healthcare professionals to obtain endorsement or support for their groups. That support becomes evident by healthcare professionals informing new patients about the group's existence and how the group may benefit them. In one study, encouragement by the cancer care team to attend self-help groups was an independent predictor of patient interest in the support group (Bui et al., 2002). In general, most healthcare professionals are positively predisposed to self-help groups but have relatively little awareness about the groups and how they operate (Gray et al., 1998). In one study of oncology nurses' perspectives about self-help groups for patients, only 20% mentioned the groups to their patients on a regular basis (Fitch, Gray, Greenberg, et al., 2001).

## Identifying Those Who Need Additional Assistance

In many cancer centers, screening programs for psychosocial distress have been implemented to help routinely identify, monitor, and refer patients who are experiencing heightened levels of emotional distress and could benefit from intervention by a psychosocial expert (Bultz et al., 2011; Jacobsen et al., 2005). Emotional distress has been widely acknowledged as the sixth vital sign, and its identification and management is a standard of quality patient care (Adler & Page, 2008; Holland et al., 2010) (see Chapter 18 on distress). The Canadian Association of Psychosocial Oncology, the National Comprehensive Cancer Network®, and the National Cancer Institute each have recommended a range of standardized screening tools for psychosocial distress on their respective websites and have suggested that patients with cancer should be screened at their initial visit, at appropriate intervals, and as clinically indicated. The actual tools being used differ among cancer centers, but the basic approach is the same: Individuals with high scores are seen immediately by a mental health professional, those with mid-range scores are called to schedule an appointment, and those with low scores are informed about available support and education programs. The use of screening procedures has been reported as useful for identifying patients with greater psychological, social, and physical impairment (Carlson & Bultz, 2003; Patrick-Miller, Much, & Axelrod, 2002). Using standardized programmatic approaches to screening for distress helps to overcome some of the stigma associated with emotional issues, identify the distress before it erupts as a crisis, and reduce costs associated with health service utilization (Zabora et al., 2001).

## Support, Education, and Therapy by Professionals

The past two decades have witnessed a remarkable increase in the amount of literature describing psychosocial interventions for patients with cancer delivered by healthcare professionals or professionals and cancer survivors working in a collaborative model. Payne (2014) reported more than 300 studies of psychological interventions have been conducted in patients with cancer since the 1980s. Interventions are provided to reduce anxiety, promote coping, and enhance quality of life. More specifically, they aim to reduce feelings of stigma, isolation, helplessness, and hopelessness while promoting understanding about cancer and its treatment, self-awareness, and personal skill development. They may focus on reducing or resolving the individual's psychosocial distress immediately (crisis intervention) or on a short-term (adjustment counseling, brief psychotherapy) or long-term (psychotherapy) basis. The most straightforward way to categorize the interventions is by mode of delivery, whether group or individual.

Group programs for patients with cancer exist in many forms and have been designed to achieve various purposes. Psychoeducational groups usually are structured, time-limited education provided in a supportive environment. Participants learn about specific topics and often gather a sense of confidence or empowerment as they learn. Participants become informed consumers and feel more capable to take control in their care. Psychotherapy groups may offer cognitive restructuring, stress management training, and behavioral training (e.g., biofeedback, hypnosis, progressive relaxation). These groups must have a licensed professional with training in psychology, behavioral medicine, or psychiatry as a leader. Support groups tend to bring individuals together for mutual learning, sharing, and understanding. These groups tend to be more open-ended in terms of time frame and agenda and provide participants an opportunity to talk about their feelings and current concerns. Some operate on a "drop-in" format. Expressive–supportive groups use art, music, or other expressive forms as an avenue to express feelings and stimulate discussions. Additionally, group programs may be offered as a workshop or as a retreat, lasting various lengths of time (e.g., day, weekend, week). Some programs include only patients, whereas others also embrace family members.

Psychosocial interventions may also be categorized broadly as mind–body techniques (e.g., yoga, mindfulness, cognitive behavioral therapy, meditation), energy-based techniques (e.g., Reiki, acupuncture, acupressure), natural products (e.g., vitamins and minerals, botanicals), and exercise interventions (e.g., walking, swimming, hiking). Mind–body techniques have been the most widely studied interventions in relation to stress and anxiety reduction and have consistently shown significant small to moderate benefits while exercise has become the focus of much recent research. Walking has been studied in detail for patients with cancer and shows significant reduction in fatigue and improvement in sleep and well-being (Payne, 2014).

Ideally, cancer centers should offer a structured psychosocial program that comprises health education, stress management, behavioral training, instructions in coping and problem-solving techniques, and support groups, especially for those newly diagnosed or in the early stages of treatment (Adler & Page, 2008). Unfortunately, significant variation remains in the availability of these programs as standard offerings in cancer centers (Jacobsen et al., 2005). Lack of qualified staff and lack of funding are critical factors influencing this variation.

Individual therapy may be more appropriate for people with an aversion to group settings, those needing crisis intervention, or those with well-entrenched problems needing in-depth psychotherapy. Individual therapy is particularly helpful for patients who use inappropriate or ineffective methods of coping with stress and resolving their illness-related problems. The individual therapy format offers the best opportunity to tailor interventions to the specific person (see Chapter 25 for information on therapeutic modalities).

Several challenges exist in trying to review the cancer literature on psychosocial interventions. Authors have reported on a wide range of techniques and have combined various interventions in their programs. Authors also are inconsistent in their use of terminology, and various definitions exist for the same word. The combination of specific techniques within similarly labeled programs frequently differs, as do the desired outcomes of interest. Some programs focus on physical symptoms (e.g., pain, fatigue) as well as psychosocial issues (e.g., anxiety, worries, family concerns), whereas others focus only on psychosocial matters. Finally, similarly named outcomes (e.g., quality of life, emotional well-being) are defined somewhat differently and measured differently from study to study. This situation makes it difficult to compare across studies, and the variability has contributed to slow uptake and clinical utilization of the research in this field. Additionally, small sample sizes, the use of specific tumor types, and the application of less rigorous methodologies (e.g., quasiexperimental) to evaluate interventions have been cited as barriers. Overall evidence has shown that psychosocial interventions are beneficial for patients, but no clear evidence supports the use of one specific model of care or framework over another. For the most part, the expressed preference clinically is for an eclectic approach to available psychosocial interventions or models and choices made on the basis of specific patient need. This is supported by several meta-analyses and systematic reviews of psychosocial intervention studies (Abbey, Stewart, & Katz, 2002; Galway et al., 2012; Hart et al., 2012).

# Conclusion

In summary, providing access to psychosocial interventions is an important part of supportive care for patients with cancer and their family members if they are to achieve quality-of-life outcomes. Systematic approaches are needed to inform patients and family members about what psychosocial services are available, to identify what type of assistance is both needed and desired by the individual, and to refer individuals to the appropriate services (professional and peer) as required. A range of psychosocial programs ought to be available so that individuals may select the type of program that best matches their style of learning, personality, and way of coping.

# References

Abbey, S., Stewart, D., & Katz, M. (2002). *Literature review: Behavioural guidelines for adjusting to medical conditions.* Toronto, Canada: Ontario Women's Health Council.

Adler, N.E., & Page, A.E.K. (Eds.). (2008). *Cancer care for the whole patient: Meeting psychosocial health needs.* Washington, DC: National Academies Press.

Agre, P., Dougherty, J., & Pirone, J. (2002). Creating a CD-ROM program for cancer-related patient education. *Oncology Nursing Forum, 29,* 573–580. doi:10.1188/02.ONF.573-580

Ankem, K. (2006). Factors influencing information needs among cancer patients: A meta-analysis. *Library and Information Science, 28,* 7–23. doi:10.1016/j.lisr.2005.11.003

Armes, J., Crowe, M., Colbourne, L., Morgan, H., Murrels, T., Oakley, C., ... Richardson, A. (2009). Patient's supportive care needs beyond the end of cancer treatment: A prospective longitudinal study. *Journal of Clinical Oncology, 27,* 6172–6179. doi:10.1200/JCO.2009.22.5151

Ashbury, F.D. (1999, March). *Literature review to determine the optimal means for design and disseminate clinical practice guidelines to persons who are "underserved."* Unpublished report submitted to Adult Health Division, Health Canada, Ottawa, Ontario.

Ashbury, F.D., Cameron, C., Mercer, S.L., Fitch, M., & Nielsen, E. (1998). One-on-one peer support and quality of life for breast cancer patients. *Patient Education and Counseling, 35,* 89–100. doi:10.1016/S0738-3991(98)00035-4

Bakker, D.A., Fitch, M.I., Gray, R., Reed, E., & Bennett, J. (2001). Patient–health care provider communication during chemotherapy treatment: The perspectives of women with breast cancer. *Patient Education and Counseling, 43,* 61–71. doi:10.1016/S0738-3991(00)00147-6

Balik, B. (2012). Patient- and family-centeredness: Growing a sustainable culture. *Health Care Quarterly, 15,* 10–12. doi:10.12927/hcq.2012.23154

Balmer, C. (2005). The information requirements of people with cancer: Where to go after the "patient information leaflet"? *Cancer Nursing, 28,* 36–44. doi:10.1097/00002820-200501000-00005

Beaunoyer, E., Arsenault, M., Lomanowska, A.M., & Guitton, M.J. (2016). Understanding online health information: Evaluation, tools, and strategies. *Patient Education and Counseling, 100,* 183–189. doi:10.1016/j.pec.2016.08.028

Borkman, T. (1990). Self-help groups at the turning point: Emerging egalitarian alliances with the formal health care system? *American Journal of Psychology, 18,* 321–332. doi:10.1007/bf00931307

Brashers, D., Goldsmith, D., & Hsieh, E. (2002). Information seeking and avoiding in health contexts. *Human Communication Research, 28,* 258–271. doi:10.1111/j.1468-2958.2002.tb00807.x

Bui, L., Last, L., Bradley, H., Law, C., Maier, B., & Smith, A. (2002). Interest and participation in support group programs among patients with colorectal cancer. *Cancer Nursing, 24,* 150–157. doi:10.1097/00002820-200204000-00012

Bultz, B., Groff, S.L., Fitch, M.I., Blais, M.C., Howes, J., Levy, K., & Mayer, C. (2011). Implementing Screening for Distress, the 6th Vital Sign: A Canadian strategy for changing practice. *Psycho-Oncology, 20,* 463–469. doi:10.1002/pon.1932

Butow, P.N., Kazemi, J.N., Beeney, L.J., Griffin, A., Dunn, S.M., & Tattersall, M.H. (1996). When the diagnosis is cancer. *Cancer, 77,* 2630–2637. doi:10.1002/(SICI)1097-0142(19960615)77:12<2630::AID-CNCR29>3.0.CO;2-S

Butow, P.N., Phillips, S.F., Schweder, J., White, K., Underhill, C., & Goldstein, D. (2012). Psycho-social well-being and supportive care needs of cancer patients living in urban and rural/regional areas: A systematic review. *Supportive Care in Cancer, 20,* 1–22. doi:10.1007/s00520-011-1270-1

Campbell, C., Craig, J., Eggert, J., & Bailey-Dorton, C. (2010). Implementing and measuring the impact of patient navigation at a comprehensive community cancer center. *Oncology Nursing Forum, 37,* 61–68. doi:10.1188/10.ONF.61-68

Canadian Cancer Society. (2002). *Measuring the performance of telephone information services: A literature review.* Toronto, Canada: Author.

Canadian Cancer Society. (2015). *Canadian Cancer Society statistics 2015.* Toronto, Canada: Author.

Cappiello, M., Cunningham, R., Knobft, T., & Erdos, D. (2007). Breast cancer survivors: Information and support after treatment. *Clinical Nursing Research, 16,* 276–293. doi:10.1177/1054773807306553

Carlson, L.E., Angen, M., Cullum, J., Goodey, E., Koopmans, J., Lamont, L., … Bultz, B.D. (2004). High levels of untreated distress and fatigue in cancer patients. *British Journal of Cancer, 90,* 2297–2304. doi:10.1038/sj.bjc.6601887

Carlson, L.E., & Bultz, B.D. (2002). Efficacy vs. cost of psychosocial interventions: An evidence-based call for action. *Oncology Exchange, 1,* 34–51.

Carlson, L.E., & Bultz, B.D. (2003). Cancer distress screening: Needs, models, and methods. *Journal of Psychosomatic Research, 55,* 403–409. doi:10.1016/S0022-3999(03)00514-2

Chan, C.W., Richardson, A., & Richardson, J. (2011). Managing symptoms of patients with advanced lung cancer during radiotherapy: Results of a randomized controlled trial. *Journal of Pain and Symptom Management, 41,* 347–357. doi:10.1016/j.jpainsymman.2010.04.024

Chan, R.J., Webster, J., & Marquart, L. (2012). Information interventions for orienting patients and their careers to cancer care facilities. *Cochrane Database of Systematic Reviews, 2012*(12). doi:10.1002/14651858.CD008273.pub2

Chien, C.-H., Liu, K.-L., Chien, H.-T., & Liu, H.-E. (2014). The effects of psychosocial strategies on anxiety and depression of patients diagnosed with prostate cancer. *International Journal of Nursing Studies, 51,* 28–38. doi:10.1016/j.ijnurstu.2012.12.019

Chou, W.Y., Liu, B., Post, S., & Hesse, B. (2011). Health-related Internet use among cancer survivors: Data from the Health Information National Trends Survey, 2003–2008. *Journal of Cancer Survivorship, 5,* 263–270. doi:10.1007/s11764-011-0179-5

Clausen, C., Strohschein, F.J., Faremo, S., Bateman, D., Posel, N., & Fleiszer, D.M. (2012). Developing an interprofessional care plan for an older adult woman with breast cancer: From multiple voices to a shared vision [Online exclusive]. *Clinical Journal of Oncology Nursing, 16,* E18–E25. doi:10.1188/12.CJON.E18-E25

Cohen, S. (2004). Social relationships and health. *American Psychologist, 59,* 676–684. doi:10.1037/0003-066X.59.8.676

Collett, A., Kent, W., & Swain, S. (2006). The role of a telephone helpline in the provision of patient information. *Nursing Standard, 20*(32), 41–44. doi:10.7748/ns.20.32.41.s47

Coulter, A. (2007). *Evidence on the effectiveness of strategies to improve patients' experiences of cancer care.* Oxford, England: Picker Institute Europe.

Coulter, A., & Ellins, J. (2007). Effectiveness of strategies for informing, educating and involving patients. *BMJ, 335,* 24–27. doi:10.1136/bmj.39246.581169.80

Cunningham, A.J., Edmonds, C.V., Phillips, C., Soots, K.I., Hedley, D., & Lockwood, G.A. (2000). A prospective longitudinal study of the relationship of psychological work to duration of survival in patients with metastatic cancer. *Psycho-Oncology, 9,* 323–339. doi:10.1002/1099-1611(200007/08)9:4<323::AID-PON465>3.0.CO;2-B

Curcio, K.R., Lambe, C., Schneider, S., & Khan, K. (2012). Evaluation of a cancer survivorship protocol: Transitioning patients to survivors. *Clinical Journal of Oncology Nursing, 16,* 400–406. doi:10.1188/12.CJON.400-406

Curtiss, C., & Haylock, P. (2006). Survivor-centered care. *American Journal of Nursing, 106*(Suppl. 3), 4–5. doi:10.1097/00000446-200603003-00002

Cyr, C., McKee, H., O'Hagan, M., & Priest, R. (2016). *Making the case for peer support.* Retrieved from http://www.mentalhealthcommission.ca/sites/default/files/2016-07/MHCC_Making_the_Case_for_Peer_Support_2016_Eng.pdf

Davison, J., Szafron, M., Gutwin, C., & Visvanathan, K. (2014). Using a web-based decision support intervention to facilitate patient-physician communication at prostate cancer treatment discussions. *Canadian Oncology Nursing Journal, 24,* 241–247.

DiMatteo, M.R., & Haskard-Zolnierek, K.B. (2011). Impact of depression on treatment adherence and survival from cancer. In D.W. Jissane, M. Mai, & N. Sartorius (Eds.), *Depression and cancer* (pp. 101–124). Oxford, England: John Wiley and Sons.

Duggan, M., Ellison, N.B., Lampe, C., Lenhart, A., & Madden, M. (2015). *Demographics of key social network platforms.* Retrieved from http://www.pewinternet.org/2015/01/09/demographics-of-key-social-networking-platforms-2/

Dunn, J., Steginga, S.K., Roseman, N., & Millichap, D. (2003). A review of peer support in the context of cancer. *Journal of Psychosocial Oncology, 21,* 55–67. doi:10.1300/J077v21n02_04

Dunn, L.B., Aouizerat, B.E., Cooper, B.A., Dodd, M., Lee, K., West, C., … Miaskowski, C. (2012). Trajectories of anxiety in oncology patients and family caregivers during and after radiation therapy. *European Journal of Oncology Nursing, 16,* 1–9. doi:10.1016/j.ejon.2011.01.003

Earle, C.C. (2006). Failing to plan is planning to fail: Improving the quality of care with survivorship care plans. *Journal of Clinical Oncology, 32,* 5112–5116. doi:10.1200/JCO.2006.06.5284

Eaton, L.H., & Tipton, J.M. (Eds.). (2009). *Putting Evidence Into Practice: Improving oncology patient outcomes.* Pittsburgh PA: Oncology Nursing Society.

Edgar, L., Greenberg, A., & Remmer, J. (2002). Providing internet lessons to oncology patients and family members: A shared project. *Psycho-Oncology, 11,* 439–446. doi:10.1002/pon.590

Epstein, R.M., & Street, R.L. (2011). The values and value of patient-centered care. *Annals of Family Medicine, 9,* 100–103. doi:10.1370/afm.1239

Eysenbach, G., Powell, J., Englesakis, M., Rizo, C., & Stern, A. (2004). Health-related virtual communities and electronic support groups: Systematic review of the effects of on-line peer-to-peer interactions. *BMJ, 328,* 1166. doi:10.1136/bmj.328.7449.1166

Faller, H., Koch, U., Brähler, E., Härter, M., Keller, M., Schulz, H., ... Mehnert, A. (2016). Satisfaction with information and unmet needs in men and women with cancer. *Journal of Cancer Survivorship, 10,* 62–70. doi:10.1007/s11764-015-0451-1

Fawzy, F.I. (1999). Psychosocial interventions for patients with cancer: What works and what doesn't. *European Journal of Cancer, 35,* 1559–1564. doi:10.1016/S0959-8049(99)00191-4

Feuerstein, M. (2007). Optimizing cancer survivorship. *Journal of Cancer Survivorship, 1,* 1–4. doi:10.1007/s11764-006-0001-y

Fillion, L., Cook, S., Veillette, A.-M., de Serres, M., Aubin, M., Rainville, F., ... Doll, R. (2012). Professional navigation: A comparative study of two Canadian models. *Canadian Oncology Nursing Journal, 22,* 257–266. doi:10.5737/1181912x224257266

Fitch, M.I., & Allard, M. (2007). Perspectives of husbands of women with breast cancer: Information needs. *Canadian Oncology Nursing Journal, 17,* 79–83. doi:10.5737/1181912x1727983

Fitch, M.I., Gray, R.E., & Franssen, E. (2000). Women's perspectives regarding the impact of ovarian cancer. *Cancer Nursing, 23,* 359–366. doi:10.1097/00002820-200010000-00006

Fitch, M.I., Gray, R.E., & Franssen, E. (2001). Perspectives on living with ovarian cancer: Older women's views. *Oncology Nursing Forum, 28,* 1433–1442.

Fitch, M.I., Gray, R.E., Godel, R., & Labreque, M. (2008). Young women's experiences with breast cancer: An imperative for tailored information and support. *Canadian Oncology Nursing Journal, 18,* 74–79. doi:10.5737/1181912x1827479

Fitch, M.I., Gray, R.E., Greenberg, M., Carroll, J., Chart, P., & Orr, V. (2001). Self-help groups: Oncology nurses' perspectives. *Canadian Oncology Nursing Journal, 11,* 76–81. doi:10.5737/1181912x1127681

Fitch, M.I., & McAndrew, A. (2011). A performance measurement tool for cancer patient information and satisfaction. *Journal of Cancer Education, 26,* 612–618. doi:10.1007/s13187-011-0260-9

Fitch, M.I., McAndrew, A., & Harth, T. (2013). Measuring trends in performance across time: Providing patient information to cancer patients. *Canadian Oncology Nursing Journal, 23,* 247–253.

Fitch, M.I., Nicoll, I., & Keller-Olman, S. (2007). Breast cancer information dissemination strategies: Finding out what works. *Canadian Oncology Nursing Journal, 17,* 206–211. doi:10.5737/1181912x174206211

Fitch, M.I., Porter, H.B., & Page, B.D. (2009). *Supportive care: A framework for person-centered care.* Ottawa, Canada: Pappin Communications.

Foley, N.M., O'Connell, E.P., Lehane, E.A., Livingstone, V., Maher, B., Kaimkhani, S., ... Corrigan, M.A. (2016). PATI: Patient-accessed tailored information: A pilot study to evaluate the effect on preoperative breast cancer patients of information delivered via a mobile telephone. *Breast, 30,* 54–58. doi:10.1016/j.breast.2016.08.012

Fox, S., & Rainie, L. (2002). *Vital decisions: A Pew Internet Health Report.* Washington, DC: Pew Internet and American Life Project.

Friedman, A., Cosby, R., Boyko, S., Hatten-Bauer, J., & Turnball, G. (2011). Effective teaching strategies and methods of delivery for patient education: A systematic review and practice guideline recommendations. *Journal of Cancer Education, 26,* 12–21. doi:10.1007/s13187-010-0183-x

Gagnon, K., & Sabus, C. (2015). Professionalism in a digital age: Opportunities and considerations for social media in health care. *Physical Therapy, 95,* 406–414. doi:10.2522/ptj.20130227

Galbraith, M.E., Hays, L., & Tanner, T. (2012). What men say about surviving prostate cancer: Complexities represented in a decade of comments. *Clinical Journal of Oncology Nursing, 16,* 65–72. doi:10.1188/12.CJON.65-72

Galway, K., Black, A., Cantwell, M., Cardwell, C.R., Mills, M., & Donnelly, M. (2012). Psychosocial interventions to improve quality of life and emotional well-being for recently diagnosed cancer patients. *Cochrane Database of Systematic Reviews, 2012*(11). doi:10.1002/14651858.CD007064.pub2

Goerling, U., Foerg, A., Sander, S., Schramm, N., & Schlag, P.M. (2011). The impact of short-term psycho-oncological interventions on the psychological outcome of cancer patients of a surgical-oncology department: A randomized controlled study. *European Journal of Cancer, 47,* 2009–2014. doi:10.1016/j.ejca.2011.04.031

Gottlieb, B.H., & Wachala, E.D. (2007). Cancer support groups: A critical review of empirical studies. *Psycho-Oncology, 16,* 379–400. doi:10.1002/pon.1078

Gould, J., Grassau, P., Manthorne, J., Gray, R.E., & Fitch, M.I. (2006). "Nothing fit me": Nationwide consultations with young women with breast cancer. *Health Expectations, 9,* 158–173. doi:10.1111/j.1369-7625.2006.00383.x

Gray, R.E., Fergus, K.D., & Fitch, M.I. (2005). Two black men with prostate cancer: A narrative approach. *British Journal of Health Psychology, 10,* 1–15. doi:10.1348/135910704x14429

Gray, R.E., Fitch, M.I., Davis, C., & Phillips, C. (1996). Breast cancer and prostate cancer self-help groups: Reflections on differences. *Psychosocial Oncology, 5,* 137–142. doi:10.1002/(SICI)1099-1611(199606)5:2<137::AID-PON222>3.0.CO;2-E

Gray, R.E., Fitch, M.I., Davis, C., & Phillips, C. (1997a). Interviews with men with prostate cancer about their self-help group experience. *Journal of Palliative Care, 13,* 15–21.

Gray, R.E., Fitch, M.I., Davis, C., & Phillips, C. (1997b). A qualitative study of breast cancer self-help groups. *Psychosocial Oncology, 6,* 279–289. doi:10.1002/(SICI)1099-1611(199712)6:4<279::AID-PON280>3.0.CO;2-0

Gray, R.E., Fitch, M.I., Phillips, C., Labrecque, M., & Fergus, K. (2000). Managing the impact of illness: The experiences of men with prostate cancer and their spouses. *Journal of Health Psychology, 5,* 525–542. doi:10.1177/135910530000500410

Gray, R.E., Greenberg, M., Fitch, M.I., Sawka, C., Hampson, A., Labrecque, M., & Moore, B. (1998). Information needs of women with metastatic breast cancer. *Cancer Prevention and Control, 2,* 57–62.

Grunfeld, E., Coyle, D., Whelan, T., Clinch, J., Reyno, L., Earle, C.C., … Glossop, R. (2004). Family caregiver burden: Results of a longitudinal study of breast cancer patients and their principal caregivers. *Canadian Medical Association Journal, 170,* 1795–1801. doi:10.1503/cmaj.1031205

Hack, T.F., Pickles, T., Bultz, B., Degner, L., Katz, A., & Davison, B. (1999). Feasibility of an audiotaped intervention for patients with cancer: A multicenter, randomized, controlled pilot study. *Journal of Psychosocial Oncology, 17,* 1–15. doi:10.1300/J077v17n02_01

Harrison, J.D., Young, J.M., Price, M.A., Butow, P.N., & Solomon, M.J. (2009). What are the unmet supportive care needs of people with cancer? A systematic review. *Supportive Care in Cancer, 17,* 1117–1128. doi:10.1007/s00520-009-0615-5

Hart, S.L., Hoyt, M.A., Diefenbach, M., Anderson, D.R., Kilbourn, K.M., Craft, L.L., … Stanton, A.L. (2012). Meta-analysis of efficacy of interventions for elevated depressive symptoms in adults diagnosed with cancer. *Journal of the National Cancer Institute, 104,* 990–1004. doi:10.1093/jnci/djs256

Hasson-Ohayon, I., Goldzweig, G., Braun, M., & Galinsky, D. (2010). Women with advanced breast cancer and their spouses: Diversity of support and psychological distress. *Psycho-Oncology, 19,* 1195–1204. doi:10.1002/pon.1678

Hawkes, A.L., Hughes, K.L., Hutchinson, S.D., & Chambers, S.K. (2010). Feasibility of brief psychological distress screening by a community-based telephone helpline for cancer patients and caregivers. *BMC Cancer, 10,* 14. doi:10.1186/1471-2407-10-14

Hibbard, J.H., & Greene, J. (2013). What the evidence shows about patient activation: Better outcomes and care experiences. *Health Affairs, 32,* 207–214. doi:10.1377/hlthaff.2012.1061

Hill-Kaycer, C.E., Vachani, C.C., Hampshire, M.K., Di Lullo, G., Jacobs, L.A., & Metz, J.M. (2013). Impact of internet-based cancer survivor care plans with health care and lifestyle behaviors. *Cancer, 119,* 3854–3860. doi:10.1002/cncr.28286

Holland, J.C., Anderson, B., Breitbart, W.S., Compas, B., Dudley, M.M., Fleishman, S., … Zevon, M.A. (2010). Distress management. *Journal of the National Comprehensive Cancer Network, 8,* 448–485.

Holland, J.C., & Bultz, B.D. (2007). The NCCN guideline for distress management: A case for making distress the sixth vital sign. *Journal of the National Comprehensive Cancer Network, 5,* 1–5.

Howell, D., Keller-Olaman, S., Oliver, T., Hack, T., Broadfield, L., Biggs, K., … Syme, A. (2015). *A pan-Canadian practice guideline: Screening, assessment and care of psychosocial distress (depression, anxiety) in adults with cancer* (Version 2.2015). Retrieved from https://www.capo.ca/wp-content/uploads/2015/11/FINAL_Distress_Guideline1.pdf

Høybye, M.T., Johansen, C., & Tjørnhøj-Thomsen, T. (2005). Online interaction. Effects of storytelling in an internet breast cancer support group. *Psycho-Oncology, 14,* 211–220. doi:10.1002/pon.837

Institute of Medicine. (2001). *Crossing the quality chasm: A new health system for the 21st century.* Washington, DC: National Academies Press.

Jacobsen, P.B., Donovan, K.A., Trask, P.C., Fleishman, S.B., Zabora, J., Baker, F., & Holland, J.C. (2005). Screening for psychologic distress in ambulatory cancer patients. *Cancer, 103,* 494–502. doi:10.1002/cncr.20940

Jones, R.B., Pearson, J., Cawsey, A.J., Bental, D., Barret, A., White, J., … Gilmour, W.H. (2006). Effect of different forms of information produced for cancer patients on their use of the information, social support, and anxiety: Randomised trial. *BMJ, 332,* 942–948. doi:10.1136/bmj.38807.571042.68

Kaasa, S., Mastekaasa, A., & Lund, E. (1989). Prognostic factors for patients with inoperable non-small cell lung cancer, limited disease. *Radiotherapy and Oncology, 15,* 235–242. doi:10.1016/0167-8140(89)90091-1

Khan, F., Amatya, B., Pallant, J.F., Rajapaksa, I., & Brand, C. (2012). Multidisciplinary rehabilitation in women following breast cancer treatment: A randomized controlled trial. *Journal of Rehabilitation Medicine, 44,* 788–794. doi:10.2340/16501977-1020

Kiesler, D.J., & Auerbach, S.M. (2006). Optimal matches of patient preferences for information, decision-making, and interpersonal behavior: Evidence, models and interventions. *Patient Education and Counseling, 61,* 319–341. doi:10.1016/j.pec.2005.08.002

Kim, H.S., Sherman, D.K., & Taylor, S.E. (2008). Culture and social support. *Annals of Psychology, 63,* 518–526. doi:10.1037/0003-066X

Kim, K.K., Bell, J.F., Bold, P., Davis, A., Ngo, V., Reed, S.C., & Joseph, J.G. (2016). A personal health network for chemotherapy care coordination: Evaluation of usability by patients. *Student Health Technology Information, 225,* 232–236.

Korber, S.F., Padula, C., Gray, J., & Powell, M. (2011). A breast cancer navigator program: Barriers, enhancers, and nursing interventions. *Oncology Nursing Forum, 38,* 44–50. doi:10.1188/11.ONF.44-50

Kroenke, C.H., Kubzansky, L.D., Schernhammer, E.S., Holmes, M.D., & Kawachi, I. (2006). Social networks, social support, and survival after breast cancer diagnosis. *Journal of Clinical Oncology, 24,* 1105–1111. doi:10.1200/JCO.2005.04.2846

Lazarus, R.S., & Folkman, S. (1984). *Stress, appraisal and coping.* New York, NY: Springer.

Lieberman, M.A., Golant, M., Giese-Davis, J., Winzlenberg, A., Benjamin, H., Humphreys, K., ... Spiegel, D. (2003). Electronic support groups for breast carcinoma: A clinical trial of effectiveness. *Cancer, 97,* 920–925. doi:10.1002/cncr.11145

Loiselle, C.G., Peters, O., Haase, K.R., Girouard, L., Körner, A., Wiljer, D., & Fitch, M.I. (2013). Virtual navigation in colorectal cancer and melanoma: An exploration of patients' views. *Supportive Care in Cancer, 21,* 2289–2296. doi:10.1007/s00520-013-1771-1

MacDonald, B.H. (2001). Quality of life in cancer care: Patients' experiences and nurses' contribution. *European Journal of Oncology Nursing, 5,* 32–41. doi:10.1054/ejon.2000.0118

Melton, L., Brewer, B., Kolva, E., Joshi, T., & Bunch, M. (2016). Increasing access to care for young adults with cancer: Results of a quality improvement program using a novel telemedicine approach to support group psychotherapy. *Palliative and Supportive Care.* Advance online publication. doi:10.1017/S1478951516000572

Miller, R. (2008). Implementing a survivorship care plan for patients with breast cancer. *Clinical Journal of Oncology Nursing, 12,* 479–487. doi:10.1188/08.CJON.479-487

Mills, M.E., & Davidson, R. (2002). Cancer patients' sources of information: Use and quality issues. *Psycho-Oncology, 11,* 371–378. doi:10.1002/pon.584

Muzzin, L.J., Anderson, N.J., Figueredo, A.T., & Gudelis, S.O. (1994). The experience of cancer. *Social Science and Medicine, 38,* 1201–1208. doi:10.1016/0277-9536(94)90185-6

Nicholas, D.R., & Veach, T.A. (2000). The psychosocial assessment of the adult cancer patient. *Professional Psychology: Research and Practice, 31,* 206–215. doi:10.1037/0735-7028.31.2.206

Padilla, G.V., & Bulcavage, L.M. (1991). Theories used in patient health education. *Seminars in Oncology Nursing, 7,* 87–96. doi:10.1016/0749-2081(91)90086-5

Patrick-Miller, L., Much, J., & Axelrod, A. (2002). Psychosocial distress screening of ambulatory oncology patients [Abstract 1519]. *Proceedings of the American Society of Clinical Oncology, 21.*

Payne, J.K. (2014). State of the science: Stress, inflammation, and cancer. *Oncology Nursing Forum, 41,* 533–540. doi:10.1188/14.ONF.533-540

Picker Institute. (2014). Principles for patient-centered care. Retrieved from http://cgp.pickerinstitute.org/?page_id=1319

Pusa, S., Persson, C., & Sundin, K. (2012). Significant others' lived experience following lung cancer trajectory—From diagnosis through and after death of a family member. *European Journal of Oncology Nursing, 16,* 34–41. doi:10.1016/j.ejon.2011.02.004

Richardson, G.E., & Johnson, B.E. (1999). The biology of lung cancer. *Seminars in Oncology, 20,* 105–127.

Rutten, L.J.F., Arora, N.K., Bakes, A.D., Aziz, N., & Rowland, J. (2005). Information needs and sources of information among cancer patients: A systematic review of literature (1980–2003). *Patient Education and Counseling, 57,* 250–261. doi:10.1016/j.pec.2004.06.006

Satin, J.R., Linden, W., & Phillips, M.J. (2009). Depression as a predictor of disease progression and mortality in cancer patients: A meta-analysis. *Cancer, 115,* 5349–5361. doi:10.1002/cncr.24561

Shaw, B.R., McTavish, F., Hawkins, R., Gustafson, D.H., & Pingree, S. (2000). Experiences of women with breast cancer: Exchanging social support over the CHESS computer network. *Journal of Health Communication, 5,* 135–159. doi:10.1080/108107300406866

Skalla, K.A., Bakitas, M., Furstenberg, C.T., Ahles, T., & Henderson, J.V. (2004). Patients' need for information about cancer therapy. *Oncology Nursing Forum, 31,* 313–319. doi:10.1188/04.ONF.313-319

Smith, C., Dickens, C., & Edwards, S. (2005). Provision of information for cancer patients: An appraisal and review. *European Journal of Cancer Care, 14,* 282–288. doi:10.1111/j.1365-2354.2005.00576.x

Stacey, D., & Legare, F. (2015). Engaging patients using an interprofessional approach to shared decision making. *Canadian Oncology Nursing Journal, 24,* 455–461.

Stanton, A.L. (2006). Psychosocial concerns and interventions for cancer survivors. *Journal of Clinical Oncology, 24,* 5132–5137. doi:10.1200/JCO.2006.06.8775

Stephens, J., Rojubally, A., MacGregor, K., McLeod, D., Speca, M., Taylor-Brown, J., ... MacKenzie, G. (2013). Evaluation of CancerChatCanada: A program of online support for Canadians affected by cancer. *Current Oncology, 20,* 39–47. doi:10.3747/co.20.1210

Street, R.L., Jr., Makoul, G., Arora, N.K., & Epstein, R.M. (2009). How does communication heal? Pathways linking clinician-patient communication to health outcomes. *Patient Education and Counseling, 74,* 295–301. doi:10.1016/j.pec.2008.11.015

Sutherland, G., Hoey, L., White, V., Jefford, M., & Hegarty, S. (2008). How does a cancer education program impact people with cancer and their family members and friends? *Journal of Cancer Education, 23,* 126–132. doi:10.1080/08858190802039177

Tattersall, M.H.N., Butow, P.N., & Clayton, J.M. (2002). Insights from cancer patient communication research. *Hematology/Oncology Clinics of North America, 16,* 731–743. doi:10.1016/S0889-8588(02)00022-9

Till, J.E. (2003). Evaluation of support groups for women with breast cancer: Importance of the navigator role. *Health and Quality of Life Outcomes, 1,* 16. doi:10.1186/1477-7525-1-16

Tyson, T. (2000). The Internet: Tomorrow's portal to non-traditional health care services. *Journal of Ambulatory Care Management, 23,* 1–7. doi:10.1097/00004479-200004000-00002

van der Molen, B. (2000). Relating information needs to the cancer experience—Jenny's story: A cancer narrative. *European Journal of Cancer Care, 9,* 41–47. doi:10.1046/j.1365-2354.2000.00191.x

Vlossak, D., & Fitch, M.I. (2008). Multiple myeloma: The patient's perspective. *Canadian Oncology Nursing Journal, 18,* 141–151. doi:10.5737/1181912x183141145

Wenzel, J., Jones, R.A., Klimmek, R., Krumm, S., Darrell, L.P., Song, D., ... Ford, J.G. (2012). Cancer support and resource needs among African American older adults. *Clinical Journal of Oncology Nursing, 16,* 372–377. doi:10.1188/12.CJON.372-377

Winzelberg, A.J., Classen, C., Alpers, G.W., Roberts, H., Koopman, C., Adams, R.E., ... Taylor, C.B. (2003). Evaluation of an internet support group for women with primary breast cancer. *Cancer, 97,* 1164–1173. doi:10.1002/cncr.11174

Zabora, J., BrintzenhofeSzoc, K., Curbow, B., Hooker, C., & Piantadosi, S. (2001). The prevalence of psychological distress by cancer site. *Psycho-Oncology, 10,* 19–28. doi:10.1002/1099-1611(200101/02)10:1<19::AID-PON501>3.0.CO;2-6

Zhang, S., O'Carroll Bantum, E., Owen, J., Bakken, S., & Elhadad, N. (2016). Online cancer communities as informatics interventions for social support: Conceptualization, characterization, and impact. *Journal of the American Medical Informatics Association, 24,* 451–459. doi:10.1093/jamia/ocw093

Zimmerman, T., Heinrichs, N., & Baucom, D.H. (2007). Does one size fit all? Moderators in psychosocial interventions for breast cancer patients: A meta-analysis. *Annals of Behavioral Medicine, 34,* 225–239. doi:10.1007/BF02874548

## APPENDIX

# Psychosocial Support Programs and Resources for People With Cancer and Their Families

*Stacey D. Green, MSN, RN, GNP-BC, AOCNP®*

Living with and surviving cancer is a complex biopsychosocial experience that varies by diagnosis, treatment, and outcome for both people with a cancer diagnosis and their family members. In addition to facing the diagnosis of cancer, those affected sometimes find their lives and families disrupted and contend with lost time from work, multiple medical visits, various treatments, an unforeseen need for travel to cancer centers, high expenses, and other issues. A cancer diagnosis may bring with it a multitude of psychosocial issues. Often, cancer survivors and their families may require financial resources, emotional support, information, education, and access to wellness promotion.

This appendix lists organizations and services that provide emotional and financial support, education, advocacy information, and wellness promotion to people who are living the cancer experience and their families. These resources may be formal or informal, online or in person, and meet different biopsychosocial needs, such as providing a forum to discuss a particular diagnosis and connecting with other cancer survivors, families, or caregivers to find information and encouragement. Some organizations provide wellness retreats or seminars for mindfulness or activities that meet the spiritual needs of those touched by cancer. Other organizations may address sexuality or provide support for cancer survivors of a specific cultural group or cater to the needs of a specific age or gender. Additionally, some organizations may mobilize financial resources. Some may charge a fee for their services, whereas other services are free. This information is subject to change over time as the funding and needs of organizations change.

This list is intended to serve as a guide to assist nurses and other members of the healthcare team in mobilizing resources for cancer survivors and their families. Although this list is comprehensive, other resources can be found by doing an online search through Google (www.google.com) or Yahoo! (www.yahoo.com). Resources exist that are limited to a local area through hospitals and clinics, places of worship, and social groups. Nurses also should familiarize themselves with these local opportunities.

Information about each organization, as it relates to the support of cancer survivors, families, and caregivers, is provided along with website and other contact information as available.

Selection criteria for inclusion in this listing of psychosocial services include organizations that appear to offer services that reach outside the local area and whose major goal is to provide support, education, or wellness promotion. Each resource was determined to have programs and services that offer people ways to discover how to enjoy living in the present, to avoid carrying unnecessary burdens, know they are not alone in their cancer journey, and learn a different meaning for hope and healing. The information provided in this list is current as of the time of publication. Inclusion in this list is not intended to be an endorsement of any organization or program.

*The author would like to acknowledge Judi Johnson, PhD, RN, FAAN, and Robin M. Lally, PhD(c), RN, MS, AOCN®, CNS, for their contributions to this chapter from the previous edition of this book.*

Appendix 533

## Psychosocial Support Programs and Resources for People Surviving Cancer and Their Families

| Program | Fees/Sponsor* | Duration/Frequency | Focus | Cancer Populations |
|---|---|---|---|---|
| **Anal Cancer** | | | | |
| **The HPV and Anal Cancer Foundation**<br>New York, NY<br>646-593-7739<br>www.analcancerfoundation.org | Free | Ongoing | Education, advocacy, and empowerment; peer-to-peer support online and in person; acceleration of prevention and research of anal cancer and human papillomavirus infection | Anyone affected by anal cancer |
| **Bone Marrow Transplant** | | | | |
| **Blood & Marrow Transplant Information Network**<br>Highland Park, IL<br>847-433-3313<br>TF: 888-597-7674<br>www.bmtinfonet.org<br>Email: help@bmtinfonet.org | Some free services; fees vary as applicable | Ongoing | Online resource directory; Caring Connections Program; facilitates communication | Bone marrow, stem cell, and cord blood recipients before, during, and after transplant |
| **The Bone Marrow Foundation**<br>New York, NY<br>212-838-3029<br>TF: 800-365-1336<br>http://bonemarrow.org<br>Email: TheBMF@BoneMarrow.org | Free | Ongoing | Active links to online resources for psychosocial matters, issues surrounding intimacy and sexuality, financial assistance, and survivor networking | Bone marrow, stem cell, and cord blood recipients, families, and caregivers before, during, and after transplant. Population-specific groups include teens and young adults, seniors, and older adult survivors. |
| **National Bone Marrow Transplant Link**<br>Southfield, MI<br>248-358-1886<br>TF: 800-546-5268<br>www.nbmtlink.org<br>Email: info@nbmtlink.org | Free | Ongoing | "Resource Guide for Bone Marrow/Stem Cell Transplant: Friends Helping Friends"; online support groups; online survivorship information | Bone marrow recipients, families, and friends |

*(Continued on next page)*

## Psychosocial Support Programs and Resources for People Surviving Cancer and Their Families *(Continued)*

| Program | Fees/Sponsor* | Duration/Frequency | Focus | Cancer Populations |
|---|---|---|---|---|
| **Brain Tumors** | | | | |
| **American Brain Tumor Association**<br>Chicago, IL<br>773-577-8750<br>TF: 800-886-2282<br>www.abta.org<br>Email: info@abta.org | Some free services; fees vary as applicable; donations accepted | Ongoing | Information, education, mentorship, and support online | Healthcare professionals, patients with brain tumors, families, and caregivers |
| **Brain Tumor Foundation**<br>New York, NY<br>212-265-2401<br>www.braintumorfoundation.org | Free | Ongoing | Live webcasts; online patient and caregiver support groups; international listing of support groups; assistance with starting local groups; insurance advocacy information | Patients with brain tumors, families, and caregivers; healthcare providers |
| **The Healing Exchange Brain Trust**<br>Everett, MA<br>http://braintrust.org | Free | Ongoing | Support to people affected by brain tumors and related conditions via online support groups with focus on specific tumor types | Patients with brain cancer, their families, and loved ones |
| **National Brain Tumor Society**<br>Newton, MA<br>617-924-9997<br>www.braintumor.org | Free | Ongoing | Blog and newsletter; telephone support network; assistance connecting with support groups nationally | Researchers, healthcare professionals, patients with brain tumors, parents of children surviving brain tumors, and their families |
| **Breast Cancer** | | | | |
| **Adelphi New York Statewide Breast Cancer Hotline and Support Program**<br>Garden City, NY<br>516-877-4320<br>TF: 800-877-8077<br>http://breast-cancer.adelphi.edu | Free; donations accepted | Ongoing | Offers emotional support and information to people with and/or concerned about breast cancer; online education, networking, and emotional support; access to counseling; virtual and live support groups; referral for access to resources | Healthcare providers, caregivers, and women surviving breast cancer |

*(Continued on next page)*

## Psychosocial Support Programs and Resources for People Surviving Cancer and Their Families *(Continued)*

| Program | Fees/Sponsor* | Duration/Frequency | Focus | Cancer Populations |
|---|---|---|---|---|
| **Breast Cancer (cont.)** | | | | |
| **African American Breast Cancer Alliance**<br>Minneapolis, MN<br>612-462-6813<br>http://aabcainc.org<br>Email: aabca@aabcainc.org | Some free services; fees vary as applicable | Ongoing | Assists African Americans diagnosed and treated for breast cancer at any life stage; offers patients and survivors support, encouragement, education, and understanding; online and live support groups; survivorship retreats and referrals | African American women and men with breast cancer, families, and caregivers; healthcare professionals |
| **After Breast Cancer Diagnosis**<br>Glendale, WI<br>414-977-1780<br>TF: 800-977-4121<br>www.abcdbreastcancersupport.org<br>Email: abcdinc@abcdmentor.org | Free | Ongoing | 24-hour hotline for access to volunteer mentors who have experienced breast cancer as a patient, family, or friend | Everyone diagnosed with breast cancer and their families and friends, regardless of ethnic background, gender, religion, or sexual orientation |
| **BreastCancer.org**<br>Ardmore, PA<br>610-642-6550<br>www.breastcancer.org | Some free services; fees vary as applicable | Ongoing | Reliable, complete, and current information about breast cancer; fosters understanding of medical issues surrounding breast cancer to assist with informed decision making; newsletter, blog, and podcasts | Women with breast cancer, their families, and friends |
| **Breast Friends**<br>Tigard, OR<br>503-598-8048<br>TF: 888-386-8048<br>www.breastfriends.org | Some free services; fees vary as applicable | Ongoing | Focus on quality of life for female patients with cancer; provides education about specific ways to offer support; programs aimed at assisting and reassuring patients, friends, and families; 24-hour telephone peer support nationwide; local face-to-face support via local affiliates to assist patients in Oregon, Washington, Florida, and Pennsylvania | Women surviving breast cancer, their families, caregivers, and friends |

*(Continued on next page)*

## Psychosocial Support Programs and Resources for People Surviving Cancer and Their Families *(Continued)*

| Program | Fees/Sponsor* | Duration/Frequency | Focus | Cancer Populations |
|---|---|---|---|---|
| **Breast Cancer *(cont.)*** | | | | |
| **His Breast Cancer Awareness**<br>www.hisbreastcancer.org | Free; donations accepted | Ongoing | Online information source for male breast cancer; education and awareness with an emphasis on possibility of men having increased risk or a positive diagnosis of breast cancer; blog, newsletter, and open discussion forum | Men at risk for or with a breast cancer diagnosis |
| **Latina Breast Cancer Agency**<br>San Francisco, CA<br>415-584-3444<br>415-584-3449 (Spanish)<br>Email: latinabca@yahoo.com | Free; donations accepted | Ongoing | Works to reduce economic, language, and cultural barriers; breast cancer screenings; follow-up diagnostic and treatment services; facilitates access to information, education, and healthcare resources; provides emotional support | Low-income, uninsured women, with a focus on Latina community, including immigrant and older adult women living in the San Francisco Bay area |
| **Living Beyond Breast Cancer**<br>Bala Cynwyd, PA<br>610-645-4567<br>TF: 855-807-6386<br>www.lbbc.org<br>Email: mail@lbbc.org | Free; donations accepted | Ongoing | Online support; quarterly newsletter; volunteer breast cancer helpline; peer and emotional support and information in a confidential setting; helpline volunteers and staff do not provide medical counseling or legal advice | Newly diagnosed, young women, those living with metastatic breast cancer, African Americans, those diagnosed with triple-negative breast cancer, and lesbian, gay, bisexual, and transgender (LGBT) people affected by breast cancer; programs for caregivers and healthcare professionals who work with people affected by breast cancer |

*(Continued on next page)*

Appendix 537

## Psychosocial Support Programs and Resources for People Surviving Cancer and Their Families (Continued)

| Program | Fees/Sponsor* | Duration/Frequency | Focus | Cancer Populations |
|---|---|---|---|---|
| **Breast Cancer (cont.)** | | | | |
| **Men Against Breast Cancer**<br>Adamstown, MD<br>TF: 866-547-6222<br>www.menagainstbreastcancer.org<br>Email: info@menagainstbreastcancer.org | Some free services; fees vary as applicable; donations accepted | Ongoing | Targeted support for men as caregivers and participants in advocacy for women surviving breast cancer; psychosocial aspects of coping with a breast cancer diagnosis in the family; mammography program for low-income and uninsured; "Partners in Survival" program workshops and online information | For partners and families of women with a breast cancer diagnosis |
| **Mothers Supporting Daughters With Breast Cancer**<br>Chestertown, MD<br>410-778-1982<br>www.mothersdaughters.org<br>Email: msdbc@verizon.net | Free; donations accepted | Ongoing | Individual, free support and mentorship; match program to connect mothers with a local volunteer whose daughter is close in age, has had the same type of breast cancer, and same type of treatment; access to information about current therapies and research and resources for breast cancer | Mothers of daughters surviving breast cancer |
| **Myself: Together Again**<br>Raleigh, NC<br>www.myselftogetheragain.org<br>Email: info@myselftogetheragain.org | Some free services; fees vary as applicable; donations accepted | Ongoing | Empowerment and education breast reconstruction following mastectomy surgery; access to real "process" images; patient advocacy and information to use throughout the breast reconstruction process; monthly newsletter | Women who are status post mastectomy for breast cancer or who are facing breast reconstruction |
| **National Breast Cancer Foundation**<br>Frisco, TX<br>www.nationalbreastcancer.org | Some free services; fees vary as applicable | Ongoing | Online source of information and encouragement through early detection, education, and support services; provides mammograms to low-income or uninsured individuals | Women living with breast cancer, their families, and caregivers; otherwise healthy women in need of breast cancer screening or educational support |

*(Continued on next page)*

## Psychosocial Support Programs and Resources for People Surviving Cancer and Their Families *(Continued)*

| Program | Fees/ Sponsor* | Duration/ Frequency | Focus | Cancer Populations |
|---|---|---|---|---|
| **Breast Cancer *(cont.)*** | | | | |
| **The Pink Fund**<br>Bloomfield Hills, MI<br>TF: 877-234-7465<br>http://thepinkfund.org<br>Email: info@pinkfund.org | Free | Ongoing | Provides short-term financial aid during treatment and recovery; helps meet basic needs, decrease stress levels, and allow patients with breast cancer to focus on healing while improving survivorship outcomes; online education about available financial resources for those affected by breast cancer | Patients with breast cancer who have lost all or part of their income during active treatment |
| **SHARE Cancer Support**<br>New York, NY<br>212-719-0364<br>TF: 844-275-7427<br>www.sharecancersupport.org | Fees vary as applicable | Ongoing | Advocacy, wellness workshops, support groups, and educational programs; run by breast and ovarian cancer survivors who know what it is like to have early-stage, recurrent, and metastatic disease; English and Spanish help available | Self-help for women surviving breast and/or ovarian cancer and their families |
| **Sharsheret**<br>Teaneck, NJ<br>201-833-2341<br>TF: 866-474-2774<br>www.sharsheret.org<br>Email: info@sharsheret.org | Some free services; fees vary as applicable; donations accepted | Ongoing | Provides 24/7 online chat and support, education, and outreach; blog and online newsletter | Jewish women surviving breast cancer, their families, and caregivers; specific information available for premenopausal women and women at any stage, including advanced disease |

*(Continued on next page)*

## Psychosocial Support Programs and Resources for People Surviving Cancer and Their Families *(Continued)*

| Program | Fees/Sponsor* | Duration/Frequency | Focus | Cancer Populations |
|---|---|---|---|---|
| **Breast Cancer *(cont.)*** | | | | |
| **Sisters Network, Inc.**<br>Houston, TX<br>713-781-0255<br>TF: 866-781-1808<br>www.sistersnetworkinc.org<br>Email: infonet@sistersnetworkinc.org | Some free services; fees vary as applicable; donations accepted | Ongoing | Committed to increasing local and national attention to the devastating impact that breast cancer has in the African American community; Breast Cancer Assistance Program provides financial assistance for medical-related lodging, co-pays, office visits, and prostheses to underserved women; provides free mammography for those who qualify; affiliate chapters in 18 states | African American women surviving breast cancer, their families, and caregivers |
| **Young Survival Coalition**<br>New York, NY<br>877-972-1011<br>www.youngsurvival.org | Free; donations accepted | Ongoing | Advocacy, education, and support for young women living with breast cancer; national organization with chapters in 36 states; connects young patients with peer survivors; assistance with finding local support groups; newsletter, networking events, and fund-raising events, including "Tour de Pink" bike ride offered annually on the East and West Coast | Young women surviving breast cancer at any stage, their families, and caregivers; healthcare providers, healthy young women, and the general public |

*(Continued on next page)*

## Psychosocial Support Programs and Resources for People Surviving Cancer and Their Families *(Continued)*

| Program | Fees/Sponsor* | Duration/Frequency | Focus | Cancer Populations |
|---|---|---|---|---|
| **Gastrointestinal/Colorectal Cancers** ||||||
| **Colorectal Cancer Alliance**<br>Washington, DC<br>202-628-0123<br>TF: 877-422-2030<br>www.ccalliance.org<br>Email: info@ccalliance.org | Some free services; fees vary as applicable; donations accepted | Ongoing | Advocacy, education, and support; promotes screening rates and survivorship; colon cancer helpline and support groups; Blue Fund offers opportunities for financial support for screening or treatment; Buddy Program provides peer support from mentors who have experienced or cared for someone affected by colorectal cancer | People surviving colon cancer, their families, friends, and caregivers; healthcare providers; healthcare organizations |
| **The Oley Foundation**<br>Albany, NY<br>518-262-5079<br>TF: 800-776-6539<br>www.oley.org | All programs are free of charge; donations accepted | Ongoing | Support, education, advocacy, and tips for maintaining health and mobility; contact lists of people living with sustained total parenteral nutrition or tube feedings; resources and charitable donations of equipment and supplies | Anyone sustained on IV or tube feeding because of gastrointestinal disease |
| **United Ostomy Associations of America, Inc.**<br>Kennebunk, ME<br>TF: 800-826-0826<br>www.uoa.org | Fees vary as applicable | Ongoing | Provision of information, advocacy, and services; organizes support groups with chapters throughout the United States, Canada, Puerto Rico, and Bermuda; online discussion forums, social networks, conferences, and visitation program | People with intestinal or urinary diversions, their families, and friends |

*(Continued on next page)*

Appendix 541

## Psychosocial Support Programs and Resources for People Surviving Cancer and Their Families *(Continued)*

| Program | Fees/ Sponsor* | Duration/ Frequency | Focus | Cancer Populations |
|---|---|---|---|---|
| **Head and Neck Cancer** | | | | |
| **Cancer Laryngectomee Trust** West Yorkshire, England +44 (0) 1422 205522 www.cancerlt.org Email: info@cancerlt.org | Some free services; fees vary as applicable | Ongoing | Provides support and understanding for people who are about to have or have had a laryngectomy; free online newsletters; book *Laryngectomy Is Not a Tragedy* available for download; based in the United Kingdom, with in-person services available to UK residents | Free help for people with cancers of the larynx who have had laryngectomies, their families, and friends |
| **International Association of Laryngectomees** Atlanta, GA TF: 866-425-3678 www.theial.com Email: webmaster@theial.com | Some free services; club dues; fees vary as applicable; donations accepted | Ongoing | A coalition of 250 member clubs and regional organizations; promotes and supports rehabilitation of individuals with laryngectomy; education and idea exchange; facilitates new club formation; fosters improvement in laryngectomee programs; improves standards for teachers of postlaryngectomy speech | People with laryngectomies and their family members |
| **Support for People With Oral and Head and Neck Cancer** Locust Valley, NY TF: 800-377-0928 www.spohnc.org Email: info@spohnc.org | Some free services; fees vary as applicable; donations accepted | Ongoing | Advocacy, awareness, psychosocial support, resources and education; publications; National Survivors Volunteer Network provides network matched volunteers who have gone through diagnosis, treatment, and recovery with patients or family members who are just beginning their journey or are recovering from side effects of oral and head and neck cancer or its treatment | People surviving head and neck cancer, their families, and friends; healthcare professionals |

*(Continued on next page)*

## Psychosocial Support Programs and Resources for People Surviving Cancer and Their Families *(Continued)*

| Program | Fees/Sponsor* | Duration/Frequency | Focus | Cancer Populations |
|---|---|---|---|---|
| **Hematologic Cancers** ||||| 
| **International Myeloma Foundation**<br>North Hollywood, CA<br>818-487-7455<br>TF: 800-452-2873 (United States and Canada)<br>www.myeloma.org<br>Email: TheIMF@myeloma.org | Some free services; fees vary as applicable; donations accepted | Ongoing | Information, education, support, and camaraderie; international webcasts, podcasts, and seminars; community workshops; maintains contact information for more than 100 support groups worldwide; online and in-person support groups | People surviving multiple myeloma, their families, caregivers, and friends; healthcare professionals |
| **Leukemia and Lymphoma Society**<br>Rye Brook, NY<br>914-949-5213<br>www.lls.org | Some free services; fees vary as applicable; donations accepted | Ongoing | Chapters throughout the United States; peer-to-peer telephone support program; family support groups; clinical trials education and matching; financial aid, including co-pay assistance and annual financial stipend available for treatment or travel | All people affected by blood-related cancers, their families, and caregivers; healthcare professionals |
| **Lymphoma Research Foundation**<br>New York, NY<br>212-349-2910<br>TF: 800-500-9976<br>www.lymphoma.org<br>Email: helpline@lymphoma.org | Some free services; fees vary as applicable; donations accepted | Ongoing | Education, support, and access to six disease-specific websites which provide visitors with information on specific lymphoma subtypes, including diagnostic information, treatment options, and free patient and caregiver resources; provides free copies of disease-specific information guides and access to patient-to-patient telephone network and online newsletters; financial assistance for people currently undergoing treatment for lymphoma | People surviving lymphoma and their families; healthcare professionals |

*(Continued on next page)*

## Psychosocial Support Programs and Resources for People Surviving Cancer and Their Families *(Continued)*

| Program | Fees/Sponsor* | Duration/Frequency | Focus | Cancer Populations |
|---|---|---|---|---|
| **Lung Cancer** | | | | |
| **American Lung Association**<br>Chicago, IL<br>312-801-7630<br>TF: 800-548-8252<br>To find nearest location (TF):<br>800-586-4872<br>www.lung.org | Free; donations accepted | Ongoing | Online education, information and support; live chat online with registered nurses, respiratory therapists, certified tobacco specialists, and counselors; survivorship and peer-to-peer information and support | All people affected by lung cancer and their families, friends, and caregivers; healthcare professionals |
| **Lung Cancer Alliance**<br>Washington, DC<br>202-463-2080<br>TF: 1-800-298-2436 (US only)<br>www.lungcanceralliance.org<br>Email: info@lungcanceralliance.org | Some free services; fees vary as applicable; donations accepted | Ongoing | Peer and professional support; in-person and telephone counseling available; access to affiliated co-pay, treatment, and travel assistance programs | People surviving lung cancer and their families, friends, and caregivers; healthcare professionals |
| **Ovarian Cancer** | | | | |
| **Familial Ovarian Cancer Registry**<br>Buffalo, NY<br>716-845-4503<br>TF: 800-682-7426<br>http://ovariancancer.com/the-registry | Fees vary as applicable; donations accepted | Ongoing | Maintains the world's largest database of genetics and family history profiles for research of familial ovarian cancer; researching methods to detect, treat, cure, and eventually prevent familial ovarian cancer | Women at risk for and/or surviving ovarian cancer |

*(Continued on next page)*

## Psychosocial Support Programs and Resources for People Surviving Cancer and Their Families *(Continued)*

| Program | Fees/ Sponsor* | Duration/ Frequency | Focus | Cancer Populations |
|---|---|---|---|---|
| **Ovarian Cancer *(cont.)*** | | | | |
| **Foundation for Women's Cancer**<br>Chicago, IL<br>312-578-1439<br>www.foundationforwomenscancer.org<br>Email: FWCinfo@sgo.org | Some free services; fees vary as applicable; donations accepted | Ongoing | Awareness, educational, and fund-raising programs; comprehensive information about gynecologic cancer risk, prevention, early detection, and optimal treatment provided by expert gynecologic oncologists and other healthcare professionals; Ovarian Cancer Survivors Course offered frequently in various locations in the United States | Women surviving gynecologic cancer, their families, friends, and caregivers; healthcare professionals |
| **Ovarian Cancer Research Fund Alliance**<br>New York, NY<br>212-268-1002<br>TF: 866-399-6262<br>www.ocrfa.org<br>Email: info@ocrfa.org | Some free services; fees vary as applicable; donations accepted | Ongoing | Education, support, and advocacy; Woman to Woman ovarian cancer survivorship and support; access to financial support links for women under treatment for ovarian cancer | Anyone affected by ovarian cancer and their families, caregivers, and friends; healthcare professionals |
| **SHARE Cancer Support**<br>New York, NY<br>212-719-0364<br>TF: 844-275-7427<br>www.sharecancersupport.org | Fee varies as applicable | Ongoing | Advocacy, wellness workshops, support groups, and educational programs; run by breast and ovarian cancer survivors who know what it's like to have early-stage, recurrent, and metastatic disease; English and Spanish help available | Self-help for women surviving breast and/or ovarian cancer and their families |

*(Continued on next page)*

## Psychosocial Support Programs and Resources for People Surviving Cancer and Their Families *(Continued)*

| Program | Fees/Sponsor* | Duration/Frequency | Focus | Cancer Populations |
|---|---|---|---|---|
| **Pain** | | | | |
| **American Chronic Pain Association**<br>Rocklin, CA<br>TF: 800-533-3231<br>https://theacpa.org<br>Email: ACPA@theacpa.org | Some free services; fees vary as applicable; donations accepted | Ongoing | Education, information, and online and in-person peer support groups; online forums; information to assist people in living well with chronic pain; several hundred support groups meet across the United States, Canada, Great Britain, and many other countries | All people experiencing chronic pain |
| **Get Palliative Care**<br>www.getpalliativecare.org | Free educational materials, blogs, referrals | Ongoing | Education, referral to palliative care professionals; provided by the Center to Advance Palliative Care | Anyone affected by serious illness |
| **National Hospice and Palliative Care Organization: Caring Info**<br>Alexandria, VA<br>703-837-1500<br>TF: 800-658-8898<br>www.caringinfo.org<br>Email: caringinfo@nhpco.org | Some free services; fees vary as applicable; donations accepted | Ongoing | Education, advocacy, and support; information designed to help make informed decisions; multiple facilitated grief support groups for adults, children, and adolescents | Anyone affected by end-of-life care issues; anyone interested in hospice or palliative care; anyone adjusting to the death of a family member or friend resulting from a variety of circumstances |
| **The Vulvar Pain Foundation**<br>Graham, NC<br>336-226-0704<br>www.thevpfoundation.org | Some free services; fees for membership vary by type | Ongoing | Education, support, and wellness activities; membership entitles women to newsletters, support group information, and other online and in-person opportunities | Women with chronic vulvar pain and related disorders |

*(Continued on next page)*

## Psychosocial Support Programs and Resources for People Surviving Cancer and Their Families *(Continued)*

| Program | Fees/Sponsor* | Duration/Frequency | Focus | Cancer Populations |
|---|---|---|---|---|
| **Pancreatic Cancer** | | | | |
| **The National Pancreas Foundation** Bethesda, MD 301-961-1508 TF: 866-726-2737 http://pancreasfoundation.org Email: info@pancreasfoundation.org | Some free services; fees vary as applicable; donations accepted | Ongoing | Provides support, education, and information; online activities and advocacy; funds cutting-edge research for new and better therapies; chapters in 18 states | People living with pancreatic cancer and other pancreatic diseases, their families, and caregivers; healthcare professionals |
| **Pancreatic Cancer Action Network** Manhattan Beach, CA 310-725-0025 TF: 877-435-8650 www.pancan.org Email: info@pancan.org | Some free services; fees vary as applicable; donations accepted | Ongoing | Advocacy, support, education, and information; Patient and Liaison Services for information and support; access to links to support groups in several states | People living with pancreatic cancer, their families, friends, and caregivers; healthcare professionals |
| **Prostate Cancer** | | | | |
| **Us TOO International** Des Plaines, IL 630-795-1002 TF: 800-808-7866 www.ustoo.org Email: ustoo@ustoo.org | Free; donations accepted | Ongoing | Serves as a resource of volunteers with peer-to-peer support and educational materials to help make informed decisions about prostate cancer detection, treatment options, and related side effects; network of chapter meetings and support groups | Men surviving prostate cancer, their families, friends, and caregivers |
| **You Are Not Alone Now** www.yananow.org Email: yananow@yananow.org | Free; donations accepted | Ongoing | Provides basic information and links to more detailed sites; online discussion forum for support and education; inspirational stories of survival and wellness; online mentors available | People living with prostate cancer, their wives, partners, and caregivers |

*(Continued on next page)*

## Psychosocial Support Programs and Resources for People Surviving Cancer and Their Families (Continued)

| Program | Fees/Sponsor* | Duration/Frequency | Focus | Cancer Populations |
|---|---|---|---|---|
| **Sarcoma** | | | | |
| **The Liddy Shriver Sarcoma Initiative**<br>http://sarcomahelp.org | Free | Inactive | Initiative is no longer active; however, information about sarcoma and links to sarcoma support groups by type and location are still available. | Everyone affected by sarcomas |
| **The Sarcoma Alliance**<br>Mill Valley, CA<br>415-381-7236<br>http://sarcomaalliance.org<br>Email: info@sarcomaalliance.org | Some free services; fees vary as applicable; donations accepted | Ongoing | Strives to improve the lives of people affected by sarcoma through accurate diagnosis, improved access to care, guidance, education and support; peer-to-peer connection and online discussion forums available | People surviving sarcoma, their families, friends, and caregivers |
| **Skin Cancer** | | | | |
| **Faces of Skin Cancer**<br>South San Francisco, CA<br>TF: 800-626-3553<br>www.facesofskincancer.org | Free | Ongoing | Online resource for education and support | People living with advanced skin cancer, their families, friends, and caregivers |
| **Melanoma Research Foundation**<br>www.melanoma.org | Free | Ongoing | Melanoma patient support groups; online support and counseling; melanoma resource center | People living with melanoma |
| **The Skin Cancer Foundation**<br>New York, NY<br>212-725-5176<br>www.skincancer.org | Free | Ongoing | Education, advocacy, and prevention; focus on all types of skin cancer and skin care; free online courses; stories from young skin cancer survivors, prevention guidelines, handouts, and activities | Anyone interested in skin cancer prevention and treatment; patients; healthcare professionals |

*(Continued on next page)*

548  Psychosocial Nursing Care Along the Cancer Continuum *(Third Edition)*

**Psychosocial Support Programs and Resources for People Surviving Cancer and Their Families** *(Continued)*

| Program | Fees/Sponsor* | Duration/Frequency | Focus | Cancer Populations |
|---|---|---|---|---|
| **Thyroid Cancer** | | | | |
| **Light of Life Foundation** <br> Manalapan, NJ <br> 609-409-0900 <br> http://lightoflifefoundation.org | Some free services; fees vary as applicable; donations accepted | Ongoing | Improves quality of life for people with thyroid cancer through continual education of the lay public and the medical community; promotes research and development to improve thyroid cancer care | All thyroid cancer survivors and healthcare professionals |
| **ThyCa: Thyroid Cancer Survivors' Association, Inc.** <br> New York, NY <br> TF: 877-588-7904 <br> www.thyca.org <br> Email: thyca@thyca.org | Free; donations accepted | Ongoing | Global face-to-face and online support groups; person-to-person matching, thyroid cancer handbooks in multiple languages; network; newsletter; free publications for patients and healthcare professionals; research grants and procedural guides | All thyroid cancer survivors, healthcare professionals, and thyroid cancer researchers |
| **All Cancers** | | | | |
| **American Cancer Society** <br> Atlanta, GA <br> TF: 800-227-2345 <br> www.cancer.org | Free; donations accepted | Ongoing | Information, education, advocacy, and support; live chat available on the website; access to help with insurance issues and cancer information specialists and nurse navigators; links to local affiliates; "I Can Cope" and "Taking Charge of Money Matters" ongoing series | Anyone touched by the experience of cancer, including patients, families, friends, and healthcare professionals |
| **CancerCare** <br> New York, NY <br> TF: 800-813-4673 <br> www.cancercare.org <br> Email: info@cancercare.org | Free; donations accepted | Ongoing; varies by site | Education, information, and emotional support from social workers and support groups via telephone, in-person, or online support groups; co-pay and other financial assistance; access to services in several eastern U.S. cities | All people surviving cancer, their families, friends, and caregivers; healthcare professionals |

*(Continued on next page)*

## Psychosocial Support Programs and Resources for People Surviving Cancer and Their Families *(Continued)*

| Program | Fees/Sponsor* | Duration/Frequency | Focus | Cancer Populations |
|---|---|---|---|---|
| **All Cancers *(cont.)*** | | | | |
| **Cancer Care Services**<br>Fort Worth, TX<br>817-921-0653<br>TF: 800-789-9944<br>www.cancercareservices.org | Some free services; fees vary as applicable; donations accepted | Ongoing; see website for details | Emotional and spiritual support; information, education, and financial assistance to those who qualify; online and peer-to-peer support groups; stress management, yoga, and visits by social workers; play therapy for children; access to cancer navigators; services also available in Spanish | All people surviving cancer and their families, caregivers, and friends; healthcare professionals |
| **Cancer Connect**<br>Ketchum, ID<br>208-727-6880<br>http://news.cancerconnect.com<br>Email: information@cancerconnect.com | Some free services; fees vary as applicable; donations accepted | Ongoing; see website for details | Education, support, and advocacy; extensive list of wellness retreats and camps nationwide and internationally located for people living with cancer | All people living with cancer, their families, friends, and caregivers |
| **Cancer Hope Network**<br>Chester, NJ<br>908-879-4039<br>TF: 877-467-3638<br>www.cancerhopenetwork.org | Free; donations accepted | Ongoing | One-on-one support from cancer survivors with same or similar cancers; matching people with similar cancer situations; free support services provided throughout 50 United States, Puerto Rico, the U.S. Virgin Islands, and Canada; online live chat | All people living with cancer, their families, friends, and caregivers |

*(Continued on next page)*

## Psychosocial Support Programs and Resources for People Surviving Cancer and Their Families *(Continued)*

| Program | Fees/Sponsor* | Duration/Frequency | Focus | Cancer Populations |
|---|---|---|---|---|
| **All Cancers *(cont.)*** | | | | |
| **Cancer Support Community**<br>Washington, DC<br>202-659-9709<br>TF: 888-793-9355<br>www.cancersupportcommunity.org<br>Email: help@cancersupportcommunity.org | Free; donations accepted | Ongoing | Emotional support, education, and encouragement; access to psychosocial oncology mental health professionals, personalized services, and education; online and in-person services and support groups; resources to start affiliate programs and individual web pages; access to online distress screening program CancerSupportSource™ | All people affected by cancer |
| **Cancer Wellness Center**<br>Northbrook, IL<br>847-509-9595<br>TF: 866-292-9355<br>www.cancerwellness.org | Free; donations accepted | Varies by location; see website for details | Provides education; community, emotional, and spiritual support; information about and access to complementary therapies; 24-hour support hotline | All cancer survivors, their families, friends, and caregivers; healthcare professionals |
| **CaringBridge**<br>Albert Lea, MN<br>651-789-2300<br>www.caringbridge.org<br>Email: customercare@caringbridge.org | Free; donations accepted | Ongoing | Offers free web pages to patients as well as a sense of community; people in a time of need can share updates, photos, and videos; connecting with friends and family who care and want to help | All people with cancer, their families, friends, and caregivers |
| **Día de la Mujer Latina y Su Familia**<br>Pearland, TX<br>281-489-1111<br>www.diadelamujerlatina.org<br>Email: info@diadelamujerlatina.org | Fees vary as applicable | Ongoing | Resource information and patient navigation for Latina women diagnosed with cancer; events provide health screenings and education; access to medical providers and community volunteers fluent in Spanish | Primarily Latina women surviving cancer and their families and caregivers |

*(Continued on next page)*

## Psychosocial Support Programs and Resources for People Surviving Cancer and Their Families *(Continued)*

| Program | Fees/Sponsor* | Duration/Frequency | Focus | Cancer Populations |
|---|---|---|---|---|
| **All Cancers** *(cont.)* | | | | |
| **Dream Foundation**<br>Santa Barbara, CA<br>TF: 888-437-3267<br>www.dreamfoundation.org | Free; donations accepted | Ongoing | National dream-granting organization for adults and their families suffering life-threatening illness; attempts to fulfill the last wishes of adults with cancer, including veterans, Spanish-speaking veterans, and disease-specific populations | Adults with a life expectancy of less than one year |
| **Hope for Two**<br>Amherst, NY<br>TF: 800-743-4471<br>www.hopefortwo.org<br>Email: info@hopefortwo.org | Free; donations accepted | Ongoing | Matches pregnant patients with cancer via phone or email with women post-partum surviving the same cancer; cancer and pregnancy registry available for questions and to offer guidance to women and/or their physicians; founding physician available to address medical questions pertaining to specific cancer and pregnancy situations | Women diagnosed with any cancer during pregnancy; open to all socioeconomic, ethnic, and religious backgrounds worldwide |
| **Imerman Angels**<br>Chicago, IL<br>TF: 866-463-7626<br>http://imermanangels.org<br>Email: info@imermanangels.org | Free | Ongoing | Provides free personalized one-on-one cancer support for cancer fighters, survivors, and their caregivers; mentorship-matching program for individuals with specific diagnoses | All people affected by cancer |
| **Livestrong Foundation**<br>Austin, TX<br>855-220-7777<br>TF: 877-236-8820<br>www.livestrong.org | Free | Ongoing | Empowerment of the cancer community; addresses unmet needs of cancer survivors through collaboration, knowledge sharing, and partnership; online support and access to education, information, and additional support resources | Anyone affected by cancer, their families, caregivers, and friends |

*(Continued on next page)*

## Psychosocial Support Programs and Resources for People Surviving Cancer and Their Families *(Continued)*

| Program | Fees/ Sponsor* | Duration/ Frequency | Focus | Cancer Populations |
|---|---|---|---|---|
| **All Cancers (cont.)** | | | | |
| **Look Good Feel Better**<br>TF: 1-800-395-5665<br>http://lookgoodfeelbetter.org<br>www.2bMe.org (for teens) | Free; donations accepted | Ongoing; sessions of 1–2 hours; frequency varies by facility | Self-help materials; one-on-one support; makeup techniques, skin and nail care, and head-covering options; nutrition, exercise, and fitness; program-specific subsites dealing with issues pertaining to women, men, and teens; Spanish materials available; international programs listed on website | Anyone undergoing cancer treatment who is interested in improving appearance from treatment-related side effects such as hair loss, pigmentation, scarring, etc. |
| **Mautner Project at Whitman-Walker**<br>Washington, DC<br>202-332-5536<br>www.whitman-walker.org/service/community-health/mautner-project<br>Email: info@whitman-walker.org | Some free services; fees vary as applicable; donations accepted | Ongoing | Emotional and practical support and bereavement groups; phone peer support; legal assistance on-site; wellness, cancer prevention, and education; cancer navigation; transportation to cancer treatment; referrals to local resources | LGBT individuals surviving cancer of any type, their partners, caregivers, and families in the Greater DC Area |
| **My Resource Search**<br>Available on Google Play and iPhone App Stores | Free | Ongoing | Provides insured and uninsured patients identification of programs to healthcare needs; individual support and solutions to healthcare barriers; direct and free access to the published tip booklets by expert case managers at Patient Advocate Foundation | People in all states facing a challenging medical diagnosis; patients, healthcare providers, and case managers who work with cancer survivors |
| **National Cancer Institute**<br>Bethesda, MD<br>TF: 800-422-6237<br>www.cancer.gov | Some free services; fees vary as applicable | Ongoing | Education, information, and support; access to resources and clinical research trial information; live chat available online; live help link access on the site | All people with cancer, their families, friends, and caregivers; healthcare professionals |

*(Continued on next page)*

Appendix 553

## Psychosocial Support Programs and Resources for People Surviving Cancer and Their Families *(Continued)*

| Program | Fees/Sponsor* | Duration/Frequency | Focus | Cancer Populations |
|---|---|---|---|---|
| **All Cancers *(cont.)*** | | | | |
| **National Coalition for Cancer Survivorship**<br>Silver Spring, MD<br>TF: 877-622-7937<br>www.canceradvocacy.org<br>Email: info@canceradvocacy.org | Some free services; fees vary as applicable; donations accepted | Ongoing | Online support, education, and information; access to educational resources, news updates, and events; online toolkit, audiotapes for coping with cancer | All people with cancer, their families, friends, and caregivers; healthcare professionals |
| **National Comprehensive Cancer Network®**<br>Fort Washington, PA<br>215-690-0300<br>www.nccn.org<br>Email: usersupport@nccn.org | Some free services; fees vary as applicable | Ongoing | Education; treatment guidelines for patients and healthcare professionals; advocacy and support; decision-making information; clinical research and clinical trials information | All people experiencing a cancer diagnosis; healthcare providers |
| **National LGBT Cancer Network**<br>New York, NY<br>212-675-2633<br>www.cancer-network.org<br>Email: info@cancer-network.org | Free; donations accepted | Ongoing 12-week cycles; see website for details | Advocacy, education, support, and understanding for the psychosocial needs of LGBT individuals; free online support, moderated by social workers; cultural competence training for healthcare professionals | LGBT people living with cancer, LGBT cancer survivors, their families, friends, and caregivers; healthcare professionals |
| **National Organization for Rare Disorders**<br>Danbury, CT<br>203-744-0100<br>www.rarediseases.org | Fees vary as applicable | Ongoing | Provides a unified voice for individuals, parents, and other caregivers seeking to help them; family counseling; information; newsletters | People with rare diseases, their families, friends, and caregivers; healthcare professionals |
| **Pathways**<br>Minneapolis, MN<br>612-822-9061<br>www.pathwaysminneapolis.org | Free; donations accepted | Ongoing extensive calendar | Provide resources and services for people with life-threatening illness to explore and experience complementary healing approaches; opportunities for psychological, emotional, and spiritual healing | Adults with life-threatening illnesses |

*(Continued on next page)*

## Psychosocial Support Programs and Resources for People Surviving Cancer and Their Families *(Continued)*

| Program | Fees/Sponsor* | Duration/Frequency | Focus | Cancer Populations |
|---|---|---|---|---|
| **All Cancers *(cont.)*** | | | | |
| **Patient Advocate Foundation**<br>Newport News, VA<br>TF: 800-532-5274<br>www.patientadvocate.org | Some free services; fees vary as applicable | Ongoing | Provides co-pay relief, mediation, and arbitration services; multiple resources assist with resolution of legal, insurance, and workplace issues; one-on-one assistance with a professional case manager to help resolve healthcare issues | All people surviving cancer, their families, and caregivers; healthcare professionals |
| **R.A. Bloch Cancer Foundation**<br>Kansas City, MO<br>816-854-5050<br>TF: 800-433-0464<br>http://blochcancer.org<br>Email: hotline@blochcancer.org | Free; donations accepted | Ongoing | Information and education; matches cancer survivors for support; access to free inspirational written materials | All people surviving cancer |
| **RESOLVE**<br>McLean, VA<br>703-556-7172<br>www.resolve.org | Some free services; fees vary as applicable | Ongoing | Dedicated to improving the lives of women and men living with infertility; charitable mission includes providing free support to anyone in need, advocating for increased access to family building options, and reducing the stigma of this disease through public education | All people experiencing infertility issues for any reason |
| **Stupid Cancer**<br>http://stupidcancer.org | Free; donations accepted | Ongoing | Online support and discussion forums; regional support groups and events; links to other online resources | Young adults surviving cancer |

*(Continued on next page)*

## Psychosocial Support Programs and Resources for People Surviving Cancer and Their Families (Continued)

| Program | Fees/Sponsor* | Duration/Frequency | Focus | Cancer Populations |
|---|---|---|---|---|
| **All Cancers (cont.)** | | | | |
| **Well Spouse Association**<br>Freehold, NJ<br>TF: 800-838-0879<br>www.wellspouse.org<br>Email: info@wellspouse.org | Some free services; fees vary as applicable; donations accepted | Ongoing | Information, advocacy, and support; provides respite weekend events and an Annual Conference organized by volunteers for members; support groups throughout the United States and Canada; online articles and information; quarterly newsletters | Spousal caregivers, partners, friends, and families of people surviving cancer |
| **Children's Support, Camps, and Retreats** | | | | |
| **Eagle Mount and Big Sky Kids**<br>Bozeman, MT<br>406-586-1781<br>406-587-8221<br>www.eaglemount.org<br>Email: eaglemount@eaglemount.org (Eagle Mount)<br>Email: bigskykids@eaglemount.org (Big Sky Kids) | Free; donations accepted | Various camps for differing age groups | Retreat at Yellowstone National Park and surrounding area; horseback riding, fly fishing, and kayaking; opportunities to meet new friends | Children and young adults (aged 5–23 years) surviving cancer |
| **Lodging and Travel** | | | | |
| **Angel Flight, Inc.**<br>Tulsa, OK<br>918-749-8992<br>www.angelflight.com<br>Email: angel@angelflight.com | Free | Air travel when and where available | Nonprofit charitable organization of pilots and volunteers; arranges free air transportation for any legitimate, charitable, medical need; transportation for financially distressed people who require non-emergency medical treatment | Individuals and healthcare organizations |

*(Continued on next page)*

### Psychosocial Support Programs and Resources for People Surviving Cancer and Their Families *(Continued)*

| Program | Fees/Sponsor* | Duration/Frequency | Focus | Cancer Populations |
|---|---|---|---|---|
| **Lodging and Travel** *(cont.)* | | | | |
| **Corporate Angel Network**<br>White Plains, NY<br>914-328-1313<br>TF: 866-328-1313<br>www.corpangelnetwork.org<br>Email: info@corpangelnetwork.org | Free | Air travel when and where available | Arranges free travel for patients with cancer across the country using empty seats on corporate jets; improves access to comprehensive cancer and academic medical centers, and reduces emotional stress, physical discomfort, and financial burden for people living with cancer | All patients with cancer, bone marrow donors, and bone marrow recipients who are ambulatory and not in need of medical care while traveling; eligibility is not based on financial need; patients may travel as often as necessary |
| **Hope Lodge**<br>TF: 800-227-2345<br>www.cancer.org/treatment/support-programs-and-services/patient-lodging/hope-lodge.html | Free | Temporary lodging | American Cancer Society program; supportive, home-like atmosphere; 31 locations throughout the United States; accommodations and eligibility requirements may vary by location | Eligible people receiving cancer treatment and their families |
| **National Association of Hospital Hospitality Houses**<br>Gresham, OR<br>TF: 800-542-9730<br>www.nahhh.org | Free or low cost | Temporary lodging | Directory of member and nonmember housing opportunities throughout the United States; provides free or low-cost lodging; provides arena for community support; facilities with shared kitchens, common living areas, and private bedrooms | Patients and families receiving treatment away from home |
| **The Patient Travel Referral Program**<br>Virginia Beach, VA<br>757-318-9145<br>TF: 800-296-1217<br>www.patienttravel.org | Free to eligible individuals; monetary and frequent-flier miles; donations accepted | No limit on number of trips | Provides information about all forms of charitable, long-distance, and medically-related transportation; provides referrals to all appropriate sources of help available in the national charitable medical transportation network | People of all ages with financial hardship needing to travel a long distance for specialized medical evaluation, diagnosis, or treatment |

*(Continued on next page)*

## Psychosocial Support Programs and Resources for People Surviving Cancer and Their Families *(Continued)*

| Program | Fees/Sponsor* | Duration/Frequency | Focus | Cancer Populations |
|---|---|---|---|---|
| **Lodging and Travel *(cont.)*** | | | | |
| **Ronald McDonald House Charities**<br>Oak Brook, IL<br>630-623-7048<br>www.rmhc.org<br>Email: info@rmhc.org | Free if unable to pay; fees may vary otherwise | Temporary lodging near medical facilities | Convenience; network of local chapters found in more than 60 countries; keeps families together by providing places that feel like home; programs tailored to meet the urgent needs of each community | Children with serious illness and their families |
| **Retreats in Variable Locations** | | | | |
| **CancerConnect**<br>Ketchum, ID<br>208-727-6880<br>http://cancerconnect.com<br>Email: information@cancerconnect.com | Some free services; fees vary as applicable; donations accepted | Ongoing; see website for details | Education, support, and advocacy; extensive list of wellness retreats and camps nationwide; internationally located for people living with cancer | All people living with cancer, their families, friends, and caregivers |
| **Casting for Recovery**<br>Manchester, VT<br>TF: 888-553-3500<br>www.castingforrecovery.org<br>Email: info@castingforrecovery.org | Free; donations accepted | Weekends (May through September) | Trips in 24 states; unique program with focus on quality of life for women with breast cancer; combines breast cancer education and peer support with the sport of fly fishing; retreats offer opportunities for inspiration, renewed energy for life, and healing connections with other women and nature | Women surviving breast cancer; open to breast cancer survivors of all ages, in all stages of treatment and recovery; free to participants |
| **The Gathering Place**<br>Westlake, OH<br>216-595-9546<br>www.touchedbycancer.org<br>Email: info@touchedbycancer.org | Free; donations accepted | Ongoing | Emotional support; educational resources; healing touch, yoga, and camping for children whose parents or loved one is a participant; bereavement and other support groups | Adults surviving cancer and their loved ones |

*(Continued on next page)*

## Psychosocial Support Programs and Resources for People Surviving Cancer and Their Families *(Continued)*

| Program | Fees/ Sponsor* | Duration/ Frequency | Focus | Cancer Populations |
|---|---|---|---|---|
| **Periodicals** | | | | |
| **Cancer Today** American Association for Cancer Research www.cancertodaymag.org | Free | Quarterly magazine and monthly online newsletter | Education, support, and motivation; up-to-date information about current options for treatment; inspirational stories of survival; free online edition | All people surviving cancer |
| **Coping With Cancer** www.copingmag.com | $19 yearly subscription for U.S. residents; $35 yearly for international residents; free online access | Six times per year | Provides information, education, support, and motivation for readers; free online edition; exclusive coverage of National Cancer Survivors Day | People whose lives have been touched by cancer |
| **CURE** www.curetoday.com | Free | Quarterly (online and print) | Provides support and information through science and personal stories; online education; newsletters | Patients with cancer, survivors, and caregivers; healthcare professionals |

*Fees indicated are those at the time of publication and are subject to change.

# Index

*The letter f after a page number indicates that relevant content appears in a figure; the letter t, in a table.*

## A

abandonment, fear of, 16–17
acceptance and commitment therapy, for smoking cessation, 438–439
active listening, 411–412
adaptation, coping and, 60–61, 77, 78f
addiction/addictive disease, 427, 431–432, 431f, 441t. *See also* substance abuse
　denial in, 292
　pain management and, 440–442
　treatment of, 437–438, 439t
Adelphi New York Statewide Breast Cancer Hotline and Support Program, 534
adenosine triphosphate (ATP) alterations, cancer-related fatigue from, 110
adjustment disorder, 250, 323
adjustment disorder with anxiety, 250
adjustment disorder with mixed anxiety and depressed mood, 250
adolescents
　body image development in, 267t, 268
　cancer-related fatigue in, 109–110
　coping responses of, 9, 72
　spiritual care for, 154
　suffering in, 173

advance care planning, 163
advanced disease. *See* terminal illness
advance directives, 466, 481–482
Affordable Care Act. *See* Patient Protection and Affordable Care Act
African American Breast Cancer Alliance, 535
African American populations
　healthcare disparities in, 98, 488
　spirituality/religiosity in, 156
After Breast Cancer Diagnosis, 535
after-death experiences, 355–357
age. *See also specific age groups*
　cancer-related fatigue and, 109
　cognitive impairment with, 48–49
　and delirium risk, 184
　spirituality/religiosity and, 155
Agency for Healthcare Research and Quality, on body image disturbance, 281
agoraphobia, 251–252
akathisia, 252, 259
ALARM model, for sexual functioning assessment, 213, 213f
alcohol use, 427–428, 429f, 430, 430f. *See also* substance abuse
　and cancer development, 432–434
　and cancer treatment, 434–436

and depression, 307
withdrawal from, 252
Alexander, Eben, 356
allodynia, 140
allogeneic hematopoietic stem cell transplantation, 220
alopecia, 10, 210, 272
alprazolam, for anxiety, 259
altered mental status, 183. *See also* delirium; dementia
altered sexual function, 203–204. *See also* body image
　assessment of, 213–214, 213f
　in patients with cancer, 204–212, 205t–206t
　case study on, 221–223
　differential diagnosis for, 214–215, 215t
　healthcare professionals' responses to, 212
　interventions for, 216–217, 216f, 218f–219f
　nursing care for, 213–221, 213f, 215t, 216f, 218f
　plan of care for, 218f
　from radiation therapy, 204, 205t–206t, 207, 209, 220
　resources for, 219f
　from surgery, 205t–206t, 207–209
Alzheimer disease, 48–49, 188. *See also* dementia
American Academy of Hospice and Palliative Medicine (AAHPM), 11

559

American Academy of Nursing, 92
American Academy of Pediatrics, 12
American Association for Marriage and Family Therapy, 219f
American Association of Sexuality Educators, Counselors and Therapists, 219f
American Brain Tumor Association, 534
American Cancer Society, 235, 548
American Chronic Pain Association, 545
American College of Surgeons Commission on Cancer (ACoS CoC), 324, 326–327, 332
American Indian or Alaska Native (AIAN) populations, healthcare disparities in, 96–97
American Lung Association, 543
American Nurses Association (ANA)
 on assisted suicide/euthanasia, 487
 on nursing ethics, 92, 480–481
 on self-care, 359
American Psychosocial Oncology Society (APOS), 324, 326
American Society of Clinical Oncology (ASCO)
 on distress, 324
 infertility counseling guidelines, 211
 on palliative care, 11
American Thoracic Society, on medically futile treatment, 483
amitriptyline, for anxiety, 259
anal cancer, resources on, 533
analgesic ladder, 144
analgesic tolerance, 440–442
androgen deprivation therapy (ADT)
 body image affected by, 275
 sexual dysfunction from, 210, 221
anemia
 cancer-related fatigue with, 110–111, 115–116
 treatment of, 115–116
Angel Flight, Inc., 555
anger, 18, 229
 as cancer response, 231–236
 case study on, 241–242
 with delirium/dementia, 196–197
 effect on cancer development, 232
 at end-of-life phase, 236
 expressions of, 231–232, 231f
 grief expressed as, 236, 341, 358
 interventions during, 238–241, 239f
 nurses' responses to, 237–238, 237t, 240–241, 241t, 419–420, 420f
 plan of care for, 239f
 from powerlessness, 385
 theories on, 229–231
animal-assisted therapy, 459
anthropologic theories, on anger, 230
anticipated post-traumatic growth, 62
anticipatory grief, 352–353
antidepressants
 for anxiety, 259–260
 for depression, 310–312, 311t
 for hot flashes, 220
 sexual function affected by, 214–215
antiemetics, anxiety from, 252, 256, 259
antihistamines, for anxiety, 259
antipsychotics, 194, 259
anxiety, 10, 247–249
 along disease trajectory, 257, 305
 assessment of, 254–257, 255f
 case study on, 260–261
 classifications of, 250–252
 cognitive impairment from, 50
 cultural influences on, 249–250
 depression with, 256, 260
 differential diagnosis for, 257
 fatigue with, 111–112
 healthcare professionals' response to, 253–254
 interventions for, 255f, 257–260
 from medical conditions, 252–253
 nursing care for, 254–260, 255f
 pain with, 140
 with patient confusion, 196
 patient history of, 68
 plan of care for, 255f
 preexisting, 251–252
 screening for, 30–31
 sexual function affected by, 215t
 in survivorship, 29–33
 symptoms of, 254–257
anxiolytic medications, 258
anxious preoccupation, 70f
appraisal-focused coping, 62, 75
approach coping, 70f
aromatase inhibitors (AIs), 219
art therapy, 459–460
Asian populations, healthcare disparities in, 97
Ask, Tell, Ask communication model, 6
assisted suicide, 484–485, 485t, 486–487
Association of Oncology Social Work, 326
attachment behavioral system, 354
attention, 45
autonomy, ethical principle of, 4–5, 145, 480–484
avoidance coping, 61–62, 64, 69, 70f
awareness, of body changes, 4

## B

baby boomers, religious affiliations of, 99
bad news, communication of, 4–6, 6f, 415–416, 415f
basal cell cancer, body image affected by, 272–273
Beck Depression Inventory, 304, 316–317
Beck Hopelessness Scale, 127t
Bedside Confusion Scale (BSCS), 192
behavioral theories, on anger, 230
behavior modification techniques, 417–419, 458–459
beneficence, 480
benzodiazepines, 194
 for anxiety, 259
 for bereavement distress, 354
bereavement
 and grief, 339–341, 352 (*See also* grief)
 involving children, 342–343, 343f
Big Sky Kids, 555

bilateral salpingo-oophorectomy (BSO), 205*t*, 207–208, 211
bioethics, defined, 479–480
biotherapy
  coping strategies for, 66*t*
  sexuality affected by, 205*t*
bladder cancer
  body image affected by, 274–275
  sexual dysfunction with, 205*t*, 209
blood-injection-injury phobias, 251–252
Blood & Marrow Transplant Information Network, 533
body betrayal, 266, 270
body changes, awareness of, 4
body image, 265–266
  and cancer, 271–276
  development of, 266–268, 267*t*
  and illness, 269–271, 269*t*
  loss of, 17 (*See also* body image disturbance)
body image disturbance
  assessment of, 276–277, 277*f*
  case study on, 281–282
  differential diagnosis for, 277
  interventions for, 277–278
  nursing care and, 276–278, 277*f*, 279*f*–280*f*
  plan of care for, 280*f*
Body Image Scale (BIS), 276
body schema, 265
The Bone Marrow Foundation, 533
bone marrow transplant (BMT)
  resources on, 533
  sexual function affected by, 209–210
brain imaging, for cognitive impairment assessment, 47–48
Brain Tumor Foundation, 534
brain tumors
  cognitive impairment from, 49–50
  resources on, 534
breast cancer
  anger suppression and, 232
  body image affected by, 273–274
  cognitive impairment with, 49
  resources on, 534–539
  sexual dysfunction with, 205*t*, 207–208, 210
BreastCancer.org, 535
Breast Friends, 535

breast reconstruction, 207
Brief Fatigue Inventory, 114*t*
Brief Symptom Inventory, 328
buprenorphine, 443
bupropion, for smoking cessation, 438
burnout, in families, 74
buspirone, for anxiety, 259

## C

CAGE substance abuse screening tool, 430, 430*f*
Canadian Association of Psychosocial Oncology, 324, 522
cancer advocacy groups, 235
cancer-associated cognitive dysfunction (CACD), 46. *See also* cognitive impairment
Cancer*Care*, 548
*Cancer Care for the Whole Patient* (IOM), 323
Cancer Care Services, 549
Cancer Communication Assessment Tool for Patients and Families (CCAT-PF), 35–36
Cancer Connect, 549, 557
Cancer Hope Network, 549
Cancer Laryngectomee Trust, 541
cancer recurrence. *See* recurrence
cancer-related fatigue (CRF), 107–108
  assessment of, 112–114, 114*t*
  case study on, 119
  epidemiology of, 108–110
  etiology of, 110–112
  nonpharmacologic interventions for, 115
  nursing management of, 116–118
  pathophysiology of, 110–111
  pharmacologic interventions for, 115
  psychosocial effects of, 112
  sexual function affected by, 209–210, 215*t*
  as source of suffering, 171
  treatment of, 114–115, 115*f*
Cancer Support Community, 80, 258, 504, 550
Cancer Survivors' Partners Unmet Needs measure, 36
*Cancer Today*, 558
Cancer Wellness Center, 550
Cancer Worry Scale, 31

caregivers. *See* families/caregivers
CaringBridge, 550
Casting for Recovery, 557
catastrophizing, 140
cervical cancer
  body image affected by, 274
  sexual dysfunction with, 207–208
chemokines, cognitive impairment and, 50
chemotherapy
  cognitive impairment with, 49–50, 187–188
  near end of life, 465
  psychosocial impact of, 10, 66*t*, 67
  sexual function affected by, 205*t*–206*t*, 207, 209–210
  substance abuse effect on, 435
chemotherapy-induced nausea and vomiting (CINV), 10
children
  anxiety in, 253
  bereavement involving, 342–343, 343*f*
  body image development in, 267*t*, 268
  cancer-related fatigue in, 109–110
  delirium in, 184
  depression in, 305
  end-of-life care for, 474–475
  guilt in, 370–371
  pain in, 142–143
  palliative care for, 12
  powerlessness in, 381
  resources for, 343, 555, 557
  response to diagnosis, 8–9
  spiritual care for, 154
  suffering in, 171–172
chlorpromazine
  for anxiety, 259
  for delirium, 194
cholinesterase inhibitors, for dementia, 194
cigarette smoking, 427–428
  and cancer development, 366*f*, 367–369, 432–433
  and cancer treatment, 434–435
  treatment for, 438–440
circadian rhythms, disruption of, 110–111
citizenship status
  and bereavement/grief, 344
  and healthcare disparities, 94–95

claustrophobia, 251–252
clonazepam, for anxiety, 259
*Code of Ethics for Nurses* (ANA), 92, 359, 480
*Code of Ethics of the American Medical Association,* 4
cognitive behavioral therapy (CBT), 81, 454
  for anxiety, 258–259
  for body image disturbance, 278–281
  for cancer-related fatigue, 118
  for families/caregivers, 504
  for smoking cessation, 438–439
  techniques used in, 417–419
cognitive functioning, defined, 45
cognitive impairment, 76
  from anxiety, 256
  assessment of, 51–52
  defined, 45
  factors contributing to, 48–51, 48f
  fear of, 53
  implications for practice, 52–53
  in oncology population, 45–48
  pain self-report with, 143, 194–196
  research limitations on, 46–47
  self-report of, 47, 51
  subjective vs. objective reports of, 47–48, 51
  during work reentry, 34
cognitive reframing, 131–132, 417–418
cognitive rehabilitation therapy, 53–54
cognitive reserve, 47
cognitive restructuring, 258
cognitive training, defined, 43
Colon Cancer Alliance, 540
colorectal cancer
  effect on body image, 275
  resources on, 540
  sexual dysfunction with, 204–207, 205t
Committee for the Study of Health Consequences of the Stress of Bereavement, 340, 349
communication
  about altered sexual function, 204, 212, 220
  about body image changes, 278, 279f
  about end-of-life care, 466–467, 467f
  about hospice, 471–472
  about suicide risk, 312, 312t
  of bad news, 4–6, 6f, 415–416, 415f
  cultural competence and, 408, 408f
  during grief/bereavement, 348–349
  near end of life, 482
  nonverbal, 409, 412–413
  of shared decision making, 416–417
  skills needed for, 409–415, 410f
complementary/alternative medicine, 115, 310, 523
complicated grief, 344, 349–352, 351f
confusion. *See* delirium
Confusion Assessment Method (CAM), 192
conscience, 366f
conscientious objection, 485t
contextual memory, 45
continuous care, 470
control
  locus of, 68–69, 379–380, 380f
  loss of, 17–19, 234, 266, 270, 379–380
coping
  and adaptation, 60–61, 77, 78f
  anger and, 232
  cultural/socioeconomic/gender dimensions of, 70–71, 73
  defined, 57–60
  denial as, 290–291
  developmental life stage affecting, 71–72
  dispositional, 59
  effect on pain perception, 140
  by families/caregivers, 74–75, 79–80, 80f, 499, 502–505
  interventions supporting, 77–82, 78f, 80f, 81t, 502–505
  over disease trajectory, 67–68
  personality traits affecting, 68–69
  as process, 65–77
  situational, 59
  social supports for, 72–74, 73t
  strategies for, 61–65
  styles of, 69, 70f
  variables influencing, 66–77, 66f, 66t
*Coping With Cancer,* 558
Corporate Angel Network, 556
corticosteroids, delirium with, 187–188
co-survivors, 34–37, 35t, 36f
counseling, 81, 118, 452–453, 504, 517t, 522. *See also* psychosocial interventions
countertransference responses, 316
cranial radiation, cognitive impairment from, 49–50
crisis intervention, 80–81, 393–396, 395f, 397–399, 398f, 517t
  across cancer continuum, 399–402
  assessment in, 395f
  cultural issues in, 396–397
  in families, 396, 396f
  research on, 401–402
cultural competence, 70, 101–102, 102t–103t, 145, 408, 408f
cultural issues
  in anxiety, 249–250
  in autonomy, 5
  in coping response, 70, 73
  in crisis intervention, 396–397
  in denial, 294
  in depression, 305
  in distress, 331
  within families, 500
  in grief/bereavement, 344–345
  influence on hope, 127–128
  in pain response/reporting, 144–145
  in spirituality/religiosity, 156, 158
  in suffering, 173
culture
  defined, 91
  in nursing literature, 92–93, 93f–94f
*CURE,* 558
cytokine dysregulation
  cancer-related fatigue from, 110
  cognitive impairment and, 50
  depression from, 304

# D

death
  crisis intervention at, 401
  denial and, 293
  family anger at, 236, 358

grief/bereavement related to, 340, 354–355, 355f, 358 (see also grief)
hastened, 315, 484–487, 485t
location of, 472–474 (see also end-of-life care)
powerlessness and, 383
Death With Dignity Act (DWDA) (1997), 315
delirium, 48, 183
  in patients with cancer, 187–188
  case study on, 198
  family/patient response to, 196–197
  healthcare professionals' responses to, 197–198
  management of, 193–196
  pathophysiology of, 185–186
  plan of care for, 195f
  presentation/prevalence of, 183–184
  risk factors/etiologies for, 184–185, 185f
  screening/assessment of, 186–187, 189–191, 190t, 192–193
  signs/symptoms of, 184
Delirium Rating Scale (DRS), 192
dementia, 48–49, 188–189
  assessment of, 189–191, 190t, 192–193
  vs. delirium, 190, 190f, 193
  etiologies of, 189
  family/patient response to, 196–197
  healthcare professionals' responses to, 197–198
  management of, 193–196
  plan of care for, 195f
  signs/symptoms of, 189
denial, 7, 61, 64, 70f, 289–290
  adaptive vs. maladaptive, 290–291, 291f, 296
  assessment of, 295
  and cancer, 292–295
  case study on, 298–299
  as coping mechanism, 290–291
  and death, 293
  healthcare professionals' response to, 294
  and illness, 291–292
  impact on family, 293–295, 297
  interventions for, 296–297, 297f–298f

nursing care and, 296–298, 297f–298f
depression, 303
  anxiety with, 256, 260
  assessment of, 303–305, 316–317
  cancer-related fatigue with, 111–112, 117–118
  case study on, 317–318
  cognitive impairment with, 48, 50
  with delirium/dementia, 196–197
  differential diagnosis for, 307–308
  in families/caregivers, 501–502
  vs. grief, 347–348
  interventions for, 308–312, 311t, 309f
  as medication side effect, 306, 307f
  with pain, 140
  patient/family history of, 306, 317
  patient history of, 68
  risk factors for, 305–307, 307f
  sexual function affected by, 215t
  in survivorship, 32
depressive disorder due to another medical condition, 304
Derogatis Interview for Sexual Functioning, 214
desensitization techniques, 258, 458–459
developmental life stages, affecting coping strategies, 71–72
dexamethasone, 252
Día de la Mujer Latina y Su Familia, 550
diagnosis
  communication of, 4–6, 6f
  crisis intervention at, 399
  postoperative, 10
  psychoeducational needs at, 518
  psychosocial impact/response to, 3–10, 32, 67, 172, 233, 369, 498
Diagnostic and Statistical Manual of Mental Disorders (DSM-V)
  on anxiety, 250–253, 255f
  on depression, 303–305
  on distress, 324
  on grief, 347–349
  on sexual dysfunction, 204

on substance abuse disorder, 428–429, 429f, 441t
diazepam, 354
diethylstilbestrol (DES), 370
dignity therapy, 161, 455
diphenhydramine, for anxiety, 259
direct action, as coping strategy, 63, 79
disengagement, 59, 75, 352
disorientation, 191
dispositional coping, 59
distress, 323–324. See also psychosocial needs/interventions
  along cancer continuum, 326
  anxiety as reaction to, 247 (see also anxiety)
  barriers to screening for, 325–329
  with cancer, 324–325
  case study on, 333–335
  fatigue with, 111–112
  interventions for, 332–333
  nursing care for, 329–333, 330f
  patterns of, 60–61, 512–515, 513f–514f
  risk factors for, 325, 325f
  screening/assessment for, 327–333, 521–522
  as sixth vital sign, 324, 326
  standards of care for, 324, 327
Distress Thermometer (NCCN), 214, 304, 327–329
diversity, in U.S. population, 92–93, 94f
donepezil, for dementia, 194
double effect, principle of, 485t, 486
Dream Foundation, 551
drug abuse, 428–429, 428t, 429f, 434–436. See also substance abuse
drug–drug interactions, 143
drug-seeking behavior, 442–443
dyadic coping, 74
dyspareunia, 207–208, 217, 219
dyspnea, as source of suffering, 171

# E

Eagle Mount, 555
educational levels, affecting coping response, 70–71
education needs, for patients/families, 36–37, 79. See also psychoeducational support

ego strength, 69, 270
embryo cryopreservation, 211
emotional distress. *See* distress
emotional expression, 64
emotional processing, 64
emotion-focused coping, 62–64
Emotion Thermometer, 328
empathic listening, 162–163
EMPATHY acronym, for nonverbal communication, 412–413
end-of-life care, 465–466
  for children, 474–475
  conversations about, 466–467, 467*f*
  denial as barrier to, 293
  ethical issues with, 481–482
  locations for, 472–474
  oncology nurse's role in, 19, 475
  *vs.* palliative care, 11
  patient anger during, 236
  powerlessness in, 383
  programs for, 469–472
  quality indicators for, 467–468, 468*t*–469*t*
endometrial cancer, sexual dysfunction with, 207–208
energy-based practices, 523
energy conservation, 118
engagement coping strategies, 58–60, 77
erectile dysfunction (ED), 203–204, 208, 210, 220–221
erythropoietin, for anemia, 115
estrogen deficits, cognitive impairment from, 50
estrogen therapy, 211, 219–220
ethics/ethical issues, 4–5, 145, 483–484
  in dealing with grief, 357
  defined, 479–484, 485*t*
  dilemmas in, 480, 485*t*
  in end-of-life care, 481–482
  in nursing practice, 92, 359, 480–481
ethnicity. *See also* cultural issues
  and healthcare disparities, 95–99, 96*f*, 488–489, 489*f*
  and spirituality/religion, 156, 158
European Organisation for Research and Treatment of Cancer, Quality of Life questionnaire, 276
euthanasia, 484–485, 485*t*, 486–487

evidence-based practices (EBP)
  for pain management, 145–146
  for spiritual support, 159–163
executive function, 45
exercise
  for anxiety, 258
  for cancer-related fatigue, 115, 117–118, 523
Explore Women's Sex (app), 219*f*
expressive suffering, 171
expressive-supportive groups, 522
extended survival, paradigm of, 28–29, 28*t*
external locus of control, 68–69

## F

Faces of Skin Cancer, 547
Familial Ovarian Cancer Registry, 543
families/caregivers, 497
  coping systems in, 74–75, 79–80, 80*f*, 499, 502–505
  crisis intervention in, 396, 396*f*
  denial and, 293–295, 297
  diagnosis responses in, 8, 498
  distress assessment in, 35–36
  guilt in, 370–373
  needs assessment in, 35, 35*t*, 498–500
  powerlessness in, 383
  presence at home death, 473–474
  quality-of-life issues with, 500–502
  recurrence responses of, 15, 20, 30–31, 499
  role in hopefulness, 129–130
  as secondary survivors, 34–37, 35*t*, 36*f*
  social/financial impact on, 36*f*
  social support dynamics of, 73
  spirituality/religiosity in, 158, 500
  suffering in, 171, 174–175
  treatment responses of, 12–13, 498–499
Family Avoidance of Communicaton About Cancer (FACC) scale, 35–36
family burnout, 74
family crisis interventions, 81
family stress theory, 59
family systems approach
  to anger management, 240

  to coping strategies, 74, 79–80, 82
family therapy, 310
fatalism, 70*f*, 99
fatigue, 10, 76, 107. *See also* cancer-related fatigue
fatigue history, 113
fear, 16–19. *See also* anxiety; recurrence
  *vs.* anxiety, 248
  of delirium/dementia, 196–197
  of opioid addiction, 141
  of pain, 16, 19, 140–141
Fear of Cancer Recurrence Inventory, 30
Fear of Progression Questionnaire (FoP-Q-SF), 30
females, altered sexual function in, 204, 205*t*–206*t*, 207–210, 217–223, 274
Female Sexual Function Index, 214
fighting spirit, 68–69, 70*f*, 78, 234
fight-or-flight response, 247–248, 256
five-year survival rates, 27
flibanserin, for decreased libido, 217
fluoxetine
  for anxiety, 260
  for smoking cessation, 438
FOCUS program, for family-based coping, 82
Foundation for Women's Cancer, 544
Frankl, Viktor, 75, 123, 170
Freud, Sigmund, 229
Functional Assessment of Chronic Illness Therapy–Fatigue (FACIT-F), 109, 114*t*
functional support, 72
futility, in medical treatment, 482–484

## G

gabapentin, for hot flashes, 220
galantamine, for dementia, 194
gastrointestinal cancer, resources on, 540
The Gathering Place, 557
gender differences
  in coping responses, 64, 71
  in health behavior, 100
  in pain response/reporting, 144
  in social support needs, 82

in spirituality/religion, 155
gender expression, defined, 100f
gender identity, defined, 100f
gender minorities
　coping responses in, 71
　healthcare disparities in, 99–101, 100f
general inpatient care, 470
generalized anxiety disorder (GAD), 251
generalized hope, 124
genetic testing, for pain management response, 144
gen Xers, religious affiliations of, 99
Get Palliative Care, 545
ginseng, for cancer-related fatigue, 115
global orientation, 191
graft-versus-host disease, vaginal stenosis with, 220
grief, 339
　anger with, 236, 341, 358
　anticipatory, 352–353
　aspects/tasks of, 341, 342f
　assessment for, 346–347
　and bereavement, 339–341, 352
　case study on, 339, 345–346, 349f, 357
　with children, 342–343, 343f
　complicated, 344, 349–352, 351f
　as coping challenge, 76–77
　cultural aspects of, 344–345
　differential diagnosis for, 347–348
　at end of life, 354–355, 355f
　expressed as anger, 236
　interventions for, 348–349, 349f, 350f–351f
　neuroanatomy of, 354
　nurses' experience of, 357–358
　nursing care for, 346–349
　professional ethics and, 357
　prolonged (See prolonged grief disorder)
　research on, 353–354
Grief Experience Inventory, 358
group cognitive training, 54
group therapy, 455
　for cancer-related fatigue, 118
　for depression, 310
　for families/caregivers, 504
guided imagery, 457–458
　for anxiety, 258

for cancer-related fatigue, 118
as spiritual support, 163
guilt, 365, 366f
　with bereavement, 341
　in cancer, 366
　case study on, 374–375
　experienced by children, 370–371
　in families/caregivers, 370–373
　interventions for, 372f
　justified, 366f, 368–369
　nurses' feelings of, 373–374
　sources of, 366–370
　survivor, 366f, 369–370
　transmission, 370
gynecologic cancer
　body image affected by, 274
　sexual dysfunction with, 205t–206t, 207–208

# H

hair loss, 10, 210, 272
haloperidol, for delirium, 194
Hamilton Rating Scale, 304, 316–317
hastened death, 315, 484–486, 485t
　legal issues in, 315, 486–487
　position statements on, 487
head and neck cancer
　body image affected by, 272, 281–282
　resources on, 541
　sexual dysfunction with, 206t, 207
The Healing Exchange Brain Trust, 534
healing paradigm, in family coping, 80, 80f
healthcare disparities, across cultures, 94–101, 96f, 100f, 488–489, 489f
healthcare power of attorney, 481–482
Healthy People 2020 initiative, 488, 489f
helplessness, 69, 70f, 379–380
hematologic cancers, resources on, 542
hero myth, 366–368, 366f
Herth Hope Index (HHI), 127, 127t, 128
Herth Hope Scale, 125, 127, 127t
heterocyclic antidepressants, 310, 311t

high-dose chemotherapy, sexual function affected by, 209–210
High Sensitivity Cognitive Screen, 47
Hinds Hopefulness Scale, 127t
Hippocratic Oath, 483, 486
His Breast Cancer Awareness, 536
Holland, Jimmie, 3
home, death at, 472–474
hope, 75–76, 78–79, 123
　assessment of, 125–128, 127t, 128f
　and honesty, 482
　loss of, 18
　in shared decision making, 416
　strategies to foster/maintain, 128–132, 128f
　theoretical/conceptual models of, 124–125, 126f
HOPE assessment, 125–126
Hope for Two, 551
hopelessness, 124, 380. See also hope
Hopelessness Scale, 313
Hope Lodge, 556
Hopkins Symptom Checklist, 304, 328
hormonal changes, cognitive impairment from, 50
hormone therapy
　coping strategies for, 66t
　sexuality affected by, 205t, 210
hospice, 469–472, 486
　barriers to, 471, 471f
　for children, 474–475
　components of, 471f
　Medicare coverage of, 470, 472, 504
Hospice and Palliative Nurses Association (HPNA), 475, 487
Hospital Anxiety and Depression Scale (HADS), 304–305, 316–317, 328
hot flashes, 210, 219
The HPV and Anal Cancer Foundation, 533
humor, use of, 129, 414–415
hyperactive delirium, 184, 186, 188
hyperalgesia, 140, 440–442, 441t, 443
hypnosis, 458
hypoactive delirium, 184, 186, 188
hypoactive sexual desire disorder (HSDD), 217

hypothalamic-pituitary-adrenal axis (HPA), disruption of, 110
hypoxia, anxiety from, 252, 258
hysterectomy, body image/sexuality affected by, 205t, 207–208, 220, 271

## I

I Can Cope program, 118, 258, 310
I Count, Too program, 343
identity, loss of, 17
Imerman Angels, 551
imipramine, for anxiety, 260
immigrant status
 and bereavement/grief, 344
 and healthcare disparities, 94–95
immune response, affected by grief, 347
immunosuppressive therapies, substance abuse effect on, 435
Impact of Cancer Scale, 30
Index of Potential Suicide, 313
infection, risk of, 10
infertility, 211
inflammatory cytokines, cognitive impairment with, 50
inflammatory processes, cancer-related fatigue from, 110
informal caregivers, defined, 8
Informant Questionnaire on Cognitive Decline in the Elderly (IQCODE), 192
information seeking, as coping strategy, 6–7, 63, 79, 502–503
informed consent, 4–5, 481
 with cognitive impairment, 53
inpatient respite care, 470
insight therapy, 453
Institute for Patient- and Family-Centered Care, 497
instrumental coping. See problem-focused coping
integrative therapies. See mind–body practices
internal locus of control, 68–69, 380f
International Association of Laryngectomees, 541
International Index of Erectile Function, 214
International Myeloma Foundation, 542
International Psycho-Oncology Society, 327
Internet, 130, 268, 385, 518–519
Interpersonal Support Evaluation List tool, 72
interprofessional cancer care, nurse's role in, 422
intimacy, effect of cancer on, 211–212. See also altered sexual function
intracytoplasmic sperm injection, 211
intrapsychic processes, 63
in vitro fertilization (IVF), 211
involuntary euthanasia, 485t
IQ, impact on cognitive impairment, 47
isolation, feelings of, 29, 129–130

## J

Joint Commission
 on distress management, 327
 on sexual minority rights, 101
 on spiritual care, 153
journaling, 418–419
justice, 480, 488–489, 489f, 490–491
justified guilt, 366f, 368–369

## K

kidney cancer, body image affected by, 274–275

## L

Latina Breast Cancer Agency, 536
learned helplessness, 379–380. See also helplessless
learning theories, on anger, 230
Leininger, Madeleine, 92
Leukemia and Lymphoma Society, 542
LGBTQ populations
 coping responses in, 71
 healthcare disparities in, 99–101
libido, decrease in, 207, 215t, 217, 220
The Liddy Shriver Sarcoma Initiative, 547
life span considerations, in diagnosis response, 8–9
life storytelling, 160–161
Light of Life Foundation, 548
listening skills, 162–163, 411–413
Livestrong Foundation, 211, 551
Living Beyond Breast Cancer, 536
locus of control, 68–69, 379–380, 380f
lodging/travel, resources for, 556–557
logotherapy, 170
long-term memory, 45, 191
Look Good Feel Better, 552
lorazepam, for anxiety, 259
loss, 76–77, 172. See also bereavement
loss of body image/self, fear of, 17. See also body image
loss of control, 17–19, 234, 266, 270, 379–380
loss of identity, fear of, 17
loss of loved ones, fear of, 17–18
loss of relationship, fear of, 17–18
lumpectomy, sexuality affected by, 205t, 207
lung cancer, 432–433
 denial with, 295
 guilt with, 366f, 367–369
 resources on, 543
 sexual dysfunction with, 206t
Lung Cancer Alliance, 543
luteinizing hormone–releasing hormone agonists, cognitive impairment with, 50, 210
lymphedema
 body image affected by, 273–274
 sexuality affected by, 207, 209
Lymphoma Research Foundation, 542

## M

magnetic resonance imaging (MRI), 47, 354
major depressive episode, 303–304, 347. See also depression
males, altered sexual function in, 203–204, 206t, 208–210, 220–221, 274–275
managed care organizations, 490–491
marijuana, 428, 442
massage therapy, 458

mastectomy, sexuality affected by, 205t, 207
mastery, as coping goal, 60
Mautner Project at Whitman-Walker, 552
meaning, search for, 75–76, 172
meaning-centered psychotherapy, 75, 163, 455–456
meaning making, 75
medically inappropriate treatment, 482–484
medical trauma, 233
Medicare Care Choices Model, 472
Medicare hospice benefit, 470, 472, 504
meditation
 for anxiety, 258
 for cancer-related fatigue, 116
 in spiritual support, 159
melanoma, body image affected by, 272–273
Melanoma Research Foundation, 547
Memorial Symptom Assessment Scale, 31–32
memory, 45, 191
Memory Impairment Screen, 192
Men Against Breast Cancer, 537
menopause, 217
 chemotherapy-induced, 210
 premature, 210–211
 radiation-induced, 209
 surgery-induced, 207, 219
mercy killing, 485t, 486. *See also* euthanasia
methadone, 443
methylphenidate
 for cancer-related fatigue, 115
 for depression, 311
metoclopramide, 252
millennials, religious affiliations of, 99
Miller Hope Scale, 127, 127t
mind–body practices, 115, 456–458, 523
mindfulness, 457
mindfulness-based stress reduction (MBSR) therapies, 159–160, 457
Mini-Cog assessment, 47, 192
Mini-Mental State Examination (MMSE), 47, 51–52, 186, 192
minority populations, 92–93, 94f

distress in, 331
pain response/management in, 144–145
social support in, 73
mixed delirium, 184, 188
monoamine oxidase inhibitors (MAOIs), for depression, 311, 311t
Montreal Cognitive Assessment (MoCA), 47, 52, 192
moral distress, 484, 485t
morphine, 440
Mothers Supporting Daughters With Breast Cancer, 537
motivational interviewing (MI)
 for cancer-related fatigue, 118
 for substance abuse treatment, 437–439, 439t
Mullan, Fitzhugh, 27–28
Multidimensional Fatigue Symptom Inventory, 114t
muscle function, impairment of, 110–111
music therapy, 258, 459
mute suffering, 171, 175
My Resource Search (app), 552
Myself: Together Again, 537
My Sex Doctor (app), 219f

## N

NANDA International, on spiritual distress, 153
National Association of Hospital Hospitality Houses, 556
National Bone Marrow Transplant Link, 533
National Brain Tumor Society, 534
National Breast Cancer Foundation, 537
National Cancer Institute (NCI), 552
 on distress screening, 522
 Office of Cancer Survivorship, 20
National Coalition for Cancer Survivorship, 235, 553
 on cognitive impairment, 45–46
National Comprehensive Cancer Network (NCCN), 553
 on body image disturbance, 281
 on cancer-related fatigue, 108, 113, 116
 on distress management, 324, 326

on distress screening, 522
 Distress Thermometer, 214, 304, 327–329
 on spiritual needs, 155
National Consensus Project for Quality Palliative Care, 468
National Hospice and Palliative Care Organization (NHPCO), 469, 545
National Hospice Study, 470
National LGBT Cancer Network, 553
National Nursing Ethics Summit (2014), 481
National Organization for Rare Disorders, 553
The National Pancreas Foundation, 546
National Patient Travel Center, 557
National Quality Forum, 468
Native Hawaiian and Other Pacific Islander (NHOPI) populations, healthcare disparities in, 96f, 98–99
nausea, sexuality affected by, 215t
near-death experiences, 355–357
Needs Assessment of Family Caregivers–Cancer (NAFC-C), 498
neurobiological theories, on anger, 230–231
neurocognitive disorders, 183. *See also* delirium; dementia
neurocognitive testing, 52
neuropsychological testing, for cognitive impairment, 47–48, 52, 192–193
neutropenia, 210
nicotine replacement therapy, 438
nicotine use, 427–428
 and cancer development, 366f, 367–369, 432–433
 and cancer treatment, 434–435
 treatment for, 438–440
nonbeneficial medical treatment, 482–484
noncompliance, 256. *See also* denial
noncontextual memory, 45
nonmaleficence, 480
nonmelanoma tumors, body image affected by, 272–273

nontherapeutic communication, 410–411
nonverbal language, 409, 412–413
North American Menopause Society, 219f
no-suicide contracts, 313
Nowotny Hope Scale, 127, 127t
nutritional evaluation/intervention, 517t
　for cancer-related fatigue, 116

## O

Office of Cancer Survivorship (NCI), 20
olanzapine, for delirium, 194
older adults
　body image in, 267t
　cancer-related fatigue in, 109
　coping responses of, 9, 72
　delirium in, 184
　depression in, 305
　distress in, 331
　grief/bereavement in, 344–345, 354
　pain in, 143–144
　powerlessness in, 381
　sexuality/intimacy in, 212
　spirituality in, 155
　suffering in, 173
The Oley Foundation, 540
Oncology Nursing Society (ONS)
　on assisted suicide/euthanasia, 487
　on caregiver burden, 503
　on cognitive training, 54
　on depression interventions, 308
　on distress management, 324, 326
　on evidence-based pain management, 145–146
　on fatigue treatment, 114, 115f
　on nursing ethics, 480–481
　on palliative care, 12
　on same-sex partnership rights, 101
opioid addiction, 430, 441t
　fear of, 141
　management of, 440–444
opioid therapy, 440–444
optimism, 69, 78
orchiectomy, 206t, 275
ospemifene, for vaginal atrophy/dyspareunia, 217–218

outcome measures, for palliative care, 12
ovarian cancer
　body image affected by, 274
　resources on, 543–544
　sexual dysfunction with, 207–208, 274
Ovarian Cancer Research Fund Alliance, 544
ovarian transposition, 209

## P

pain, 76, 137–139
　addiction and, 440–442
　anxiety from, 252, 258
　cultural effects on, 144–145
　depression from, 307
　effect on hope, 129
　fear of, 16, 19, 140–141
　in infants/children, 142–143
　nonverbal signs of, 143
　in older adults, 143–144
　physical effects of, 139–140, 139f
　psychological effects of, 140–141
　and quality of life, 139–142, 139f
　resources on, 545
　self-report of, 138, 143, 194–196
　sexuality affected by, 209, 215t, 217
　social effects of, 139f, 141–142
　as source of suffering, 171
　spiritual effects of, 139f, 142
pain facilitation syndrome, with addiction, 440
pain management, 517t
　with delirium/dementia, 194–196
　evidence-based, 145–146
　standards/best practices for, 138, 138f, 327
　in substance abusers, 443–444
palliative care
　defined, 11, 485t
　at end of life, 469, 486
　as nursing specialty, 475
　outcome measures for, 12
　pediatric, 12, 474–475
　psychosocial impact of, 11–12
palliative coping. See emotion-focused coping
*Palliative Nursing: Scope and Standards of Practice* (HPNA), 475

palliative sedation, 485t, 486
palliative surgery, 10
pancreatic cancer
　anxiety with, 252–253
　resources on, 546
Pancreatic Cancer Action Network, 546
panic disorder, 251, 256, 258
paraneoplastic syndromes, anxiety from, 252
paroxetine, for anxiety, 260
particularized hope, 124
pastoral counseling, 459
Pathways, 553
Patient Advocate Foundation, 554
patient-controlled analgesia, 443
Patient Health Questionnaire-9, 304
patient pathway, over disease trajectory, 512–515, 513f–514f
Patient Protection and Affordable Care Act (ACA), 95, 490
Patient-Reported Outcomes Measurement Information System, 328
Patient Self-Determination Act (1991), 481–482
patterns of distress, over disease trajectory, 60–61
peer groups. See support groups
pelvic exenteration, 208, 274
penectomy, 275
penile cancer, body image affected by, 274–275
People Living Through Cancer, 554
periodicals, 558–559
peripheral neuropathy, 210
person-centered care, defined, 512
pet therapy, 459
phenothiazines, anxiety from, 259
pheochromocytoma, panic symptoms from, 252
phobias, 251–252, 258
phosphodiesterase type 5 (PDE5) inhibitors, for decreased libido, 217, 220–221
physical activity
　for anxiety, 258
　for cancer-related fatigue, 115, 117–118, 523
physical dependence, 441t. See also addiction

physical/practical support, to patients/caregivers, 504–505, 517t
physical restraints, use of, 196
physician-assisted suicide (PAS), 484–485
The Pink Fund, 538
Piper Fatigue Scale (PFS), 112, 114t
place of death, 472–473
PLISSIT model, for sexual counseling, 216, 216f
polypharmacy, 143
positron-emission tomography (PET) scans, for cognitive impairment assessment, 47
post-traumatic growth, 64–65
anticipated, 62
post-traumatic stress disorder (PTSD), 253, 349
powerlessness, 63, 379–381
across age continuum, 381
assessment of, 384
and cancer, 382–383
case study on, 387–388
differential diagnosis for, 384
in families, 383
and illness, 381–382
interventions for, 385, 386f
nurses' experience of, 387
research on, 383–384
prayer, 161–162, 162f, 346
prednisone, 252
prescription drug abuse, 428, 428t
presence ("being there"), 162–163, 175
primary appraisal, of stressor, 62
principle of double effect, 485t, 486
problem-focused coping, 62–63, 69, 79
problem-solving techniques, 240, 417
prochlorperazine, 252, 256
progesterone therapy, 219–220
prolonged grief disorder (PGD), 344, 348–351, 353–354
prostate cancer
body image affected by, 274–275
cognitive impairment with, 50
resources on, 546
sexual dysfunction with, 204, 206t, 208–210, 221
prostatectomy, 204, 208–209, 275
pseudoaddiction, 441t, 442–443

psychoanalysis, 453–454
psychoanalytic theories
on anger, 229–230
on guilt, 367
psychodynamic therapy, 453
psychoeducational support, 452, 517t, 518–520, 520f, 522
for anxiety, 258–259
for cancer-related fatigue, 118
as coping strategy, 72–73, 79
for depression, 310
for families/caregivers, 36–37, 503
for powerlessness, 385
Psychological Distress Inventory, 328
psychosocial, defined, 511
psychosocial distress. See distress
psychosocial needs/interventions
for anger, 240
for anxiety, 258
for body image disturbance, 277–278
for cancer-related fatigue, 118
for depression, 308–309
emergence of, 326
for families/caregivers, 503–504
goals of, 323
screening for, 521–522
to support coping, 77–82, 78f, 80f, 81t
types of, 452–460, 515–523, 516f, 517t, 520f
psychosocial oncology, defined, 3
psychotherapy, 81, 453–456, 504, 517t, 522–523. See also psychosocial interventions
for anxiety, 258
for depression, 308–309

# R

R.A. Bloch Cancer Foundation, 554
race, and healthcare disparities, 95–99, 96f, 144–145, 488–489, 489f
radiation therapy
body image affected by, 273, 275
cognitive impairment with, 49–50
psychosocial impact of, 10–11, 66t, 67
sexual dysfunction from, 204, 205t–206t, 207, 209, 220

substance abuse effect on, 435
rational suicide, 316, 317f
Reasons for Living Inventory, 313
rebound anxiety, 259
recognition phase, before diagnosis, 4
recurrence
anger at, 235–236
crisis intervention in, 400
fear of, 20, 29–31, 33, 67, 325
guilt and, 369
oncology nurse's response to, 15–16
psychosocial impact of, 13–15, 81–82, 172
reentry phase, distress during, 325
reframing, 131–132, 417–418
relaxation therapy, 456
for anxiety, 258
for cancer-related fatigue, 118
for depression, 309
as spiritual support, 163
religion/religiosity, 75, 99, 151–152, 346
factors related to, 155–158
vs. spirituality, 152
traditions/rituals in, 161–162
religious support, 152–153, 346
rationale for, 153–154
remission, 172, 400. See also survivorship
resiliency, 69, 79
RESOLVE, 554
restorative therapy, for cancer-related fatigue, 116–117
restraints, use of, 196
retroperitoneal lymph node dissection (RPLND), 209
risperidone, for delirium, 194
rivastigmine, for dementia, 194
role modeling, 78
role-play techniques, 419
Ronald McDonald House Charities, 557
routine home care, 470

# S

same-sex partnership rights, 101. See also sexual minorities
sarcoma, resources on, 547
The Sarcoma Alliance, 547
Saunders, Dame Cicely, 469
Schedule of Attitudes toward Hastened Death, 313

Schilder, Paul Ferdinand, 265
Schwartz Cancer Fatigue Scale, 114t
Screener and Opioid Assessment for Patients with Pain–
search for meaning, 75–76, 172
seasons of survival, paradigm of, 28–29, 28t
secondary appraisal, of stressor, 62
secondary cancer survivors, caregivers as, 34–37, 35t, 36f
selective estrogen receptor modulators (SERMs), 217–218
selective serotonin reuptake inhibitors (SSRIs)
  for anxiety, 259–260
  for depression, 310, 311t
  for hot flashes, 220
self-blame, 366f, 368
self-care, for caregivers, 358–359
self-efficacy, as coping skill, 62, 140
self-forgiveness therapy, 163
self-help groups. *See* support groups
serotonin–norepinephrine reuptake inhibitors (SNRIs)
  for anxiety, 259
  for depression, 310, 311t
Seven-Minute Screen, 192
Seven-Stage Crisis Intervention Model, 393. *See also* crisis intervention
Sexual Adjustment Questionnaire, 214
sexual dysfunction. *See* altered sexual function
Sexual Health Guide (app), 219f
sexuality
  alterations in, 112, 203 (*see also* altered sexual function)
  communication about, 204, 212, 220
  principles about, 204
Sexuality Information and Education Council of the United States, 219f
sexual minorities
  coping responses in, 71
  healthcare disparities in, 99–101, 100f
sexual orientation, defined, 100f
sexual response cycle, 213, 213f

SHARE Cancer Support, 538, 544
shared decision making, 416–417, 481–482, 485t
Sharsheret, 538
short-term memory, 45, 191
sildenafil, 220–221
Sisters Network, Inc., 539
situational coping, 59
sixth vital sign, distress as, 324, 327
skin cancer
  body image affected by, 272–273
  resources on, 547
The Skin Cancer Foundation, 547
sleep hygiene, 117, 310
sleep–wake disturbances/disorders, 110–111
  with delirium/dementia, 191
  in families/caregivers, 501–502
smoking, 427–428
  and cancer development, 366f, 367–369, 432–433
  and cancer treatment, 434–435
smoking cessation, 438–440
Snyder Hope Scale, 127t
social learning theories
  on anger, 230
  on helplessness, 379–380
social media, 130, 268, 385, 518–519
social skills, in professional interactions, 409, 410f. *See also* communication
social supports
  as coping strategy, 72–74, 73t
  domains of, 72
  to foster/maintain hope, 129–130
  gender differences and, 82
Society for Cognitive Rehabilitation, 53
Society for Sex Therapy and Research, 219f
Society of Critical Care Medicine, on medically futile treatment, 483
sociocultural theories, on anger, 230
socioeconomic status
  affecting coping response, 70–71
  distress and, 331
sorrow, fear of, 19

sperm banking, 211
SPIKES model, of communicating bad news, 5–6m415, 415f
spirituality, 75, 151–152
  effect of pain on, 142
  factors related to, 155–158
  in families/caregivers, 158, 500
  health beliefs affected by, 157–158
  hope fostered by, 130–131
  *vs.* religiosity, 152
spiritual needs, 154–155, 156t
spiritual screening/assessment, 159, 160f, 500
spiritual support, 152–153, 346
  evidence-based approaches to, 159–163
  nurse's role in, 163, 163f
  rationale for, 153–154
squamous cell carcinoma, body image affected by, 273
stages of change, 438, 439t. *See also* motivational interviewing
*Statement on the Scope and Standards of Oncology Nursing Practice* (ONS), 480–481
St. Christopher's Hospice, 469
stepped care approach, to psychosocial interventions, 77
steroid-induced anxiety, 252, 256
steroids, 252, 256
stoic acceptance, 70f
Stoner Hope Scale, 126, 127t
stress
  anxiety as reaction to, 247–248 (*See also* anxiety)
  and caregiver outcomes, 499
  cognitive impairment from, 50
  and depression, 306 (*see also* depression)
  as precipitator of addiction relapse, 432, 442
stress-coping framework, 61–65
stress management training, 118
stress theory, 249
structural support, 72
Stupid Cancer, 554
substance abuse. *See also* opioid addiction
  and cancer development, 432–434
  and cancer treatment, 434–436
  clinician education on, 444
  and depression, 307
  epidemiology of, 427–429, 428t, 429f

in oncology populations, 429–430
pain management with, 442–444
terminology of, 441t–442t
substance-induced anxiety disorder, 252
suffering, 169–171
  across disease trajectory, 172
  across life span, 172–173
  among oncology professionals, 176–177
  case study on, 177
  cultural influence on, 173
  fear of, 16, 19
  nursing interventions for, 175–176, 176f
  and quality of life, 170
  sources of, 171–172
suicide, 485t
  assessment/intervention for, 312–316, 312t, 309f, 314t–315t
  rational, 316, 317f
  and spirituality/religiosity, 157
  with uncontrolled pain, 140
Suicide Probability Scale, 313
Suicide Risk Measure, 313
sundowning, 191
Support for People With Oral and Head and Neck Cancer, 541
support groups, 517t, 520–522
  for anger management, 240
  for anxiety, 258–259
  for cancer-related fatigue, 118
  for families/caregivers, 504–505
  for grief/bereavement, 358–359
  hope fostered by, 130
  nurses' roles in, 420–421, 421f
  for powerlessness, 385
supportive care, defined, 511, 516f
Supportive Care Needs Survey–Partners and Caregivers, 36
supportive psychotherapy, 454
Support Person's Unmet Needs Survey, 502
surgery. *See also specific surgical procedures*
  body image affected by, 273, 275
  psychosocial impact of, 9–10, 66t, 67
  sexuality affected by, 205t–206t, 207–209

substance abuse effect on, 434–435
survivor guilt, 366f, 369–370
survivors, defined, 20, 27. *See also* survivorship
survivorship, 27
  anger in, 235
  crisis intervention in, 400
  distress in, 325
  guilt in, 366f, 369–370
  models of, 28–29, 28t
  oncology nurse's role in, 21
  powerlessness in, 382
  psychosocial impact of, 19–21
  recurrence anxiety in, 29–31, 33
  symptom persistence in, 31–33, 33f
  work reentry during, 33–34, 34f
survivorship care plans, 31
symptom clusters
  in children/adolescents, 109–110
  with pain, 140
symptom management, 12, 517t
symptom persistence, in survivorship, 31–33, 33f
systematic desensitization, 258, 458–459
Systemic–Transactional Model, of dyadic coping, 74

# T

targeted therapies, psychosocial impact of, 10
terminal illness. *See also* end-of-life care
  anger with, 236
  anxiety with, 258
  crisis intervention in, 400–401
  delirium with, 188
  denial with, 293
  depression with, 305–306
  psychosocial impact of, 16–19, 67, 172, 499
testicular cancer
  body image affected by, 274–275
  sexual dysfunction with, 204, 206t, 209
*Textbook of the Principles and Practice of Nursing*, 92
therapeutic communication, 411
therapeutic dependence, 442–443, 442t

thioridazine, for delirium, 194
thought-stopping techniques, 418
The Three C's framework, 278
thrombocytopenia, 210
ThyCa: Thyroid Cancer Survivors' Association, Inc., 548
thyroid cancer, resources on, 548
Time Opinion Survey, 126
tobacco use, 427–428
  and cancer development, 366f, 367–369, 432–434
  and cancer treatment, 434–435
  treatment for, 438–440
  tolerance, 442t. *See also* addiction
transgender populations, healthcare disparities in, 101
transmission guilt, 370
travel/lodging, resources for, 556–557
treatment phase
  crisis intervention in, 400
  oncology nurse's role in, 13
  psychosocial impact of, 9–13, 66t, 67, 172, 233–235, 498–499
tricyclic antidepressants
  for anxiety, 259–260
  for depression, 310–311
Tylor, Edward Burnett, 91
type C personality, 232

# U

United Ostomy Associations of America, Inc., 540
unknown, fear of, 16
urinary incontinence, after prostatectomy, 208
U.S. Preventive Services Task Force (USPSTF), depression screening recommendations, 214, 304
Us TOO International, 546
uterine cancer, body image affected by, 274

# V

vaginal atrophy, 217–219
vaginal dilators, 220
vaginal dryness, 207, 219
vaginal fibrosis, 207, 220
vaginal reconstruction, 208

vaginal shortening/narrowing, 207, 209, 220
vaginal stenosis, 220
varenicline, for smoking cessation, 438
venlafaxine, for hot flashes, 220
violence, 241. *See also* anger
Visual Analogue Fatigue Scale, 114*t*
visualization, 309, 458. *See also* guided imagery
visuospatial ability, 45
voluntary euthanasia, 485*t*
vulvar cancer, 208, 274
The Vulvar Pain Foundation, 545
vulvectomy, sexuality affected by, 205*t*, 208

# W

Well Spouse Association, 555
*When Children Die: Improving Palliative and End-of-Life Care for Children and Their Families* (IOM), 474
work reentry, during survivorship, 33–34, 34*f*
World Health Organization (WHO), on sexual health, 204

# Y

yoga, 457
  for anxiety, 258
  for cancer-related fatigue, 116–117
  in spiritual support, 159, 163
You Are Not Alone Now, 546
young adults
  body image development in, 267*t*
  coping responses of, 9, 72
  spirituality in, 154–155
  suffering in, 173
Young Survival Coalition, 539

# Z

Zung Self-Rating Depression Scale, 304